DROP
A SIZE
CARB
and
CALORIE
counter

Other titles by the same author:

Body Blitz
Carb Curfew
Drop a Size in Two Weeks Flat!
Drop a Size for Life

The UK's No.1 DIET and FITNESS EXPERT

Joanna Hall MSc

DROP
A SIZE
CARB
and
CALORIE
counter

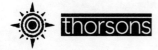

Thorsons
An Imprint of HarperCollins*Publishers*
77–85 Fulham Palace Road,
Hammersmith, London W6 8JB

The website address is: www.thorsonselement.com

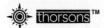

and Thorsons are trademarks of
HarperCollins*Publishers* Ltd

First published by Thorsons 2004

10 9 8 7 6 5 4 3 2 1

© Joanna Hall 2004

Joanna Hall asserts the moral right to be
identified as the author of this work

Joanna Hall's website adress is: www.joannahall.com

Branded food data supplied by Weight Loss Resources

A catalogue record of this book is
available from the British Library

ISBN 0 00 717528 0

Printed and bound in Great Britain by
Clays Ltd, St Ives plc

CONTENTS

Section Three: Brand Name Foods   127

HOW TO USE THIS BOOK

The *Drop a Size Calorie and Carb Counter* has been split into three sections to make it simple and easy to use.

Section One: The Carb Curfew Plan outlines the principles of the Carb Curfew – my easy-to-use strategy for achieving and maintaining weight loss. It also features plenty of tips and pointers on improving your health whilst you achieve your fat loss goals.

Section Two: Basic and Generic Foods details not only the calorie value of basic foods, but also their protein, carbohydrate, fat, fibre and sodium contents. Included in this section are the basic ingredients of meals – for instance rice, vegetables, meat and poultry and so on – as well as store cupboard ingredients and various other everyday foods. You will find the values for both raw and cooked ingredients, so you can analyse recipes and cooking favourites. Where popular, widely available dishes are featured, such as a one-crust apple pie, the values given are averages.

Section Three: Brand Name Foods features branded foods – the supermarket favourites, specialist ranges and processed convenience foods that may be a regular feature in your shopping basket. I've included the nutritional breakdown as the standard 'per 100 gram' and 'per serving'; just as you would find on food labels. Since even a basic product, like bread, can vary in the amount of carbohydrate or fat it contains, I have included a variety of different manufacturers. The nutritional value of two brands can be surprisingly different and, as consumers, we can be quite particular about our favourite brand of foods. While I have tried to include as many products as possible, there are bound to be some foods that you regularly eat that are not listed. So to help you judge for yourself how healthy these are, section one includes information on how to decipher food labels.

All the foods featured are categorized and listed alphabetically so in order to find a particular food, first decide if it a generic food such as chicken or a branded item such as Sweet Chilli Chicken Fillets by Waitrose then simply look up the relevant category from the list of contents on pages v–vii.

In total, I have detailed the overall calorie value and macronutrient content of over 5000 foods. However, while vitamins and minerals are vital components in our daily diet, I have not included the proportions of vitamins and minerals found in these foods in this book – it would simply have been too big! While they provide no direct energy to the body in the form of calories, vitamins and minerals do have a very important role to play in the health of your body. To help ensure you are getting an adequate supply of vitamins and minerals, check out the guide on page 53. This quick reference table will help you see the benefits fruits, vegetables and other foods provide for your body. It's important to bear in mind that food doesn't just provide the calories to get us through the day, but can directly affect our health, looks and energy.

The following notes will help you get the most accurate information from the book.

1. Food items listed in the Basic and Generic Foods section are listed 'per 100g'. Sodium is listed in milligrams. All other listings are in grams.

2. Food items in the Brand Name Foods section are listed 'per serving' and 'per 100g'. For each item, the figures are given 'per serving/per 100g'. The categories are clearly given at the top of each column on every page.

3. You can find restaurant and fast food meals in Eating Out and Fast Food in Section Three. Sandwiches are listed separately in Section Three.

Abbreviations

Brand Foods:

COU = Marks & Spencer Count on Us

TTD = Sainsbury's Taste the Difference

BGTY = Sainsbury's Be Good to Yourself

GFY = Asda Good for You

In the nutritional tables:

N = negligible	tbsp = tablespoon
Tr = trace	tsp = teaspoon

INTRODUCTION

Hello, and welcome to my *Drop a Size Calorie and Carb Counter*. I am always being asked about the calorie value of different foods and what the best foods are for Carb Curfew suppers – so I've put everything you need to know in one place. The idea is not to overwhelm you with lots of different figures, but to give you concise information, whether you want to lose weight or just stay within a healthy weight range.

Traditionally, calorie-counting books are used as a way of helping us monitor the amount of energy we are getting from our food and drink. To lose weight, the number of calories you eat has to be fewer than the number of calories your body burns off through exercise and your daily activities. But it's not all about numbers: eating the right type of nutrients can increase your energy levels and maximize health. Unfortunately, we often forget this in our efforts to keep weight under control and, as a result, we opt for low calorie but nutritionally poor foods. Even though your first motivation for picking up this book may be to help you count and cut calories, you'll soon find the information helps you realize your weight loss goals *and* improve your health, by enabling you to make wiser food choices. For example, you'll learn that energy-dense foods such as fats, and specifically saturated fats, are associated with an increased risk of heart disease, while nutritionally poor foods, such as processed, carbo-hydrate-rich foods that are high in sugar, can play havoc with your blood sugar levels and energy levels, and foods high in salt can affect your blood pressure.

This little book isn't just about counting calories for weight loss, but about counting your carbs and being aware of the nutrients required for a healthy body, too! So as well as lots of weight management tips, you'll also find plenty of health tips too. This calorie and carb counter is an invaluable companion to any weight loss programme but it will be especially useful for those following my Carb Curfew plan. It has been fascinating researching all the material and has been a real eye opener for me, too.

Be active!

Joanna

THE CARB CURFEW PLAN

CARB CURFEW – HOW IT CAME ABOUT

As a weight management specialist, my studies and expertise led me to work with individuals and organizations in the United States, Australia and in the UK. During my travels, I became increasingly aware that many people out there were putting a lot of effort into reaching their weight loss goals, but their hard work appeared to be going un-rewarded. The scales were not moving in the right direction, their clothes were not feeling looser and their energy levels were not as high as they should be – but most galling of all, they were experiencing all of this while putting their real lives on hold! Yes, they were following recognized dietary advice to cut fat intake as a means of reducing overall calorie intake, and they were taking some physical exercise, but instead of feeling trimmer, lighter and full of energy, they didn't seem to be reaping the benefits.

What I began to realize, as I researched my Master's degree in sports science, was that following a low-fat diet wasn't the sole solution to weight loss. Yes, sticking to a low fat intake is still sensible dietary advice – one gram of fat alone provides 9 calories (the equivalent of nearly 45 calories per teaspoon) – but my studies have shown that for successful weight loss, you need to address your *total* calorie intake plus the proportion of carbohydrates and protein you are eating. Reducing fat alone won't work. What's more, my research revealed that people who were cutting the amount of fat in their diets were compensating for the 'loss' by filling up on 'non' or 'low-fat' starchy carbohydrates such as bread, pasta, rice, potatoes and cereal. This meant, quite simply, that while their fat intake was going down, their overall calorie intake was going up. A recent study from the centre for disease control and prevention reported a 22 per cent jump in the calories we consumed between 1971 and 2000. This increase in calories was directly attributed to increased carbohydrate intake despite a reduction in the percentage of fat we consumed over the same period. It seems people are eating more 'non-fat' starches under the misapprehension that because these starches contained little or no fat this automatically translates into little or no calories! This is what motivated me to develop the Carb Curfew – a tool that can help people achieve successful weight loss and healthy nutrition. The Carb Curfew Plan helps you redress your nutritional and calorie balance without having to count every calorie, or put your life on hold.

So what is the Carb Curfew?

The Carb Curfew means no bread, pasta, rice, potatoes or cereal after 5 p.m. As a result, your evening meal now becomes based around lean meat, fish, pulses, vegetables, fruit, low-fat dairy products and essential fats. It is not about cutting out all starchy carbs, as starch provides a valuable source of muscle fuel for our bodies. Instead, to ensure you get the right balance of nutrients at the right time, I recommend you eat some starchy wholegrain carbs at breakfast (try porridge with semi-skimmed milk and a piece of fruit, or boiled egg and wholemeal toast), lunch (for example, a small jacket potato with tuna or an open chicken sandwich) and in your mid-afternoon snack if you wish, but avoid them after 5 p.m.

WHAT ARE THE BENEFITS OF FOLLOWING THE CARB CURFEW?

There are several great bonuses to implementing my Carb Curfew:

- ✪ It will help you cut your calorie intake without you having to obsess over calories.
- ✪ It will reduce bloatedness.
  When we eat starchy carbs, they are stored in the body in the form of glycogen. Glycogen is an important muscle fuel, but for every unit of glycogen stored in the body it is necessary to also store three units of water. This helps to explain why it is common to feel very bloated and uncomfortable in your clothes after eating a starch-heavy meal, such as pasta.
- ✪ It will boost your energy levels.
  Since you will be eating more fruit and vegetables, you will be putting more vital nutrients into your body and these are essential in the breakdown of macronutrients (i.e. carbs, protein and fat) to release energy. Plus many of my clients say how much more energetic they feel as a result of not eating so many starchy carbs.
- ✪ It helps you reach your five-a-day fruit and veg quota.
  The absence of starchy carbs in your evening meal will encourage you fill up your plate with these important foods.

In essence then, Carb Curfew is a strategy that allows you to get the right balance of calories and nutrients at the right time of day.

THE CARB CURFEW PLAN – A LIFESTYLE, NOT A DIETARY REGIME

To me, successful weight management is all about having a strategy that fits with your life – if you have to press the pause button while you go on a diet, you can bet your bottom dollar your weight loss is not going to last long term. I developed Carb Curfew as a tool to help people achieve their weight loss goals, while boosting their energy levels, changing their shape and getting on with their lives. One of the main reasons people tell me it works is because they feel they have made a positive lifestyle change without too much effort – they feel in control and not 'on a diet'. The Carb Curfew has helped thousands of people, and it can help you, too.

THE PLAN

The Carb Curfew Plan consists of five steps, each of which plays a different role in helping you achieve and maintain your ideal weight and body fat goals. The plan has been tried and tested by my weight management clients over the past 10 years – and it works! The five steps are:

1. **Use the Carb Curfew:** By not eating certain starchy carbohydrates after 5 p.m. you will lose weight and boost your energy levels. It is a strategy that allows you to cut your overall calorie intake and get the right balance of nutrients at the right time of the day. For example, eating starchy carbs with protein at lunchtime, instead of in your evening meal, will help

you beat your mid-afternoon sugar cravings – a challenge to those of us with even the strongest willpower – and boost your energy and brainpower for the rest of the day.

2. **Drink more water:** If you drink less than eight glasses of water a day you may be chronically dehydrated. This can affect your energy levels, and cause you to misinterpret tiredness as a need to eat more food. By drinking a minimum of two litres of water a day, you will fuel yourself with energy, curb your hunger and enhance your nutrient absorption.

3. **Figure out your fats:** This is not about cutting all fat from the diet, as some fat is essential for our health, rather, it is about reducing your overall fat intake, and specifically saturated fat, while at the same time increasing the good sources of fat in your diet.

4. **Be consistent:** The good news is the best way to lose weight is not to deprive yourself of all those things in life you love, but instead to stick to the 80–20 rule. You don't have to be 'good' 100 per cent of the time – if you can stick to the Carb Curfew plan for just 80 per cent of the time, you will have succeeded. Being consistent means you can actually eat a little more and you will still lose weight and body fat, and, more importantly, you are not setting yourself up for guilt and 'failure'.

5. **Move more, more often:** Most of us know we have to take regular exercise to lose weight. But we also know how hard it is to find the time to fit structured exercise sessions into our increasingly busy lives – so it's hardly surprising even the best intentions often fall by

the wayside. Well, the good news is that simply moving your body more often, in daily physical activities, is an important part of the exercise formula. It's important to try and make time for some regular, prolonged exercise when you can, but it is the combination of structured exercise with informal daily activity that really helps you on the road to feeling healthier, more energetic and to achieving your weight and body fat goals.

WEIGHT LOSS BASICS

If you are serious about losing weight and your motivation for using this book is to get your body size down then you need to get your head around some simple weight loss basics. Successful weight management is not just about getting excess body fat off, but keeping it off. Fad diets may help you drop the pounds, but the results will only be temporary, and your short-term smaller size can be at the cost of optimal health. So let's get back to basics and look at what you need to do:

1. DECREASE YOUR CALORIE INTAKE

To lose weight, you must create a negative calorie balance. In other words, the amount of energy that you consume from food and drinks must be less than the amount of energy that you expend in exercise and your everyday life. Exercise, as you have seen, is an important step in the Carb Curfew plan, and it is vitally important for long-term successful weight management and your health! However, for maximum success, you will also need to look at the 'energy in' side of the equation – in other words, what you eat. Generally, women need 1400–1800 calories a day and men 1600–2100, depending on their activity levels. To lose weight I recommend 1200–1500 calories for women and 1500–1800 for men, again subject to activity levels. Safe weight loss should focus on losing no more than 1–2 pounds of weight a week. This steady rate of weight loss helps to ensure that what is lost is not lean muscle but fat. According to most nutritional experts, to lose 1–2 pounds per week, you should consume 500 fewer calories than normal each day, which equates to about 3500 calories less per week.

2. MONITOR YOUR PORTION SIZES

If you are confused by what exactly is an adequate portion, you're not alone! Studies have shown that in the fast food, restaurant and packaged food industries, the average portion has increased by as much as eight-fold over the past 20 years, so it isn't any wonder that many of us serve bigger-than-necessary helpings on our own plates at home. Getting your portion sizes right is important no matter what sort of food you are eating – an excess of carrots or healthy brown rice is still extra calories, even though it may be healthier than a giant size portion of chips! This is one of the most overlooked aspects of weight loss – so be wary not to fall into this trap. (You will find more information on portion sizes on page 31.)

3. KEEP A FOOD JOURNAL

Keeping a record of the foods that you eat can help make you more aware of your calorie consumption and where there is room for improvement. Many of my clients find keeping a food diary helps them stay on track with the Carb Curfew eating plan. On page 38 we look at how you can be your own Carb Curfew coach, which will help you see, at a glance, how to get the right nutrients at the right time of the day.

4. FOCUS ON BODY COMPOSITION

Standing on the bathroom scales is one of the most emotionally-fraught things you can do when you're trying to lose weight – will it result in elation, frustration or disillusionment? But standing on the scales can give you a false picture of how your body shape is changing. A typical set of bathroom scales will only tell you the number of kilos or pounds you have gained or lost – not how your body has changed shape, and it may be that decreased fat and increased muscle tone actually lead to a slight increase in weight. Furthermore, scales often show mere shifts in water retention, which are temporary and do not reflect changes in the level of body fat.

Instead of simply relying on bathroom scales, assess your weight using the body mass index, or BMI. This will help you determine whether you are close to a healthy body weight or if you have a more significant amount of body fat to lose. To determine your BMI, measure your height in metres and your weight in kilos, and then divide your weight by your height squared ($W/H^2 = BMI$). So, for example, if you weigh 76kg and are 1.70m tall, you multiply 1.7 by 1.7 to give you 2.89, then divide 76 by 2.89. This gives a BMI of 26.29, which, as you can see from the categories below, would put you within the overweight range.

BMI categories

Underweight = under 20

Normal weight = 20–24.9

Overweight = 25–29.9

Very overweight = 30+

Once you're on the road to a healthier weight, I suggest you judge your progress by taking your body measurements on a weekly basis and, if you wish, measuring your body fat. This can be done using skin fold callipers or, more conveniently, a body fat monitor – these are similar to bathroom scales but they determine your percentage body fat. Taking your measurements and monitoring your body fat gives a truer idea of what is going on in your body than traditional bathroom scales. Remember also to check your BMI occasionally to ensure you are moving towards your goal weight. You can do this quickly and easily at my website www.joannahall.com.

FOOD GROUPS

To help you get to grips with your diet let's look at the main food groups and their relevance to health and weight loss.

Foods contain some or all of the six main nutrient groups – carbohydrates, proteins, fats, vitamins, minerals and water. As a rule of thumb, the main macronutrient in a particular food determines whether that food will be classified as a carbohydrate, protein or fat. For example, butter is considered a fat as it contains a lot of fat – but it is also made up of some protein, vitamins, minerals and water and very little carbohydrate. Meat is considered a protein as it contains a lot of protein, as well as water, some fat, vitamins and minerals and very little carbohydrate. Wholemeal bread, in contrast, is considered a carbohydrate as it contains a lot of carbohydrate, as well as vitamins and minerals, some protein and fat and very little water.

The amount of carbohydrate, protein and fat in a food determines the calorie value, as these energy-producing nutrients all supply a certain amount of energy per gram. Fat supplies the most energy, at 9 calories per gram, while carbohydrates and proteins each provide 4 calories per gram (alcohol also provides calories – 7 kcals per gram – but it is referred to as a non-nutrient since it doesn't offer the body any beneficial nutrition).

Before we look at each of the food groups featured in the nutritional tables let me remind you that eating should be pleasurable! Think in terms of having a good overall diet – avoid blacklisting foods, instead enjoy higher calorie value foods in moderation. Use the 80/20 rule – that way you won't feel as if you're on a diet.

Carbohydrates

What they are

Carbohydrates form the backbone of our diet. Fruit, vegetables, simple sugars such as biscuits and cakes, and starchy carbs such as potatoes, rice and bread are all carbohydrate-rich foods. Carbohydrates, which provide the main fuel for our bodies, have traditionally been described as being either simple or complex. This refers to their chemical structure, and is a useful rough guide to how quickly carbohydrates raise blood sugar levels. Basically, simple carbohydrates such as sugars, some fruits, cakes and biscuits, provide a quick increase in blood sugar levels, while complex carbohydrates such as brown rice and wholegrains raise them at a slower rate. Recently, a more precise classification – the Glycaemic index – has become widely adopted. This classifies individual carbohydrates according to the speed at which the body breaks them down and converts them to glucose to use as energy. The faster the food breaks down the higher the Glycaemic index, or GI, of that food. Foods with a high GI factor are rapidly digested and absorbed and quickly raise blood sugar levels. Low GI foods are broken down and digested more slowly so ensuring a slow and sustained release of glucose. You will find more information about this in the Drop a Size books series.

What they do

Carbohydrate-rich foods supply the body with its primary source of fuel – glucose. Glucose is a type of sugar that the body can easily use and transport – when we talk about blood sugars we are actually talking about our blood glucose levels. Glucose can also be stored in the muscles as glycogen and is the main source of fuel for the nervous system and brain. Carbohydrates must be present for us to burn body fat, so following a completely carb-free diet can actually encourage your body to burn muscle, as opposed to fat, as a source of fuel. Long term this may have a detrimental effect on your metabolism resulting in your body burning less calories. However, it's important to remember that *excess* calories from carbohydrates will be converted to and stored as body fat in the fat cells.

The problem with sugar

The only negative health effect of sugars that has been conclusively demonstrated is their association with dental cavities. Surprisingly, there is no proven scientific relationship between sugar intake and excess weight, but what we do know is that consuming too many calories contributes to obesity and that most foods which are high in sugar are also high in calories. There is also some preliminary evidence to support a link between high sugar intake and increased blood triglycerides (fats) in overweight individuals.

For all of the above reasons, it is advisable to limit your intake of sugary foods. Carbohydrates are of course made up of sugars but these naturally occurring sugars are far preferable to the refined and processed sugars added to many foods. Unfortunately, food labels often just list total sugars and not distinguish between added and naturally occurring sugars, but most of know what the worst offenders are – desserts, soft drinks, sweets and so on.

However, don't forget that sugar is also added to products like beans and savoury sauces, so it makes sense to check out the sugar content of foods that feature regularly in your diet – using my calorie and carb counter, you may just be able to find a similar product that has a lower sugar content.

Tips for those with a sweet tooth

- ✪ Split a dessert with a friend or take half home to enjoy another day.
- ✪ Don't ban sweets from your child's diet (or your own for that matter) – by occasionally allowing sweets, children will develop the habit of not overdoing it.
- ✪ Limit your intake of soft drinks to one a day and if ordering from a take away, opt for the smaller size.
- ✪ Learn to think unprocessed sugar sources first before processed foods. In other words, fresh fruit before sweets!
- ✪ While few people have trouble enjoying fruit as a snack, some individuals do seem to find it difficult to digest fruit after a meal. If this applies to you, mix pureed fruit with natural bio yoghurt for dessert. One of my favourites is pureed apple with cinnamon, a little nutmeg and natural bio yoghurt.

How much carbohydrate do we need?

Some health bodies and nutritionists recommend that we get a certain percentage of our total energy from carbohydrates – usually between 50 and 65 per cent. However, in the light of the need to reduce our overall calorie intake it may be more helpful to look at this another way and follow the more recent guidelines based on body weight. These recommend 4–5g of carbohydrate per kilogram of body weight for healthy, active people. In addition, there is a growing support for the need to reduce the amount of carbohydrate in the diet. My Carb Curfew plan is a simple way to do this without compromising the overall quality of your diet.

Fats

What they are

The fat in our food is the most concentrated source of energy, providing more than twice as many calories per gram as either protein or carbohydrate. Foods such as butter, oils, nuts, cheese and coconuts are all rich sources of fat.

Why we need them

It is important to stress that some fat is important for good health. Certain foods that contain fat supply the fat-soluble vitamins A, D, E, K and some essential fats that the body cannot make for itself. Fat also helps the body to transport some important antioxidants as well as helping to produce key hormones that regulate various body processes. If we were to cut out all fat in the diet, we would be depriving ourselves of some very important nutrients.

THE DIFFERENT TYPES OF FAT

All fats provide nine calories per gram. However, the health qualities of each fat are quite different and they perform different functions in the body. So while it is sensible to decrease overall intake of fat, the type of fat that we eat is also very important. There are three main subgroups of fats: saturated, polyunsaturated and monounsaturated. Each of these groups of fats has a different chemical structure and this can have a direct impact on how our body processes them.

Saturated fats

These are the least healthy. Eating too much saturated fat is associated with an increased risk of heart disease. These fats have little functional role in the body and when we consume too much saturated fat, the simplest thing for our body to do with it is transport it to the fat cells and dump it there. Quite simply, if the calories from fat are not being burnt off through physical exercise the fat cells welcome the saturated fat we eat with open arms and our fat cells get bigger and bigger, our clothes get tighter and tighter and our health risks get higher and higher. Saturated fats include butter, lard, cheese and the fat on meat.

Polyunsaturated fats

These are generally found in vegetable oils and fish. In contrast to saturated fats, polyunsaturated fats help to improve blood cholesterol levels. They are sub-divided into two groups:

✪ Omega-3 essential fatty acids. These are found mainly in oily fish such as salmon, herring, sardines, trout, pilchards and mackerel, and in flax seed and pumpkin seeds. They are thought to help to prevent atherosclerosis, and are also believed to lower blood pressure and triglycerides, a form of blood fat. This makes the blood less sticky and hence less susceptible to blood clots. Eating three servings of oily fish a week, or using flaxseed oil as part of your salad dressing, will help you hit your omega-3 fatty acid quota.

✪ Omega-6 essential fatty acids. These are found mainly in hemp, pumpkin, sunflower, safflower sesame and corn oil. About half of the oils found in these seeds are from omega-6 fatty acids. Omega-6 fatty acids, like their omega-3 cousins, have an important function in the body. They are involved in preventing blood clots, lowering blood pressure, helping to maintain the water balance in the body and helping the body to stabilize blood sugar levels. However, excessive consumption of omega-6 fatty acids may reduce HDL (good) cholesterol levels, as well as increasing the damage done by 'free radicals' linked to cancer.

Health tips

✪ If you use flaxseed oil, ensure you store it in the fridge as light damages its health properties.

✪ Polyunsaturated fats can become damaged when heated at high temperatures. It is therefore advisable to avoid cooking at high temperatures with these fats – instead use monounsaturated fats (see below).

Monounsaturated fats

These have been termed the most 'healthy' fats, partly because research has shown that the Mediterranean diet, with its high olive oil content, is associated with the lowest risk of heart disease. However, bear in mind that a tablespoon of olive oil has the same number of calories as a tablespoon of melted lard! So the total amount of fat is still important. Monounsaturated fats are liquid at room temperature and are better for cooking with than polyunsaturated oils because they are more stable (this simply means that their chemical structure is not adversely affected by heat). Sources of monounsaturated fat include olive oil and rapeseed oil (also known as canola oil).

Since fats contain twice as many calories as carbohydrates or protein, it is easy to see why they have become the easy scapegoat. However, when you consider the many people who have followed a low-fat diet yet are still overweight, it is obvious that the body converts not only the fat in our food into fat on the body, but also the excess carbohydrates and protein. This is why the Centres for Disease Control and Prevention urge us to address total calorie intake. Using the Carb Curfew is a simple way to do this.

Trans fats

You may well have come across the term trans fats or hydro-genated fats. These fats have no functional health role to play in the body and have been shown to be detrimental to our health. They often start out as more healthy polyunsat-urated oil, but processing at a very high temperature (generally in order to turn them from an oil into a solid fat) changes their chemical structure, damaging them and making them less stable. The consumption of trans or hydrogenated fats is associated with an increased risk of cancers and heart disease. The majority of margarines are made from hydrogenated fats and they are also found in numerous processed foods. Look for the word hydro-genated on your food labels and you have found trans fats!

As you can see, fat is important in the diet and it should not be outlawed, but use this table as a healthy pointer to keep your body on track. Let's not make food complicated – let's enjoy it!

Good fats, bad fats at a glance

Type of fat	Typical sources	Health rating
Monounsaturated fat	Olive oil	Excellent
	Canola (rapeseed) oil	
	Olives	
	Avocados	
Polyunsaturated	Corn oil	Good
	Sunflower oil	
	Sesame oil	
	Nuts and seeds	
Saturated fats	Butter	Unhealthy
	Lard	
	Meat	
	Eggs	
	Dairy products	
Hydrogenated fats	Vegetable shortening	Bad
	Margarine	
	Palm oil	

How much fat do we need?

According to new dietary recommendations, fat should constitute no more than 30 per cent of one's total calories and of this only 10 per cent or less should come from saturated sources. If you are following a 1600-calorie intake diet this equates to 50– 60 grams per day (a figure recommended by the American Dietary Association). However, in my experience with weight loss clients, reducing your calorie intake to around 1200–1400 calories initially and aiming for a fat intake of 40 grams a day (predominantly from essential fats) is advisable and a good rule of thumb. Remember, ensure you choose essential healthy fats and avoid saturated fats as far as possible.

Take home message

- ⊙ A balanced diet includes some fat every day.
- ⊙ Eat foods that contain the essential fatty acids. Essential fatty acids are abundant in fish, nuts and nut oils and seeds, flaxseed, olive and canola oil. Try to eat at least three servings of oily fish a week.
- ⊙ Decrease your saturated fat intake. Animal sources of fat are generally high in saturated fat.
- ⊙ Choose the healthiest fat possible. All fats increase the calorie value of your diet but less healthy fat-laden foods, such as margarine, can be replaced with foods rich in more beneficial omega-3 fats. Remember, a teaspoon of butter and a teaspoon of flaxseed oil both contain 45 calories and 5 grams of fat, but the flaxseed oil has many more health benefits.

Proteins

What they are

Proteins are made up of chains of amino acids. There are hundreds of amino acids in nature, but only 20 are important to we humans. Of these, eight are considered 'essential', as we cannot manufacture them in the body and therefore need to derive them from the foods we eat. Meat, fish, pulses and dairy products are all foods with a high protein content.

Protein and vegetarians

If you eat a variety of foods it is not difficult to get all your essential amino acids, however, if you are a vegetarian or vegan, you will need to take more care with your protein intake, as individual plant protein sources such as legumes, nuts, seeds and grains do not contain all the essential amino acids. It is therefore important to combine different sources of plant proteins in order to obtain all the essential amino acids.

What they do

Proteins make up part of every cell in the body and are essential for tissue repair, maintenance and growth. A regular supply of protein is required in the diet to compensate for the continual loss that occurs due to maintenance and growth processes. Protein can be divided into two groups: dairy products, which includes milk, cheese and yogurt, and non-dairy sources such as meat, fish, eggs, pulses and beans. The important role that protein plays in repairing the body means that it is much harder for the body to store excess protein as body fat in the cells.

How much do we need?

The Foods Standards Agency recommends we obtain 15 per cent of our energy from protein, which, in grams, will be dependent on the number of calories you take in overall. This figure is adequate for health purposes, but a higher absolute intake of protein a day is preferable if you are restricting your calorie intake with the aim of losing weight.

In this situation, 15 per cent is considered to be on the low side. Another way of determining your protein needs is by body weight. Guidelines suggest aiming for 0.75 grams of protein per kilogram of body weight. However, it is important that you obtain your protein from healthy sources such as fish, lean meat and nuts and seeds, and that you keep up a balanced intake of fruit and vegetables.

Exercise and Protein

If you are very athletic or involved in regular intense exercise you will have a greater protein demand, as protein is required for muscle repair and recovery after training. However, studies have shown that you only need between 1.2 and 1.4 grams per kilogram of body weight to meet the average requirements of a strength or endurance training programme – any amount over and above this does not provide any additional benefit.

Sodium

What it is

Sodium is a calorie-free mineral that finds its way into the diet in the form of salt. However, we're not just talking about the saltshaker here. Salt finds its way into our diet through the numerous refined and packaged foods we eat, so even if you don't add salt to your food, you'd be surprised how much salt you are consuming through processed foods. It is estimated about 75 per cent of the salt in our diet comes from processed foods.

Why we need it

We do need a certain amount of salt for our bodies to function smoothly – to keep nerve pathways working and to maintain our muscles. But too much salt has been clearly linked with hypertension (it raises blood pressure), which in turn increases the risk of heart disease or stroke – Britain's biggest killer. It is currently thought that we are consuming in the region of 9 grams of salt a day, which is about 2 teaspoons. The Food Standards Agency is so alarmed by this figure that it is lobbying the food industry to reduce the amount of salt in processed food.

How much do we need?

Everyone should lower their sodium intake to 1,500mg daily, about half the average intake (half a teaspoon of salt contains about 1,200mg of sodium). So bear in mind just how much is added to the diet through processed food and read those labels! Also, try cooking with spices, herbs, lemon and salt-free seasoning blends to reduce sodium intake – and go easy on the saltshaker.

Healthy tip

While table salt (sodium chloride) is responsible for raising blood pressure and causing heart problems, natural sea salt is health-promoting, since it contains many minerals, including magnesium and calcium. It is the healthy alternative to sodium chloride, so use it when cooking and on food instead of table salt. Up to 6g per day is considered safe.

How to measure how much salt you are eating

In Section Two, featuring basic foods, the sodium content for each entry is given. However, because food manufacturers are not always forthcoming with this information, it is not featured for branded foods. You will, of course, find that many of your favourite foods do list the salt or sodium content. Where the sodium content is given you can calculate the amount of salt simply by multiplying the sodium content by 2.5.

Here's an example of a food label:

Typical Values per pack
Energy Kcal: 230
Sodium g: 0.92

The equivalent amount of salt will therefore be 2.3g (0.92 x 2.5 = 2.3g). Since the recommendation is that we eat no more than 6 grams daily, this one food item would provide nearly half of the recommended intake in one go. Interestingly, this food label is not from a packet of smoked bacon or bag of ready salted crisps but from a pre-packed three bean salad – which you wouldn't generally consider a salty food. So it pays to read your labels and get sodium savvy!

If, like me, maths is not your strong point, then you can judge whether something is a high or low sodium food using the following criteria:

0.5g sodium or more per 100g is a lot of sodium
0.1g sodium or less per 100g is a little sodium

Watch out for sneaky sodium

Check food labels for other forms of sodium that are used as flavour enhancers and preservatives – for example, monosodium glutamate and sodium bicarbonate. These are found in savoury foods, soups, sauces and meat products.

Children and sodium

Accurate information on the amount of salt our children are eating is not currently available, however it is estimated that, on a body weight basis, the average salt intake of children is higher than that of adults. The maximum amount of salt babies and children should be consuming varies with age:

Up to 6 months – less than 1g a day
7–12 months – 1g a day
1–3 years – 2g a day
4–6 years – 3g a day
7–10 years – 5g a day

From the age of 11, children should be having no more than 6g a day. This is the same level recommended for adults.

TAKE HOME MESSAGE

✪ Eat more of foods that contain potassium – fruits, vegetables, lentils, pulses, fresh meat and fish, eggs, unsalted nuts, potatoes, pasta and rice. Potassium balances the effect of salt on the body.

- ❂ Avoid very salty foods – for example, processed, cured or pickled foods such as bacon, gammon, sausages, canned meat, packet soups, soy sauce, bottled sauces such as ketchup or chutneys, crisps, salted or roasted nuts and crackers. Also go easy on salt-heavy fast food such as hamburgers and chips.
- ❂ Stop adding table salt to food once it is served.

Dietary fibre

What it is

Dietary fibre is mainly derived from plant cell walls. There are two types of dietary fibre, soluble and insoluble. Soluble fibre dissolves in water and forms a gel. Found in fruits, vegetables, legumes and oat bran, it helps reduce cholesterol when eaten as part of a diet low in saturated fat. Soluble fibre can also help control blood sugar. Insoluble fibre does not dissolve in water, but instead absorbs water as it passes through the body. Found in fruits, vegetables, wholegrains and wheat bran, it adds fecal bulk and helps speed up the rate at which food passes through the digestive system.

WHY YOU NEED IT

A high fibre diet is a good idea for many reasons – it can give your energy levels a boost, and it helps lower the risk of diabetes, heart disease and possibly cancer. And probably most important to you right now – it can help you control your weight. Fibre slows digestion and makes you feel full, which is just the ticket for helping you to slim down.

How much do we need?

It will take a minimum of six servings of fruits and veggies and three servings of wholegrains daily to reach the recommended intake. Studies show that certain fibres lower cholesterol, normalize blood sugar in diabetics and, of course, help with regularity. Regularity appears to be such an important function of our daily lives that not only does it have an impact on our bowel health but also on our moods!

A word about water

In my opinion, no natural resource is undervalued as much as water and no nutrient will have a greater immediate impact on your energy levels. If you drink less than eight glasses of water a day, your body may be chronically dehydrated. You will lack energy and your brain will misinterpret this tiredness as a need to eat more food. By addressing your hydration levels you will provide the body with the right environment for metabolic processes to take place – and you should feel less compelled to reach for a sugar or caffeine fix.

Why is water important?

Water is crucial to everything that happens in our bodies. Water is especially important for weight management, because it swells food cells and helps our body take up vital nutrients. Water also makes us feel more satisfied and full. It bulks up food, stretching the stomach wall and sending messages to the brain telling us we are full. In addition, the water content in blood helps the absorption and transportation of all the nutrients, vitamins and mineral in the body, and flushes waste products away. When you make the change to a healthier eating plan your body will initially produce more toxins, which will need to be flushed away with water.

A few common questions

IS IT BETTER TO EAT 3 LARGER MEALS OR 6 SMALLER MEALS A DAY?

The number of times you eat per day is a personal preference and dependent upon your lifestyle. While eating three meals a day is the way most of us were brought up to eat, many of us now work longer hours, spend more time away from home and eat on the run, necessitating a more 'snacky' style of eating. Often known as 'grazing', this generally consists of eating smaller, but more frequent, meals. When the smaller meals or snacks are nutritionally sound and amount to the same number of calories as three larger meals, this strategy works well (research demonstrating that five or more meals per day are more beneficial has been conducted in controlled environments) but, unfortunately, people frequently end up consuming more calories and less nutritious food than they would if they stuck to the more traditional pattern. Whichever style of eating most suits your lifestyle, the important thing to remember for weight loss is that total number of calories is still important, which is why Carb Curfew can be an effective and an easy to implement healthy eating strategy when you're on the road or eating on the hoof.

Weight loss tip – follow the 100 calories snacking rule

It is a good rule of thumb to restrict the calorie value of your snacks to 100 calories. This allows you to quantify the snack and gives you a specific number to work to. This book will help you identify healthier 100-calorie snack choices, such as low-calorie fruits and vegetables and low-fat dairy foods, such as yoghurt. This calorie amount also gives an indication of the ideal portion size for your chosen snack.

WHAT IS A PORTION?

In my research for this book, I came across a wide discrepancy in portion sizes. What I found even more alarming was that, at present, there is no uniform portion sizing, even within food manufacturers. For example, a serving of pasta salad in a pre-packed lunch may be detailed on the front of the pack as having X number of calories but the actual serving that this relates to may be a third or even half of the container, not the entire thing. While unification of portion size would be very helpful across all foods, it would be even more helpful if individual manufacturers kept a level of consistency in their ranges. So until that occurs, please take a moment to turn over the label and see what exactly the label is referring to when it says 'per serving'!

To make matters worse, according to the *Journal of the American Dietetic Association*, many of today's most popular packaged foods and beverages are actually two to five times larger than they were when these foods were first introduced in the marketplace! Thanks to supersized portions, it's estimated that we are eating 150 calories per day more than we were 20 years ago. That adds up to an extra 15 pounds per person per year. Whatever way you look at it, portion control goes hand in hand with weight control and learning to downsize is one way to prevent your waistline from expanding. However, knowing exactly what is a portion can be a challenge – the chart below will help you size up your servings.

Food	What a serving should look like
Peanut butter (1 tbsp/30g) 16g fat/190 calories	size of a jaffa cake
Dry white spaghetti (50g/2oz) 0.9g fat/171 calories	the diameter of a 10p
Bagel (1 small) 1g fat/190 calories	size of a 150g can of tuna
One muffin (bran) 5g fat/179 calories	size of a tennis ball

Mashed potatoes (½ cup)   half a cricket ball
9g fat/112 calories

Swiss cheese (30g/1oz)   pair of dice
9g fat/115 calories

Meat, chicken, fish (100g/4oz)   a deck of cards
7.5g fat/165 calories (average)

Low-fat vanilla ice cream (½ cup)   half an orange
3g fat/92 calories

Dry-roasted peanuts 28g   one and a half golf balls
14g fat/168 calories

Low-fat muesli (½ cup)   a fist
3g fat/186 calories

Crisps 28g   half of a grapefruit
10g fat/152 calories

Navigating your way round a food label

Whilst the tables in this book feature a vast number of foods, they cannot conceivably feature everything, so it is important to know how to read a food label.

These days, all packaged foods are required to carry detailed labels explaining the nutritional value of the product. Here is an example of what you may see when you take a look at a food label.

Average values	per 100g	per 300g serving
Energy	305kj	915kj
	70kcal	210kcal
Protein	6.1g	18.3g
Carbohydrate	9.6g	28.8g
of which sugars	0.8g	2.4g
Fat	1.9g	5.7g
of which saturates	0.6g	1.8g
Fibre	1.2g	3.6g
Sodium	0.25g	0.75g

What to look for

- ✪ The amount of energy in a product is shown as kcal and kj. Kcal and kilocalories are the same as calories. Kj or kilojoules is simply another way of measuring energy. Although kilojoules is the more scientifically correct term to describe the amount of energy, most of us refer to calories, so for simplicity ignore the kj information and just concentrate on the calorie info.

- ✪ You will see that the information is presented in per 100g and per serving. I always advise looking at the 'per serving' information, because you have to do less arithmetic and this amount will be closer to what you will actually be putting in your mouth. But a word of warning: not all serving sizes are the same across all brands and products, and bear in mind that the package might say 'serves 2' when you were planning to eat the whole pack – so be vigilant!

- ✪ Look at the total amount of calories. In this example, the food will provide 210 calories per serving.

✪ Look at the total amount of fat per serving. This product will provide you with 5.7 grams per serving.

✪ Look at the amount of saturated fat. 1.8 grams of the *total* amount of fat in this product is saturated fat.

✪ Look at the amount of sodium. Remember, this is *not* the same as the amount of salt in the product as sodium is only a component of salt. The general rule is that any packaged food has had salt added. If the sodium content per 100g is greater than 0.2g the food is high in salt.

✪ Check out the fibre content. Natural wholegrain unprocessed foods will have a higher content of dietary fibre than a lot of pre-prepared foods.

✪ Look at the carbohydrate and sugar values. Sugar can be added to our foods but can also be found naturally in the foods we eat, such as fruit and milk. Nutrition experts advise that we restrict the intake of added sugars, but not of the latter.

✪ Finally, check out the list of ingredients. Avoid ingredients such as hydrogenated or partially hydrogenated vegetable oils and trans fats. As a rule of thumb the higher up the ingredient list these fats figure, the more of them there will be in the product.

MISLEADING LABELS

As well as nutritional facts, food labels tell us about their contents by using terms such as 'low-fat' and 'sugar-free'. While this can be useful, it can also be misleading. A 'low-fat' cheese, for example, may well be 'low fat' for a cheese but is rarely a low fat food! And a sugar-free label on a product that is normally sweet is often a warning sign that it contains artificial sweeteners and a host of other additives that are hardly health promoting.

'Cholesterol free' is another label that causes confusion – do not to fall into the trap of thinking that cholesterol free means fat free. A peanut butter label may well read 'cholesterol free' but it's far from fat free (oh, and by the way, it never had cholesterol in it in the first place!). When it comes to cereals, some manufacturers proclaim 'No added fat' on their packets of muesli or wholesome cereals, yet the natural grains have been processed with coconut or palm oils, which are high in saturated fat.

So what's the answer? Don't just rely on terms like 'low fat' or 'reduced fat' that are flashed on the front of food packets, look at the nutritional information that is often displayed in much smaller print.

Here's a good example of why it pays to delve a bit deeper. The nutritional information below is from a muesli bar that had the words '87% fat free' flashed across the front.

Typical values	Per 100g	Per 75g bar
Energy	400 calories	300 calories
Protein	6.4g	4.8g
Carbohydrates	67.2g	50.4g
Fat	12.8g	9.6g
Dietary Fibre	4.4g	3.3g

Given its claim to be '87% fat free' you would assume that this means only 13 per cent of its calories come from fat. Wrong! In actual fact, what 87% fat free means is that of 100g of the product, less than 13g – that's weight not calories – comes from fat. In calorie terms, this means a total of about 26 per cent of the calories in the bar come directly from fat.

Here's why: a gram of fat gives 9 calories, while protein and carbohydrate provide 4 calories per gram. So of the total calories contained in this bar, 87 calories come from fat (9.6 grams of fat multiplied by 9 calories), which is equivalent to 26 per cent of the calories coming directly from fat!

Although clever calculations mean food labels can bend the truth, now that you can decipher food labels for yourself you can be more responsible for what you put in your mouth.

Travellers beware

Being savvy about food is a demanding business. Just when you've got to grips with food labels, ingredients and terminology, you find that it's all different when you leave UK soil. For example, what does your calorie-counting book mean when it says 'muffin?' Is it a relatively healthy English muffin or a potentially calorie-laden American one? Does 'chips' refer to fried potatoes or crisps? Ensure that you are looking up and evaluating the right product.

What's more, if you are checking labels, be aware that in Europe and Australia, the more common energy term used is kilojoules, not kilocalories. To calculate calories from kilojoules, simply divide by 4.2.

BE YOUR OWN CARB CURFEW COACH

Those of us who are struggling with weight issues and searching for ways to improve our eating habits often lump foods into 'good' or 'bad' categories. Consequently, processed foods advertised as 'no fat', 'low fat' or 'reduced fat' find their way into our shopping trolley, while healthy foods such as nuts and avocados, which are a rich source of healthy fat, are banished to the 'bad' food category, never to win a place in our weekly shop. Looking at the big picture of your eating is important, and keeping a food diary allows you to look at your diet as a whole, shifting the emphasis away from individual foods and allowing you to establish healthy eating patterns. To help you achieve a healthy diet here are some tips for becoming your own healthy eating Carb Curfew coach.

FRUIT AND VEGETABLES

✪   **ARE FRUIT AND VEG PREDOMINANT IN YOUR DIET?**

These foods are not only naturally low in fat but are also a great source of dietary fibre. Fibre adds no calories to your diet, yet creates a feeling of fullness. This means you need less of other foods and you're getting all the benefits of a natural source of vitamins, minerals and antioxidants.

The World Health Organization recommends we eat *at least* five portions of fruit and vegetables a day, but a recent survey revealed that as a nation we are eating less than three portions a day!

But what exactly is a portion? Well, one serving of fruit and vegetables is about 80g. That equates to roughly a bowl of salad, three tablespoons of carrots or peas, half a fresh pepper or a medium tomato, apple or orange. So, unfortunately, the slice of tomato in our sandwiches does not equal a portion, and sorry, potatoes don't count – they're a starchy carb. Aim to have as much variety as possible and remember, a glass of fruit or vegetable juice counts too – but only once, no matter how much you drink. Use the quick reference table below to check you are hitting your daily quota – if you're eating less than five a day, add in one more at a time, gradually building up to at least five.

One portion equals ...

✿	Apple, orange or banana	1 fruit
✿	Very large fruit e.g. melon, pineapple	1 large slice
✿	Small fruits e.g. plums, kiwi, satsuma	2 fruits
✿	Raspberries, strawberries, grapes	1 cupful
✿	Fresh fruit salad, stewed or canned fruit	2–3 tablespoons
✿	Dried fruit	½–1 tablespoon
✿	Fruit juice	1 glass (150ml)
✿	Vegetables, raw, cooked, frozen or canned	2 tablespoons
✿	Salad	1 dessert-bowl full

DAIRY PRODUCTS

✪ **ARE THE DAIRY FOODS YOU EAT LABELLED NON-FAT OR LOW-FAT?**

Sticking to non- or low-fat items reduces your total fat intake as well as your consumption of saturated fat, and there is just as much calcium in, say, skimmed milk as there is in the full-fat version. Calcium is crucial to your bone health too, so aim to consume dairy products daily.

RED AND WHITE MEAT

✪ **IF YOU EAT RED MEAT, DO YOU TRIM OFF THE VISIBLE FAT?**

✪ **DO YOU SELECT LEAN CUTS?**

✪ **WHEN EATING POULTRY ARE YOU EATING PRIMARILY THE WHITE MEAT WITHOUT THE SKIN?**

Skinless white poultry is lower in fat than the dark poultry with the skin on.

COOKING METHODS

✪ **DO YOUR PREPARATION AND COOKING METHODS AID IN REDUCING YOUR TOTAL FAT INTAKE, ESPECIALLY FROM SATURATED SOURCES?**

✪ **DO YOU COOK YOUR FOODS IN WAYS THAT ADD EXTRA FAT?**

If so, check out the alternatives opposite.

Cooking Method	Healthier Options
Frying	Bake, steam, grill
Stir-frying	Blanch vegetables first and then flash stir-fry in a little olive oil
Stewing and casseroling	Brown off the meat first in a small amount of liquid, or prepare dish a day ahead of serving and skim off fat from the top of the dish
Deep-fat frying	Experiment with microwaving and en papillote, a method where food is wrapped in greaseproof paper or foil and baked in the oven. This works well with vegetables and seafood – adding a little liquid such as citrus juices or wine and herbs can help keep food moist as well as adding flavour
Roasting	Can be a no-fat cooking method – use a trivet to help fat drain away from food. If basting is required try brushing with oil to reduce the quantity used and mix with balsamic and sherry vinegar to make a small amount of oil go further

GRAINS

✪ **ARE YOU OPERATING THE CARB CURFEW?**

✪ **ARE YOU EATING SOME SOURCES OF CARBS AT BREAKFAST AND LUNCH?**

✪ **ARE YOUR CARB SOURCES WHOLEGRAIN, RATHER THAN PROCESSED?**

Carbs are naturally low in fat but they can be high in calories so be wary of serving yourself a hefty portion. Also bear in mind that eating large quantities will make you feel sleepy, possibly triggering a sugar craving, and that, regardless of their source, excess calories are converted into fat. Following the Carb Curfew is a quick and effective way of getting a better balance of carbs in your diet.

Your daily Carb Curfew coach record

You can use a daily checklist to help you put the Carb Curfew plan into action. Begin by copying out the chart and checklists below into a handy notebook that you can carry around with you. (Yes, as you've probably noticed, there is an exercise checklist but don't worry, I'll give you some guidance on exercise in the next few pages.) You may want to copy out a week's worth at a time to motivate yourself, or do it every day on the way to the office – whatever works for you.

This is what you then need to do:

1. Simply remember to fill it in when you eat, and not at the end of the day – you will end up forgetting!
2. Tally up your calories by looking at the nutritional charts in sections B and C.
3. Be sure to include all foods and beverages eaten and drunk.
4. Estimate portion sizes to the best of your ability i.e. large, medium or small. Be honest!
5. Include food preparation information whenever possible (e.g. grilled, fried, roasted, baked, steamed).

NUTRITION CHECKLIST

Have I followed the Carb Curfew?	YES/NO
Have I drunk two litres of water?	YES/NO
Have I watched my fat intake?	YES/NO
Have I had five portions of fruit and vegetables?	YES/NO

EXERCISE CHECKLIST

Have I accumulated 30 minutes of physical activity?	YES/NO
Have I completed a structured exercise session today?	YES/NO

By filling in a food diary like this you can see where you're going wrong – and right; where you can make improvements and how you can consolidate the progress you are making.

Daily Carb Curfew Counter Record

DAY:		DATE:	
Meal	Time	Food/Beverage	Calories
BREAKFAST			
LUNCH			
DINNER (Remember to operate Carb Curfew)			
SNACKS			

Nutrition checklist

Have I followed the Carb Curfew?	YES/NO
Have I drunk two litres of water?	YES/NO
Have I watched my fat intake?	YES/NO
Have I had five portions of fruit and vegetables?	YES/NO

Exercise checklist

Have I accumulated 30 minutes of physical activity?	YES/NO
Have I completed a structured exercise session today?	YES/NO

Health tip

Remember that while your main motivation for losing weight may be to look better, even a moderate decrease in weight of 5–10 per cent can result in improved health and relief from medical conditions. Focusing on small changes over time results in long-term reduction in weight and associated risk factors.

EXERCISE

If you are really serious about controlling your weight and wanting to optimize your health, the total amount of calories you expend through exercise is crucial. You can expend energy in two simple ways: by accumulating physical activity throughout the day, and by taking more structured exercise. Building more physical activity into your life requires a little thought, but once you find ways of injecting bouts of activity into your normal lifestyle, you'll find it comes easily – and you'll soon feel the benefit. The advantage of accumulating physical activity over the course of the day is that you don't need to plan it, you don't have to wear any particular fitness kit and you can do it at the drop of a hat – provided you seize the opportunity. This is a vital skill to learn and I call it navigating your 24.

Navigating the 24

Do you remember a time when you always got up to change the TV channel, you walked to collect your take-away, or quickly nipped to the shops on foot for that ½ litre of milk? Well, all of these activities are part of daily life. Modern society is good at providing us with labour-saving devices and saving us time – but if we don't use the time to move our bodies more we become increasingly sedentary. Physical inactivity has become such a concern for the government that it has set up an initiative to get 70 per cent of the population taking 30 minutes of exercise five times a week by the year 2020.

Navigating your 24 to include more activity shouldn't be difficult – all you have to do is not labour save but labour spend! Here are some examples you may be able to fit into your day:

- ✪ Don't email colleagues in the building – get up and talk to them. An American study recently reported that using email for 5 minutes out of every hour in your working day will cause a pound of weight gain a year – that's 10lbs of surplus fat in the next decade!
- ✪ Put all your small labour-saving devices in a box out of use for a week. Lock up your TV remote, DVD controller, sound system remote, whatever you have that allows you to keep still, banish it for a week.
- ✪ Stop wearing your mobile phone like it's a part of your body. Leave it in the other room, so you have to get up and move to answer it.

✪ Whether at home or in the office commit to always use the toilet on another floor. The average person goes to the toilet four times a day so try doing that every day, every week for a month.

✪ Walk down as well as up the stairs in the office. We're all aware that we should take the stairs whenever we can but did you know that the additional impact your body absorbs when walking downstairs can safeguard against osteoporosis.

✪ Do a chore at lunchtime. Everyone has errands to run at lunchtime – be savvy and plan an errand that involves you physically moving – post that letter, pay that cheque in at the bank. Breaking up your activity into three 10-minute bouts has been shown to have positive health benefits, helping to counter over 20 diseases – now that's a great payoff for three bouts of 10 minutes!

✪ Play interval games with the kids. If you have children of different ages don't let that be a deterrent to your activity plans. On walks take it in turns with your partner or friends to push the buggy while one of you runs with the older ones then swap over to catch your breath. The kids will get a great workout and an important health message too.

Structured exercise

Structured exercise involves putting on your trainers and getting a little bit hot and sweaty. In a balanced, structured exercise programme, both aerobic (cardiovascular) exercise and resistance training are needed to optimize the way your body burns energy. I am always being asked which exercise is best for burning calories. Well, aerobic endurance exercise that uses the large muscles of your body in a continuous rhythmic fashion is great for burning calories. However, you also need some form of resistance training as this helps maintain muscle mass, which keeps your body burning calories (it takes far more calories to maintain a pound of muscle than a pound of fat).

Successful long-term weight management is about moving your body on a regular basis so it is vital that you find something that you enjoy – otherwise you're just not going to keep it up. However, it is also a good idea to vary the form of exercise you are doing regularly, to avoid overuse injury and maintain interest.

A great way to optimize the number of calories you burn in endurance exercise is to vary the intensity with various interval training schemes.

INTERVAL TRAINING

Interval training combines segments of high intensity work with moderate to light intensity work. It is highly effective and can be a useful form of exercise to complement an active lifestyle, helping you to improve your fitness and aiding weight management. The specific design of the interval training programme depends on how fit you are, how long you plan to exercise for and what your specific aims are. The sample interval training programme outlined below is designed to enhance the body's calorie burning capacity. It's easy, as you are the one in control – you choose the form of exercise you wish to do and the appropriate level of intensity and you're away! Choose something you enjoy doing such as walking, jogging, cycling, rowing, stair climbing or elliptical training.

Sample interval programme:

- ✪ Always start gradually with a 3–5 minute warm up of light intensity cardiovascular activity to prepare the lungs, heart and muscles for the workout to follow.
- ✪ After the warm up, train for 4 minutes at a high intensity followed by 4 minutes at a moderate to light intensity.
- ✪ Alternate these 4-minute intervals for the entire workout to enhance the calorie-burning cellular systems. During the high intensity interval, you should feel 'comfortably challenged'. During the moderate intensity interval you should feel 'somewhat challenged'.
- ✪ Start with a 20-minute workout duration and progress up to 60 minutes over several weeks, according to your fitness.

For variety, regularly alternate the interval programme with a continuous CV exercise programme.

The key is to challenge your body. However, this doesn't mean pushing it to extremes – even walking on a treadmill and varying the gradient of the interval can push your cardiovascular system, whether you're doing interval training or a continuous CV workout. As long as you can hear your body saying 'oh, that feels a bit harder – what's going on here?' you can be sure that you have provided a challenge, which is essential in order for your body to get fitter and improve the stamina of your heart and lungs. Always start doing exercise when you are well hydrated – otherwise your body will find it harder to exercise.

RESISTANCE TRAINING

At present the type of resistance training technique best for burning calories is unknown – the most important thing you can do is incorporate some sort of resistance training into your schedule two to three times a week. This not only helps to increase muscle tone and boost metabolism, but also strengthens bones and soft tissues. The traditional method of strength training, with weights, sets and repetitions is great, but don't panic if you don't know what to do, even everyday tasks, such as gardening, cleaning or carrying heavy shopping bags count as light resistance work. Exercises that tone and use your own body weight, such as Pilates and Yoga, work too!

Metabolism and calorie expenditure

You often hear larger people say 'I've got a slow metabolism' to explain their excess weight, but the truth is, the larger and heavier you are, the higher your metabolism. A 9-stone person jogging for 15 minutes will burn fewer calories than a 12-stone person jogging for the same amount of time, as the heavier jogger has to expend more energy to propel themselves forward. That's why it is impossible to say that an hour of aerobics burns a specific number of calories – it depends on the person participating in the class.

Eating that means exercising this long ...

The following estimates are based on a person weighing 10 stone/64kgs. If you are heavier, you will burn the necessary number of calories more quickly. If you are lighter, you will need a little longer to reach the calorie expenditure given.

Food:	Burger King chicken sandwich
Cals:	659
Activity:	Downhill skiing
Time to burn it off:	1 hour 6 minutes

Food:	KFC chicken drumstick
Cals:	195
Activity:	Skipping
Time to burn it off:	18 minutes

Food:	Slice of Domino's cheese and tomato pizza
Cals:	125
Activity:	Running
Time to burn it off:	10 minutes

Food:	Banana
Cals:	62
Activity:	Swimming
Time to burn it off:	13 minutes

Food:	Sirloin steak (112g)
Cals:	248
Activity:	Cycling
Time to burn it off:	36 minutes

GUIDE TO VITAMINS AND MINERALS

Having briefly touched on the importance of vitamins and minerals earlier, this chart is designed to provide a practical guide to the vitamin and mineral content of some popular foods. I have tried to present the information in the most useful way possible, by showing you which foods contain specific vitamins and minerals in reasonable amounts, rather than by telling you all about, say, vitamin A and then telling you where you can find it. To get the most out of your diet, vary the types of foods you eat regularly. For example, swap green grapes for red ones; swap your daily serving of broccoli for kale once in a while and so on. Fruits and vegetables are all unique in the types and amounts of micronutrients and phytochemicals they contain so eating a wide variety will increase your chances of getting all the nutrients your body needs.

If you eat	you get this/ these vitamin(s)	which help your body in the following ways
Dairy Products	Vitamin A (retinol), Vitamin D (calciferol)	**Vitamin A:** Maintenance of healthy growth, development, vision, cells in the skin, gut and respiratory tract **Vitamin D:** Aids in bone and tooth formation, and helps maintain heart action and nervous system
Green leafy vegetables	Vitamin A (beta-carotene), Vitamin E (alpha-tocopherol), Vitamin B2 (riboflavin), Vitamin K, folic acid (folacin, folate)	**Vitamin A:** Maintenance of healthy growth, development, vision, cells in the skin, gut and respiratory tract **Vitamin E:** Protects blood cells, body tissue and essential fatty acids from harmful destruction in the body **Vitamin B2:** Helps the body release energy from protein, fats and carbohydrates during metabolism **Vitamin K:** Essential for blood clotting functions **Folic acid:** Aids in genetic material development such as DNA; involved in red blood cell production and strengthens the immune system
All vegetables	Vitamin B1 (thiamine), Vitamin C (ascorbic acid), pantothenic acid	**Vitamin B1:** Maintenance of healthy nervous system, heart and growth. Necessary for the conversion of carbohydrates to energy **Vitamin C:** Essential for structure of bones, cartilage, muscle and blood vessels; helps maintain capillaries and gums; stimulates the immune system and aids in absorption of iron **Pantothenic acid:** Helps in the release of energy from fats and carbohydrates

If you eat	you get this/ these vitamin(s)	which help your body in the following ways
Legumes	Biotin, pantothenic acid	**Biotin:** Involved in metabolism of protein, fats and carbohydrates **Pantothenic acid:** Helps in the release of energy from fats and carbohydrates
Dried peas, beans and lentils	Folic acid (folacin, folate)	**Folic acid:** Aids in genetic material development such as DNA; involved in red blood cell production and strengthens the immune system
Fruits	Vitamin K, pantothenic acid	**Vitamin K:** Essential for blood clotting functions **Pantothenic acid:** Helps in the release of energy from fats and carbohydrates
Citrus fruits, berries	Vitamin C (ascorbic acid)	**Vitamin C:** Essential for structure of bones, cartilage, muscle and blood vessels; helps maintain capillaries and gums; stimulates the immune system and aids in absorption of iron
Yellow and orange fruits	Vitamin A (beta-carotene)	**Vitamin A:** Maintenance of healthy growth, development, vision, cells in the skin, gut and respiratory tract
Fortified cereals and oatmeals	Vitamin B1 (thiamine), Vitamin A, Vitamin E (alpha-tocopherol), Vitamin B3 (niacin), biotin	**Vitamin B1:** Maintenance of healthy nervous system, heart and growth. Necessary for the conversion of carbohydrates to energy **Vitamin A:** Maintenance of healthy growth, development, vision, cells in the skin, gut and respiratory tract **Vitamin E:** Protects blood cells, body tissue and essential fatty acids from harmful destruction in the body

If you eat	you get this/ these vitamin(s)	which help your body in the following ways
		Vitamin B3: Involved in carbohydrate, protein and fat metabolism **Biotin:** Involved in metabolism of protein, fats and carbohydrates
Grain products, vegetable oils, nuts	Vitamin E (alpha-tocopherol), Vitamin K, biotin	**Vitamin E:** Protects blood cells, body tissue and essential fatty acids from harmful destruction in the body **Vitamin K:** Essential for blood clotting functions **Biotin:** Involved in metabolism of protein, fats and carbohydrates
Whole grains	Vitamin B1 (thiamine), Vitamin B2 (riboflavin), Vitamin B6 (pyridoxine), biotin, pantothenic acid	**Vitamin B1:** Maintenance of healthy nervous system, heart and growth. Necessary for the conversion of carbohydrates to energy **Vitamin B2:** Helps the body release energy from protein, fats and carbohydrates during metabolism **Vitamin B6:** Aids in both glucose and protein metabolism and energy production, and maintains healthy nervous system. Important in the resistance to infection **Biotin:** Involved in metabolism of protein, fats and carbohydrates **Pantothenic acid:** Helps in the release of energy from fats and carbohydrates
Rice and pasta	Vitamin B1 (thiamine)	**Vitamin B1:** Maintenance of healthy nervous system, heart and growth. Necessary for the conversion of carbohydrates to energy

If you eat	you get this/ these vitamin(s)	which help your body in the following ways
Organ meats	Vitamin A (retinol), Vitamin B1 (thiamine), Vitamin B2 (riboflavin), biotin, folic acid (folacin, folate)	**Vitamin A:** Maintenance of healthy growth, development, vision, cells in the skin, gut and respiratory tract **Vitamin B1:** Maintenance of healthy nervous system, heart and growth. Necessary for the conversion of carbohydrates to energy **Vitamin B2:** Helps the body release energy from protein, fats and carbohydrates during metabolism **Biotin:** Involved in metabolism of protein, fats and carbohydrates **Folic acid:** Aids in genetic material development such as DNA; involved in red blood cell production and strengthens the immune system
Meats	Vitamin B1 (thiamine), Vitamin B3 (niacin), Vitamin B6 (pyridoxine), Vitamin B12 (cobalamin), pantothenic acid	**Vitamin B1:** Maintenance of healthy nervous system, heart and growth. Necessary for the conversion of carbohydrates to energy **Vitamin B3:** Involved in carbohydrate, protein and fat metabolism **Vitamin B6:** Aids in both glucose and protein metabolism and energy production, and maintains healthy nervous system. Important in the resistance to infection **Vitamin B12:** Aids cell development, functioning of the nervous system and the metabolism of protein and fat **Pantothenic acid:** Helps in the release of energy from fats and carbohydrates
Poultry	Vitamin B3 (niacin),	**Vitamin B3:** Involved in carbohydrate, protein and fat metabolism

If you eat	you get this/these vitamin(s)	which help your body in the following ways
	Vitamin B6 (pyridoxine)	**Vitamin B6:** Aids in both glucose and protein metabolism and energy production, and maintains healthy nervous system. Important in the resistance to infection
Fish	Vitamin B3 (niacin), Vitamin B6 (pyridoxine), Vitamin D	**Vitamin B3:** Involved in carbohydrate, protein and fat metabolism **Vitamin B6:** Aids in both glucose and protein metabolism and energy production, and maintains healthy nervous system. Important in the resistance to infection **Vitamin D:** Aids in bone and tooth formation, and helps maintain heart action and nervous system
Seafood	Vitamin B12 (cobalamin)	**Vitamin B12:** Aids cell development, functioning of the nervous system and the metabolism of protein and fat

If you eat	you get this/ these mineral(s)	which help your body in the following ways
Milk and milk products	Calcium, phosphorus	**Calcium:** Essential for healthy bone structure and teeth formation. Important in muscle contraction and in the transmission of nerve impulses **Phosphorus:** Important role in the final delivery of energy to all cells including muscles. Helps create the structure of bones and teeth. Essential to the normal functioning of B group vitamins
Eggs	Zinc, phosphorus	**Zinc:** Involved in digestion and metabolism, important in development of reproductive system, and aids in healing **Phosphorus:** Important role in the final delivery of energy to all cells including muscles. Helps create the structure of bones and teeth. Essential to the normal functioning of B group vitamins
Green vegetables	Magnesium	**Magnesium:** Involved in most body processes including repair and maintenance, hormonal activity, acid/alkaline balance, and the metabolism of carbohydrates, minerals and sugar
Vegetables (particularly potatoes /tomatoes)	Potassium	**Potassium:** Maintenance of body fluids; controls activity of heart muscle, nervous system and kidneys
Legumes	Copper, iron	**Copper:** Necessary for the formation of red blood cells, the production of energy and adrenal hormones.

If you eat	you get this/ these mineral(s)	which help your body in the following ways
		Important in the production of collagen, which is responsible for health of skin, cartilage and bones **Iron:** Essential in red blood cell formation. Improves blood quality, and increases resistance to stress and disease
Fruits (particularly banana/ oranges)	Potassium	**Potassium:** Maintenance of body fluids; controls activity of heart muscle, nervous system and kidneys
Whole grains	Zinc, manganese, magnesium, chromium	**Zinc:** Involved in digestion and metabolism, important in development of reproductive system, and aids in healing **Manganese:** Involved in enzyme activation, carbohydrate and fat production, sex hormone production, and skeletal development. Important role in maintenance of healthy brain function **Magnesium:** Involved in most body processes including repair and maintenance, hormonal activity, acid/alkaline balance, and the metabolism of carbohydrates, minerals and sugar **Chromium:** Important in regulating blood-sugar levels, it increases effectiveness of insulin and stimulates glucose metabolism
Grains	Phosphorus, selenium	**Phosphorus:** Important role in the final delivery of energy to all cells including muscles. Helps create the

If you eat	you get this/ these mineral(s)	which help your body in the following ways
		structure of bones and teeth. Essential to the normal functioning of B group vitamins **Selenium:** Protects body tissues against oxidative damage from normal metabolic processing and pollution. Important for immune system function and liver function, and can help protect against heart and circulatory diseases
Nuts	Copper, manganese, magnesium	**Copper:** Necessary for the formation of red blood cells, the production of energy and adrenal hormones. Important in the production of collagen, which is responsible for health of skin, cartilage and bones **Manganese:** Involved in enzyme activation, carbohydrate and fat production, sex hormone production, and skeletal development. Important role in maintenance of healthy brain function **Magnesium:** Involved in most body processes including repair and maintenance, hormonal activity, acid/alkaline balance, and the metabolism of carbohydrates, minerals and sugar
Corn oil, clams, brewer's yeast	Chromium	**Chromium:** Important in regulating blood-sugar levels, it increases effectiveness of insulin and stimulates glucose metabolism
Seafood	Iodine, selenium, zinc	**Iodine:** Component of hormone thyroxine which controls metabolism

If you eat	you get this/ these mineral(s)	which help your body in the following ways
		Selenium: Protects body tissues against oxidative damage from normal metabolic processing and pollution. Important for immune system function and liver function, and can help protect against heart and circulatory diseases **Zinc:** Involved in digestion and metabolism, important in development of reproductive system, and aids in healing
Oysters	Copper	**Copper:** Necessary for the formation of red blood cells, the production of energy and adrenal hormones. Important in the production of collagen, which is responsible for health of skin, cartilage and bones
Organ meats	Copper, iron, selenium, zinc (liver)	**Copper:** Necessary for the formation of red blood cells, the production of energy and adrenal hormones. Important in the production of collagen, which is responsible for health of skin, cartilage and bones **Iron:** Essential in red blood cell formation. Improves blood quality, and increases resistance to stress and disease **Selenium:** Protects body tissues against oxidative damage from normal metabolic processing and pollution. Important for immune system function and liver function, and can help protect against heart and circulatory diseases

If you eat	you get this/ these mineral(s)	which help your body in the following ways
		Zinc: Involved in digestion and metabolism, important in development of reproductive system, and aids in healing
Meats	Iron, phosphorous	**Iron:** Essential in red blood cell formation. Improves blood quality, and increases resistance to stress and disease **Phosphorus:** Important role in the final delivery of energy to all cells including muscles. Helps create the structure of bones and teeth. Essential to the normal functioning of B group vitamins
Lean meats	Potassium, selenium, zinc	**Potassium:** Maintenance of body fluids; controls activity of heart muscle, nervous system and kidneys **Selenium:** Protects body tissues against oxidative damage from normal metabolic processing and pollution. Important for immune system function and liver function, and can help protect against heart and circulatory diseases **Zinc:** Involved in digestion and metabolism, important in development of reproductive system, and aids in healing
Poultry	Phosphorus	**Phosphorus:** Important role in the final delivery of energy to all cells including muscles. Helps create the structure of bones and teeth. Essential to the normal functioning of B group vitamins

If you eat	you get this/ these mineral(s)	which help your body in the following ways
Fish	Phosphorus	**Phosphorus:** Important role in the final delivery of energy to all cells including muscles. Helps create the structure of bones and teeth. Essential to the normal functioning of B group vitamins

BASIC AND GENERIC FOOD

kcal/100g	protein/100g	carb/100g	fat/100g	fibre/100g	sodium/100g

Please note the serving size in this section is 100 grams. Values for sodium are given in milligrams. All other values are given in grams.

CEREALS AND CEREAL-BASED FOODS

Biscuits (savoury and sweet)

Brandy snaps

437	2.5	64.0	20.3	0.8	250

Chocolate biscuits, fully coated

524	5.7	67.4	27.6	2.1	160

Cream crackers

440	9.5	68.3	16.3	2.2	610

Crispbread, rye

321	9.4	70.6	2.1	11.7	220

Digestive biscuits, chocolate

493	6.8	66.5	24.1	2.2	450

Digestive biscuits, plain

471	6.3	68.6	20.9	2.2	600

Gingernut biscuits

456	5.6	79.1	15.2	1.4	330

Jaffa cakes

363	3.5	67.8	10.5	Tr	130

Melting moments

549	3.3	55.2	36.5	1.2	370

Oatcakes

441	10.0	63.0	18.3	0	1230

Rusks, plain

408	6.5	82.8	7.9	0	66

Rusks, low sugar

414	8.6	77.8	9.7	0	110

Rusks, flavoured

401	6.8	78.1	9.0	0	87

Rusks, wholemeal

411	8.3	76.5	10.1	0	23

Sandwich biscuits

513	5.0	69.2	25.9	0	220

	kcal/100g	protein/100g	carb/100g	fat/100g	fibre/100g	sodium/100g
Semi-sweet biscuits						
	457	6.7	74.8	16.6	1.7	410
Short-sweet biscuits						
	469	6.2	62.2	23.4	1.5	360
Shortbread						
	498	5.9	63.9	26.1	1.9	230
Wafer biscuits, filled						
	535	4.7	66.0	29.9	1.4	70
Water biscuits						
	440	10.8	75.8	12.5	3.1	470
Wholemeal crackers						
	413	10.1	72.1	11.3	4.4	700

Breads

	kcal/100g	protein/100g	carb/100g	fat/100g	fibre/100g	sodium/100g
Breadsticks						
	392	11.2	72.5	8.4	2.8	860
Brown bread, average						
	218	8.5	44.3	2.0	3.5	540
Chapatis, made with fat						
	328	8.1	48.3	12.8	0	130
Chapatis, made without fat						
	202	7.3	43.7	1.0	0	120
Croissants						
	360	8.3	38.3	20.3	1.6	390
Currant bread						
	289	7.5	50.7	7.6	0	290
Currant bread, toasted						
	323	8.4	56.8	8.5	0	330
Granary bread						
	235	9.3	46.3	2.7	4.3	580
Hamburger bun						
	264	9.1	48.8	5.0	1.5	550
Malt bread						
	268	8.3	56.8	2.4	0	280
Milk bread						
	296	9.0	48.5	8.7	1.9	460
Naan bread						
	336	8.9	50.1	12.5	1.9	380

	kcal/100g	protein/100g	carb/100g	fat/100g	fibre/100g	sodium/100g
Papadums, raw						
	272	20.6	46.0	1.9	0	2850
Papadums, fried						
	369	17.5	39.1	16.9	0	2420
Pitta bread, white						
	265	9.2	57.9	1.2	2.2	520
Rolls, brown, crusty						
	255	10.3	50.4	2.8	3.5	570
Rolls, brown, soft						
	268	10.0	51.8	3.8	3.5	560
Rolls, morning						
	269	10.4	53.3	3.1	1.5	530
Rolls, white, crusty						
	280	10.9	57.6	2.3	1.5	640
Rolls, white, soft						
	268	9.2	51.6	4.2	1.5	560
Rolls, wholemeal						
	241	9.0	48.3	2.9	5.9	460
Rye bread						
	219	8.3	45.8	1.7	4.4	580
Soda bread						
	258	7.7	54.6	2.5	2.1	420
Tortillas, made with wheat flour						
	262	7.2	59.7	1.0	2.4	280
Wheatgerm bread, average						
	232	9.2	42.5	2.5	3.3	570
White bread, average						
	235	8.4	49.3	1.9	5.3	520
White bread, French stick						
	270	9.6	55.4	2.7	1.5	570
Wholemeal bread, average						
	215	9.2	41.6	2.5	5.8	550
Wholemeal bread, toasted						
	252	10.8	48.7	2.9	5.9	640

Cakes (large)

	kcal/100g	protein/100g	carb/100g	fat/100g	fibre/100g	sodium/100g
Battenburg cake						
	370	5.9	50.0	17.5	0	440

	kcal/100g	protein/100g	carb/100g	fat/100g	fibre/100g	sodium/100g
Cake mix						
	331	4.7	77.2	2.5	0	510
Cake mix, made-up						
	250	5.3	77.2	3.3	0	370
Cherry cake						
	394	5.1	61.7	15.8	1.1	310
Chocolate cake						
	456	7.4	50.4	26.4	0	430
Chocolate cake, with butter icing						
	481	5.7	50.9	29.7	0	420
Coconut cake						
	434	6.7	51.2	23.8	2.5	460
Crispie cakes						
	464	5.6	73.1	18.6	0.3	450
Fruit cake, rich						
	341	3.8	59.6	11.0	1.7	200
Fruit cake, rich, retail						
	322	4.9	50.7	12.5	1.7	220
Fruit cake, rich, iced						
	356	4.1	62.7	11.4	1.7	140
Fruit cake, wholemeal						
	363	6.0	52.8	15.7	2.4	310
Gingerbread						
	379	5.7	64.7	12.6	1.2	200
Lardy cake						
	375	6.7	53.7	16.3	1.8	270
Madeira cake						
	393	5.4	58.4	16.9	0.9	380
Sponge cake						
	459	6.4	52.4	26.3	0.9	350
Sponge cake, fatless						
	294	10.1	53.0	6.1	0.9	82
Sponge cake, jam-filled						
	302	4.2	64.2	4.9	1.8	420
Sponge cake, with butter icing						
	490	4.5	52.4	30.6	0.6	360
Swiss roll						
	276	7.2	55.5	4.4	0.8	130

	kcal/100g	protein/100g	carb/100g	fat/100g	fibre/100g	sodium/100g

Cakes (small)

Chelsea buns

	366	7.8	56.1	13.8	1.7	330

Choux buns

	381	5.4	17.6	32.5	0.7	210

Cream horns

	435	3.8	25.8	35.8	0.9	200

Crumpets, fresh

	177	6.0	38.6	0.9	1.8	720

Crumpets, toasted

	199	6.7	43.4	1.0	2.0	810

Currant buns

	296	7.6	52.7	7.5	0	230

Custard tarts, individual

	277	6.3	32.4	14.5	1.2	130

Danish pastries

	374	5.8	51.3	17.6	1.6	190

Doughnuts, custard-filled

	358	6.2	43.3	19.0	0	200

Doughnuts, jam

	336	5.7	48.8	14.5	0	180

Doughnuts, ring

	397	6.1	47.2	21.7	3.1	230

Doughnuts, ring, iced

	383	4.8	55.1	17.5	0	170

Eccles cake

	475	3.9	59.3	26.4	1.6	240

Eclairs, fresh

	373	4.1	37.9	23.8	0.5	150

Eclairs, frozen

	396	5.6	26.1	30.6	0.8	73

Fancy iced cakes, individual

	407	3.8	68.8	14.9	0	250

Halva

	615	14.8	54.2	31.9	0	190

Hot cross buns

	310	7.4	58.5	6.8	1.7	120

	kcal/100g	protein/100g	carb/100g	fat/100g	fibre/100g	sodium/100g
Jam tarts						
	380	3.3	62.0	14.9	1.6	230
Mince pies, individual						
	423	4.3	59.0	20.4	2.1	310
Muffins						
	283	10.1	49.6	6.3	2.0	130
Muffins, bran						
	272	7.8	45.6	7.7	7.7	770
Pancakes, Scotch						
	292	5.8	43.6	11.7	1.4	430
Rock cakes						
	396	5.4	60.5	16.4	1.5	390
Rum baba						
	223	3.5	32.2	8.1	0.8	120
Scones, cheese						
	363	10.1	43.2	17.8	1.6	760
Scones, fruit						
	316	7.3	52.9	9.8	0	710
Scones, plain						
	362	7.2	53.8	14.6	1.9	770
Scones, potato						
	296	5.1	39.1	14.3	1.6	730
Scones, wholemeal						
	326	8.7	43.1	14.4	5.2	730
Scones, wholemeal, fruit						
	324	8.1	47.2	12.8	4.9	650
Tartlets, strawberry						
	206	2.5	26.2	10.8	1.2	160
Teacakes, fresh						
	296	8.0	52.5	7.5	0	270
Teacakes, toasted						
	329	8.9	58.3	8.3	0	300
Vanilla slices						
	330	4.5	40.2	17.9	0.8	230
Waffles						
	334	8.7	39.6	16.7	1.5	580

	kcal/100g	protein/100g	carb/100g	fat/100g	fibre/100g	sodium/100g

Cereals (grains)

Barley, pearl, raw

	360	7.9	83.6	1.7	0	3

Barley, pearl, boiled

	120	2.7	27.6	0.6	0	1

Barley, whole grain, raw

	301	10.6	64.0	2.1	14.8	4

Bran, wheat

	206	14.1	26.8	5.5	36.4	28

Buckwheat

	364	8.1	84.9	1.5	2.1	1

Bulgur wheat

	353	9.7	76.3	1.7	0	5

Couscous

	227	5.7	51.3	1.0	0	0

Oatmeal, raw

	401	12.4	72.8	8.7	6.8	33

Oatmeal, quick cook, raw

	375	11.2	66.0	9.2	7.1	9

Porridge Oats, raw

	368	11	62	8	7	33

Rice, brown, raw

	357	6.7	81.3	2.8	1.9	3

Rice, brown, boiled

	141	2.6	32.1	1.1	0.8	1

Rice, pilau

	217	2.7	25.7	11.5	0.6	110

Rice, risotto, plain

	224	3.0	34.4	9.3	0.4	410

Rice, savoury, raw

	415	8.4	77.4	10.3	0	1440

Rice, savoury, cooked

	142	2.9	26.3	3.5	1.4	490

Rice, white, basmati, raw

	359	7.4	79.8	0.5	0	0

Rice, white, easy cook, raw

	383	7.3	85.8	3.6	0.4	4

	kcal/100g	protein/100g	carb/100g	fat/100g	fibre/100g	sodium/100g
Rice, white, easy cook, boiled						
	138	2.6	30.9	1.3	0.1	1
Rice, white, flaked, raw						
	346	6.6	77.5	1.2	0	0
Rice, white, fried						
	131	2.2	25.0	3.2	0.6	56
Wheatgerm						
	302	26.7	44.7	9.2	15.6	5

Cereals (packet)

	kcal/100g	protein/100g	carb/100g	fat/100g	fibre/100g	sodium/100g
All-Bran						
	252	15.1	43.0	3.4	24.5	1480
Bran Buds						
	273	13.1	52.0	2.9	20.0	510
Bran Flakes						
	319	10.2	69.7	1.9	11.3	910
Corn Flakes						
	355	7.9	84.9	0.6	0.9	1110
Crunchy Nut Corn Flakes						
	398	7.4	88.6	4.0	0.8	770
Frosties						
	382	5.3	95.4	0.4	0.5	740
Fruit 'n' Fibre						
	352	8.1	73.1	5.1	7.0	560
Grapenuts						
	346	10.5	79.9	0.5	0	590
Honey Smacks						
	371	7.0	89.1	1.0	4.7	320
Muesli, Swiss-style						
	364	10.6	71.1	5.9	6.1	380
Muesli, with no added sugar						
	366	10.5	67.1	8.1	7.7	29
Nutri-Grain						
	379	9.8	68.3	9.3	8.9	500
Puffed Wheat						
	321	14.2	67.3	1.3	5.6	4
Ready Brek						
	389	12.4	69.5	8.7	7.2	23

	kcal/100g	protein/100g	carb/100g	fat/100g	fibre/100g	sodium/100g
Rice Krispies						
	369	6.1	89.7	0.9	0.5	1260
Ricicles						
	383	4.3	96.3	0.5	0.3	880
Shredded Wheat						
	325	10.6	68.3	3.0	9.8	8
Shreddies						
	331	10.0	74.1	1.5	9.5	550
Special K						
	380	15.3	82.5	1.0	2.0	1150
Sugar Puffs						
	324	5.9	84.5	0.8	3.2	9
Sultana Bran						
	302	8.5	67.7	1.6	10.0	610
Weetabix						
	342	10.7	74.9	2.0	9.7	370
Weetaflake						
	342	10.7	74.9	2.0	9.8	370

Desserts (cereal-based)

	kcal/100g	protein/100g	carb/100g	fat/100g	fibre/100g	sodium/100g
Apple pie, one crust						
	197	1.8	31.4	8.0	1.6	120
Apple pie, pastry top and bottom						
	266	2.9	35.8	13.3	1.7	200
Arctic roll						
	200	4.1	33.3	6.6	0	150
Bakewell tart						
	456	6.3	43.5	29.7	1.9	290
Blackcurrant pie, pastry top and bottom						
	262	3.1	34.5	13.3	4.8	200
Bread and butter pudding						
	160	6.2	17.5	7.8	0.3	150
Bread pudding						
	297	5.9	49.7	9.6	1.2	310
Christmas pudding						
	291	4.6	49.5	9.7	1.7	200
Crumble, with pie filling						
	210	1.9	36.3	7.3	1.2	100

	kcal/100g	protein/100g	carb/100g	fat/100g	fibre/100g	sodium/100g
Crumble, apple						
	207	1.8	36.6	6.9	1.6	68
Flan, pastry, with fruit						
	118	1.4	19.3	4.4	0.7	60
Flan, sponge, with fruit						
	112	2.8	23.3	1.5	0.6	27
Flan case, pastry						
	544	7.1	56.7	33.6	1.8	400
Flan case, sponge						
	295	9.8	53.6	6.1	0.8	83
Fruit pie, one crust						
	186	2.0	28.7	7.9	1.7	120
Fruit pie, pastry top and bottom						
	260	3.0	34.0	13.3	1.8	200
Lemon meringue pie						
	319	4.5	45.9	14.4	10.7	200
Pancakes, sweet						
	301	5.9	35.0	16.2	0.8	53
Queen of puddings						
	213	4.8	33.1	7.8	0.2	140
Rice pudding, canned						
	89	3.4	14.0	2.5	0.2	50
Sponge pudding, with dried fruit						
	331	5.4	48.1	14.3	1.2	270
Sponge pudding, with jam or treacle						
	333	5.1	48.7	14.4	1.0	290
Sponge pudding, canned						
	285	3.1	45.4	11.4	0.8	340
Spotted dick						
	327	4.2	42.7	16.7	1.0	390
Suet pudding						
	335	4.4	40.5	18.3	0.9	420
Treacle tart						
	368	3.7	60.4	14.1	1.1	360
Trifle						
	160	3.6	22.4	6.3	0.5	54
Trifle, with Dream Topping						
	148	3.7	22.9	4.7	0.5	56

	kcal/100g	protein/100g	carb/100g	fat/100g	fibre/100g	sodium/100g
Trifle, with fresh cream						
	166	2.4	19.5	9.2	0.5	63

Flours and Starches

	kcal/100g	protein/100g	carb/100g	fat/100g	fibre/100g	sodium/100g
Chapati flour, brown						
	333	11.5	73.7	1.2	0	39
Chapati flour, white						
	335	9.8	77.6	0.5	0	15
Cornflour						
	354	0.6	92.0	0.7	0.1	52
Cornmeal, unsifted						
	353	9.3	71.5	3.8	0	1
Rice flour						
	366	6.4	80.1	0.8	2.0	5
Rye flour, whole						
	335	8.2	75.9	2.0	11.7	1
Sago, raw						
	355	0.2	94.0	0.2	0.5	3
Semolina, raw						
	350	10.7	77.5	1.8	2.1	12
Tapioca, raw						
	359	0.4	95.0	0.1	0.4	4
Wheat flour, brown						
	323	12.6	68.5	1.8	6.4	4
Wheat flour, white, breadmaking						
	341	11.5	75.3	1.4	3.1	3
Wheat flour, white, plain						
	341	9.4	77.7	1.3	3.1	3
Wheat flour, wholemeal						
	310	12.7	63.9	2.2	9.0	3

Pasta and Noodles

	kcal/100g	protein/100g	carb/100g	fat/100g	fibre/100g	sodium/100g
Lasagne, raw						
	346	11.9	74.8	2.0	3.1	10
Lasagne, boiled						
	100	3.0	22.0	0.6	0.9	1
Macaroni, raw						
	348	12.0	75.8	1.8	3.1	11

	kcal/100g	protein/100g	carb/100g	fat/100g	fibre/100g	sodium/100g
Macaroni, boiled						
	86	3.0	18.5	0.5	0.9	1
Macaroni, canned in cheese sauce						
	138	4.5	16.4	6.5	0.4	560
Macaroni cheese						
	174	7.1	13.3	10.6	0.5	320
Noodles, egg, raw						
	391	12.1	71.7	8.2	2.9	180
Noodles, egg, boiled						
	62	2.2	13.0	0.5	0.6	15
Noodles, fried						
	153	1.9	11.3	11.5	0.5	84
Noodles, plain, raw						
	388	11.7	76.1	6.2	2.9	2
Noodles, plain, boiled						
	62	2.4	13.0	0.4	0.7	1
Noodles, rice, dried						
	360	4.9	81.5	0.1	0	12
Ravioli, canned in tomato sauce						
	70	3.0	10.3	2.2	0.9	490
Spaghetti, white, raw						
	342	12.0	74.1	1.8	2.9	3
Spaghetti, white, boiled						
	104	3.6	22.2	0.7	1.2	Tr
Spaghetti, wholemeal, raw						
	324	13.4	66.2	2.5	8.4	130
Spaghetti, wholemeal, boiled						
	113	4.7	23.2	0.9	3.5	45
Spaghetti, canned in tomato sauce						
	64	1.9	14.1	0.4	0.7	420
Vermicelli, raw						
	355	8.7	78.3	0.4	0	8

Pastries (sweet and savoury)

	kcal/100g	protein/100g	carb/100g	fat/100g	fibre/100g	sodium/100g
Cheese pastry, cooked						
	498	13.2	37.2	33.9	1.5	560
Choux pastry, cooked						
	325	8.5	29.8	19.8	1.2	360

	kcal/100g	protein/100g	carb/100g	fat/100g	fibre/100g	sodium/100g
Flaky pastry, cooked						
	560	5.6	45.9	40.6	1.8	460
Puff pastry, frozen, raw						
	373	5.7	37.0	23.5	0	310
Samosas, meat						
	593	5.1	17.9	56.1	1.2	33
Samosas, vegetable						
	472	3.1	22.3	41.8	1.8	200
Shortcrust pastry, cooked						
	521	6.6	54.2	32.3	2.2	480
Shortcrust pastry, frozen, raw						
	440	4.5	44.3	28.4	1.9	160
Wholemeal pastry, cooked						
	499	8.9	44.6	32.9	6.3	410

DAIRY PRODUCTS

Cheese

	kcal/100g	protein/100g	carb/100g	fat/100g	fibre/100g	sodium/100g
Brie						
	319	19.3	Tr	26.9	0	700
Caerphilly						
	375	23.2	0.1	31.3	0	480
Camembert						
	297	20.9	Tr	23.7	0	650
Cheese spread, plain						
	276	13.5	4.4	22.8	0	1060
Cheese spread, flavoured						
	258	14.2	4.4	20.5	0	1130
Cheddar, average						
	412	25.5	0.1	34.4	0	670
Cheddar, English						
	412	25.5	0.1	34.4	0	670
Cheddar-type, reduced-fat						
	261	31.5	Tr	15.0	0	670
Cheddar, vegetarian						
	425	25.8	Tr	35.7	0	670
Cheshire						
	379	24.0	0.1	31.4	0	550

	kcal/100g	protein/100g	carb/100g	fat/100g	fibre/100g	sodium/100g
Cheshire-type, reduced-fat						
	269	32.7	Tr	15.3	0	470
Cottage cheese, plain						
	98	13.8	2.1	3.9	0	380
Cottage cheese, plain, reduced-fat						
	78	13.3	3.3	1.4	0	380
Cream cheese						
	439	3.1	Tr	47.4	0	300
Danish blue						
	347	20.1	Tr	29.6	0	1260
Derby						
	402	24.2	0.1	33.9	0	580
Double Gloucester						
	405	24.6	0.1	34.0	0	590
Edam						
	333	26.0	Tr	25.4	0	1020
Edam-type, reduced-fat						
	229	32.6	Tr	10.9	0	N
Emmental						
	382	28.7	Tr	29.7	0	450
Feta						
	250	15.6	1.5	20.2	0	1440
Fromage frais, plain						
	113	6.8	5.7	7.1	0	31
Fromage frais, fruit						
	131	6.8	13.8	5.8	0	35
Fromage frais, very low fat						
	58	7.7	6.8	0.2	0	33
Gouda						
	375	24.0	Tr	31.0	0	910
Gruyère						
	409	27.2	Tr	33.3	0	670
Lancashire						
	373	23.3	0.1	31.0	0	590
Leicester						
	401	24.3	0.1	33.7	0	630
Lymeswold						
	425	15.6	Tr	40.3	0	560

	kcal/100g	protein/100g	carb/100g	fat/100g	fibre/100g	sodium/100g
Mozzarella						
	289	25.1	Tr	21.0	0	610
Parmesan						
	452	39.4	Tr	32.7	0	1090
Processed cheese, plain						
	330	20.8	0.9	27.0	0	1320
Processed cheese, smoked						
	303	20.5	0.2	24.5	0	1270
Ricotta						
	144	9.4	2.0	11.0	0	100
Roquefort						
	375	19.7	Tr	32.9	0	1670
Soft cheese, full-fat						
	313	8.6	Tr	31.0	0	330
Soft cheese, goat's milk						
	198	13.1	1.0	15.8	0	470
Soya cheese						
	319	18.3	Tr	27.3	0	600
Stilton, blue						
	411	22.7	0.1	35.5	0	930
Stilton, white						
	362	19.9	0.1	31.3	0	770
Wensleydale						
	377	23.3	0.1	31.5	0	520

Cream

	kcal/100g	protein/100g	carb/100g	fat/100g	fibre/100g	sodium/100g
Cream, fresh, clotted						
	586	1.6	2.3	63.5	0	18
Cream, fresh, double						
	449	1.7	2.7	48.0	0	37
Cream, fresh, half						
	148	3.0	4.3	13.3	0	49
Cream, fresh, single						
	198	2.6	4.1	19.1	0	49
Cream, fresh, soured						
	205	2.9	3.8	19.9	0	41
Cream, fresh, whipping						
	373	2.0	3.1	39.3	0	40

	kcal/100g	protein/100g	carb/100g	fat/100g	fibre/100g	sodium/100g
Cream, UHT, canned spray						
	309	1.9	3.5	32.0	0	33
Dessert Top						
	291	2.4	6.0	28.8	Tr	50
Elmlea, double						
	450	2.4	2.3	48.0	Tr	42
Elmlea, single						
	195	3.0	3.5	19.0	Tr	54
Elmlea, whipping						
	315	2.4	2.3	33.0	Tr	42

Desserts (dairy-based)

	kcal/100g	protein/100g	carb/100g	fat/100g	fibre/100g	sodium/100g
Cornetto						
	260	3.7	34.5	12.9	0	91
Crème caramel						
	109	3.0	20.6	2.2	0	70
Custard, canned						
	95	2.6	15.4	3.0	0	67
Dream Topping						
	626	6.0	39.8	50.4	0	130
Milk puddings						
	128	3.9	19.7	4.3	0.1	60
Mousse, chocolate, rich						
	178	4.7	26.0	6.9	0	N
Rice pudding, canned						
	89	3.4	14.0	2.5	0	50

Eggs

	kcal/100g	protein/100g	carb/100g	fat/100g	fibre/100g	sodium/100g
Hen's egg, whole, raw						
	147	12.5	Tr	10.8	0	140
Hen's egg, white, raw						
	36	9.0	Tr	Tr	0	190
Hen's egg, yolk, raw						
	339	16.1	Tr	30.5	0	50
Hen's egg, boiled						
	147	12.5	Tr	10.8	0	140
Hen's egg, fried, with fat						
	179	13.6	Tr	13.9	0	160

	kcal/100g	protein/100g	carb/100g	fat/100g	fibre/100g	sodium/100g
Hen's egg, fried, without fat						
	174	15.0	Tr	12.7	0	170
Hen's egg, poached						
	147	12.5	Tr	10.8	0	140
Hen's egg, scrambled, with milk						
	247	10.7	0.6	22.6	0	1030
Hen's eggs scrambled, without milk						
	160	13.8	Tr	11.6	0	150
Scotch eggs, retail						
	251	12.0	13.1	17.1	0	670

Milk

	kcal/100g	protein/100g	carb/100g	fat/100g	fibre/100g	sodium/100g
Buttermilk						
	37	3.4	5.0	0.5	0	56
Channel Island milk, whole, pasteurised						
	78	3.6	4.8	5.1	0	54
Condensed milk, skimmed, sweetened						
	267	10.0	60.0	0.2	0	150
Condensed milk, whole, sweetened						
	333	8.5	55.5	10.1	0	140
Dried milk, skimmed						
	348	36.1	52.9	0.6	0	550
Evaporated milk, whole						
	151	8.4	8.5	9.4	0	180
Flavoured milk						
	68	3.6	10.6	1.5	0	61
Goat's milk, pasteurised						
	60	3.1	4.4	3.5	0	42
Semi-skimmed milk, average						
	46	3.3	5.0	1.6	0	55
Sheep's milk, raw						
	95	5.4	5.1	6.0	0	44
Skimmed milk, average						
	33	3.3	5.0	0.1	0	54
Skimmed milk, UHT						
	32	3.4	4.9	0.1	0	51
Soya milk, plain						
	32	2.9	0.8	1.9	0	32

	kcal/100g	protein/100g	carb/100g	fat/100g	fibre/100g	sodium/100g

Soya milk, flavoured

	40	2.8	3.6	1.7	0	61

Whole milk, average

	66	3.2	4.8	3.9	0	55

Whole milk, pasteurised

	66	3.2	4.8	3.9	0	55

Sauces (dairy-based)

Cheese sauce, made with whole milk

	197	8.0	9.0	14.6	0	450

Cheese sauce, made with semi-skimmed milk

	179	8.1	9.1	12.6	0	450

Cheese sauce, made with skimmed milk

	168	8.1	9.1	11.3	0	450

Onion sauce, made with whole milk

	99	2.8	8.3	6.5	0	430

Onion sauce, made with semi-skimmed milk

	86	2.9	8.4	5.0	0.4	435

Onion sauce, made with skimmed milk

	77	2.9	8.4	4.0	0.4	430

White sauce packet mix

	355	9.0	60.0	10.5	0	4160

White sauce packet mix, made up with whole milk

	93	3.9	9.4	4.7	0	400

White sauce packet mix, made up with semi-skimmed milk

	73	4.0	9.6	2.4	0	400

White sauce packet mix, made up with skimmed milk

	59	4.0	9.6	0.9	0	400

Spreads

Butter

	737	0.5	Tr	81.7	0	750

Margarine

	739	0.2	1.0	81.6	0	800

Dairy/fat spread

	662	0.4	Tr	73.4	0	760

	kcal/100g	protein/100g	carb/100g	fat/100g	fibre/100g	sodium/100g

Yoghurt

Drinking yoghurt

	62	3.1	13.1	Tr	0	47

Greek yoghurt, cow's

	115	6.4	2.0	9.1	0	71

Greek yoghurt, sheep's

	106	4.4	5.6	7.5	0	150

Low-fat yoghurt, flavoured

	90	3.8	17.9	0.9	Tr	65

Low-fat yoghurt, fruit

	90	4.1	17.9	0.7	0	64

Low-fat yoghurt, plain

	51	5.1	7.5	0.8	0	83

Soya yoghurt

	72	5.0	3.9	4.2	0	N

Whole milk yoghurt, fruit

	105	5.1	15.7	2.8	0	82

Whole milk yoghurt, goat's

	63	3.5	3.9	3.8	0	39

Whole milk yoghurt, plain

	79	5.7	7.8	3.0	0	80

FISH AND SEAFOOD

Fish (see also Oily Fish)

Bass, Sea, raw

	100	19.3	0	2.5	0	69

Bream, Sea, raw

	96	17.5	0	2.9	0	110

Caviare, bottled in brine, drained

	92	10.9	0	5.4	0	2120

Cod, raw

	80	18.3	0	0.7	0	60

Cod, baked

	96	21.4	Tr	1.2	0	340

Cod, baked, weighed with bones and skin

	82	18.2	Tr	1.0	0	290

	kcal/100g	protein/100g	carb/100g	fat/100g	fibre/100g	sodium/100g
Cod, poached						
	94	20.9	Tr	1.1	0	110
Cod, steamed						
	83	18.6	0	0.9	0	65
Cod, steamed, weighed with bones and skin						
	67	15.1	0	0.7	0	53
Cod, in batter, fried in blended oil						
	247	16.1	11.7	15.4	0	160
Cod, in batter, fried in sunflower oil						
	247	16.1	11.7	15.4	0	160
Cod, in parsley sauce, frozen, boiled						
	84	12.0	2.8	2.8	0	260
Coley, raw						
	82	18.3	0	1.0	0	86
Dover sole, raw						
	89	18.1	0	1.8	0	100
Fish cakes, grilled						
	154	9.9	19.7	4.5	0	600
Fish fingers, cod, grilled						
	200	14.3	16.6	8.9	0.7	440
Fish fingers, cod, fried in blended oil						
	238	13.2	15.5	14.1	0.6	450
Haddock, raw						
	81	19.0	0	0.6	0	67
Haddock, grilled						
	104	24.3	0	0.8	0	86
Haddock, grilled, weighed with bones						
	97	22.6	0	0.7	0	80
Haddock, poached						
	113	17.7	1.1	4.3	0	99
Haddock, steamed						
	89	20.9	0	0.6	0	73
Haddock, in batter, fried in blended oil						
	232	17.1	10.0	14.0	0.4	180
Haddock, smoked, raw						
	81	19.0	0	0.6	0	760
Haddock, smoked, poached						
	134	18.7	1.1	6.1	0	770

	kcal/100g	protein/100g	carb/100g	fat/100g	fibre/100g	sodium/100g
Haddock, smoked, poached, weighed with bones and skin						
	121	16.8	1.0	5.5	0	690
Halibut, raw						
	103	21.5	0	1.9	0	60
Halibut, grilled						
	121	25.3	0	2.2	0	71
Halibut, grilled, weighed with bones and skin						
	95	19.7	0	1.7	0	55
Halibut, poached						
	154	24.7	1.1	5.7	0	100
Halibut, poached, weighed with bones and skin						
	142	22.7	1.0	5.3	0	96
Lemon sole, raw						
	83	17.4	0	1.5	0	95
Lemon sole, grilled						
	97	20.2	0	1.7	0	110
Lemon sole, grilled, weighed with bones and skin						
	62	12.9	0	1.1	0	71
Monkfish, grilled						
	96	22.7	0	0.6	0	26
Monkfish, grilled, weighed with bones						
	74	17.5	0	0.4	0	20
Mullet, Red, raw						
	109	18.7	0	3.8	0	91
Mullet, Red, grilled						
	121	20.4	0	4.4	0	110
Mullet, Red, grilled, weighed with bones and skin						
	57	9.6	0	2.1	0	50
Plaice, raw						
	79	16.7	0	1.4	0	120
Plaice, grilled						
	96	20.1	0	1.7	0	140
Plaice, grilled, weighed with bones and skin						
	70	14.7	0	1.2	0	110
Plaice, in batter, fried in blended oil						
	257	15.2	12.0	16.8	0.5	210
Swordfish, raw						
	109	18.0	0	4.1	0	130

	kcal/100g	protein/100g	carb/100g	fat/100g	fibre/100g	sodium/100g
Swordfish, grilled						
	139	22.9	0	5.2	0	170
Swordfish, grilled, weighed with bones and skin						
	123	20.4	0	4.6	0	150
Trout, rainbow, raw						
	125	19.6	0	5.2	0	45
Trout, rainbow, grilled						
	135	21.5	0	5.4	0	55
Trout, rainbow, grilled, weighed with bones and skin						
	98	15.7	0	3.9	0	40
Tuna, raw						
	136	23.7	0	4.6	0	47
Tuna, canned in brine, drained						
	99	23.5	0	0.6	0	320
Tuna, canned in oil, drained						
	189	27.1	0	9.0	0	290
Whiting, raw						
	81	18.7	0	0.7	0	90

Oily Fish

	kcal/100g	protein/100g	carb/100g	fat/100g	fibre/100g	sodium/100g
Anchovies, canned in oil, drained						
	280	25.2	0	19.9	0	3930
Herring, raw						
	190	17.8	0	13.2	0	120
Herring, grilled						
	181	20.1	0	11.2	0	160
Herring, grilled, weighed with bones and skin						
	123	13.7	0	7.6	0	110
Herring, in oatmeal, fried in vegetable oil						
	234	23.1	1.5	15.1	0	160
Herring, canned in tomato sauce						
	193	12.8	3.2	14.4	0	380
Kipper, raw						
	229	17.5	0	17.7	0	830
Kipper, grilled						
	255	20.1	0	19.4	0	940
Kipper, grilled, weighed with bones						
	161	12.7	0	12.2	0	590

	kcal/100g	protein/100g	carb/100g	fat/100g	fibre/100g	sodium/100g
Mackerel, raw						
	220	18.7	0	16.1	0	63
Mackerel, fried in blended oil						
	272	24.0	0	19.5	0	81
Mackerel, grilled						
	239	20.8	0	17.3	0	63
Mackerel, grilled, weighed with bones and skin						
	220	19.1	0	15.9	0	58
Mackerel, smoked						
	354	18.9	0	30.9	0	750
Mackerel, canned in brine, drained						
	237	19.0	0	17.9	0	270
Mackerel, canned in tomato sauce						
	206	16.4	1.4	15.0	0	250
Pilchards, canned in tomato sauce						
	144	16.7	1.1	8.1	0	290
Salmon, raw						
	180	20.2	0	11.0	0	45
Salmon, grilled						
	215	24.2	0	13.1	0	54
Salmon, grilled, weighed with bones and skin						
	176	19.8	0	10.7	0	44
Salmon, steamed						
	194	21.8	0	11.9	0	49
Salmon, steamed, weighed with bones and skin						
	150	16.8	0	9.2	0	37
Salmon, smoked						
	142	25.4	0	4.5	0	1880
Salmon, pink, canned in brine, flesh only, drained						
	153	23.5	0	6.6	0	430
Salmon, pink, canned in brine, flesh and bones, drained						
	153	23.5	0	6.6	0	440
Salmon, red, canned in brine, flesh only, drained						
	167	21.6	0	9.0	0	430
Salmon, red, canned in brine, flesh and bones, drained						
	153	23.5	0	6.6	0	440
Sardines, raw						
	165	20.6	0	9.2	0	120

	kcal/100g	protein/100g	carb/100g	fat/100g	fibre/100g	sodium/100g
Sardines, grilled						
	195	25.3	0	10.4	0	140
Sardines, grilled, weighed with bones						
	119	15.4	0	6.3	0	85
Sardines, canned in brine, drained						
	172	21.5	0	9.6	0	530
Sardines, canned in oil, drained						
	220	23.3	0	14.1	0	450
Sardines, canned in tomato sauce						
	162	17.0	1.4	9.9	0	350
Whitebait, in flour, fried						
	525	19.5	5.3	47.5	0.2	230

Seafood

	kcal/100g	protein/100g	carb/100g	fat/100g	fibre/100g	sodium/100g
Crab, boiled						
	128	19.5	Tr	5.5	0	420
Crab, boiled, weighed with shell						
	45	6.8	Tr	1.9	0	150
Crab, canned in brine, drained						
	77	18.1	Tr	0.5	0	550
Crabsticks						
	68	10.0	6.6	0.4	0	700
Lobster, boiled						
	103	22.1	Tr	1.6	0	330
Lobster, boiled, weighed with shell						
	37	8.0	Tr	0.6	0	120
Mussels, raw						
	74	12.1	2.5	1.8	0	290
Mussels, boiled						
	104	16.7	3.5	2.7	0	360
Mussels, boiled, weighed with shells						
	28	4.5	0.9	0.7	0	96
Octopus, raw						
	83	17.9	Tr	1.3	0	N
Oysters, raw						
	65	10.8	2.7	1.3	0	510
Oysters, raw, weighed with shells						
	9	1.5	0.4	0.2	0	71

	kcal/100g	protein/100g	carb/100g	fat/100g	fibre/100g	sodium/100g
Prawns, raw						
	76	17.6	0	0.6	0	190
Prawns, boiled						
	99	22.6	0	0.9	0	1590
Prawns, boiled, weighed with shells						
	37	8.6	0	0.3	0	600
Prawns, frozen, raw						
	79	18.3	0	0.6	0	780
Scallops, steamed						
	118	23.2	3.4	1.4	0	180
Scampi, in breadcrumbs, frozen, fried in blended oil						
	237	9.4	20.5	13.6	0	660
Shrimps, boiled, weighed with shells						
	39	7.9	Tr	0.8	0	1270
Shrimps, frozen						
	73	16.5	Tr	0.8	0	380
Squid, raw						
	81	15.4	1.2	1.7	0	110
Squid, in batter, fried in blended oil						
	195	11.5	15.7	10.0	0.5	88

FRUIT AND NUTS

Fruit (fresh, dried and canned)

	kcal/100g	protein/100g	carb/100g	fat/100g	fibre/100g	sodium/100g
Apples, cooking, raw, peeled						
	35	0.3	8.9	0.1	1.6	2
Apples, cooking, weighed with skin and core						
	26	0.2	6.4	0.1	1.1	1
Apples, cooking, stewed without sugar						
	33	0.3	8.1	0.1	1.5	4
Apples, cooking, baked without sugar, flesh and skin						
	45	0.5	11.2	0.1	2.0	3
Apples, eating, average, raw						
	47	0.4	11.8	0.1	1.8	3
Apples, eating, average, raw, peeled						
	45	0.4	11.2	0.1	1.6	3
Apricots, fresh						
	31	0.9	7.2	0.1	1.7	2

	kcal/100g	protein/100g	carb/100g	fat/100g	fibre/100g	sodium/100g
Apricots, stewed without sugar						
	27	0.7	6.2	0.1	1.5	1
Apricots, dried						
	188	4.8	43.4	0.7	7.7	56
Apricots, canned in syrup						
	63	0.4	16.1	0.1	0.9	10
Apricots, canned in juice						
	34	0.5	8.4	0.1	0.9	5
Apricots, ready-to-eat						
	158	4.0	36.5	0.6	6.3	14
Avocado, average, weighed with skin and stone						
	134	1.3	1.3	13.8	2.4	4
Banana chips						
	511	1.0	59.9	31.4	1.7	5
Bananas, weighed with skin						
	62	0.8	15.3	0.2	0.7	1
Blackberries, raw						
	25	0.9	5.1	0.2	3.1	2
Blackberries, stewed without sugar						
	21	0.8	4.4	0.2	2.6	1
Blackcurrants, raw						
	28	0.9	6.6	Tr	3.6	3
Cherries, raw						
	48	0.9	11.5	0.1	0.9	1
Cherries, glace						
	251	0.4	66.4	Tr	0.9	27
Cherry pie filling						
	82	0.4	21.5	Tr	0.4	30
Clementines, segments only						
	37	0.9	8.7	0.1	1.2	4
Cranberries						
	15	0.4	3.4	0.1	3.0	2
Currants						
	267	2.3	67.8	0.4	1.9	14
Damsons, raw						
	38	0.5	9.6	Tr	1.8	2
Dates, raw						
	124	1.5	31.3	0.1	1.8	7

	kcal/100g	protein/100g	carb/100g	fat/100g	fibre/100g	sodium/100g
Dates, raw, weighed with stones						
	107	1.3	26.9	0.1	1.5	6
Dates, dried						
	270	3.3	68.0	0.2	4.0	10
Dates, dried, weighed with stones						
	227	2.8	57.1	0.2	3.4	8
Dried mixed fruit						
	268	2.3	68.1	0.4	2.2	48
Figs, raw						
	43	1.3	9.5	0.3	1.5	3
Figs, dried						
	227	3.6	52.9	1.6	7.5	62
Figs, ready-to-eat						
	209	3.3	48.6	1.5	6.9	57
Fruit cocktail, canned in juice						
	29	0.4	7.2	Tr	1.0	3
Fruit cocktail, canned in syrup						
	57	0.4	14.8	Tr	1.0	3
Fruit pie filling						
	77	0.4	20.1	Tr	1.0	43
Gooseberries, cooking, raw						
	19	1.1	3.0	0.4	2.4	2
Grapefruit, raw						
	30	0.8	6.8	0.1	1.3	3
Grapefruit, raw, weighed with peel and pips						
	20	0.5	4.6	0.1	0.9	2
Grapefruit, canned in juice						
	30	0.6	7.3	Tr	0.4	10
Grapefruit, canned in syrup						
	60	0.5	15.5	Tr	0.6	10
Grapes, average						
	60	0.4	15.4	0.1	0.7	2
Grapes, weighed with pips						
	57	0.4	14.6	0.1	0.7	2
Guava, raw						
	26	0.8	5.0	0.5	3.7	5
Kiwi fruit						
	49	1.1	10.6	0.5	1.9	4

	kcal/100g	protein/100g	carb/100g	fat/100g	fibre/100g	sodium/100g
Kiwi fruit, weighed with skin						
	42	1.0	9.1	0.4	1.6	3
Kumquats, raw						
	43	0.9	9.3	0.5	3.8	6
Lemons, whole, without pips						
	19	1.0	3.2	0.3	N	5
Mandarin oranges, canned in juice						
	32	0.7	7.7	Tr	0.3	6
Mandarin oranges, canned in syrup						
	52	0.5	13.4	Tr	0.2	6
Mangoes, ripe, raw						
	57	0.7	14.1	0.2	2.6	2
Mangoes, ripe, raw, weighed with skin and stone						
	39	0.5	9.6	0.1	1.8	1
Mangoes, ripe, canned in syrup						
	77	0.3	20.3	Tr	0.7	3
Melon, average						
	24	0.6	5.5	0.1	0.7	24
Melon, average, weighed whole						
	15	0.4	3.4	0.1	0.4	15
Melon, Canteloupe-type						
	19	0.6	4.2	0.1	1.0	8
Melon, Galia						
	24	0.5	5.6	0.1	0.4	31
Melon, Honeydew						
	28	0.5	6.6	0.1	0.6	32
Melon, watermelon						
	31	0.5	7.1	0.3	0.1	2
Mixed peel						
	231	0.3	59.1	0.9	4.8	280
Nectarines, segments only						
	40	1.4	9.0	0.1	1.2	1
Olives, in brine						
	103	0.9	Tr	11.0	2.9	2250
Olives, in brine, weighed with stones						
	82	0.7	Tr	8.8	2.3	1800
Oranges, weighed with peel and pips						
	26	0.8	5.9	0.1	1.2	3

	kcal/100g	protein/100g	carb/100g	fat/100g	fibre/100g	sodium/100g
Passion fruit						
	36	2.6	5.8	0.4	3.3	19
Paw-paw, raw						
	36	0.5	8.8	0.1	2.2	5
Peaches, raw						
	33	1.0	7.6	0.1	1.5	1
Peaches, dried						
	219	3.4	53.0	0.8	7.3	6
Peaches, canned in juice						
	39	0.6	9.7	Tr	0.8	12
Peaches, canned in syrup						
	55	0.5	14.0	Tr	0.9	4
Pears, average, raw						
	40	0.3	10.0	0.1	2.2	3
Pears, average, stewed without sugar						
	35	0.3	9.1	0.1	1.5	2
Pears, dried						
	207	1.6	52.4	0.5	8.3	15
Pears, canned in juice						
	33	0.3	8.5	Tr	1.4	3
Pears, canned in syrup						
	50	0.2	13.2	Tr	1.1	3
Pineapple, raw						
	41	0.4	10.1	0.2	1.2	2
Pineapple, dried						
	276	2.5	67.9	1.3	8.1	13
Pineapple, canned in juice						
	47	0.3	12.2	Tr	0.5	1
Pineapple, canned in syrup						
	64	0.5	16.5	Tr	0.7	2
Plums, average, raw						
	36	0.6	8.8	0.1	1.6	2
Plums, average, raw, weighed with stones						
	34	0.5	8.3	0.1	1.5	2
Plums, average, stewed without sugar						
	30	0.5	7.3	0.1	1.3	2
Plums, canned in syrup						
	59	0.3	15.5	Tr	0.8	6

	kcal/100g	protein/100g	carb/100g	fat/100g	fibre/100g	sodium/100g
Plums, Victoria, raw						
	39	0.6	9.6	0.1	1.8	2
Plums, Victoria, raw, weighed with stones						
	37	0.5	9.0	0.1	1.7	2
Plums, yellow, raw, weighed with stones						
	24	0.5	5.7	0.1	1.0	1
Pomegranate, weighed with skin						
	33	0.9	7.7	0.1	2.2	1
Prunes						
	160	2.8	38.4	0.5	6.5	12
Prunes, weighed with stones						
	134	2.4	32.3	0.4	5.5	10
Prunes, stewed without sugar						
	81	1.4	19.5	0.3	2.9	6
Prunes, canned in juice						
	79	0.7	19.7	0.2	2.4	18
Prunes, canned in syrup						
	90	0.6	23.0	0.2	2.8	18
Prunes, ready-to-eat						
	141	2.5	34.0	0.4	5.7	11
Prunes, ready-to-eat, weighed with stones						
	121	2.1	29.2	0.3	4.9	9
Raisins						
	272	2.1	69.3	0.4	2.0	60
Raspberries, raw						
	25	1.4	4.6	0.3	2.5	3
Raspberries, stewed without sugar						
	24	1.4	4.4	0.3	2.4	2
Raspberries, canned in syrup						
	88	0.6	22.5	0.1	1.5	4
Redcurrants, raw						
	21	1.1	4.4	Tr	3.4	2
Redcurrants, stewed without sugar						
	17	0.9	3.8	Tr	2.9	1
Rhubarb, raw						
	7	0.9	0.8	0.1	1.4	3
Rhubarb, stewed without sugar						
	7	0.9	0.7	0.1	1.3	1

	kcal/100g	protein/100g	carb/100g	fat/100g	fibre/100g	sodium/100g
Rhubarb, canned in syrup						
	31	0.5	7.6	Tr	0.8	4
Satsumas, weighed with peel						
	26	0.6	6.0	0.1	0.9	3
Sharon fruit						
	73	0.8	18.6	Tr	1.6	5
Strawberries, raw						
	27	0.8	6.0	0.1	1.1	6
Sultanas						
	275	2.7	69.4	0.4	2.0	19
Tangerines, segments						
	35	0.9	8.0	0.1	1.3	2

Fruit Juices

	kcal/100g	protein/100g	carb/100g	fat/100g	fibre/100g	sodium/100g
Lemon juice, fresh						
	7	0.3	1.6	Tr	0.1	1
Lime juice, fresh						
	9	0.4	1.6	0.1	0.1	1
Mango juice, canned						
	39	0.1	9.8	0.2	Tr	9
Orange juice, freshly squeezed						
	33	0.6	8.1	Tr	0.1	2
Orange juice, unsweetened						
	36	0.5	8.8	0.1	0.1	10
Passion fruit juice						
	47	0.8	10.7	0.1	Tr	19
Pineapple juice, unsweetened						
	41	0.3	10.5	0.1	Tr	8
Pineapple juice concentrate, unsweetened						
	184	1.3	47.5	0.1	Tr	14
Prune juice						
	57	0.5	14.4	0.1	Tr	12

Nuts and Seeds

	kcal/100g	protein/100g	carb/100g	fat/100g	fibre/100g	sodium/100g
Almonds						
	612	21.1	6.9	55.8	7.4	14
Bombay mix						
	503	18.8	35.1	32.9	6.2	770

	kcal/100g	protein/100g	carb/100g	fat/100g	fibre/100g	sodium/100g
Brazil nuts						
	682	14.1	3.1	68.2	4.3	3
Cashew nuts, plain						
	573	17.7	18.1	48.2	3.2	15
Cashew nuts, roasted and salted						
	611	20.5	18.8	50.9	3.2	290
Chestnuts						
	170	2.0	36.6	2.7	4.1	11
Chestnuts, dried						
	319	3.7	69.0	5.1	7.7	21
Coconut, fresh						
	351	3.2	3.7	36.0	7.3	17
Coconut, creamed block						
	669	6.0	7.0	68.8	N	30
Coconut, desiccated						
	604	5.6	6.4	62.0	13.7	28
Coconut cream						
	350	4.0	5.9	34.7	0	4
Coconut milk						
	22	0.3	4.9	0.3	Tr	110
Hazelnuts						
	650	14.1	6.0	63.5	6.5	6
Macadamia nuts, salted						
	748	7.9	4.8	77.6	5.3	280
Mixed nuts						
	607	22.9	7.9	54.1	6.0	300
Mixed nuts and raisins						
	481	14.1	31.5	34.1	4.5	24
Peanut butter, smooth						
	623	22.6	13.1	53.7	5.4	350
Peanut butter, wholegrain						
	606	24.9	7.7	53.1	6.0	370
Peanuts, plain						
	564	25.6	12.5	46.1	6.2	2
Peanuts, dry-roasted						
	600	25.5	10.3	49.8	6.4	790
Peanuts, roasted and salted						
	602	24.5	7.1	53.0	6.0	400

	kcal/100g	protein/100g	carb/100g	fat/100g	fibre/100g	sodium/100g
Peanuts, raisins and chocolate chips						
	441	12.3	45.9	24.5	3.1	52
Peanuts and raisins						
	435	15.3	37.5	26.0	4.4	27
Pecan nuts						
	689	9.2	5.8	70.1	4.7	1
Pine nuts						
	688	14.0	4.0	68.6	1.9	1
Pistachio nuts, roasted and salted, weighed with shells						
	331	9.9	4.6	30.5	3.3	290
Pumpkin seeds						
	569	24.4	15.2	45.6	5.3	18
Quinoa						
	309	13.8	55.7	5.0	0	61
Sesame seeds						
	598	18.2	0.9	58.0	7.9	20
Sunflower seeds						
	581	19.8	18.6	47.5	6.0	3
Sunflower seeds, toasted						
	602	20.5	19.3	49.2	6.2	3
Tahini paste						
	607	18.5	0.9	58.9	8.0	20
Trail mix						
	432	9.1	37.2	28.5	4.3	27
Walnuts						
	688	14.7	3.3	68.5	3.5	7

MEAT, POULTRY AND GAME

Meat

	kcal/100g	protein/100g	carb/100g	fat/100g	fibre/100g	sodium/100g
Beef, average, trimmed lean, raw						
	136	22.5	0	5.1	0	63
Beef, braising steak, raw, lean						
	139	21.8	0	5.7	0	64
Beef, braising steak, raw, lean meat with fat						
	160	20.7	0	8.6	0	60
Beef, braising steak, braised, lean						
	225	34.4	0	9.7	0	62

	kcal/100g	protein/100g	carb/100g	fat/100g	fibre/100g	sodium/100g
Beef, braising steak, braised, lean meat with fat						
	246	32.9	0	12.7	0	60
Beef, braising steak, slow-cooked, lean						
	197	31.4	0	7.9	0	53
Beef, brisket, raw, lean						
	139	21.1	0	6.1	0	59
Beef, brisket, raw, lean meat with fat						
	218	18.4	0	16.0	0	50
Beef, brisket, boiled, lean						
	225	31.4	0	11.0	0	50
Beef, brisket, boiled, lean meat with fat						
	268	27.8	0	17.4	0	46
Beef, fillet steak, raw, lean						
	140	21.2	0	6.1	0	44
Beef, fillet steak, raw, lean meat with fat						
	155	20.9	0	7.9	0	43
Beef, fillet steak, fried, lean						
	184	28.2	0	7.9	0	68
Beef, fillet steak, grilled, lean						
	188	29.1	0	8.0	0	70
Beef, fillet steak, grilled, lean meat with fat						
	200	28.7	0	9.5	0	67
Beef, flank, raw, lean						
	175	22.7	0	9.3	0	64
Beef, flank, raw, lean meat with fat						
	266	0	19.7	20.8	0	54
Beef, flank, pot-roasted, lean						
	253	31.8	0	14.0	0	51
Beef, fore-rib/rib-roast, raw, lean						
	145	21.5	0	6.5	0	61
Beef, fore-rib/rib-roast, microwaved, lean						
	243	35.0	0	11.4	0	60
Beef, fore-rib/rib-roast, microwaved, lean meat with fat						
	306	30.4	0	20.5	0	60
Beef, fore-rib/rib-roast, roasted, lean						
	236	33.3	0	11.4	0	57
Beef, mince, raw						
	225	19.7	0	16.2	0	80

	kcal/100g	protein/100g	carb/100g	fat/100g	fibre/100g	sodium/100g
Beef, mince, stewed						
	209	21.8	0	13.5	0	73
Beef, mince, extra lean, raw						
	174	21.9	0	9.6	0	90
Beef, mince, extra lean, stewed						
	177	24.7	0	8.7	0	75
Beef, rump steak, raw, lean						
	125	22.0	0	4.1	0	60
Beef, rump steak, raw, lean meat with fat						
	174	20.7	0	10.1	0	56
Beef, rump steak, barbecued, lean						
	176	31.2	0	5.7	0	78
Beef, rump steak, fried, lean						
	183	30.9	0	6.6	0	78
Beef, rump steak, grilled, lean						
	177	31.0	0	5.9	0	74
Beef, sirloin joint, roasted, lean						
	188	32.4	0	6.5	0	55
Beef, sirloin joint, roasted, lean meat with fat						
	233	29.8	0	12.6	0	53
Beef, sirloin steak, raw, lean						
	135	23.5	0	4.5	0	70
Beef, sirloin steak, fried, lean						
	189	28.8	0	8.2	0	69
Beef, sirloin steak, grilled rare, lean						
	166	26.4	0	6.7	0	63
Beef, sirloin steak, grilled rare, lean meat with fat						
	216	25.1	0	12.8	0	60
Beef, sirloin steak, grilled medium-rare, lean meat with fat						
	213	24.8	0	12.6	0	60
Beef, sirloin steak, grilled well-done, lean						
	225	33.9	0	9.9	0	81
Beef, sirloin steak, grilled well-done, lean meat with fat						
	257	31.8	0	14.4	0	76
Beef, stewing steak, raw, lean						
	122	22.6	0	3.5	0	69
Beef, stewing steak, raw, lean meat with fat						
	146	22.1	0	6.4	0	66

	kcal/100g	protein/100g	carb/100g	fat/100g	fibre/100g	sodium/100g
Beef, stewing steak, pressure cooked, lean						
	199	35.1	0	6.5	0	60
Beef, stewing steak, pressure cooked, lean meat with fat						
	217	34.0	0	9.0	0	60
Beef, stewing steak, stewed, lean						
	185	32.0	0	6.3	0	54
Beef, stewing steak, stewed, lean meat with fat						
	203	29.2	0	9.6	0	51
Beef, topside, raw, lean						
	116	23.0	0	2.7	0	77
Beef, topside, raw, lean meat with fat						
	198	20.4	0	12.9	0	67
Beef, topside, microwaved, lean						
	181	35.0	0	4.6	0	60
Beef, topside, microwaved, lean meat with fat						
	228	32.1	0	11.1	0	55
Beef, topside, roasted medium-rare, lean						
	175	32.2	0	5.1	0	66
Beef, topside, roasted medium-rare, lean meat with fat						
	222	29.9	0	11.4	0	62
Beef, topside, roasted well-done, lean						
	202	36.2	0	6.3	0	62
Beef, topside, roasted well-done, lean meat with fat						
	244	32.8	0	12.5	0	57
Lamb, average, trimmed of most fat, raw						
	518	13.3	0	51.6	0	36
Lamb, average, trimmed of most fat, cooked						
	568	15.4	0	56.3	0	72
Lamb, best end neck cutlets, raw, lean meat with fat						
	316	16.3	0	27.9	0	58
Lamb, breast, raw, lean						
	179	19.6	0	11.2	0	86
Lamb, breast, raw, lean meat with fat						
	287	16.2	0	24.7	0	69
Lamb, breast, roasted, lean						
	273	26.7	0	18.5	0	93
Lamb, breast, roasted, lean meat with fat						
	359	22.4	0	29.9	0	85

	kcal/100g	protein/100g	carb/100g	fat/100g	fibre/100g	sodium/100g
Lamb, chump chops, raw, lean meat with fat						
	242	18.3	0	18.8	0	56
Lamb, chump chops, raw, lean meat with fat, weighed with bone						
	211	15.9	0	16.4	0	49
Lamb, chump chops, fried, lean						
	213	28.1	0	11.2	0	74
Lamb, chump chops, fried, lean, weighed with fat and bone						
	135	17.7	0	7.1	0	47
Lamb, leg, average, raw, lean meat with fat						
	187	19.0	0	12.3	0	58
Lamb, leg chops, grilled, lean meat with fat						
	221	28.3	0	12.0	0	71
Lamb, leg joint, roasted, lean						
	210	30.8	0	9.6	0	82
Lamb, leg joint, roasted, lean meat with fat						
	236	29.7	0	13.0	0	82
Lamb, leg steaks, grilled, lean						
	198	29.2	0	9.0	0	70
Lamb, leg steaks, grilled, lean meat with fat						
	231	28.0	0	13.2	0	71
Lamb, leg, whole, roasted medium, lean						
	203	29.7	0	9.4	0	63
Lamb, leg, whole, roasted medium, lean meat with fat						
	240	28.1	0	14.2	0	64
Lamb, leg, whole, roasted well done, lean						
	208	31.3	0	9.2	0	62
Lamb, leg, whole, roasted well done, lean meat with fat						
	242	29.8	0	13.6	0	64
Lamb, loin chops, raw, lean meat with fat						
	277	17.6	0	23.0	0	63
Lamb, loin chops, raw, lean meat with fat, weighed with bone						
	216	13.7	0	17.9	0	49
Lamb, loin chops, grilled, lean						
	213	29.2	0	10.7	0	80
Lamb, loin chops, grilled, lean, weighed with fat and bone						
	130	17.8	0	6.5	0	49
Lamb, loin chops, grilled, lean meat with fat						
	305	26.5	0	22.1	0	81

kcal/100g	protein/100g	carb/100g	fat/100g	fibre/100g	sodium/100g

Lamb, loin chops, grilled, lean meat with fat, weighed with bone

| 247 | 21.5 | 0 | 17.9 | 0 | 66 |

Lamb, loin chops, roasted, lean

| 257 | 34.4 | 0 | 13.3 | 0 | 91 |

Lamb, loin chops, roasted, lean, weighed with fat and bone

| 144 | 19.3 | 0 | 7.4 | 0 | 51 |

Lamb, loin chops, roasted, lean meat with fat

| 359 | 29.1 | 0 | 26.9 | 0 | 85 |

Lamb, loin chops, roasted, lean meat with fat, weighed with bone

| 316 | 22.4 | 0 | 20.7 | 0 | 75 |

Lamb, loin joint, raw, lean meat with fat

| 307 | 16.9 | 0 | 26.6 | 0 | 61 |

Lamb, loin joint, raw, lean meat with fat, weighed with bone

| 236 | 13.0 | 0 | 20.5 | 0 | 47 |

Lamb, mince, raw

| 196 | 19.1 | 0 | 13.3 | 0 | 69 |

Lamb, mince, stewed

| 208 | 24.4 | 0 | 12.3 | 0 | 59 |

Lamb, rack of, raw, lean meat with fat, weighed with bone

| 204 | 12.5 | 0 | 17.1 | 0 | 44 |

Lamb, rack of, roasted, lean

| 225 | 27.1 | 0 | 13.0 | 0 | 77 |

Lamb, rack of, roasted, lean meat with fat

| 363 | 23.0 | 0 | 30.1 | 0 | 75 |

Lamb, shoulder, raw, lean meat with fat

| 235 | 17.6 | 0 | 18.3 | 0 | 63 |

Lamb, shoulder, raw, lean meat with fat, weighed with bone

| 188 | 14.1 | 0 | 14.6 | 0 | 50 |

Lamb, shoulder, diced, kebabs, grilled, lean meat with fat

| 288 | 28.5 | 0 | 19.3 | 0 | 87 |

Lamb, shoulder joint, roasted, lean

| 235 | 28.4 | 0 | 13.5 | 0 | 75 |

Lamb, shoulder joint, roasted, lean meat with fat

| 282 | 25.9 | 0 | 19.8 | 0 | 74 |

Lamb, shoulder, whole, roasted, lean

| 218 | 27.2 | 0 | 12.1 | 0 | 80 |

Lamb, shoulder, whole, roasted, lean meat with fat

| 298 | 24.7 | 0 | 22.1 | 0 | 80 |

	kcal/100g	protein/100g	carb/100g	fat/100g	fibre/100g	sodium/100g
Lamb, shoulder, whole, roasted, lean meat with fat, weighed with bone						
	235	19.5	0	17.5	0	63
Lamb, stewing, raw, lean meat with fat						
	203	22.5	0	12.6	0	66
Lamb, stewing, raw, lean meat with fat, weighed with bone						
	136	15.1	0	8.4	0	44
Lamb, stewing, stewed, lean						
	240	26.6	0	14.8	0	49
Lamb, stewing, stewed, lean meat with fat						
	279	24.4	0	20.1	0	50
Pork, trimmed of most fat, raw						
	548	10.1	0	56.4	0	47
Pork, belly joint/slices, raw, lean meat with fat						
	258	19.1	0	20.2	0	69
Pork, belly joint/slices, raw, lean meat with fat, weighed with bone						
	238	17.6	0	18.6	0	75
Pork, belly joint, roasted, lean meat with fat						
	293	25.1	0	21.4	0	90
Pork, belly slices, grilled, lean meat with fat						
	320	27.4	0	23.4	0	97
Pork, chump chops, raw, lean meat with fat						
	194	20.1	0	12.6	0	54
Pork, chump chops, raw, lean meat with fat, weighed with bone						
	194	17.3	0	9.8	0	43
Pork, chump steaks, raw, lean meat with fat						
	151	21.3	0	7.3	0	56
Pork, diced, raw, lean						
	122	21.4	0	4.0	0	70
Pork, diced, raw, lean meat with fat						
	147	20.5	0	7.2	0	68
Pork, diced, casseroled, lean						
	184	31.7	0	6.4	0	37
Pork, diced, casseroled, lean meat with fat						
	184	30.8	0	6.8	0	37
Pork, diced, kebabs, grilled, lean						
	179	34.1	0	4.7	0	80
Pork, diced, kebabs, grilled, lean meat with fat						
	189	33.6	0	6.1	0	81

	kcal/100g	protein/100g	carb/100g	fat/100g	fibre/100g	sodium/100g
Pork, diced, slow-cooked, lean						
	169	30.0	0	5.4	0	41
Pork, fillet, raw, lean meat with fat						
	147	22.0	0	6.5	0	53
Pork, fillet slices, grilled, lean						
	170	33.6	0	4.0	0	67
Pork, fillet slices, grilled, lean meat with fat						
	178	33.2	0	5.0	0	67
Pork, leg joint, raw, lean						
	107	21.7	0	2.2	0	65
Pork, leg joint, raw, lean meat with fat						
	213	19.0	0	15.2	0	60
Pork, leg joint, raw, lean meat with fat, weighed with bone						
	185	16.5	0	13.2	0	52
Pork, leg joint, roasted medium, lean						
	182	33.0	0	5.5	0	69
Pork, leg joint, roasted medium, lean meat with fat						
	215	30.9	0	10.2	0	70
Pork, leg joint, roasted well done, lean						
	185	34.7	0	5.1	0	74
Pork, leg joint, roasted well done, lean meat with fat						
	259	30.1	0	15.4	0	71
Pork, loin chops, raw, lean meat with fat						
	270	18.6	0	21.7	0	53
Pork, loin chops, raw, lean meat with fat, weighed with bone						
	227	15.7	0	18.2	0	45
Pork, loin chops, grilled, lean						
	184	31.6	0	6.4	0	66
Pork, loin chops, grilled, lean meat with fat						
	257	29.0	0	15.7	0	70
Pork, loin chops, roasted, lean						
	241	37.5	0	10.1	0	70
Pork, loin chops, roasted, lean meat with fat						
	301	31.9	0	19.3	0	68
Pork, loin chops, roasted, lean meat with fat, weighed with bone						
	229	24.2	0	14.7	0	51
Pork, loin joint, roasted, lean						
	182	30.1	0	6.8	0	61

	kcal/100g	protein/100g	carb/100g	fat/100g	fibre/100g	sodium/100g
Pork, loin joint, roasted, lean meat with fat						
	253	26.3	0	16.4	0	61
Pork, loin steaks, raw, lean meat with fat						
	225	19.9	0	16.1	0	56
Pork, mince, raw						
	164	19.2	0	9.7	0	66
Pork, mince, stewed						
	191	24.4	0	10.4	0	61
Pork, spare rib chops, raw, lean meat with fat						
	186	18.5	0	12.4	0	62
Pork, spare rib chops, raw, lean meat with fat, weighed with bone						
	147	14.6	0	9.8	0	49
Pork, spare ribs, raw, lean meat with fat						
	195	18.7	0	13.4	0	98
Pork, steaks, raw, lean						
	120	22.4	0	3.4	0	60
Pork, steaks, raw, lean meat with fat						
	169	21.0	0	9.4	0	58
Pork, steaks, grilled, lean						
	169	33.9	0	3.7	0	76
Pork, steaks, grilled, lean meat with fat						
	198	32.4	0	7.6	0	76
Veal, escalope, raw						
	106	22.7	0	1.7	0	59
Veal, escalope, fried						
	196	33.7	0	6.8	0	86
Veal, mince, raw						
	144	20.3	0	7.0	0	83
Veal, mince, stewed						
	205	26.3	0	11.1	0	74

Offal

	kcal/100g	protein/100g	carb/100g	fat/100g	fibre/100g	sodium/100g
Kidney, lamb, raw						
	91	17.0	0	2.6	0	150
Kidney, pig, raw						
	86	15.5	0	2.7	0	200
Liver, calf, raw						
	104	18.3	0	3.4	0	71

	kcal/100g	protein/100g	carb/100g	fat/100g	fibre/100g	sodium/100g

Liver, chicken, raw

	92	17.7	0	2.3	0	76

Liver, lamb's, raw

	137	20.3	0	6.2	0	73

Poultry and Game

Chicken, dark meat, raw

	109	20.9	0	2.8	0	90

Chicken, light meat, raw

	106	24.0	0	1.1	0	60

Chicken, meat, average, raw

	108	22.3	0	2.1	0	77

Chicken, leg quarter, raw, meat and skin

	193	18.3	0	13.3	0	80

Chicken, leg quarter, raw, meat and skin, weighed with bone

	133	12.6	0	9.2	0	55

Chicken, wing quarter, raw, meat and skin

	193	20.3	0	12.4	0	60

Chicken, wing quarter, raw, meat and skin, weighed with bone

	127	13.4	0	8.2	0	40

Chicken, corn-fed, raw, dark meat only

	143	19.5	0	7.2	0	80

Chicken, breast, casseroled, meat only

	114	28.4	0	5.2	0	60

Chicken, breast, grilled without skin, meat only

	148	32.0	0	2.2	0	55

Chicken, breast, grilled with skin, meat only

	147	29.8	0	3.1	0	60

Chicken, breast, grilled, meat and skin

	173	28.9	0	6.4	0	61

Chicken, meat, average, roasted

	177	27.3	0	7.5	0	80

Chicken, drumsticks, roasted, meat and skin

	185	25.8	0	9.1	0	130

Chicken, leg quarter, roasted, meat and skin

	236	20.9	0	16.9	0	95

Chicken, wing quarter, roasted, meat and skin

	226	24.8	0	14.1	0	100

	kcal/100g	protein/100g	carb/100g	fat/100g	fibre/100g	sodium/100g
Duck, raw, meat only						
	137	19.7	0	6.5	0	110
Duck, raw, meat, fat and skin						
	388	13.1	0	37.3	0	73
Duck, roasted, meat only						
	195	25.3	0	10.4	0	96
Duck, roasted, meat, fat and skin						
	423	20.0	0	38.1	0	87
Goose, raw, meat, fat and skin						
	361	16.5	0	32.8	0	61
Goose, roasted, meat, fat and skin						
	301	27.5	0	21.2	0	80
Grouse, roasted, meat only						
	128	27.6	0	2.0	0	110
Pheasant, roasted, meat only						
	220	27.9	0	12.0	0	66
Poussin, raw, meat and skin, weighed with bone						
	117	11.1	0	8.1	0	40
Turkey, dark meat, raw						
	104	20.4	0	2.5	0	90
Turkey, light meat, raw						
	105	24.4	0	0.8	0	50
Turkey, meat, average, raw						
	105	22.6	0	1.6	0	68
Turkey, mince, stewed						
	176	28.6	0	6.8	0	45
Turkey, breast, fillet, grilled, meat only						
	155	35.0	0	1.7	0	90
Turkey, dark meat, roasted						
	177	29.4	0	6.6	0	110
Turkey, light meat, roasted						
	153	33.7	0	2.0	0	50
Turkey, meat, average, roasted						
	166	31.2	0	4.6	0	90
Turkey, skin, dry, roasted						
	481	29.9	0	40.2	0	110
Venison, raw						
	103	22.2	0	1.6	0	55

	kcal/100g	protein/100g	carb/100g	fat/100g	fibre/100g	sodium/100g
Venison, roasted						
	165	35.6	0	2.5	0	52

MISCELLANEOUS

Everyday Store Cupboard Items

	kcal/100g	protein/100g	carb/100g	fat/100g	fibre/100g	sodium/100g
Bournvita powder						
	377	8.7	79.0	5.1	0	460
Breadcrumbs, manufactured						
	354	10.1	78.5	2.1	2.2	400
Brown sauce, sweet						
	98	1.2	22.2	0.1	0	1420
Chilli sauce						
	79	1.3	17.7	0.8	0	2620
Chutney, mango, sweet						
	189	0.7	48.3	0.1	0	1300
Chutney, tomato						
	128	1.2	31.0	0.2	1.3	410
Cocoa powder						
	312	18.5	11.5	21.7	0	950
Coffee Compliment						
	554	3.0	58.1	36.0	0	800
Coffeemate						
	540	2.7	57.3	34.9	0	200
Cranberry sauce						
	151	0.2	39.9	0.1	0	Tr
Drinking chocolate powder						
	366	5.5	77.4	6.0	0	250
Gravy, instant granules						
	462	4.4	40.6	32.5	0	6330
Horlicks powder						
	378	12.4	78.0	4.0	0	460
Horseradish sauce (average creamed and plain)						
	153	2.5	17.9	8.4	2.5	910
Instant dessert powder						
	391	2.4	60.1	17.3	0	1100
Jelly, made with water						
	61	1.2	15.1	0	0	5

	kcal/100g	protein/100g	carb/100g	fat/100g	fibre/100g	sodium/100g
Mayonnaise, retail						
	691	1.1	1.7	75.6	0	450
Mayonnaise, retail, reduced-calorie						
	288	1.0	8.2	28.1	0	940
Mincemeat						
	274	0.6	62.1	4.3	0	18
Mint sauce						
	101	1.6	21.5	Tr	0	690
Molasses						
	266	0	68.8	0.1	0	37
Oil, corn						
	899	Tr	0	99.9	0	Tr
Oil, grapeseed						
	899	Tr	0	99.9	0	Tr
Oil, hazelnut						
	899	Tr	0	99.9	0	Tr
Oil, olive						
	899	Tr	0	99.9	0	Tr
Oil, peanut						
	899	Tr	0	99.9	0	Tr
Oil, sesame						
	898	0.2	0	99.7	0	2
Oil, sunflower						
	899	Tr	0	99.9	0	Tr
Oil, vegetable, blended, average						
	899	Tr	0	99.9	0	Tr
Oil, walnut						
	899	Tr	0	99.9	0	Tr
Ovaltine powder						
	358	9.0	79.4	2.7	0	160
Piccalilli						
	84	1.0	17.6	0.5	1.0	1340
Pickle, sweet						
	141	0.6	36.0	0.1	1.2	1610
Popcorn, candied						
	480	2.1	77.6	20.0	0	56
Popcorn, plain						
	593	6.2	48.7	42.8	0	4

	kcal/100g	protein/100g	carb/100g	fat/100g	fibre/100g	sodium/100g
Redcurrant jelly						
	240	0.3	63.8	Tr	0	10
Relish, burger/chilli/tomato						
	114	1.2	27.6	0.1	1.3	480
Salad cream						
	348	1.5	16.7	31.0	0	1040
Salad cream, reduced-calorie						
	194	1.0	9.4	17.2	0	N
Sugar, brown (average value, light and dark)						
	362	0.1	101.3	0	0	31
Sugar, white						
	394	Tr	105	0	0	5
Stuffing mix, dried						
	338	9.9	67.2	5.2	4.7	1460
Stuffing mix, dried, made-up						
	97	2.8	19.3	1.5	1.3	420
Suet, vegetable						
	836	1.2	10.1	87.9	0	10
Syrup, golden						
	298	0.3	79.0	0	0	270
Syrup, golden, pouring						
	296	Tr	79.0	0	0	340
Syrup, maple						
	262	0	67.2	0.2	0	9
Tartare sauce						
	299	1.3	17.9	24.6	Tr	800
Tomato ketchup						
	115	1.6	28.6	0.1	0.9	1630
Tomato puree, with salt						
	76	5.0	14.2	0.3	2.8	240
Tomatoes, sun-dried in oil						
	495	3.3	5.4	51.3	N	1000
Yeast extract						
	180	40.7	3.5	0.4	0	4300

Drinks (alcoholic)

Bitter						
	30	0.3	2.2	Tr	0	6

	kcal/100g	protein/100g	carb/100g	fat/100g	fibre/100g	sodium/100g
Bitter, low-alcohol						
	13	0.2	2.1	0	0	7
Champagne						
	76	0.3	1.4	0	0	4
Cider, dry						
	36	Tr	2.6	0	0	7
Cider, sweet						
	42	Tr	4.3	0	0	7
Lager, average						
	29	0.3	Tr	Tr	0	7
Lager, alcohol-free						
	7	0.4	1.5	Tr	0	2
Lager, low alcohol, average						
	10	0.2	1.5	0	0	12
Lager, premium						
	59	0.3	2.4	Tr	0	7
Port						
	157	0.1	12.0	0	0	4
Shandy						
	11	Tr	3.0	0	0	7
Sherry, dry						
	116	0.2	1.4	0	0	10
Sherry, medium						
	116	0.1	5.9	0	0	27
Sherry, sweet						
	136	0.3	6.9	0	0	13
Spirits, 40% volume (average brandy, gin, rum, whisky and vodka)						
	222	Tr	Tr	0	0	Tr
Stout/Guinness						
	30	0.4	1.5	Tr	0	6
Wine, red						
	68	0.1	0.2	0	0	7
Wine, rose, medium						
	71	0.1	2.5	0	0	4
Wine, white, dry						
	66	0.1	0.6	0	0	4
Wine, white, medium						
	74	0.1	3.0	0	0	11

	kcal/100g	protein/100g	carb/100g	fat/100g	fibre/100g	sodium/100g
Wine, white, sparkling						
	74	0.3	5.1	0	0	5
Wine, white, sweet						
	94	0.2	5.9	0	0	13

VEGETABLES AND PULSES

Potatoes and Potato Products

	kcal/100g	protein/100g	carb/100g	fat/100g	fibre/100g	sodium/100g
Chips, crinkle cut, frozen, fried in corn oil						
	290	3.6	33.4	16.7	2.2	78
Chips, French fries, cooked in oil						
	280	3.3	34.0	15.5	2.1	310
Chips, microwave, cooked						
	221	3.6	32.1	9.6	2.9	40
Chips, oven, frozen, baked						
	162	3.2	29.8	4.2	2.0	53
Chips, retail, fried in vegetable oil						
	239	3.2	30.5	12.4	2.2	35
Chips, straight-cut, frozen, fried in corn oil						
	273	4.1	36.0	13.5	2.4	29
Instant potato powder, raw						
	320	8.4	74.9	0.6	5.8	1090
Instant potato powder, made up with water						
	57	1.5	13.5	0.1	1	200
Potato croquettes, fried in blended oil						
	214	3.7	21.6	13.1	1.3	420
Potato flour						
	328	9.1	75.6	0.9	5.7	31
Potatoes, new, average, raw						
	70	1.7	16.1	0.3	1	11
Potatoes, new, boiled in salted water						
	75	1.5	17.8	0.3	1.1	26
Potatoes, new, in skins, boiled in salted water						
	66	1.4	15.4	0.3	1.5	26
Potatoes, new, canned, re-heated, drained						
	63	1.5	15.1	0.1	0.8	250
Potatoes, new, chipped, fried in corn oil						
	228	4.4	33.3	9.5	1.7	17

	kcal/100g	protein/100g	carb/100g	fat/100g	fibre/100g	sodium/100g
Potatoes, old, average, raw						
	75	2.1	17.2	0.2	1.3	7
Potatoes, old, baked, flesh and skin						
	136	3.9	31.7	0.2	2.7	12
Potatoes, old, baked, flesh only						
	77	2.2	18.0	0.1	1.4	7
Potatoes, old, boiled in salted water						
	72	1.8	17.0	0.1	1.2	64
Potatoes, old, roast in corn oil						
	149	2.9	25.9	4.5	1.8	9
Potato waffles, frozen, cooked						
	200	3.2	30.3	8.2	2.3	430

Pulses, Beans and Lentils

	kcal/100g	protein/100g	carb/100g	fat/100g	fibre/100g	sodium/100g
Aduki beans, dried, raw						
	272	19.9	50.1	0.5	11.1	5
Aduki beans, dried, boiled						
	123	9.3	22.5	0.2	5.5	2
Baked beans, canned in tomato sauce						
	81	4.8	15.1	0.6	3.5	550
Baked beans, canned in tomato sauce, reduced-sugar						
	74	5.4	12.8	0.6	3.8	550
Barbecue beans, canned in sauce						
	77	5.3	14.0	0.4	0	500
Beansprouts, mung, raw						
	31	2.9	4.0	0.5	1.5	5
Beansprouts, mung, boiled						
	25	2.5	2.8	0.5	1.3	57
Beansprouts, mung, stir-fried in blended oil						
	72	1.9	2.5	6.1	0.9	3
Beansprouts, mung, canned, drained						
	10	1.6	0.8	0.1	0.7	80
Blackeye beans, dried, raw						
	311	23.5	54.1	1.6	8.2	16
Blackeye beans, dried, boiled						
	116	8.8	19.9	0.7	3.5	5
Broad beans, raw, fresh						
	59	5.7	7.2	1.0	6.1	1

	kcal/100g	protein/100g	carb/100g	fat/100g	fibre/100g	sodium/100g
Broad beans, boiled						
	48	5.1	5.6	0.8	5.4	110
Broad beans, frozen, boiled						
	81	7.9	11.7	0.6	6.5	8
Broad beans, canned, re-heated, drained						
	87	8.3	12.7	0.7	5.2	290
Butter beans, dried, raw						
	290	19.1	52.9	1.7	16.0	40
Butter beans, dried, boiled						
	103	7.1	18.4	0.6	5.2	9
Butter beans, canned, re-heated, drained						
	77	5.9	13.0	0.5	4.6	420
Chickpea flour						
	313	19.7	49.6	5.4	10.7	39
Chickpeas, whole, dried, raw						
	320	21.3	49.6	5.4	10.7	39
Chickpeas, whole, dried, boiled						
	121	8.4	18.2	2.1	4.3	5
Chickpeas, split, dried, raw						
	325	22.7	49.6	5.4	0	39
Chickpeas, split, dried, boiled						
	114	7.7	17.4	2.0	0	5
Chickpeas, canned, re-heated, drained						
	115	7.2	16.1	2.9	4.1	220
Chilli beans, canned, re-heated						
	70	4.9	12.2	0.5	3.9	590
Green beans/French beans, raw						
	24	1.9	3.2	0.5	2.2	Tr
Green beans/French beans, boiled in salted water						
	22	1.8	2.9	0.5	2.4	66
Green beans/French beans, canned, re-heated, drained						
	22	1.5	4.1	0.1	2.6	340
Haricot beans, dried, raw						
	286	21.4	49.7	1.6	17.0	43
Haricot beans, dried, boiled in unsalted water						
	95	6.6	17.2	0.5	6.1	15
Lentils, green and brown, whole, dried, raw						
	297	24.3	48.8	1.9	8.9	12

	kcal/100g	protein/100g	carb/100g	fat/100g	fibre/100g	sodium/100g
Lentils, green and brown, whole, dried, boiled						
	105	8.8	16.9	0.7	3.8	3
Lentils, red, split, dried, raw						
	318	23.8	56.3	1.3	4.9	36
Lentils, red, split, dried, boiled						
	100	7.6	17.5	0.4	1.9	12
Miso						
	203	13.3	23.5	6.2	N	3650
Mung beans, whole, dried, raw						
	279	23.9	46.3	1.1	10.0	12
Mung beans, whole, dried, boiled						
	91	7.6	15.3	0.4	3.0	2
Mung beans, dahl, dried, raw						
	291	26.8	46.3	1.1	0	12
Mung beans, dahl, dried, boiled						
	92	7.8	15.3	0.4	0	2
Pinto beans, dried, raw						
	327	21.1	57.1	1.6	0	10
Pinto beans, dried, boiled						
	137	8.9	23.9	0.7	0	1
Re-fried beans						
	107	6.2	15.3	1.1	0	420
Red kidney beans, dried, raw						
	266	22.1	44.1	1.4	15.7	18
Red kidney beans, dried, boiled						
	103	8.4	17.4	0.5	6.7	2
Red kidney beans, canned, re-heated, drained						
	100	6.9	17.8	0.6	6.2	390
Soya beans, dried, raw						
	370	35.9	15.8	18.6	15.7	5
Soya beans, dried, boiled						
	141	14.0	5.1	7.3	6.1	1
Tempeh						
	166	20.7	6.4	6.4	4.3	6
Tofu, soya bean, steamed						
	73	8.1	0.7	4.2	N	4
Tofu, soya bean, steamed then fried						
	261	23.5	2.0	17.7	N	12

	kcal/100g	protein/100g	carb/100g	fat/100g	fibre/100g	sodium/100g

Vegetables

Alfalfa sprouts, raw

24	4.0	0.4	0.7	1.7	6

Artichoke, globe, raw

18	2.8	2.7	0.2	N	27

Artichoke, globe, boiled, weighed as served

8	1.2	1.2	0.1	N	6

Artichoke, Jerusalem, boiled

41	1.6	10.6	0.1	3.5	3

Asparagus, raw

25	2.9	2.0	0.6	1.7	1

Asparagus, boiled, weighed as served

13	1.6	0.7	0.4	0.7	29

Asparagus, boiled

26	3.4	1.4	0.8	1.4	60

Asparagus, canned, re-heated, drained

24	3.4	1.5	0.5	2.9	340

Aubergine, raw

15	0.9	2.2	0.4	2.0	2

Aubergine, fried in corn oil

302	1.2	2.8	31.9	2.3	2

Bamboo shoots, canned, drained

11	1.5	0.7	0.2	1.7	4

Beetroot, raw

36	1.7	7.6	0.1	1.9	66

Beetroot, boiled in salted water

46	2.3	9.5	0.1	1.9	110

Beetroot, pickled, drained

28	1.2	5.6	0.2	1.7	120

Breadfruit, raw

95	1.3	23.1	0.3	N	1

Breadfruit, boiled

119	1.6	29.0	0.4	N	1

Broccoli, green, raw

33	4.4	1.8	0.9	2.6	8

Broccoli, green, boiled

24	3.1	1.1	0.8	2.3	150

	kcal/100g	protein/100g	carb/100g	fat/100g	fibre/100g	sodium/100g
Broccoli, green, frozen, boiled						
	31	3.3	2.5	0.9	3.6	13
Broccoli, purple sprouting, raw						
	35	3.9	2.6	1.1	3.5	10
Broccoli, purple sprouting, boiled						
	19	2.1	1.3	0.6	2.3	66
Brussels sprouts, raw						
	42	3.5	4.1	1.4	4.1	6
Brussels sprouts, boiled						
	35	2.9	3.5	1.3	3.1	73
Brussels sprouts, frozen, boiled						
	35	3.5	2.5	1.3	4.3	73
Cabbage, raw, average						
	26	1.7	4.1	0.4	2.4	5
Cabbage, boiled						
	16	1.0	2.2	0.4	1.8	120
Cabbage, Chinese, raw						
	12	1.0	1.4	0.2	1.2	7
Cabbage, red, raw						
	21	1.1	3.7	0.3	2.5	8
Cabbage, red, boiled						
	15	0.8	2.3	0.3	2.0	130
Cabbage, Savoy, raw						
	27	2.1	3.9	0.5	3.1	5
Cabbage, Savoy, boiled						
	17	1.1	2.2	0.5	2.0	120
Cabbage, white, raw						
	27	1.4	5.0	0.2	2.1	7
Cabbage, white, boiled						
	14	1.0	2.2	0.2	1.5	110
Carrot juice						
	24	0.5	5.7	0.1	N	51
Carrots, old, raw						
	35	0.6	7.9	0.3	2.4	25
Carrots, old, boiled						
	24	0.6	4.9	0.4	2.5	120
Carrots, young, raw						
	30	0.7	6.0	0.5	2.4	40

kcal/100g	protein/100g	carb/100g	fat/100g	fibre/100g	sodium/100g
Carrots, young, boiled in salted water					
22	0.6	4.4	0.4	2.3	130
Carrots, frozen, boiled					
22	0.4	4.7	0.3	2.3	35
Carrots, canned, re-heated, drained					
20	0.5	4.2	0.3	1.9	370
Cauliflower, raw					
34	3.6	3.0	0.9	1.8	9
Cauliflower, boiled					
28	2.9	2.1	0.9	1.6	60
Cauliflower, frozen, boiled					
20	2.0	2.0	0.5	1.2	7
Celeriac, raw					
18	1.2	2.3	0.4	3.7	91
Celeriac, boiled					
15	0.9	1.9	0.5	3.2	160
Celery, raw					
7	0.5	0.9	0.2	1.1	60
Celery, boiled					
8	0.5	0.8	0.3	1.2	160
Chard, Swiss, raw					
19	1.8	2.9	0.2	N	210
Chard, Swiss, boiled					
20	1.9	3.2	0.1	N	180
Chicory, raw					
11	0.5	2.8	0.6	0.9	1
Chicory, boiled					
7	0.6	2.1	0.3	1.1	150
Courgette, raw					
18	1.8	1.8	0.4	0.9	1
Courgette, boiled					
19	2.0	2.0	0.4	1.2	1
Courgette, fried in corn oil					
63	2.6	2.6	4.8	1.2	1
Cucumber, raw					
10	0.7	1.5	0.1	0.6	3
Curly kale, raw					
33	3.4	1.4	1.6	3.1	43

	kcal/100g	protein/100g	carb/100g	fat/100g	fibre/100g	sodium/100g
Curly kale, boiled						
	24	2.4	1.0	1.1	2.8	100
Endive, raw						
	13	1.8	1.0	0.2	2.0	10
Fennel, Florence, raw						
	12	0.9	1.8	0.2	2.4	11
Fenugreek leaves, raw						
	35	4.6	4.8	0.2	0	76
Garlic, raw						
	98	7.9	16.3	0.6	4.1	4
Gherkins, raw						
	12	1.0	1.8	0.1	0.8	11
Gherkins, pickled, drained						
	14	0.9	2.6	0.1	1.2	690
Ginger root, raw						
	38	1.4	7.2	0.6	0	10
Horseradish, raw						
	62	4.5	11.0	0.3	6.2	8
Kohl rabi, raw						
	23	1.6	3.7	0.2	2.2	4
Kohl rabi, boiled in salted water						
	18	1.2	3.1	0.2	1.9	110
Leeks, raw						
	22	1.6	2.9	0.5	2.2	2
Leeks, boiled						
	21	1.2	2.6	0.7	1.7	81
Lettuce, average, raw						
	14	0.8	1.7	0.5	0.9	3
Lettuce, Cos, raw						
	16	1.0	1.7	0.6	1.2	1
Lettuce, Iceberg, raw						
	13	0.7	1.9	0.3	0.6	2
Mange-tout peas, raw						
	32	3.6	4.2	0.2	2.3	2
Mange-tout peas, boiled						
	26	3.2	3.3	0.1	2.2	42
Mange-tout peas, stir-fried in blended oil						
	71	3.8	3.5	4.8	2.4	2

	kcal/100g	protein/100g	carb/100g	fat/100g	fibre/100g	sodium/100g
Marrow, raw						
	12	0.5	2.2	0.2	0.5	1
Marrow, boiled						
	9	0.4	1.6	0.2	0.6	100
Mixed vegetables, frozen, boiled						
	42	3.3	6.6	0.5	N	96
Mixed vegetables, canned, re-heated, drained						
	38	1.9	6.1	0.8	1.7	380
Mixed vegetables, stir-fry type, frozen, fried in oil						
	64	2.0	6.4	3.6	N	11
Mushrooms, common, raw						
	13	1.8	0.4	0.5	1.1	5
Mushrooms, common, fried in corn oil						
	157	2.4	0.3	16.2	1.5	4
Mushrooms, common, canned, re-heated, drained						
	12	2.1	Tr	0.4	1.3	360
Mushrooms, Chinese, dried, raw						
	284	10.0	59.9	1.8	N	38
Mushrooms, oyster, raw						
	8	1.6	Tr	0.2	0	77
Mushrooms, shiitake, dried, raw						
	296	9.6	63.9	1.0	N	13
Mushrooms, straw, canned, drained						
	15	2.1	1.2	0.2	N	260
Mustard and cress, raw						
	13	1.6	0.4	0.6	1.1	19
Mustard leaves, raw						
	27	2.5	3.6	0.3	0	25
Okra, raw						
	31	2.8	3.0	1.0	4.0	8
Okra, boiled						
	28	2.5	2.7	0.9	3.6	5
Okra, stir-fried in corn oil						
	269	4.3	4.4	26.1	6.3	13
Onions, raw						
	36	1.2	7.9	0.2	1.4	3
Onions, baked						
	103	3.5	22.3	0.6	3.9	8

	kcal/100g	protein/100g	carb/100g	fat/100g	fibre/100g	sodium/100g
Onions, boiled						
	17	0.6	3.7	0.1	0.7	2
Onions, fried in corn oil						
	164	2.3	14.1	11.2	3.1	4
Onions, dried, raw						
	313	10.2	68.6	1.7	12.1	170
Onions, pickled, drained						
	24	0.9	4.9	0.2	1.2	450
Parsnip, raw						
	64	1.8	12.5	1.1	4.6	10
Parsnip, boiled						
	66	1.6	12.9	1.2	4.7	120
Peas, raw						
	83	6.9	11.3	1.5	4.7	1
Peas, boiled						
	79	6.7	10.0	1.6	4.5	94
Peas, canned, re-heated, drained						
	80	5.3	13.5	0.9	5.1	250
Peas, dried, raw						
	303	21.6	52.0	2.4	13.0	38
Peas, dried, boiled						
	109	6.9	19.9	0.8	5.5	13
Peas, frozen, raw						
	66	5.7	9.3	0.9	5.1	3
Peas, frozen, boiled						
	69	6.0	9.7	0.9	5.1	94
Peas, marrowfat, canned, re-heated, drained						
	100	6.9	17.5	0.8	4.1	420
Peas, mushy, canned, re-heated						
	81	5.8	13.8	0.7	1.8	340
Peas, processed, canned, re-heated, drained						
	99	6.9	17.5	0.7	4.8	380
Peas, split, dried, raw						
	328	22.1	58.2	2.4	6.3	38
Peas, split, dried, boiled						
	126	8.3	22.7	0.9	2.7	14
Pease pudding, canned, re-heated, drained						
	93	6.8	16.1	0.6	1.8	290

	kcal/100g	protein/100g	carb/100g	fat/100g	fibre/100g	sodium/100g
Peppers, capsicum, chilli, green, raw						
	20	2.9	0.7	0.6	N	7
Peppers, capsicum, chilli, red, raw						
	26	1.8	4.2	0.3	N	12
Peppers, capsicum, green, raw						
	15	0.8	2.6	0.3	1.6	4
Peppers, capsicum, red, raw						
	32	1.0	6.4	0.4	1.6	4
Peppers, capsicum, yellow, raw						
	26	1.2	5.3	0.2	1.7	4
Petit pois, canned, drained						
	45	5.2	4.9	0.6	4.3	230
Plantain, raw						
	117	1.1	29.4	0.3	1.3	4
Plantain, boiled						
	112	0.8	28.5	0.2	1.2	4
Plantain, ripe, fried in oil						
	267	1.5	47.5	9.2	2.3	3
Pumpkin, raw						
	13	0.7	2.2	0.2	1.0	Tr
Pumpkin, boiled						
	13	0.6	2.1	0.3	1.1	76
Quorn, mycoprotein						
	86	11.8	2.0	3.5	4.8	240
Radicchio, raw						
	14	1.4	1.7	0.2	1.8	7
Radish, red, raw						
	12	0.7	1.9	0.2	0.9	11
Radish, white/mooli, raw						
	15	0.8	2.9	0.1	0	27
Radish leaves, raw						
	33	3.5	3.5	0.5	0	110
Runner beans, raw						
	22	1.6	3.2	0.4	2.0	Tr
Runner beans, boiled						
	18	1.2	2.3	0.5	1.9	110
Salsify, raw						
	27	1.3	10.2	0.3	3.2	5

	kcal/100g	protein/100g	carb/100g	fat/100g	fibre/100g	sodium/100g
Salsify, boiled						
	23	1.1	8.6	0.4	3.5	120
Sauerkraut						
	9	1.1	1.1	Tr	2.2	590
Seakale, boiled						
	8	1.4	0.6	Tr	0	4
Shallots, raw						
	20	1.5	3.3	0.2	1.4	10
Spinach, raw						
	25	2.8	1.6	0.8	2.1	140
Spinach, boiled						
	19	2.2	0.8	0.8	2.1	210
Spinach, frozen, boiled						
	21	3.1	0.5	0.8	2.1	16
Spinach, canned, drained						
	19	2.8	0.8	0.5	1.6	200
Spring greens, raw						
	33	3.0	3.1	1.0	3.4	20
Spring greens, boiled						
	20	1.9	1.6	0.7	2.6	79
Spring onions, bulbs and tops, raw						
	23	2.0	3.0	0.5	1.5	7
Squash, acorn, raw						
	40	0.8	9.0	0.1	2.3	3
Squash, acorn, baked						
	56	1.1	12.6	0.1	3.2	4
Squash, butternut, raw						
	36	1.1	8.3	0.1	1.6	4
Squash, butternut, baked						
	32	0.9	7.4	0.1	1.4	4
Squash, spaghetti, raw						
	26	0.6	4.6	0.6	2.3	17
Squash, spaghetti, baked						
	23	0.7	4.3	0.3	2.1	18
Sugar-snap peas, raw						
	34	3.4	5.0	0.2	1.5	4
Sugar-snap peas, boiled						
	33	3.1	4.7	0.3	1.3	62

	kcal/100g	protein/100g	carb/100g	fat/100g	fibre/100g	sodium/100g
Swede, raw						
	24	0.7	5.0	0.3	1.9	15
Swede, boiled						
	11	0.3	2.3	0.1	0.7	120
Sweetcorn, baby, fresh and frozen, boiled in salted water						
	24	2.5	2.7	0.4	2.0	59
Sweetcorn, baby, canned, drained						
	23	2.9	2.0	0.4	1.5	1140
Sweetcorn, kernels, raw						
	93	3.4	17.0	1.8	1.5	1
Sweetcorn, kernels, boiled						
	111	4.2	19.6	2.3	2.2	15
Sweetcorn, kernels, canned, re-heated, drained						
	122	2.9	26.6	1.2	1.4	270
Sweetcorn, on-the-cob, whole, boiled						
	66	2.5	11.6	1.4	1.3	9
Sweet potato, raw						
	87	1.2	21.3	0.3	2.4	40
Sweet potato, baked						
	115	1.6	27.9	0.4	3.3	52
Sweet potato, boiled						
	84	1.1	20.5	0.3	2.3	32
Sweet potato, steamed						
	84	1.1	20.4	0.3	2.3	35
Tomatoes, raw						
	17	0.7	3.1	0.3	1.0	9
Tomatoes, cherry, raw						
	18	0.8	3.0	0.4	1.0	13
Tomatoes, fried in corn oil						
	91	0.7	5.0	7.7	1.3	10
Tomatoes, grilled						
	49	2.0	8.9	0.9	2.9	26
Tomatoes, canned, whole contents						
	16	1.0	3.0	0.1	0.7	39
Tomato juice						
	14	0.8	3.0	Tr	0.6	230
Turnip, raw						
	23	0.9	4.7	0.3	2.4	15

	kcal/100g	protein/100g	carb/100g	fat/100g	fibre/100g	sodium/100g
Turnip, boiled						
	12	0.6	2.0	0.2	1.9	120
Water chestnuts, raw						
	46	1.4	10.4	0.2	N	12
Water chestnuts, canned, drained						
	31	0.9	7.4	Tr	N	11
Watercress, raw						
	22	3.0	0.4	1.0	1.5	49
Yam, raw						
	114	1.5	28.2	0.3	1.3	2
Yam, boiled						
	133	1.7	33.0	0.3	1.4	72
Yam, steamed						
	114	1.5	28.2	0.3	1.3	17

SECTION THREE

BRAND NAME FOODS

	kcal serv/100g	prot serv/100g	carb serv/100g	fat serv/100g	fibre serv/100g

BISCUITS, BREADS, CAKES AND OTHER BAKED GOODS

Biscuits, Abbey Crunch, McVitie's*, 1 biscuit/9g

43/477	0.5/6	6.6/72.8	1.6/17.9	0.2/2.5

Biscuits, All Butter Viennese, Marks & Spencer*, 1 biscuit/7g

40/571	0.5/7.1	5/71.4	2.2/31.4	0.1/1.4

Biscuits, Amaretti, Doria*, 1 biscuit/4g

17/433	0.2/6	3.4/84.8	0.3/7.8	0/0

Biscuits, Belgian Chocolate, Selection, Finest, Tesco*, 1 biscuit/10g

52/515	0.6/6	6.2/62	2.7/27	0.3/3

Biscuits, Bisc & M&Ms, Masterfoods*, 1 biscuit/25g

132/527	1.5/5.8	14.8/59.2	7.4/29.6	0/0

Biscuits, Bisc & Twix, Masterfoods*, 1 bar/27g

140/520	1.4/5.2	16.5/61.1	7.6/28.3	0/0

Biscuits, Biscotti, Starbucks*, 1 biscuit/27g

100/370	2/7.4	15/55.6	4/14.8	0/0

Biscuits, Boasters, Hazelnut & Choc Chip, McVitie's*, 1 biscuit/16g

88/549	1.1/7	8.9/55.5	5.3/33.3	0.4/2.4

Biscuits, Bourbon Creams, Sainsbury's*, 1 biscuit/13g

60/476	0.7/5.7	8.9/70.4	2.4/19.1	0.2/1.7

Biscuits, Bourbon Creams, Tesco*, 1 biscuit/14g

68/485	0.8/5.6	9.5/67.8	3/21.3	0.3/2.2

Biscuits, Butter Crinkle Crunch, Fox's*, 1 biscuit/11g

51/464	0.7/6.2	7.6/69.4	2/18	0/0

Biscuits, Caramel Crunch, Go Ahead, McVitie's*, 1 bar/24g

106/440	1.1/4.7	18.4/76.6	3.3/13.8	0.2/0.8

Biscuits, Chocolate Caramel Crunch Shortcake, Go Ahead, McVitie's*, 1 biscuit/24g

106/443	1.2/4.8	18.4/76.8	3.4/14.1	0.2/0.8

Biscuits, Chocolate Fingers, Milk, Extra Crunchy, Cadbury's*, 1 biscuit/5g

25/505	0.3/6.6	3.3/66.2	1.2/23.6	0/0

Biscuits, Chocolate Viennese Sandwich, Fox's*, 1 biscuit/14g

76/542	1/6.9	8/57.4	4.4/31.6	0.2/1.6

Biscuits, Classic Creams, Fox's*, 1 biscuit/14g

72/516	0.6/4.4	9.1/65.2	3.6/25.8	0.2/1.7

Biscuits, Classic, Milk Chocolate, Fox's*, 1 biscuit/13g

67/517	0.8/6.1	8.4/64.9	3.1/24	0.2/1.6

kcal serv/100g	prot serv/100g	carb serv/100g	fat serv/100g	fibre serv/100g
Biscuits, Club, Fruit, Jacob's*, 1 biscuit/25g				
124/496	1.4/5.6	15.6/62.2	6.3/25	0.6/2.3
Biscuits, Club, Milk Chocolate, Jacob's*, 1 biscuit/24g				
123/511	1.4/5.8	15/62.6	6.3/26.4	0.5/2
Biscuits, Club, Mint, Jacob's*, 1 biscuit/24g				
124/517	1.3/5.6	15/62.5	6.5/27.2	0.4/1.7
Biscuits, Club, Orange, Jacob's*, 1 biscuit/24g				
125/519	1.3/5.6	14.9/62.2	6.6/27.6	0.4/1.7
Biscuits, Custard Creams, Crawfords*, 1 biscuit/11g				
57/517	0.6/5.9	7.6/69.2	2.7/24.1	0.2/1.5
Biscuits, Digestive, Crawfords*, 1 biscuit/12g				
58/484	0.9/7.1	8.3/68.8	2.4/20	0.4/3.4
Biscuits, Digestive, McVitie's*, 1 biscuit/15g				
74/495	1.1/7	10.1/67.6	3.3/21.9	0.4/2.8
Biscuits, Digestive, Milk Chocolate Homewheat, McVitie's*, 1 biscuit/17g				
86/505	1.2/6.8	11.2/65.8	4.1/23.9	0.4/2.3
Biscuits, Digestive, Milk Chocolate, BGTY, Sainsbury's*, 1 biscuit/17g				
77/480	1.2/7.4	11.6/72.5	2.8/17.8	0.4/2.6
Biscuits, Digestive, Milk Chocolate, GFY, Asda*, 1 biscuit/17g				
79/466	1.2/7	11.7/69	3.1/18	0.4/2.6
Biscuits, Digestive, Milk Chocolate, Tesco*, 1 biscuit/17g				
85/499	1.2/6.9	10.8/63.7	4.1/24.1	0.4/2.4
Biscuits, Digestive, Plain Chocolate Homewheat, McVitie's*, 1 biscuit/17g				
86/507	1/6.1	11.2/65.6	4.1/24.4	0.5/2.8
Biscuits, Digestive, Plain Chocolate, Tesco*, 1 biscuit/17g				
85/499	1.1/6.2	10.8/63.5	4.1/24.4	0.5/2.8
Biscuits, Echo, Fox's*, 1 bar/25g				
128/510	2/7.8	14.9/59.5	6.7/26.7	0.3/1.2
Biscuits, Fruit Shortcake, McVitie's*, 1 biscuit/8g				
39/483	0.5/5.9	5.6/69.6	1.6/20.1	0.2/2.1
Biscuits, Ginger Nuts, McVitie's*, 1 biscuit/12g				
57/473	0.7/5.6	9/75.3	2/16.6	0.2/1.7
Biscuits, Ginger, Traditional, Fox's*, 1 biscuit/8.2g				
32/404	0.4/4.4	5.6/70.1	0.9/11.7	0.1/1.4
Biscuits, Golden Crunch Creams, Fox's*, 1 biscuit/13g				
66/511	0.6/4.3	8.5/65.6	3.3/25.7	0.2/1.2
Biscuits, Hob Nobs, McVitie's*, 1 biscuit/14g				
68/485	1.1/7.7	8.9/63.6	3.1/22.1	0.7/4.7

kcal serv/100g	prot serv/100g	carb serv/100g	fat serv/100g	fibre serv/100g
Biscuits, Hob Nobs, Milk Chocolate, McVitie's*, 1 biscuit/16g				
79/496	1.2/7.3	10.1/63	3.8/24	0.6/3.7
Biscuits, Jam Rings, Crawfords*, 1 biscuit/12g				
56/470	0.7/5.5	8.8/73	2.1/17.2	0.2/1.9
Biscuits, Jammie Dodgers, Burton's*, 1 biscuit/19g				
85/448	0.9/4.8	13.1/68.8	3.2/16.7	0.3/1.7
Biscuits, Malted Milk, Tesco*, 1 biscuit/8g				
39/488	0.6/7.2	5.2/65.6	1.8/21.9	0.2/2
Biscuits, Nice, Asda*, 1 biscuit/8g				
38/480	0.5/6	5.4/68	1.7/21	0.2/2.4
Biscuits, Nice, Tesco*, 1 biscuit/8g				
39/485	0.5/6.5	5.4/68	1.7/20.8	0.2/2.4
Biscuits, Party Rings, Fox's*, 1 biscuit/6g				
27/453	0.3/4.3	4.7/77.8	0.8/13.8	0.1/1.3
Biscuits, Rich Tea, McVitie's*, 1 biscuit/8.3g				
38/475	0.6/7.5	6.1/76.3	1.2/15.5	0.2/2.3
Biscuits, Shortcake, Crawfords*, 1 biscuit/10.3g				
52/518	0.6/6.4	6.8/68.1	2.4/24.4	0.2/2
Biscuits, Shortcake, Dairy Milk Chocolate, Cadbury's*, 1 bar/49g				
252/515	3.7/7.5	29/59.2	13.5/27.5	0/0
Biscuits, Shortcake, Snack, Cadbury's*, 1 biscuit/8g				
42/525	0.6/7	5.1/64.2	2.1/26.6	0/0
Biscuits, Strawberry Mallows, Go Ahead, McVitie's*, 1 biscuit/18g				
69/385	0.8/4.3	12.7/70.6	1.7/9.5	0.2/0.9
Biscuits, Viscount* Mint, 1 biscuit/16g				
83/521	0.8/4.8	10/62.7	4.5/27.9	0.2/1.3
Biscuits, Water, Carr's*, 1 biscuit/8g				
35/436	0.7/9.3	6.1/76.7	0.7/9.2	0/0
Bread, Amazing Grain, Nimble*, 1 slice/22g				
49/224	2.4/10.7	9.1/41.3	0.4/1.8	1.5/7
Bread, Bagel, Cinnamon & Raisin, New York Bagel Co*, 1 bagel/85g				
240/282	8.9/10.5	47.6/56	1.5/1.8	1.9/2.2
Bread, Bagel, Onion, New York Bagel Co*, 1 bagel/85g				
233/274	9.4/11.1	45.8/53.9	1.4/1.6	1.8/2.1
Bread, Bagel, Original, New York Bagel Co*, 1 bagel/85g				
230/271	9.5/11.2	45.2/53.2	1.3/1.5	1.9/2.2
Bread, Brown, Danish, Weight Watchers*, 1 slice/19g				
38/200	1.6/8.6	7.2/37.7	0.3/1.6	1.8/9.6

	kcal serv/100g	prot serv/100g	carb serv/100g	fat serv/100g	fibre serv/100g
Bread, Brown, Good Health, Warburton's*, 1 slice/34.8g					
	79/226	3.6/10.3	13.9/39.6	1/2.9	2.5/7.2
Bread, Ciabatta, Finest, Tesco*, ¼ ciabatta/70g					
	185/264	6.5/9.3	29.8/42.5	4.4/6.3	1.6/2.3
Bread, Ciabatta, Garlic, Finest, Tesco*, 1 serving/65g					
	200/307	5/7.7	26.8/41.3	8/12.3	1.2/1.8
Bread, Ciabatta, Half, TTD, Sainsbury's*, ½ ciabatta/133g					
	346/260	11.8/8.9	63.4/47.7	4.9/3.7	2.9/2.2
Bread, Ciabatta, Italian-Style, Safeway*, ¼ loaf/75g					
	194/258	6.7/8.9	35.8/47.7	2.6/3.5	1.7/2.2
Bread, Fruit Loaf, Rich, Soreen*, ¹⁄₁₀th loaf/30g					
	93/310	2.2/7.4	18.2/60.7	1.2/4.1	0/0
Bread, Garlic Baguette, Asda*, ¼ baguette/42g					
	158/375	3.7/8.9	18.2/43.3	7.8/18.5	0.5/1.2
Bread, Garlic Baguette, BGTY, Sainsbury's*, 1 serving/28g					
	93/333	2.5/9.1	14/49.9	3.5/12.6	0.7/2.4
Bread, Garlic Baguette, GFY, Asda *, ¼ baguette/42.5g					
	120/280	3.9/9	18.5/43	3.4/8	0.9/2
Bread, Garlic Baguette, Healthy Eating, Tesco*, 1 serving/42g					
	111/264	3.4/8	17.3/41.1	3.2/7.5	1.1/2.6
Bread, Garlic Baguette, Italiano, Tesco*, 1 slice/19g					
	63/334	1.3/7.1	8.3/43.8	2.8/14.5	0.4/2.2
Bread, Garlic Baguette, Sainsbury's*, 1 serving/50g					
	196/391	4.5/8.9	24.3/48.6	9.6/19.2	1.2/2.3
Bread, Garlic Bread, Pizza Express*, 1 serving/100g					
	278/278	7.5/7.5	43/43	9.9/9.9	0/0
Bread, Granary, COU, Marks & Spencer*, 1 slice/25g					
	62/246	2.9/11.7	11.3/45.1	0.5/2.1	1.4/5.7
Bread, Naan, Garlic & Coriander, Asda*, ½ naan/74g					
	260/352	5.2/7	33.3/45	11.8/16	1.7/2.3
Bread, Naan, Garlic & Coriander, Mini, Asda*, 1 naan/49.7g					
	165/330	3.5/7	22/44	7/14	0.6/1.2
Bread, Naan, Garlic & Coriander, Mini, Sainsbury's*, 1 naan/50g					
	148/295	4.3/8.6	22.1/44.2	4.7/9.3	1.9/3.7
Bread, Naan, Garlic & Coriander, Mini, Tesco*, 1 naan/60g					
	178/296	4.6/7.6	28.2/47	5.2/8.6	1.5/2.5
Bread, Naan, Garlic & Coriander, Tesco*, 1 naan/150g					
	374/249	10.7/7.1	54.8/36.5	12.5/8.3	3.2/2.1

kcal serv/100g	prot serv/100g	carb serv/100g	fat serv/100g	fibre serv/100g
Bread, Naan, Mini, Plain, Tesco*, 1 naan/60g				
175/292	5.6/9.3	28.6/47.6	4.3/7.2	1.5/2.5
Bread, Naan, Plain, Sharwood's*, 1 bread/120g				
294/245	12.1/10.1	51.7/43.1	4.3/3.6	4.1/3.4
Bread, Naan, Plain, Tesco*, 1 naan/150g				
429/286	11.7/7.8	71.4/47.6	10.8/7.2	3.8/2.5
Bread, Pitta Pockets, Sainsbury's*, 1 serving/75g				
188/250	6.4/8.5	39/52	0.8/1	2.6/3.5
Bread, Pitta, Brown, Organic, Waitrose*, 1 pitta/61g				
138/226	3.9/6.4	29/47.5	0.9/1.4	4/6.6
Bread, Pitta, Garlic & Coriander, Asda*, 1 bread/57g				
149/261	4.6/8	30.2/53	1.1/1.9	0/0
Bread, Pitta, White, Marks & Spencer*, 1 pitta/61g				
156/255	5.4/8.9	31.5/51.6	1.5/2.4	0/0
Bread, Pitta, White, Sainsbury's*, 1 pitta/59g				
151/256	5.6/9.5	30.7/52	0.6/1.1	1.4/2.3
Bread, Pitta, White, Tesco*, 1 pitta/56g				
147/262	5.7/10.1	28.7/51.2	1.1/1.9	1.5/2.6
Bread, Pitta, Wholemeal, Asda*, 1 pitta/56g				
128/229	6.2/11	23/41	1.3/2.3	0/0
Bread, Pitta, Wholemeal, Sainsbury's*, 1 pitta/59g				
146/247	7.3/12.4	27.1/46	0.9/1.5	3.1/5.3
Bread, Pitta, Wholemeal, Tesco*, 1 pitta/60g				
151/251	7.1/11.9	27.8/46.4	1.2/2	4/6.6
Bread, Pitta, Wholemeal, Tesco*, 1 pitta/62g				
138/222	5.6/9.1	26.4/42.5	1.1/1.7	3.6/5.8
Bread, Pumpernickel Rye, Kelderman*, 1 slice/50g				
93/185	3/6	19/38	0.5/1	0/0
Bread, Rolls, Best of Both, Hovis*, 1 roll/29g				
68/235	2.8/9.8	11.5/39.5	1.2/4.2	1.2/4.2
Bread, Rye with Sesame Seeds, Ryvita*, 1 slice/9g				
31/339	0.9/10.5	5.3/58.5	0.6/7	1.4/16
Bread, White, Danish, Weight Watchers*, 1 slice/19g				
42/222	1.7/8.7	8.3/43.9	0.2/1.3	0.5/2.8
Bread, White, Good Health, Warburton's*, 1 slice/38g				
84/220	3.6/9.4	15.8/41.6	0.7/1.8	1.6/4.1
Bread, White, Medium-Sliced, Nimble*, 1 slice/20g				
46/232	1.9/9.7	8.9/44.3	0.4/1.8	0.6/2.9

kcal serv/100g	prot serv/100g	carb serv/100g	fat serv/100g	fibre serv/100g

Bread, White, Medium-Sliced, Weight Watchers*, 1 slice/12g

| 27/226 | 1.2/10.3 | 5.1/42.6 | 0.2/1.6 | 0.4/3.6 |

Bread, Wholemeal, Nimble*, 1 slice/20g

| 43/216 | 2.2/11.2 | 7.4/36.9 | 0.5/2.7 | 1.4/6.9 |

Bread, Wholemeal, with Pumpkin & Sunflower Seeds, Tesco*, 1 slice/25g

| 61/243 | 2.8/11 | 8.3/33.1 | 1.9/7.4 | 1.3/5.2 |

Breadsticks, Grissini Italian, Sainsbury's*, 1 breadstick/5g

| 20/408 | 0.6/11.6 | 3.6/72.9 | 0.4/7.8 | 0.1/2.9 |

Buns, Belgian, Tesco*, 1 bun/125g

| 451/361 | 5.5/4.4 | 70.9/56.7 | 16.1/12.9 | 3.4/2.7 |

Buns, Hot Cross, Sainsbury's*, 1 bun/70g

| 205/293 | 5.3/7.6 | 37.2/53.2 | 3.9/5.5 | 1.5/2.1 |

Buns, Iced Finger, Tesco*, 1 finger/69g

| 241/349 | 4.4/6.4 | 40.2/58.3 | 6.9/10 | 1.2/1.7 |

Cake, Apple Bakes, Go Ahead, McVitie's*, 1 cake/35g

| 129/368 | 1/2.8 | 26.1/74.7 | 2.9/8.3 | 0.4/1.2 |

Cake, Apple Sponge, Marks & Spencer*, 1 portion/63g

| 178/283 | 2.4/3.8 | 20.2/32 | 10.3/16.4 | 0.4/0.7 |

Cake, Banana Loaf, Waitrose*, 1 slice/70g

| 236/337 | 3.5/5 | 38.6/55.2 | 7.5/10.7 | 1.2/1.7 |

Cake, Banana, Date & Walnut Slices, BGTY, Sainsbury's*, 1 slice/28g

| 78/280 | 1.5/5.3 | 15.7/56.1 | 1.4/4.9 | 0.6/2.2 |

Cake, Birthday, Marks & Spencer*, 1 serving/60g

| 240/400 | 1.4/2.3 | 42.5/70.9 | 7.1/11.9 | 0.5/0.8 |

Cake, Brownie, Pret A Manger*, 1 av pack/50g

| 328/656 | 3.6/7.2 | 40.5/81 | 16.9/33.8 | 0.5/1 |

Cake, Butterfly, Mr Kipling*, 1 cake/29g

| 114/392 | 1.3/4.4 | 12.6/43.4 | 6.4/22.2 | 0.2/0.6 |

Cake, Caramel Slice, Marks & Spencer*, 1 slice/64g

| 304/475 | 3.1/4.9 | 38.7/60.4 | 16.1/25.2 | 1.7/2.6 |

Cake, Carrot & Orange Slices, Healthy Eating, Tesco*, 1 slice/29g

| 75/257 | 0.9/3 | 16.4/56.4 | 0.8/2.7 | 0.6/1.9 |

Cake, Carrot & Orange, Finest, Tesco*, 1 serving/50g

| 171/342 | 2.1/4.1 | 24.6/49.1 | 7.2/14.3 | 0.5/1 |

Cake, Carrot & Walnut, Marks & Spencer*, ⅙ cake/82g

| 279/340 | 4.8/5.8 | 28.5/34.8 | 16/19.5 | 1.2/1.5 |

Cake, Carrot Slices, BGTY, Sainsbury's*, 1 slice/27g

| 81/313 | 0.9/3.4 | 17.9/68.7 | 0.7/2.7 | 0.6/2.4 |

kcal serv/100g	prot serv/100g	carb serv/100g	fat serv/100g	fibre serv/100g
Cake, Carrot, Entenmann's*, 1 serving/40g				
156/391	1.6/4.1	19/47.4	8.2/20.5	0.6/1.5
Cake, Carrot, Pret A Manger*, 1 av pack/120g				
288/240	3.5/2.9	49.9/41.6	8.3/6.9	0.2/0.2
Cake, Cherry Bakewell, Mr Kipling*, 1 cake/45g				
186/414	1.8/3.9	26.7/59.3	8.1/17.9	0.5/1.2
Cake, Choc Chip Bar, Go Ahead, McVitie's*, 1 bar/28g				
100/356	1.8/6.4	15.9/56.9	3.4/12.1	0.3/1
Cake, Chocolate Brownie, Fudge, Entenmann's*, ⅛ cake/55g				
168/306	2.2/4	34.5/62.7	2.4/4.4	0.8/1.5
Cake, Chocolate Brownie, Slices, Marks & Spencer*, 1 brownie/36g				
158/440	1.9/5.3	18.4/51.1	8.7/24.1	0.5/1.3
Cake, Chocolate Brownie, Waitrose*, 1 brownie/45g				
192/426	2.8/6.3	25/55.6	8.9/19.8	1.2/2.7
Cake, Chocolate Indulgence, Finest, Tesco*, 1 slice/52g				
203/390	2/3.8	24.9/47.8	10.6/20.4	0.2/0.4
Cake, Chocolate Victoria Sponge, Co-Op*, 1 slice/61g				
201/330	3.1/5	25.6/42	9.8/16	0.6/1
Cake, Christmas, Rich Fruit, All Iced, Sainsbury's*, 1⁄16 cake/85g				
307/361	3.4/4	56.5/66.4	7.6/8.9	1.3/1.5
Cake, Classic Lemon Drizzle, Marks & Spencer*, ⅙ cake/67.5g				
255/375	3.2/4.7	37.4/55	10.4/15.3	0.4/0.6
Cake, Coconut Macaroons, Sainsbury's*, 1 macaroon/33g				
144/436	1.6/4.8	21.5/65.1	5.7/17.3	0.5/1.6
Cake, Coffee, Iced, Marks & Spencer*, 1 slice/33g				
135/410	1.5/4.4	18/54.5	6.5/19.6	0.5/1.6
Cake, Cream Slices, Marks & Spencer*, 1 slice/80g				
310/387	1.8/2.3	36.6/45.7	18.3/22.9	0.5/0.6
Cake, Crispy Fruit Slices, Forest Fruit, Go Ahead, McVitie's*, 1 biscuit/14g				
56/400	0.8/5.5	10.2/73	1.2/8.8	0.5/3.7
Cake, Custard Slices, Tesco*, 1 slice/108g				
320/296	2.6/2.4	40.5/37.5	16.4/15.2	0.5/0.5
Cake, Fairy, Iced, Somerfield*, 1 cake/15.1g				
59/392	0.7/4.9	9.4/62.9	2/13.4	0.2/1.4
Cake, Fondant Fancies, Sainsbury's*, 1 cake/27g				
95/353	0.6/2.4	17.7/65.7	2.4/9	0.1/0.4
Cake, Fruit Slice, Value, Tesco*, 1 slice/22.6g				
85/372	0.9/4	11.2/48.7	4.1/17.7	0.3/1.3

kcal serv/100g	prot serv/100g	carb serv/100g	fat serv/100g	fibre serv/100g
Cake, Ginger, Jamaica Bar, McVitie's*, 1 mini cake/33g				
128/388	1.2/3.5	19.9/60.2	4.9/14.7	0.4/1.2
Cake, Ginger, Marks & Spencer*, ⅛ cake/41g				
156/380	2.6/6.3	25.5/62.3	4.7/11.5	0.7/1.7
Cake, Jaffa Cake Bar, McVitie's, 1 bar/31g				
126/408	1.2/3.9	18.3/59	5.4/17.4	0/0
Cake, Jaffa Cakes, McVitie's*, 1 biscuit/12g				
46/384	0.5/4.4	8.8/73.3	1/8.1	0.2/1.3
Cake, Jaffa Cakes, Mini, McVitie's*, 1 cake/5.9g				
26/441	0.3/5.1	5/83.1	0.6/10.2	0.1/1.7
Cake, Lemon Slices, Healthy Eating, Tesco*, 1 slice/26g				
86/329	0.9/3.4	18/69.1	0.7/2.6	0.8/3
Cake, Mini Rolls, Cadbury's*, 1 roll/26g				
113/434	1.4/5.5	14.5/55.6	5.4/20.6	0.2/0.6
Cake, Mini Rolls, Chocolate, Tesco*, 1 roll/31g				
137/442	1.9/6	17.5/56.3	6.6/21.4	0.2/0.8
Cake, Pecan Pie, Pret A Manger*, 1 av pack/70g				
333/476	4.3/6.1	31.1/44.4	21.2/30.3	0.5/0.7
Cake, Victoria Sponge, Fresh Cream, Tesco*, 1 slice/46.7g				
157/334	1.8/3.9	19.2/40.8	8.1/17.3	0.3/0.7
Chapatis, Patak's*, 1 chapatis/42g				
121/287	3.2/7.5	22.3/53.1	2.7/6.4	1.3/3.2
Cookies, All-Butter Chocolate Chunk, Marks & Spencer*, 1 cookie/26g				
130/500	1.4/5.2	16.2/62.4	6.6/25.2	0.7/2.6
Cookies, Big Milk Chocolate Chunk, Cookie Coach Co*, 1 cookie/35g				
174/497	2.2/6.2	21.5/61.4	8.8/25.1	0/0
Cookies, Choc Chip, Asda*, 1 cookie/11g				
56/506	0.6/5	6.9/63	2.9/26	0.2/1.8
Cookies, Choc Chip, Maryland*, 1 cookie/11g				
56/511	0.7/6.2	7.5/68	2.6/23.9	0/0
Cookies, Choc Chip, McVitie's*, 1 cookie/10g				
45/453	0.5/5.2	7.6/75.5	1.5/14.5	0.2/1.7
Cookies, Chocolate Chip, Sainsbury's*, 1 cookie/11g				
56/508	0.7/6.2	7.4/67	2.6/23.9	0.1/1.3
Cookies, Chocolate, Half-Coated Triple, Finest, Tesco*, 1 cookie/25g				
129/517	1.5/5.8	14.7/58.8	7.2/28.7	0.6/2.2
Cookies, Cranberry & Orange, Go Ahead, McVitie's*, 1 cookie/17g				
77/452	0.9/5.3	13.3/78	2.2/13.2	0.4/2.4

kcal serv/100g	prot serv/100g	carb serv/100g	fat serv/100g	fibre serv/100g
Cookies, Fruit, Giant, Cookie Coach Co*, 1 cookie/60g				
280/466	2.9/4.9	37.2/62	13.2/22	0/0
Cookies, Real Chocolate Chip, Weight Watchers*, 2 cookies/23g				
98/427	1.2/5.3	15.2/66.1	3.6/15.7	0.4/1.6
Crispbread, Dark Rye, Ryvita*, 1 serving/9g				
27/303	0.9/9.9	5.6/62	0.2/1.7	1.7/18.5
Crispbread, Multigrain, Ryvita*, 1 slice/11g				
37/335	1.3/11.5	6.4/58.5	0.7/6.1	1.8/16.2
Crispbread, Original, Ryvita*, 1 crispbread/9g				
27/305	0.8/9.4	5.7/63.3	0.1/1.6	1.6/17.4
Crispbread, Sesame, Ryvita*, 28g				
95/339	2.9/10.5	16.4/58.5	2/7	4.5/16
Croissant, All-Butter, Finest, Tesco*, 1 croissant/77g				
328/426	6.6/8.6	34.6/44.9	18.2/23.6	1.5/1.9
Croissant, All-Butter, Sainsbury's*, 1 croissant/44g				
196/446	4.1/9.3	16.8/38.2	12.5/28.4	0.9/2
Croissant, All-Butter, Tesco*, 1 croissant/77g				
297/386	5/6.5	31.1/40.4	17/22.1	1.5/1.9
Croissant, Chocolate, Pret A Manger*, 1 croissant/70g				
322/460	6.5/9.3	24.9/35.6	21.9/31.3	0/0
Crumpets, Asda*, 1 crumpet/45g				
94/208	2.7/6	19.8/44	0.4/0.9	0/0
Crumpets, Less Than 1% Fat, Warburton's*, 1 crumpet/45.6g				
71/155	2.6/5.6	14.6/31.7	0.3/0.7	0/0
Crumpets, Mother's Pride*, 1 crumpet/48g				
90/187	2.7/5.6	18.7/38.9	0.5/1	0.8/1.7
Crumpets, Sainsbury's*, 1 crumpet/44g				
91/207	2.5/5.6	19.4/44	0.4/0.9	0.2/0.5
Crumpets, Tesco*, 1 crumpet/46g				
92/201	2.8/6	19.6/42.6	0.3/0.7	0.8/1.8
Crumpets, Warburton's*, 1 crumpet/50g				
89/178	3.6/7.1	17.9/35.8	0.4/0.7	0/0
Danish Pastry, Apple & Sultana, Tesco*, 1 pastry/72g				
293/407	3.9/5.4	32.4/45	16.4/22.8	1/1.4
Danish Pastry, Danish Apple Bar, Sara Lee*, ⅙ bar/70g				
160/229	3/4.3	29.5/42.1	4/5.7	1.2/1.7
Danish Pastry, Pecan, Marks & Spencer*, 1 serving/67g				
287/428	4.2/6.2	30.2/45	17.4/26	0.9/1.3

kcal serv/100g	prot serv/100g	carb serv/100g	fat serv/100g	fibre serv/100g
Doughnuts, Cream & Jam, Tesco*, 1 doughnut/90g				
324/360	3.7/4.1	35.7/39.7	18.5/20.5	1.2/1.3
Fig Rolls, Go Ahead, McVitie's*, 1 roll/15g				
55/365	0.6/4.2	11.5/76.8	0.7/4.6	0.4/2.9
Fig Rolls, Jacob's*, 1 biscuit/17g				
61/357	0.6/3.5	11.5/67.7	1.4/8	0.7/3.9
Flapjack, All-Butter, Sainsbury's*, 1 flapjack/35g				
156/446	2/5.7	19.1/54.5	8/22.8	0.9/2.7
Flapjack, Crazy Raizin, The Fabulous Bakin' Boys*, 1 pack/90g				
378/420	5.4/6	54/60	15.3/17	3.6/4
Flapjack, Weight Watchers*, 1 slice/30g				
109/364	2/6.5	21.3/71	1.8/6	1.2/3.9
Krisprolls, Cracked Wheat, Original, Pogen*, 1 piece/10g				
38/380	1.2/12	6.7/67	0.7/7	0.9/9
Melba Toast, Original, Van Der Meulen*, 1 slice/3g				
12/399	0.4/12.8	2.4/80.5	0.1/2.9	0.1/3.9
Muffin, Blueberry, Asda*, 1 muffin/77.3g				
272/353	3.9/5	34.7/45	13.1/17	1/1.3
Muffin, Blueberry, Sainsbury's*, 1 muffin/75g				
242/322	4.1/5.4	35/46.7	9.5/12.6	1.7/2.2
Muffin, Blueberry, Tesco*, 1 muffin/70g				
279/398	3.4/4.8	27.8/39.7	17.1/24.4	0.9/1.3
Muffin, Chocolate Chip, American-Style, Sainsbury's*, 1 muffin/75g				
328/437	4.4/5.9	39.3/52.4	17/22.7	0.5/0.6
Muffin, Classic Blueberry, Starbucks*, 1 muffin/129g				
438/337	5.7/4.4	51.6/39.7	23/17.7	1.8/1.4
Muffin, Double Chocolate Chip, Sainsbury's*, 1 muffin/72.0g				
290/403	3.5/4.8	36/50	14.7/20.4	1.4/1.9
Muffin, Double Chocolate Chip, Tesco*, 1 muffin/72g				
302/419	4.4/6.1	34.6/48	16.2/22.5	1/1.4
Muffin, Double Chocolate, Mini, Tesco*, 1 muffin/28g				
116/414	1.8/6.3	12.8/45.7	6.4/23	0.4/1.4
Muffin, English, Marks & Spencer*, 1 muffin/60g				
135/225	6.7/11.2	26.2/43.7	1.1/1.9	1.7/2.9
Muffin, Skinny Blueberry, Starbucks*, 1 muffin/129g				
306/236	4.8/3.7	61.2/47.2	4.1/3.2	2.2/1.7
Muffin, Skinny Peach & Raspberry, Starbucks*, 1 muffin/120.2g				
286/238	6.1/5.1	55.8/46.5	4.4/3.7	1.7/1.4

kcal serv/100g	prot serv/100g	carb serv/100g	fat serv/100g	fibre serv/100g
Muffin, White, Tesco*, 1 muffin/60g				
143/238	6.1/10.2	25.2/42	1.9/3.2	1.3/2.1
Pain Au Chocolat, Marks & Spencer*, 1 pain/60g				
210/350	3.5/5.9	22.8/38	11.5/19.2	1/1.6
Pain Au Chocolate, Tesco*, 1 pain/56g				
235/420	3.9/7	26/46.5	12.8/22.9	0.8/1.4
Pancake, Scotch, BGTY, Sainsbury's*, 1 pancake/30g				
76/252	1.6/5.3	14.6/48.5	1.2/4.1	0.4/1.3
Pastry, Filo, Sainsbury's*, 1 sheet/33g				
104/315	3/9.2	20.5/62.1	1.4/4.1	0.3/0.8
Pretzels, American-Style, Salted, Sainsbury's*, 1 serving/50g				
191/381	4.8/9.6	40.9/81.8	2/4	2.6/5.2
Pretzels, New York-Style, Salted, Mini, Shapers, Boots*, 1 bag/25g				
94/375	2.5/10	19.8/79	0.5/2.1	1.1/4.2
Pretzels, Salt & Cracked Black Pepper, COU, Marks & Spencer*, 1 pack/25g				
95/380	2.4/9.7	20.8/83.3	0.6/2.4	0.7/2.7
Profiteroles, Classic French, Sainsbury's*, 1 serving/90g				
284/316	5.9/6.6	30.3/33.7	15.5/17.2	0.1/0.1
Rice Cakes, Apple & Cinnamon Flavour, Kallo*, 1 cake/11g				
41/376	0.7/6.2	9.1/83.1	0.2/2.2	0.4/3.9
Rice Cakes, Caramel Flavour, Kallo*, 1 cake/9.9g				
38/383	0.6/6.2	7.9/78.9	0.5/4.8	0.4/3.9
Rice Cakes, Caramel Flavour, Tesco*, 1 cake/35g				
133/379	1.9/5.5	28.9/82.7	1/2.9	0.3/0.9
Rice Cakes, Dark Chocolate, Organic, Kallo*, 1 cake/12g				
57/471	0.8/6.8	6.9/57.2	2.9/24.1	0.9/7.4
Rice Cakes, Lightly Salted, Thick-Slice, Low-Fat, Kallo*, 1 cake/8g				
30/372	0.6/8	6.3/78.7	0.2/2.8	0.4/5.1
Rice Cakes, Low-Fat, Kallo*, 1 cake/10g				
38/375	0.6/6.2	8.3/83.1	0.2/2.2	0.4/3.9
Rice Cakes, Oat, Lightly Salted, Thick Slice, Kallo*, 1 cake/7.6g				
28/356	0.8/10.6	6/75	0.4/5.5	0.7/9
Rice Cakes, Ryvita*, 1 cake/7g				
28/395	0.6/8.8	5.7/82.1	0.2/3.4	0.1/1.3
Rice Cakes, Salt 'n' Vinegar, Jumbo, Tesco*, 1 cake/8.8g				
28/306	0.8/8.4	5.6/62.5	0.7/7.5	0.5/6
Rice Cakes, Savoury with Yeast Extract, Kallo*, 1 slice/11g				
40/364	1.4/12.7	7.9/72	0.3/2.8	0.5/4.7

kcal serv/100g	prot serv/100g	carb serv/100g	fat serv/100g	fibre serv/100g
Rice Cakes, Slightly Salted, Thick-Slice, Organic, Kallo*, 1 cake/8g				
30/372	0.6/8	6.3/78.7	0.2/2.8	0.4/5.1
Rice Cakes, Thin-Slice, Organic, Kallo*, 1 cake/5g				
19/372	0.4/8	3.9/78.7	0.1/2.8	0.3/5.1
Scone, All-Butter, Tesco*, 1 scone/41g				
126/308	3/7.2	21.4/52.3	3.2/7.8	0.7/1.6
Scone, Cheese, Marks & Spencer*, 1 scone/60g				
237/395	6.2/10.3	23.3/38.9	13.1/21.9	1/1.6
Scone, Sultana, Finest, Tesco*, 1 scone/70g				
225/321	6.2/8.9	32.7/46.7	7.6/10.9	1.5/2.1
Shortbread, Chocolate & Caramel, TTD, Sainsbury's*, 1 serving/55g				
245/446	2.6/4.7	24.8/45	15.2/27.7	0.7/1.3
Shortbread, Fingers, All-Butter, Royal Edinburgh Bakery*, 1 biscuit/17g				
88/519	1/5.8	10.3/60.3	4.8/28.3	0.3/1.8
Shortbread, Fingers, All-Butter, Tesco*, 1 finger/13g				
67/519	0.8/5.8	7.8/60.3	3.7/28.3	0.2/1.8
Shortbread, Fingers, Asda*, 1 finger/18g				
93/519	1/5.8	10.9/60.3	5.1/28.3	3.2/18
Shortbread, Fingers, Highland, Sainsbury's*, 1 finger/20g				
106/528	1.1/5.6	11.6/57.8	6.1/30.5	0.4/1.9
Taco, Shells, Old El Paso*, 1 taco/12g				
57/478	0.9/7.4	7.3/60.8	2.7/22.8	0/0
Teacakes, Chocolate, Marks & Spencer*, 1 cake/17g				
73/430	0.9/5	11.1/65.4	2.8/16.7	0.2/1
Teacakes, Chocolate, Tunnock's*, 1 cake/22g				
91/413	1.2/5.3	13.4/61	4/18.1	0/0
Teacakes, Jam, Burton's*, 1 cake/10g				
43/429	0.4/3.6	6.6/66	1.7/16.7	0.1/1
Teacakes, Tesco*, 1 cake/61g				
163/267	4.8/7.8	31.2/51.1	2.1/3.5	1.5/2.4
Tortillas, Flour, Asda*, 1 serving/34g				
106/311	2.7/8	18.4/54	2.4/7	0.9/2.5
Tortillas, Flour, Old El Paso*, 2 tortillas/81g				
277/342	8.1/10	48.6/60	5.3/6.6	0/0
Tortillas, Plain Flour, Tesco*, 1 serving/63g				
171/272	4.3/6.9	30.4/48.2	3.6/5.7	1.3/2
Tortillas, Plain, Wheat Flour, Sainsbury's*, 1 tortilla/56g				
175/313	4.8/8.6	30.2/53.9	3.9/7	1.4/2.5

	kcal serv/100g	prot serv/100g	carb serv/100g	fat serv/100g	fibre serv/100g
Tortillas, Soft Flour, Discovery*, 1 serving/39g					
	122/313	3.4/8.6	21/53.9	2.7/7	1/2.5
Tortillas, Wrap, Marks & Spencer*, 1 wrap/44g					
	134/305	3.6/8.1	22.8/51.8	3.7/8.4	1.3/2.9
Tortillas, Wrap, Tomato & Herb, Tesco*, 1 serving/63g					
	165/262	5/7.9	28.4/45.1	3.5/5.5	1.3/2.1
Wafers, Caramel, Tunnock's*, 1 biscuit/26g					
	118/454	1.2/4.6	17.7/68	5.2/20.1	0/0
Wafers, Pink, Crawfords*, 1 biscuit/7g					
	36/521	0.2/2.5	4.8/68.6	1.9/26.5	0.1/1.1

CEREALS

Advantage, Weetabix*, 1 serving/30g					
	105/350	3.1/10.2	21.6/72	0.7/2.4	2.7/9
All Bran, Kellogg's, 1 serving/40g					
	108/270	5.2/13	18/45	1.6/4	11.6/29
All Bran, Apricot Bites, Kellogg's*, 1 serving/45g					
	126/280	4.5/10	25.2/56	1.4/3	7.7/17
All Bran Flakes, Kellogg's*, 1 serving/40g					
	128/320	4/10	26.4/66	1/2.5	6/15
All Bran Splitz, Kellogg's*, 1 serving/40g					
	130/325	3.6/9	27.6/69	0.8/2	3.6/9
Alpen, Caribbean Crunch, Weetabix*, 1 serving/40g					
	155/388	3.5/8.8	27.2/67.9	3.6/9	1.8/4.6
Alpen, Crunchy Bran, Weetabix*, 1 serving/40g					
	120/299	4.7/11.8	20.9/52.3	1.9/4.7	9.9/24.8
Alpen, No Added Sugar, Weetabix*, 1 serving/40g					
	143/357	4.8/12.1	24.5/61.3	2.8/7.1	3.6/9
Alpen, Nutty Crunch, Weetabix*, 1 serving/40g					
	159/398	4.3/10.7	25.4/63.6	4.5/11.2	2.6/6.5
Alpen, Original, Weetabix*, 1 serving/40g					
	146/365	4/10	26.4/66	2.7/6.8	3.1/7.7
Alpen, Strawberry, Weetabix*, 1 serving/40g					
	144/359	3.8/9.4	27.8/69.5	1.9/4.8	3.2/7.9
Alpen, Wheat Flakes, Weetabix*, 1 serving/40g					
	140/350	4.1/10.2	28.8/72	1/2.4	3.6/9

kcal serv/100g	prot serv/100g	carb serv/100g	fat serv/100g	fibre serv/100g
Apple & Cinnamon Flakes, Marks & Spencer*, 1 serving/30g				
111/370	1.8/6	24.8/82.7	0.6/1.9	1/3.4
Apple & Cinnamon, Crisp, Sainsbury's*, 1 serving/50g				
217/433	3.1/6.2	34.6/69.1	7.4/14.7	1.7/3.4
Apple, Blackberry & Raspberry Flakes, GFY, Asda*, 1 serving/40g				
138/344	3.6/9	29.2/73	0.7/1.8	4.4/11
Apricot Bites, Kellogg's*, 1 serving/45g				
126/280	5.4/12	23/51	1.6/3.5	9.5/21
Apricot Wheats, Asda*, 1 serving/50g				
165/330	3.9/7.8	35.5/71	0.8/1.5	4/8
Apricot Wheats, Whole Grain, Sainsbury's*, 1 serving/50g				
165/330	3.9/7.8	35.7/71.4	0.8/1.5	4/8
Balance, with Red Fruit, Sainsbury's*, 1 serving/40g				
148/369	4/9.9	31.2/78.1	0.8/1.9	1.2/3.1
Banana, Papaya & Honey Oat, Crunchy, Waitrose*, 1 serving/40g				
170/426	3.8/9.6	27.9/69.8	4.8/12	2.2/5.5
Berries, Cherries & Flakes, COU, Marks & Spencer*, 1 serving/40g				
152/380	3.4/8.5	32.9/82.2	0.8/1.9	1.3/3.2
Blueberry & Cranberry, Oat Crunchy, Waitrose*, 1 serving/60g				
262/437	4.8/8	40.2/67	9.1/15.2	4.4/7.4
Bran Flakes, Asda*, 1 serving/47g				
157/333	5.2/11	30.6/65	1.5/3.2	6.6/14
Bran Flakes, Basics, Somerfield*, 1 serving/50g				
154/308	6.2/12.3	29.5/58.9	1.3/2.6	9.7/19.3
Bran Flakes, Co-Op*, 1 serving/30g				
99/330	3.3/11	19.5/65	0.9/3	4.5/15
Bran Flakes, Harvest Home, Nestle*, 1 serving/30g				
99/331	3.1/10.2	20.1/67.1	0.7/2.4	4.2/14.1
Bran Flakes, Healthwise, Kellogg's*, 1 serving/40g				
128/320	4/10	26.4/66	1/2.5	6/15
Bran Flakes, Honey & Nut, Safeway*, 1 serving/47g				
168/358	4.5/9.6	32.9/70	2.1/4.4	5.2/11
Bran Flakes, Honey Nut, Asda*, 1 serving/50g				
179/358	4.8/9.6	35/70	2.2/4.4	5.5/11
Bran Flakes, Honey Nut, Morrisons*, 1 serving/40g				
57/143	1.5/3.8	11.2/28	0.7/1.8	1.8/4.4
Bran Flakes, Honey Nut, Sainsbury's*, 1 serving/40g				
143/358	3.8/9.6	28/70	1.8/4.4	4.4/11

kcal serv/100g	prot serv/100g	carb serv/100g	fat serv/100g	fibre serv/100g
Bran Flakes, Honey Nut, Tesco*, 1 serving/40g				
143/358	3.8/9.6	28/70	1.8/4.4	4.4/11
Bran Flakes, Kellogg's*, 1 serving/30g				
99/330	3/10	19.8/66	0.8/2.5	4.5/15
Bran Flakes, Morrisons*, 1 serving/25g				
83/331	2.8/11.1	16.2/64.6	0.8/3.2	3.6/14.5
Bran Flakes, Oat with Apple & Raisin, Kellogg's*, 1 serving/40g				
140/350	4/10	26.4/66	2/5	4/10
Bran Flakes, Organic, Tesco*, 1 serving/30g				
99/330	3.1/10.2	20.1/67	0.7/2.4	4.2/14.1
Bran Flakes, Safeway*, 1 serving/40g				
132/331	4.1/10.2	26.8/67.1	1/2.4	5.6/14.1
Bran Flakes, Tesco*, 1 serving/30g				
99/331	3.1/10.2	20.1/67.1	0.7/2.4	4.2/14.1
Bran Flakes, Value, Tesco*, 1 serving/50g				
160/320	5.7/11.4	31.6/63.2	1.2/2.4	8.6/17.1
Bran Flakes, Waitrose*, 1 serving/30g				
100/333	3/10.1	20.3/67.7	0.7/2.4	3.8/12.7
Bran Flakes, Whole Grain, Sainsbury's*, 1 serving/30g				
99/331	3.1/10.2	20.1/67.1	0.7/2.4	4.2/14.1
Cheerios, Honey Nut, Nestle*, 1 serving/40g				
150/374	2.8/7	31.6/78.9	1.4/3.4	2.1/5.2
Cheerios, Nestle*, 1 serving/30g				
170/567	6.7/22.3	28.5/95	3.2/10.7	2/6.7
Cheerios, Whole Grain, Nestle*, 1 serving/30g				
110/366	2.4/8.1	22.4/74.6	1.2/3.9	2/6.5
Choco Corn Flakes, Asda*, 1 serving/50g				
187/374	3/6	43/86	0.4/0.7	1.3/2.6
Choco Corn Flakes, Kellogg's*, 1 serving/30g				
114/380	1.8/6	24.9/83	0.8/2.5	0.9/3
Choco Crackles, Morrisons*, 1 serving/30g				
115/383	1.7/5.5	25.4/84.8	0.7/2.4	0.6/1.9
Choco Flakes, Tesco*, 1 serving/30g				
112/374	1.7/5.6	25.9/86.3	0.2/0.7	0.8/2.6
Choco Hoops, Co-Op*, 1 serving/30g				
116/385	2.1/7	24/80	1.2/4	1.5/5
Choco Rice, Somerfield*, 1 serving with 125ml milk/155g				
176/114	5.9/3.8	31.7/20.5	2.8/1.8	0.6/0.4

	kcal serv/100g	prot serv/100g	carb serv/100g	fat serv/100g	fibre serv/100g
Choco Snaps, Tesco*, 1 serving/30g					
	114/379	1.7/5.5	25.2/83.9	0.7/2.4	0.7/2.3
Chocolate Cereal, Tesco*, 1 serving/40g					
	169/423	3.2/8	26.5/66.3	5.6/14	2.4/6
Chocolate Corn Flakes, Mini Bites, Marks & Spencer*, 1 bite/8g					
	38/475	0.5/6.2	5.3/66.5	1.7/20.7	0.1/1
Cinnamon & Apple, Sensations, Asda*, 1 serving/30g					
	112/373	3/10	21.6/72	1.5/5	2.1/7
Cinnamon Grahams, Nestle*, 1 serving/40g					
	166/416	1.8/4.6	30/75.1	4.4/10.9	1.7/4.2
Clusters, Nestle*, 1 serving/40g					
	153/382	4/10	28.1/70.2	2.7/6.8	3.4/8.5
Coco Pops Crunchers, Kellogg's*, 1 serving/30g					
	114/380	2.1/7	24.3/81	1.1/3.5	0.9/3
Coco Pops, Kellogg's*, 1 serving/30g					
	114/380	1.5/5	25.5/85	0.8/2.5	0.8/2.5
Corn Flakes, Banana Crunch, Kellogg's*, 1 serving/40g					
	159/398	2.4/6	32/80	2.8/7	1/2.5
Corn Flakes, Crunchy Nut, Kellogg's*, 1 serving/30g					
	117/390	2.1/7	24.6/82	1.1/3.5	0.9/3
Corn Flakes, Kellogg's*, 1 serving/30g					
	111/370	2.4/8	24.6/82	0.2/0.8	0.9/3
Corn Pops, Kellogg's*, 1 serving/40g					
	152/380	2.4/6	34.8/87	0.4/1	0.8/2
Country Crisp Four Nut Combo, Jordans*, 1 serving/50g					
	240/480	4.5/8.9	27.1/54.2	12.7/25.3	3/5.9
Country Crisp Wild About Berries, Jordans*, 1 serving/50g					
	222/443	3.8/7.5	34/68	7.9/15.7	1.6/3.1
Country Crisp with Strawberries, Jordans*, 1 serving/40g					
	174/435	3/7.4	25.8/64.5	6.6/16.4	3.2/8
Country Crisp with Whole Raspberries, Jordans*, 1 serving/40g					
	174/435	3/7.4	25.8/64.5	6.6/16.4	3.2/8
Cranberry Wheats, Tesco*, 1 serving/40g					
	130/325	2.9/7.3	28.4/70.9	0.6/1.4	3.1/7.7
Cranberry, Cherry & Almond, Dorset Cereals*, 1 serving/25g					
	89/355	2.3/9.2	15.1/60.5	2.1/8.5	2.1/8.4
Crispy Rice & Wheat Flakes, Asda*, 1 serving/50g					
	185/370	5.5/11	39/78	0.8/1.5	1.6/3.2

	kcal serv/100g	prot serv/100g	carb serv/100g	fat serv/100g	fibre serv/100g
Crunchy Bran Curls, Weetabix*, 1 serving/40g					
	120/299	4.7/11.8	20.9/52.3	1.9/4.7	9.9/24.8
Crunchy Cereal, Safeway*, 1 serving/45g					
	207/459	4.1/9.2	29.4/65.4	8/17.8	2.8/6.3
Crunchy Choco, Crisp & Square, Tesco*, 1 serving/50g					
	212/423	4/8	33.2/66.3	7/14	3/6
Crunchy Nut Clusters, Kellogg's*, 1 serving/40g					
	178/444	2.8/7	27.2/68	6.4/16	1.6/4
Crunchy Nut, Red, Kellogg's*, 1 serving/40g					
	164/410	2.8/7	29.2/73	4/10	1.2/3
Crunchy Oat with Raisins, Almonds & Honey, Tesco*, 1 serving/50g					
	213/425	4.6/9.1	31.4/62.8	7.7/15.3	2.4/4.7
Crunchy Oat, Golden Sun, Lidl*, 1 serving/50g					
	206/411	4.3/8.6	32.5/65	6.5/12.9	3.1/6.2
Crunchy Raisin & Coconut, Organic, Jordans*, 1 serving/40g					
	168/419	3.2/8.1	26.5/66.3	5.4/13.5	2.6/6.4
Eat my Shorts, Kellogg's*, 1 serving/30g					
	173/577	6/20	31/103.3	3/10	0.6/2
Fibre 1 Nestle*, 1 serving/40g					
	107/267	4.3/10.8	20.1/50.2	1/2.6	12.2/30.5
Fibre Bran, Safeway*, 1 serving/48.3g					
	124/259	6.4/13.3	20.8/43.4	1.7/3.6	14.9/31
Fitness & Fruits, Nestle*, 1 serving/40g					
	140/350	2.2/5.6	30.8/77	0.9/2.2	2.2/5.6
Flakes & Grains, Exotic Fruit, BGTY, Sainsbury's*, 1 serving/30g					
	113/377	2/6.8	22.9/76.4	1.5/4.9	1.8/5.9
Flakes & Orchard Fruits, BGTY, Sainsbury's*, 1 serving/40g					
	154/385	5.2/13	32.2/80.6	0.5/1.2	1.8/4.5
Force, Nestle*, 1 serving/40g					
	138/344	4.2/10.6	28.1/70.3	0.9/2.3	3.7/9.2
Frosted Flakes, Sainsbury's*, 1 serving/30g					
	112/374	1.5/4.9	26.3/87.8	0.1/0.4	0.7/2.4
Frosted Flakes, Tesco*, 1 serving/30g					
	112/374	1.5/4.9	26.3/87.8	0.1/0.4	0.7/2.4
Frosted Wheats, Kellogg's*, 1 serving/30g					
	102/340	3/10	21.6/72	0.6/2	2.7/9
Frosties, Caramel, Kellogg's*, 1 serving/30g					
	113/377	1.5/5	26.4/88	0.2/0.6	0.6/2

	kcal serv/100g	prot serv/100g	carb serv/100g	fat serv/100g	fibre serv/100g
Frosties, Chocolate, Kellogg's*, 1 serving/40g					
	160/400	2/5	33.6/84	1.8/4.5	0.8/2
Frosties, Kellogg's*, 1 serving/30g					
	114/380	1.5/5	26.4/88	0.2/0.6	0.6/2
Fruit & Fibre, Asda*, 1 serving/30g					
	112/372	2.7/9	19.8/66	2.4/8	2.4/8
Fruit & Fibre, Flakes, Waitrose*, 1 serving/40g					
	140/350	3.3/8.2	26.3/65.7	2.4/6	4/10.1
Fruit & Fibre, Harvest Morn, Aldi*, 1 serving/40g					
	149/372	3.6/8.9	27.6/68.9	2.7/6.8	3.2/8
Fruit & Fibre, Morrisons*, 1 serving/30g					
	110/366	2.6/8.8	20/66.5	2.2/7.2	2.6/8.5
Fruit & Fibre, Organic, Sainsbury's*, 1 serving/40g					
	147/367	4/10	29/72.4	1.6/4.1	3.1/7.8
Fruit & Fibre, Safeway*, 1 serving/40g					
	143/358	3.6/9	26.6/66.4	2.6/6.4	3.6/9
Fruit & Fibre, Sainsbury's*, 1 serving/30g					
	108/361	2.4/8.1	20.6/68.5	1.8/6.1	2.7/8.9
Fruit & Fibre, Tesco*, 1 serving/30g					
	113/375	2.6/8.5	19.9/66.3	2.5/8.4	2.3/7.8
Fruit 'n' Fibre, Kellogg's*, 1 serving/50g					
	175/350	4.5/9	34.5/69	2.3/4.5	4.5/9
Fruit Nuts & Flakes, Marks & Spencer*, 1 serving/30g					
	117/391	2.7/9.1	20.9/69.6	2.6/8.5	1.1/3.5
Golden Grahams, Nestle*, 1 serving/40g					
	152/381	2.2/5.6	32.6/81.6	1.4/3.6	1.3/3.2
Golden Nuggets, Nestle*, 1 serving/40g					
	152/381	2.5/6.2	35/87.4	0.3/0.7	0.6/1.5
Golden Puffs, Sainsbury's*, 1 serving/28g					
	107/383	1.8/6.6	24.2/86.3	0.3/1.2	0.8/3
Grape Nuts, Kraft*, 1 serving/30g					
	104/345	3.2/10.5	21.8/72.5	0.6/1.9	2.6/8.6
Harvest Crunch, Nut, Quaker*, 1 serving/40g					
	184/459	3.2/8	25/62.5	7.8/19.5	2.4/6
Harvest Crunch, Real Red Berries, Quaker*, 1 serving/50g					
	224/447	3.5/7	33/66	8.5/17	2.3/4.5
Harvest Crunch, Soft Juicy Raisins, Quaker*, 1 serving/50g					
	221/442	3/6	33.5/67	8/16	2/4

kcal serv/100g	prot serv/100g	carb serv/100g	fat serv/100g	fibre serv/100g
Hawaiian Crunch, Mornflake*, 1 serving/60g				
247/411	4.9/8.1	40.1/66.8	7.4/12.4	4.1/6.8
High-Fibre Bran, Asda*, 1 serving/50g				
137/273	6.5/13	22/44	2.5/5	14.5/29
High-Fibre Bran, Co-Op*, 1 serving/40g				
108/270	5.2/13	17.6/44	2/5	11.6/29
High-Fibre Bran, New, Tesco*, 1 serving/30g				
73/242	4.2/14	11.5/38.4	1.1/3.5	9.3/31
High-Fibre Bran, Sainsbury's*, 1 serving/40g				
114/286	5.4/13.4	20.3/50.7	1.3/3.3	9.4/23.6
High-Fibre Bran, Tesco*, 1 serving/40g				
108/271	5.2/13	17.4/43.6	2/5	11.6/29
High-Fibre Bran, Waitrose*, 1 serving/40g				
112/281	5.8/14.4	18.9/47.2	1.5/3.8	10.4/26
Honey Loops, Kellogg's*, 1 serving/30g				
111/370	2.4/8	23.1/77	0.9/3	2.1/7
Honey Nut & Flakes, Marks & Spencer*, 1 serving/40g				
164/411	3.9/9.8	29.4/73.4	3.5/8.7	1/2.6
Honey Raisin & Almond, Crunchy, Waitrose*, 1 serving/40g				
170/425	4.2/10.5	27.5/68.8	4.8/12	2.3/5.7
Hot Cereal, Flaxomeal*, 1 serving/40g				
130/325	21/52.5	1/2.5	6/15	12/30
Hot Oats, Instant, Tesco*, 1 serving/30g				
107/356	3.5/11.5	17.6/58.8	2.5/8.3	2.7/8.9
Hot Oats, Safeway*, 1 serving/20g				
71/356	2.3/11.6	11.8/58.8	1.7/8.3	1.8/8.9
Hunny B's, Kellogg's*, 1 serving/28g				
106/380	1.7/6	23.2/83	0.7/2.5	0.8/3
Just Right, Kellogg's*, 1 serving/40g				
144/360	2.8/7	31.2/78	1/2.5	1.8/4.5
Malt Bites, Safeway*, 1 serving/40g				
137/343	4/10	27.7/69.2	1.2/2.9	4/10
Malted Wheaties, Asda*, 1 serving/50g				
171/342	5/10	34.5/69	1.5/2.9	5/10
Malties, Sainsbury's*, 1 serving/40g				
137/343	4/10	27.7/69.2	1.2/2.9	4/10

kcal serv/100g	prot serv/100g	carb serv/100g	fat serv/100g	fibre serv/100g

Malty Flakes with Cranberry & Apple Cereal, BGTY, Sainsbury's*, 1 serving/40g

| 142/356 | 3.8/9.4 | 30.5/76.2 | 0.6/1.5 | 1.5/3.7 |

Malty Flakes with Peach & Raspberry, BGTY, Sainsbury's*, 1 serving/40g

| 146/364 | 4.3/10.8 | 30.6/76.4 | 0.7/1.7 | 1.3/3.3 |

Malty Flakes with Red Berries, Tesco*, 1 serving/30g

| 111/369 | 3/9.9 | 23.4/78.1 | 0.6/1.9 | 0.9/3.1 |

Malty Flakes, Tesco*, 1 serving/40g

| 148/371 | 4.4/11 | 31.4/78.4 | 0.6/1.5 | 1.7/4.3 |

Maple & Pecan, Crisp, Asda*, 1 serving/30g

| 135/451 | 2.4/8 | 18.6/62 | 5.7/19 | 1.8/6 |

Maple & Pecan, Crisp, Tesco*, 1 serving/60g

| 277/461 | 4.9/8.2 | 36.4/60.6 | 12.4/20.6 | 3.7/6.2 |

Maple & Pecan, Luxury Crunchy, Jordans*, 1 serving/50g

| 224/448 | 5/9.9 | 30/59.9 | 9.4/18.7 | 3.3/6.5 |

Maple & Pecan, Sainsbury's*, 1 serving/60g

| 318/530 | 8/13.3 | 41.8/69.7 | 13.2/22 | 3.2/5.3 |

Minibix, Banana, Weetabix*, 1 serving/40g

| 148/370 | 3.5/8.8 | 29.2/73 | 2/5 | 3.2/8.1 |

Minibix, Chocolate, Weetabix*, 1 serving/39g

| 149/383 | 3.3/8.4 | 28.6/73.3 | 2.4/6.2 | 2.6/6.7 |

Minibix, Fruit & Nut, Weetabix*, 1 serving/40g

| 141/353 | 3.5/8.8 | 28.5/71.2 | 1.5/3.8 | 3.2/8.1 |

Minibix, Honey, Weetabix*, 1 serving/40g

| 144/359 | 3.5/8.8 | 30.4/76.1 | 0.9/2.2 | 0/0 |

Minibix, Weetabix*, 1 serving/40g

| 134/335 | 3.5/8.8 | 28.5/71.2 | 1.5/3.8 | 3.2/8.1 |

Muesli, 12 Fruit & Nut, Sainsbury's*, 1 serving/50g

| 166/332 | 4.1/8.1 | 32.1/64.2 | 2.4/4.7 | 3.9/7.8 |

Muesli, BGTY, Sainsbury's*, 1 serving/64.8g

| 211/324 | 4.4/6.7 | 46/70.8 | 1/1.6 | 4/6.2 |

Muesli, COU, Marks & Spencer*, 1 serving/60g

| 201/335 | 4.6/7.6 | 42.1/70.2 | 1.5/2.5 | 4.9/8.1 |

Muesli, Creamy Tropical Fruit, Finest, Tesco*, 1 serving/80g

| 283/354 | 5.8/7.2 | 55/68.8 | 4.5/5.6 | 5.5/6.9 |

Muesli, Crunchy Bran, Nature's Harvest*, 1 serving/50g

| 176/352 | 4.4/8.8 | 31.5/62.9 | 5/9.9 | 3.2/6.4 |

	kcal serv/100g	prot serv/100g	carb serv/100g	fat serv/100g	fibre serv/100g
Muesli, Crunchy, Organic, Sainsbury's*, 1 serving/40g					
	168/420	4.2/10.6	24.8/62	5.8/14.4	3.7/9.2
Muesli, De Luxe, No Added Salt or Sugar, Sainsbury's*, 1 serving/40g					
	161/403	4.8/11.9	23/57.6	5.6/13.9	3.4/8.4
Muesli, Eat Smart, Safeway*, 1 serving/40g					
	134/335	3.5/8.7	27.4/68.6	1.1/2.8	3/7.4
Muesli, Fruit & Bran, Unsweetened, Marks & Spencer*, 1 serving/40g					
	128/320	3.2/8.1	27.2/68	1.1/2.7	3.8/9.4
Muesli, Fruit & Fibre, COU, Marks & Spencer*, 1 serving/40g					
	130/325	3/7.5	29.8/74.5	1.1/2.8	3/7.5
Muesli, Fruit & Nut, Iceland*, 1 serving/30g					
	105/350	2.8/9.3	18.3/61	2.3/7.5	2.4/8.1
Muesli, Fruit & Nut, Jordans*, 1 serving/50g					
	189/378	3.7/7.3	30.3/60.6	5.9/11.8	3.4/6.7
Muesli, Fruit & Nut, Luxury, Co-Op*, 1 serving/40g					
	150/375	3.2/8	25.6/64	4/10	2.4/6
Muesli, Fruit & Nut, Luxury, Marks & Spencer*, 1 serving/50g					
	175/349	3.9/7.7	31.1/62.2	3.9/7.7	3.7/7.3
Muesli, Fruit & Nut, Luxury, Waitrose*, 1 serving/40g					
	145/363	3.6/9	24.1/60.3	3.8/9.5	2.6/6.5
Muesli, Fruit & Nut, Marks & Spencer*, 1 serving/40g					
	128/320	3/7.4	29.8/74.5	1.1/2.8	3/7.4
Muesli, Fruit & Nut, Organic, Marks & Spencer*, 1 serving/50g					
	167/333	4.1/8.2	30.8/61.6	3/6	3.8/7.6
Muesli Fruit & Nut, Sainsbury's*, 1 serving/30g					
	121/402	3.1/10.4	15.4/51.3	5.2/17.2	2.8/9.2
Muesli Fruit & Nut, Tesco*, 1 serving/65g					
	237/365	4.8/7.4	37.6/57.9	7.5/11.5	5.2/8
Muesli Fruit Sensation, Marks & Spencer*, 1 serving/50g					
	158/315	3/6	33/66	1.5/3	3.7/7.4
Muesli, Fruit, 55%, Asda*, 1 serving/35g					
	111/318	2.1/6	23.5/67	1/2.9	2.5/7
Muesli, Fruit, GFY, Asda*, 1 serving/50g					
	152/304	4/8	32/64	0.9/1.8	5/10
Muesli, Fruit, Healthy Eating, Tesco*, 1 serving/40g					
	129/322	2.8/7	26.6/66.6	1.7/4.2	2.8/6.9
Muesli, Fruit, Sainsbury's*, 1 serving/40g					
	132/330	3.2/8.1	25.7/64.3	1.8/4.5	3.8/9.6

kcal serv/100g	prot serv/100g	carb serv/100g	fat serv/100g	fibre serv/100g
Muesli, Fruit, Tesco*, 1 serving/50g				
167/333	3.5/7	33/66	2.1/4.2	3.5/6.9
Muesli, Fruit, The Best, Safeway*, 1 serving/40g				
138/346	2.1/5.3	28.5/71.3	1.7/4.3	2/5
Muesli, Gluten-Free, Nature's Harvest, Holland & Barrett*, 1 serving/60g				
234/390	8.5/14.1	32.5/54.1	7.8/13	2/3.3
Muesli, Golden Sun, Lidl*, 1 serving/40g				
144/360	3.2/8	24/60	3.9/9.8	3/7.5
Muesli, Luxury Fruit, Perfectly Balanced, Waitrose*, 1 serving/50g				
162/324	3.6/7.1	33.2/66.4	1.7/3.3	3.5/7
Muesli, Luxury Fruit, Safeway*, 1 serving/40g				
139/347	2.8/7.1	29.7/74.3	0.4/1	0.9/2.2
Muesli, Luxury Fruit, Sainsbury's*, 1 serving/50g				
162/324	3.6/7.1	33.2/66.4	1.7/3.3	3.5/7
Muesli, Luxury Fruit, Waitrose*, 1 serving/30g				
101/337	2.3/7.7	19.9/66.3	1.4/4.5	2.1/6.9
Muesli, Luxury, Dorset Cereals*, 1 serving/28g				
92/328	2.4/8.4	17.6/63	1.8/6.5	2.5/9
Muesli, Luxury, Jordans*, 1 serving/40g				
154/384	3.8/9.6	23.4/58.4	5/12.5	3.3/8.2
Muesli, Luxury, Sainsbury's*, 1 serving/40g				
144/359	3.4/8.5	22.8/57.1	4.3/10.7	3.1/7.7
Muesli, Natural, Jordans*, 1 serving/40g				
141/352	4.2/10.4	25/62.4	2.7/6.7	3.6/8.9
Muesli, No Added Sugar or Salt, Organic, Jordans*, 1 serving/50g				
191/381	5/9.9	31.2/62.3	5.1/10.2	4.7/9.3
Muesli, No Added Sugar, Waitrose*, 1 serving/40g				
146/364	4.8/12	26/64.9	2.5/6.3	2.7/6.7
Muesli, Organic, Jordans*, 1 serving/40g				
150/374	4.4/10.9	21.7/54.2	5/12.6	4.2/10.5
Muesli, Organic, Waitrose*, 1 serving/50g				
179/358	5.4/10.8	29.6/59.1	4.4/8.7	3.9/7.8
Muesli, Organic, Whole Earth*, 1 serving/25g				
87/347	2.6/10.5	15.3/61	1.6/6.4	2/8
Muesli, Original, Holland & Barrett*, 1 serving/30g				
105/351	3.3/11.1	18.4/61.2	2.5/8.4	2.1/7.1
Muesli, Original, Sainsbury's*, 1 serving/60g				
226/376	5.6/9.3	39.4/65.7	5/8.4	4.3/7.1

	kcal serv/100g	prot serv/100g	carb serv/100g	fat serv/100g	fibre serv/100g
Muesli, Special, Jordans*, 1 serving/40g					
	143/358	3.4/8.4	24.3/60.8	3.6/9	3.2/8.1
Muesli, Swiss Style, Co-Op*, 1 serving/40g					
	148/370	4.4/11	26.8/67	2.4/6	2.4/6
Muesli, Swiss Style, No Added Salt Or Sugar, Sainsbury's*, 1 serving/40g					
	143/358	4.3/10.7	25.7/64.3	2.6/6.4	2.8/7
Muesli, Swiss Style, No Added Sugar or Salt, Asda*, 1 serving/50g					
	182/363	5.5/11	32/64	3.5/7	4/8
Muesli, Swiss Style, SmartPrice, Asda*, 1 serving/60g					
	222/370	5.4/9	42/70	3.6/6	6/10
Muesli, Swiss-Style, Somerfield*, 1 serving/50g					
	180/359	5.5/11	32/64	3.3/6.5	4/8
Muesli, Swiss-Style, Tesco*, 1 serving/40g					
	141/353	4.4/10.9	26/65.1	2.2/5.4	3.3/8.2
Muesli, Swiss-Style, Waitrose*, 1 serving/40g					
	146/364	4.1/10.2	26.4/66.1	2.6/6.5	3/7.6
Muesli, Tropical Fruit, Holland & Barrett*, 1 bowl/60g					
	197/328	4.5/7.5	41.9/69.8	1.9/3.2	3.1/5.1
Muesli, Tropical, Tesco*, 1 serving/50g					
	173/346	3.9/7.8	34.1/68.2	2.4/4.7	4.6/9.1
Muesli, Unsweetened Wholewheat, Safeway*, 1 serving/50g					
	180/360	3.9/7.7	34/68	3.2/6.3	3.6/7.2
Muesli, Unsweetened, Marks & Spencer*, 1 serving/40g					
	129/322	3.2/8.1	27.2/68	1.1/2.7	3.8/9.4
Muesli, Value, Tesco*, 1 serving/50g					
	171/342	3.8/7.5	33.8/67.6	2.3/4.6	4.3/8.6
Muesli, Wholewheat, Co-Op*, 1 serving/40g					
	140/350	4.4/11	24.4/61	2.8/7	2.8/7
Muesli, Wholewheat, No Added Salt or Sugar, Sainsbury's*, 1 serving/40g					
	140/351	3.3/8.2	23.6/58.9	3.7/9.2	3.2/8.1
Muesli, Wholewheat, No Added Sugar & Salt, Tesco*, 1 serving/40g					
	152/379	3.8/9.6	24.1/60.2	4.4/11.1	3.2/8.1
Muesli, Wholewheat, No Added Sugar, Tesco*, 1 serving/40g					
	154/386	3.8/9.5	23.6/59.1	5/12.4	3/7.4
Muesli, Wholewheat, Sainsbury's*, 1 serving/40g					
	136/339	3.4/8.5	24.2/60.6	2.8/6.9	3/7.6
Multi Fruit & Flake, COU, Marks & Spencer, 1 serving/39g					
	142/365	2.5/6.5	31.9/81.8	0.4/1.1	1.6/4

kcal serv/100g	prot serv/100g	carb serv/100g	fat serv/100g	fibre serv/100g
Multi Fruit & Flake, Perfectly Balanced, Waitrose*, 1 serving/40g				
134/335	3.3/8.2	27.5/68.8	1.2/3	5.6/14
Multigrain Flakes with Apple, Eat Smart, Safeway*, 1 serving/45g				
160/355	3.6/8	33.6/74.7	1.1/2.5	3.2/7
Multigrain, Start, Kellogg's*, 1 serving/40g				
144/360	3.2/8	31.6/79	0.8/2	2.4/6
Natural Wheatgerm, Jordans*, 1 serving/40g				
138/345	10.6/26.5	15.8/39.6	3.6/9	5.5/13.7
Natures Wholegrains, Jordans*, 1 serving/25g				
98/390	2.4/9.4	15.4/61.7	2.9/11.7	1.9/7.7
Oat & Bran Flakes, Sainsbury's*, 1 serving/50g				
172/344	6.3/12.6	30/60	3/5.9	7.5/15
Oat Bran, Crispies, Quaker*, 1 serving/40g				
153/383	4.4/11	27.6/69	2.6/6.5	3.6/9
Oat Krunchies, Quaker*, 1 serving/30g				
118/393	2.9/9.5	21.6/72	2.1/7	1.7/5.5
Oat with Tropical Fruits, Crunchy, Tesco*, 1 serving/35g				
157/448	3/8.7	23.1/66	5.8/16.6	1.1/3.2
Oat, Crunchy, Sainsbury's*, 1 serving/50g				
227/453	4.1/8.2	29.7/59.3	10.2/20.3	3.3/6.6
Oatbran Flakes, Nature's Path*, 1 serving/30g				
124/414	2.6/8.7	24.9/83	1.4/4.7	2/6.7
Oatmeal, Instant, Quaker*, 1 serving/35g				
126/360	4.8/13.6	20/57	3/8.7	3.4/9.7
Oatso Simple, Apple & Cinnamon, Quaker*, 1 sachet/38g				
136/358	3/8	25.8/68	2.1/5.5	1/2.5
Oatso Simple, Baked Apple Flavour, Quaker*, 1 serving/38g				
141/370	3/8	26.6/70	2.36/6	2.1/5.5
Oatso Simple, Berry Burst, Quaker*, 1 serving/38g				
141/370	3/8	26.6/70	2.3/6	2.5/6.5
Oatso Simple, Country Honey, Quaker*, 1 serving/36g				
134/373	3.1/8.5	24.8/69	2.3/6.5	2.2/6
Oatso Simple, Fruit Muesli, Quaker*, 1 sachet/39g				
140/360	2.9/7.5	26.9/69	2.3/6	2.7/7
Oatso Simple, Golden Syrup Flavour, Quaker*, 1 serving/39g				
142/364	2.9/7.5	27.3/70	2.1/5.5	2/5
Oatso Simple, Quaker*, 1 serving/27g				
100/372	3/11	16.7/62	2.3/8.5	1.9/7

kcal serv/100g	prot serv/100g	carb serv/100g	fat serv/100g	fibre serv/100g
Orange, Banana, Strawberry Flakes & Grains, BGTY, Sainsbury's*, 1 serving/35g				
130/370	2.9/8.4	28.2/80.6	0.5/1.5	1.6/4.7
Perfect Balance, Weight Watchers*, 1 serving/30g				
90/300	2.3/7.8	19/63.3	0.5/1.7	4.7/15.6
Porage Oats, Scot's, Quaker*, 1 serving/30g				
110/368	3.3/11	18.6/62	2.4/8	2.1/7
Porridge Oats & Bran, Co-Op*, 1 serving/40g				
141/353	5/12.5	24/60	2.8/7	4.8/12
Porridge Oats & Bran, Somerfield*, 1 serving/40g				
154/385	4.8/12	27.2/68	2.8/7	0/0
Porridge Oats, Quick & Easy, Morrisons*, 1 serving/28g				
103/367	3.3/11.8	17.4/62	2.2/8	2/7
Porridge, Instant, Quakers*, 1 serving/34g				
125/368	4.4/12.8	22.7/66.7	2.6/7.6	1.7/5
Porridge, Quick, Marks & Spencer*, 1 serving/40g				
159/398	6.2/15.5	22/55.1	5.1/12.8	2.4/5.9
Porridge, Weight Watchers*, 1 pack/220g				
114/52	2.4/1.1	20.9/9.5	2.4/1.1	2/0.9
Precise, Sainsbury's*, 1 serving/40g				
148/371	2.6/6.4	32/79.9	1.2/2.9	1.4/3.5
Puffed Rice, Kallo*, 1 serving/25g				
95/380	2/8	20/80	0.8/3	2.3/9
Puffed Wheat, Quaker*, 1 serving/15g				
49/328	2.3/15.3	9.4/62.4	0.2/1.3	0.8/5.6
Puffed Wheat, Tesco*, 1 serving/28g				
104/373	3.9/13.9	20.2/72.2	0.9/3.2	1.6/5.7
Quaker Oats Crunch, Quaker*, 1 serving/40g				
178/445	3.2/8	26.6/66.5	6.4/16	2/5
Quaker Oats, Quaker*, 1 serving/30g				
110/368	3.3/11	18.6/62	2.4/8	2.1/7
Raisin & Almond, Crunchy, Jordans*, 1 serving/56g				
230/411	4.7/8.4	37/66	7/12.5	2.8/5
Raisin Wheats, Kellogg's*, 1 serving/30g				
96/320	2.7/9	20.7/69	0.6/2	2.7/9
Raisin Wheats, Sainsbury's*, 1 serving/50g				
166/332	4.1/8.2	35.8/71.5	0.8/1.5	4/8

kcal serv/100g	prot serv/100g	carb serv/100g	fat serv/100g	fibre serv/100g

Raisin, Bran Flakes, Asda*, 1 serving/50g

| 166/331 | 3.5/7 | 34.5/69 | 1.5/3 | 5/10 |

Raisin, Honey & Almond Crunch, Asda*, 1 serving/60g

| 265/442 | 4.8/8 | 37.2/62 | 10.8/18 | 3.6/6 |

Ready Brek, Banana, Weetabix*, 1 serving/40g

| 146/365 | 3.6/8.9 | 27.2/68 | 2.6/6.4 | 2.7/6.7 |

Ready Brek, Chocolate, Weetabix*, 1 serving/40g

| 144/360 | 3.8/9.6 | 25.5/63.7 | 3/7.4 | 3.2/8.1 |

Ready Brek, Strawberry, Weetabix*, 1 serving/40g

| 146/365 | 3.5/8.7 | 27.4/68.6 | 2.5/6.2 | 2.7/6.8 |

Ready Brek, Weetabix*, 1 serving/40g

| 142/356 | 4.6/11.6 | 23.5/58.8 | 3.3/8.3 | 3.6/8.9 |

Red Berry & Almond Luxury Crunch, Jordans*, 1 serving/40g

| 176/441 | 3.3/8.2 | 24.2/60.5 | 7.4/18.5 | 2.6/6.6 |

Rice & Wheat Flake, Special Choice, Waitrose*, 1 serving/30g

| 111/370 | 3.4/11.4 | 23.3/77.7 | 0.5/1.5 | 1/3.2 |

Rice Krispies, Honey, Kellogg's*, 1 serving/30g

| 114/380 | 1.2/4 | 26.7/89 | 0.2/0.7 | 0.3/1 |

Rice Krispies, Kellogg's*, 1 serving/30g

| 111/370 | 1.8/6 | 25.5/85 | 0.3/1 | 0.5/1.5 |

Rice Pops, Blue Parrot Cafe, Sainsbury's*, 1 serving/30g

| 111/370 | 2.2/7.2 | 24.7/82.3 | 0.4/1.3 | 0.7/2.2 |

Rice Pops, Organic, Dove's Farm*, 1 serving/30g

| 107/357 | 2/6.8 | 25.8/86.1 | 0.2/0.8 | 0.6/2 |

Rice Pops, Sainsbury's*, 1 serving/30g

| 113/378 | 2.2/7.4 | 25.3/84.2 | 0.4/1.3 | 0.5/1.5 |

Rice Snaps, Asda*, 1 serving/28g

| 105/376 | 2/7 | 23.5/84 | 0.4/1.3 | 0.4/1.5 |

Rice Snaps, Harvest Home, Nestle*, 1 serving/25g

| 95/378 | 1.9/7.4 | 21.1/84.2 | 0.3/1.3 | 0.4/1.5 |

Rice Snaps, Healthy Eating, Tesco*, 1 pack/25g

| 93/370 | 1.8/7.2 | 20.6/82.3 | 0.3/1.3 | 0.6/2.2 |

Rice Snaps, Tesco*, 1 serving/30g

| 113/378 | 2.2/7.3 | 25.3/84.2 | 0.4/1.3 | 0.5/1.5 |

Ricicles, Kellogg's*, 1 serving/30g

| 114/380 | 1.2/4 | 26.7/89 | 0.2/0.7 | 0.3/1 |

Right Balance, Morrisons*, 1 serving/50g

| 181/362 | 3.5/6.9 | 39.3/78.6 | 1.1/2.2 | 2.7/5.3 |

kcal serv/100g	prot serv/100g	carb serv/100g	fat serv/100g	fibre serv/100g
Shredded Wheat, Bitesize, Nestle*, 1 serving/50g				
168/335	5.8/11.5	33.9/67.7	1.1/2.2	5.8/11.6
Shredded Wheat, Fruitful, Nestle*, 1 serving/50g				
177/353	4.2/8.4	33.5/66.9	2.9/5.8	5.2/10.3
Shredded Wheat, Honey Nut, Nestle*, 1 serving/40g				
151/378	4.4/10.9	27.5/68.8	2.6/6.6	4.2/10.4
Shredded Wheat, Nestle*, 1 piece/22g				
72/325	2.5/11.2	14.3/65.2	0.5/2.1	2.7/12.4
Shreddies, Coco, Nestle*, 1 serving/50g				
177/353	4/8	38.1/76.1	1/1.9	4.6/9.2
Shreddies, Frosted, Kellogg's*, 1 serving/50g				
162/323	0.4/0.7	39.3/78.5	0.9/1.8	2.4/4.7
Shreddies, Frosted, Nestle*, 1 serving/50g				
178/356	3.7/7.3	39.3/78.5	0.7/1.4	4.2/8.3
Shreddies, Frosted, Variety Pack, Nestle*, 1 pack/45g				
163/363	3/6.7	36.5/81.1	0.6/1.3	3.1/6.8
Shreddies, Malt Wheats, Tesco*, 1 serving/45g				
151/335	3.7/8.3	31.8/70.7	0.9/2.1	4.4/9.7
Shreddies, Nestle*, 1 serving/45g				
154/343	4.4/9.8	32.3/71.7	0.9/1.9	5/11.2
Smart Start, Kellogg's*, 1 serving/70g				
252/360	4.2/6	60.2/86	0.7/1	2.8/4
Smoothies, Strawberry, Quaker*, 1 sachet/29g				
117/402	1.9/6.5	19.4/67	3.5/12	1.6/5.5
Special K, Apricot & Peach, Kellogg's*, 1 serving/30g				
111/369	4.5/15	22.5/75	0.3/1	0.9/3
Special K, Kellogg's*, 1 serving/30g				
111/370	4.5/15	22.5/75	0.3/1	0.8/2.5
Special K, Red Berries, Kellogg's*, 1 serving/30g				
111/370	4.2/14	22.2/74	0.3/1	0.9/3
Start Right, Asda*, 1 serving/40g				
150/376	3.2/8	29.6/74	2.4/6	2/5
Strawberry & Almond Crunch, Marks & Spencer*, 1 serving/40g				
186/465	3.2/8	26.4/66	7.4/18.6	2/4.9
Sugar Puffs, Quaker*, 1 serving/30g				
116/387	2/6.5	26/86.5	0.3/1	0.9/3
Sultana Bran, Asda*, 1 serving/30g				
98/327	2.7/9	19.8/66	0.9/3	3.3/11

kcal serv/100g	prot serv/100g	carb serv/100g	fat serv/100g	fibre serv/100g
Sultana Bran, Co-Op*, 1 serving/40g				
130/325	3.6/9	26.4/66	1.2/3	4.4/11
Sultana Bran, Healthwise, Kellogg's*, 1 serving/40g				
128/320	3.6/9	26.4/66	0.8/2	5.2/13
Sultana Bran, Healthy Eating, Tesco*, 1 serving/48g				
156/326	3.9/8.1	33.1/69	0.9/1.9	4.7/9.8
Sultana Bran, Morrisons*, 1 serving/30g				
98/325	2.6/8.8	19.7/65.8	0.9/3	3.4/11.4
Sultana Bran, Safeway*, 1 serving/50g				
162/324	4.1/8.2	34.3/68.6	1/1.9	5.8/11.6
Sultana Bran, Sainsbury's*, 1 serving/30g				
97/324	2.5/8.2	20.6/68.6	0.6/1.9	3.5/11.6
Sultana Bran, Somerfield*, 1 serving/30g				
97/324	2.5/8.2	20.6/68.6	0.6/1.9	3.5/11.6
Super High Fibre, Dorset Cereals*, 1 serving/60g				
214/357	4.8/8	36.1/60.1	5.6/9.4	5/8.4
Superfast Oats, Mornflake*, 1 serving/40g				
144/359	4.4/11	24.2/60.4	3.2/8.1	3.4/8.5
Triple Chocolate Crisp, Sainsbury's*, 1 serving/40g				
180/451	3.1/7.7	25.5/63.8	7.3/18.3	2.4/6
Tropical Fruit & Bran Multiflakes, COU, Marks & Spencer*, 1 serving/40g				
140/350	2.8/7.1	32.5/81.2	1/2.6	0/0
Tropical, Crunchy, Jordans*, 1 serving/40g				
170/425	3.4/8.5	26.3/65.8	5.7/14.2	2.5/6.2
Tropicana, Weight Watchers*, 1 serving/50g				
120/240	2.5/5.1	26/52	0.5/1	3.5/7
Weetabix*, 2 biscuits/37.5g				
128/340	4.2/11.2	25.4/67.6	1/2.7	3.9/10.5
Weetabix, Organic, Weetabix*, 2 biscuits/35g				
117/335	3.8/10.9	23.2/66.2	1.1/3	4/11.3
Weetos, Weetabix*, 1 serving/30g				
115/384	1.9/6.2	23.5/78.4	1.5/5	1.7/5.6
Wheat Biscuits, Healthy Eating, Tesco*, 2 biscuits/55g				
191/348	6.1/11	38.5/70	1.5/2.7	4.4/8
Wheat Biscuits, Nature's Own, Organic, Weetabix*, 1 biscuit/17g				
58/339	1.8/10.3	11.8/69.2	0.4/2.4	1.8/10.4
Wheat Biscuits, Somerfield*, 2 biscuits/37.5g				
129/339	4.3/11.2	25.7/67.6	1/2.7	4/10.5

	kcal serv/100g	prot serv/100g	carb serv/100g	fat serv/100g	fibre serv/100g

Wheat Biscuits, Value, Tesco*, 2 biscuits/30g

103/342	4.1/13.7	20.9/69.5	0.3/1	2.3/7.5

Wheat Bisks, Asda*, 1 serving/29g

99/340	3.2/11	19.7/68	0.8/2.7	2.9/10

Wholewheat Biscuits, Sainsbury's*, 1 biscuit/36g

122/340	4/11.2	24.3/67.6	1/2.7	3.8/10.5

Yoghurt & Raspberry, Crisp, Sainsbury's*, 1 serving/45g

199/442	3.4/7.5	29.7/66	7.4/16.4	2.4/5.4

CHEESE, CREAM, MILK AND YOGHURT

Cheese Singles, 50% Less Fat, BGTY, Sainsbury's*, 1 slice/20g

38/190	3.6/18	1.4/7	2/10	0/0

Cheese Singles, Healthy Eating, Tesco*, 1 slice/20g

39/194	4.3/21.7	0.8/4.2	2/10	0/0

Cheese Slices, 97% Fat-Free, Kraft*, 1 slice/20g

31/155	4.7/23.3	2/9.9	0.5/2.3	0/0

Cheese Slices, Bavarian Smoked, Asda*, 1 slice/18g

50/277	3.1/17	0.1/0.4	4.1/23	0/0

Cheese Slices, Better For You, Morrisons*, 1 slice/20g

39/196	4.2/21	1.1/5.4	2/10	0/0

Cheese Slices, Cheddar, Mature, Marks & Spencer*, 1 slice/30g

124/412	7.7/25.5	0/0.1	10.3/34.4	0/0

Cheese Slices, Cheddar, Mild, Tesco*, 1 slice/30g

123/410	7.5/25	0/0.1	10.3/34.4	0/0

Cheese Slices, Dairylea, Kraft*, 1 slice/25g

76/305	3.3/13	2/8	6.1/24.5	0/0

Cheese Slices, Half-Fat, Asda*, 1 slice/20g

39/194	4.1/20.6	1.1/5.4	2/10	0/0

Cheese Slices, Light, Dairylea, Kraft*, 1 slice/25g

55/220	4.6/18.5	1.8/7	3.1/12.5	0/0

Cheese Slices, Light, Thick, Dairylea, Kraft*, 1 slice/25g

51/205	4.3/17.3	2.2/8.6	2.6/10.5	0/0

Cheese Slices, Lightlife, Leerdammer*, 1 slice/20g

55/273	6.1/30.6	0/0	3.3/16.4	0/0

Cheese Slices, Low-Fat, Healthy Living, Tesco*, 1 slice/27g

52/193	9.7/36.1	1.6/6	0.7/2.7	0/0

	kcal serv/100g	prot serv/100g	carb serv/100g	fat serv/100g	fibre serv/100g

Cheese Straws, Cheddar, Marks & Spencer*, 1 straw/11g

59/535	1.6/14.9	4.4/40.1	3.8/34.9	0.3/2.4

Cheese Strips, Dairylea, Kraft*, 1 pack/21g

72/345	4.9/23.5	0.1/0.4	5.7/27	0/0

Cheese Triangles, Big Portions, Laughing Cow*, 1 triangle/18g

48/269	1.8/10	1.2/6.5	4.1/22.5	0/0

Cheese Triangles, Chunky, Light, Dairylea, Kraft*, 1 triangle/23g

37/161	3.1/13.5	1.6/6.9	2/8.7	0/0

Cheese Triangles, Healthy Eating, Tesco*, 1oz/28g

52/187	4.7/16.8	1.8/6.4	2.9/10.5	0/0

Cheese Triangles, Light, Dairylea, Kraft*, 1 triangle/23g

43/185	3.3/14.5	1.7/7.6	2.5/11	0/0

Cheese Triangles, Light, Laughing Cow*, 1 triangle/17.5g

25/143	2.3/13	1.2/7	1.2/7	0/0

Cheese, 15% Fat, Sainsbury's*, 1 serving/100g

261/261	31.5/31.5	0.1/0.1	15/15	0/0

Cheese, Babybel, Fromageries Bel*, 1 cheese/20g

62/308	4.6/23	0/0	4.8/24	0/0

Cheese, Babybel, Light, Mini, Fromageries Bel*, 1 mini cheese/20g

43/214	5.3/26.5	0/0	2.4/12	0/0

Cheese, Brie, 50% Less Fat, Sainsbury's*, 1 serving/30g

62/207	7.7/25.6	0/0.1	3.5/11.6	0/0

Cheese, Brie, Continental, Healthy Eating, Tesco*, 1 serving/50g

85/170	10/20	0/0	5/10	0/0

Cheese, Cheddar, 3% Fat, Marks & Spencer*, 1oz/28g

48/172	10.1/36.2	0/0.1	0.8/2.8	0/0

Cheese, Cheddar, Half-Fat, Tesco*, 1oz/28g

73/259	8.7/30.9	0/0.1	4.2/15	0/0

Cheese, Cheddar, Mature, 16% Fat, BGTY, Sainsbury's*, 1 serving/100g

260/260	29.3/29.3	0.1/0.1	15.8/15.8	0/0

Cheese, Cheddar, Mature, GFY, Asda*, 1 serving/28g

73/259	8.7/31	0/0	4.2/15	0/0

Cheese, Cheestrings, Golden Vale*, 1 stick/21g

69/328	5.9/28	0/0	5/24	0/0

Cheese, Cottage, BGTY, Sainsbury's*, 1oz/28g

25/91	3.4/12.1	2.4/8.4	0.3/0.9	0.1/0.2

Cheese, Cottage, Healthy Choice, Asda*, 1oz/28g

25/88	3.6/13	1.1/4	0.6/2	0/0

	kcal serv/100g	prot serv/100g	carb serv/100g	fat serv/100g	fibre serv/100g

Cheese, Cottage, Less Than 5% Fat, Sainsbury's*, ½ pot/125g

131/105	15.4/12.3	5.5/4.4	5.3/4.2	0/0

Cheese, Cottage, Natural, Healthy Eating, Tesco*, 1 pot/125g

98/78	14.9/11.9	4.5/3.6	2.3/1.8	0/0

Cheese, Cottage, Virtually Fat Free, Sainsbury's*, 1oz/28g

22/80	3.6/12.9	1.8/6.5	0.1/0.3	0/0

Cheese, Cottage, with Chargrilled Vegetables, BGTY, Sainsbury's*, 1oz/28g

25/88	3.4/12.1	2.2/7.8	0.3/0.9	0.2/0.6

Cheese, Cottage, with Crunchy Vegetables, Healthy Eating, Tesco*, 1 pot/125g

91/73	12.4/9.9	6.3/5	1.9/1.5	0.3/0.2

Cheese, Cottage, with Onion & Chive, BGTY, Sainsbury's*, 1 serving/50g

42/83	6.2/12.4	3.2/6.4	0.5/0.9	0.1/0.1

Cheese, Cottage, with Onion & Chive, GFY, Asda*, 1 serving/50g

43/85	6/12	2.2/4.4	1/1.9	0.1/0.1

Cheese, Cottage, with Onion & Chives, Marks & Spencer*, 1 serving/100g

90/90	11.9/11.9	4.3/4.3	2.8/2.8	0.1/0.1

Cheese, Cottage, with Pineapple, BGTY, Sainsbury's*, 1oz/28g

24/84	2.9/10.5	2.5/8.9	0.2/0.7	0/0.1

Cheese, Cottage, with Pineapple, GFY, Asda*, 1 serving/200g

184/92	20/10	18/9	3.2/1.6	0.4/0.2

Cheese, Cottage, with Pineapple, Healthy Eating, Tesco*, 1oz/28g

21/75	2.8/10.1	1.5/5.3	0.4/1.5	0/0.1

Cheese, Cottage, with Pineapple, Healthy Living, Tesco*, ½ pot/125g

119/95	12.5/10	11.3/9	2.5/2	0.3/0.2

Cheese, Cottage, with Pineapple, Sainsbury's*, ½ pot/125g

121/97	12.4/9.9	8.5/6.8	4.3/3.4	2.6/2.1

Cheese, Cottage, with Pineapple, Shape*, 1oz/28g

20/73	2.7/9.8	2.2/8	0.1/0.2	0/0.1

Cheese, Cottage, with Pineapple, Tesco*, 1 serving/150g

158/105	13.7/9.1	14.7/9.8	5/3.3	0.2/0.1

Cheese, Dolcelatte, Tesco*, 1oz/28g

108/385	4.8/17.3	0.1/0.2	9.8/35	0.3/1.1

Cheese, Dutch Edam, 50% Less Fat, BGTY, Sainsbury's*, 1 serving/30g

69/231	9.6/31.9	0/0.1	3.4/11.4	0/0

Cheese, Edam Hard, Medium-Fat, Healthy Eating, Tesco*, 1 serving/100g

229/229	32.6/32.6	0.1/0.1	10.9/10.9	0/0

kcal serv/100g	prot serv/100g	carb serv/100g	fat serv/100g	fibre serv/100g
Cheese, Edam, Slices, Asda*, 1 serving/100g				
316/316	25/25	0/0	24/24	0/0
Cheese, Feta, Marks & Spencer*, 1 serving/20g				
62/310	3/15	0.4/2	5.4/26.8	0/0
Cheese, Feta, Tesco*, 1 serving/70g				
212/303	11.9/17	1.8/2.5	17.5/25	0/0
Cheese, Goat's, French Chevre Blanc, Sainsbury's*, 1 serving/50g				
163/326	11.5/23	0/0	13/26	0/0
Cheese, Goat's, French, Fresh, Finest, Tesco*, 1 serving/40g				
66/166	4.6/11.5	1.1/2.8	4.8/12.1	0/0
Cheese, Goat's, French, Mild, Sainsbury's*, 1 serving/30g				
48/160	3.3/11	1/3.2	3.5/11.5	0/0
Cheese, Goat's, Organic, Marks & Spencer*, 1oz/28g				
77/275	4.2/14.9	0.7/2.5	6.4/22.8	0/0.1
Cheese, Gorgonzola, Creamy, Marks & Spencer*, 1oz/28g				
92/330	5.3/19	0/0.1	7.3/26	0/0
Cheese, Gorgonzola, Somerfield*, 1oz/28g				
95/338	5.9/21	0/0	7.8/28	0/0
Cheese, Mature, Healthy Eating, Tesco*, 1oz/28g				
73/259	8.7/30.9	0/0.1	4.2/15	0/0
Cheese, Mature, Low-Fat, Weight Watchers*, 1 serving/40g				
75/188	14.4/36.1	2.3/5.8	0.9/2.3	0/0
Cheese, Mild, Low-Fat, Weight Watchers*, ⅕ pack/40g				
73/182	13.7/34.2	0/0.1	2/5	0/0
Cheese, Mild, Value, Tesco*, 1 serving/25g				
103/410	6.3/25	0/0.1	8.6/34.4	0/0
Cheese, Mozzarella, Grated Italian, Sainsbury's*, 1 serving/25g				
74/294	6.1/24.5	0.2/0.6	5.4/21.5	0/0.1
Cheese, Mozzarella, Half-Fat, Healthy Eating, Tesco*, 1 serving/125g				
231/185	25/20	0.9/0.7	12.5/10	0/0
Cheese, Mozzarella, Italian, Tesco*, 1 serving/50g				
134/268	9/18	1/2	10/20	0/0
Cheese, Mozzarella, Light, BGTY, Sainsbury's*, 1oz/28g				
48/172	5.3/19	0.4/1.5	2.8/10	0/0
Cheese, Parmesan Shavings, Asda*, 1 serving/25g				
97/388	8.3/33	0/0	7.1/28.4	0/0
Cheese, Parmesan, Continental Fresh, Grated, Tesco*, 1 tbsp/6g				
25/415	2/34	0/0.1	1.9/31	0/0

kcal serv/100g	prot serv/100g	carb serv/100g	fat serv/100g	fibre serv/100g

Cheese, Parmesan, Freshly Grated, Parmigiano Reggiano*, 1 serving/10g

| 39/388 | 3.3/33 | 0/0.1 | 2.8/28.4 | 0/0.1 |

Cheese, Port Salut, Marks & Spencer*, 1oz/28g

| 90/322 | 5.9/21 | 0.3/1 | 7.3/26 | 0/0 |

Cheese, Quark, Asda*, 1 serving/20g

| 12/61 | 2.2/11 | 0.8/3.9 | 0/0.2 | 0/0 |

Cheese, Quark, Sainsbury's*, 1 serving/16g

| 11/67 | 2/12.3 | 0.7/4.1 | 0/0.2 | 0/0.1 |

Cheese, Red Leicester, Asda*, 1 serving/15g

| 60/402 | 3.6/24 | 0/0.1 | 5.1/34 | 0/0 |

Cheese, Red Leicester, BGTY, Sainsbury's*, 1 serving/50g

| 130/259 | 15.5/31 | 0.1/0.1 | 7.5/15 | 0/0 |

Cheese, Red Leicester, Half-Fat, Asda*, ¼ pack/75g

| 194/259 | 23.3/31 | 0/0 | 11.3/15 | 0/0 |

Cheese, Red Leicester, Tesco*, 1oz/28g

| 112/399 | 6.7/23.8 | 0/0.1 | 9.4/33.7 | 0/0 |

Cheese, Ricotta, Italian, Tesco*, 1 serving/50g

| 63/125 | 5.3/10.5 | 1.4/2.8 | 4/8 | 0/0 |

Cheese, Roule, French, Sainsbury's*, 1 serving/30g

| 96/321 | 2.6/8.5 | 0.9/3 | 9.2/30.5 | 0/0 |

Cheese, Soft, Creamy, with Onion & Chives, BGTY, Sainsbury's*, 1 serving/20g

| 23/115 | 2.7/13.5 | 0.8/4 | 1/5 | 0.2/1 |

Cheese, Soft, Extra Light, Low-Fat, BGTY, Sainsbury's*, 1oz/28g

| 31/111 | 3.1/11 | 1.2/4.3 | 1.5/5.5 | 0.1/0.4 |

Cheese, Soft, Extra Light, Philadelphia, Kraft*, 1 serving/30g

| 30/101 | 3.3/11 | 0.9/3 | 1.5/5 | 0.2/0.6 |

Cheese, Soft, Extra Light, Tesco*, 1oz/28g

| 36/128 | 4.2/15 | 1/3.5 | 1.7/6 | 0/0 |

Cheese, Soft, Less Than 5% Fat, Marks & Spencer*, 1oz/28g

| 31/111 | 3.6/13 | 1.2/4.2 | 1.3/4.5 | 0.1/0.3 |

Cheese, Soft, with Chives, Light, Philadelphia, Kraft*, 1 serving/15g

| 28/185 | 1.1/7.5 | 0.5/3.4 | 2.3/15.5 | 0/0.3 |

Cheese, Soft, with Cracked Pepper, Marks & Spencer*, 1 serving/40g

| 44/110 | 5.2/13 | 1.7/4.2 | 1.8/4.5 | 0.1/0.3 |

Cheese, Soft, with Garlic & Herb, Extra Light, Healthy Eating, Tesco*, 1 serving/50g

| 63/126 | 6.8/13.5 | 2.8/5.6 | 2.8/5.5 | 0/0 |

	kcal serv/100g	prot serv/100g	carb serv/100g	fat serv/100g	fibre serv/100g

Cheese, Soft, with Onion & Chives, Extra Light, Tesco*, 1 serving/30g

36/121	3.9/12.9	1.5/5	1.7/5.5	0/0

Cream, Clotted, Fresh, Waitrose*, 1 serving/28g

157/560	0.4/1.5	0.7/2.5	16.9/60.5	0/0

Cream, Double, Asda*, 1 tbsp/13g

58/449	0.2/1.7	0.3/2.6	6.2/48	0/0

Cream, Double, Elmlea*, 1 serving/25ml

87/349	0.6/2.4	1/3.9	9/36	0.1/0.3

Cream, Double, Fresh, Marks & Spencer*, 1 tbsp/15ml

67/445	0.3/1.7	0.4/2.6	7.1/47.5	0/0

Cream, Double, Fresh, Sainsbury's*, 1 tbsp/15ml

67/445	0.3/1.7	0.4/2.6	7.1/47.5	0/0

Cream, Double, Tesco*, 1 tbsp/15ml

68/450	0.3/1.7	0.4/2.7	7.2/48	0/0

Cream, Extra Thick Double, Tesco*, 1 tbsp/15ml

68/450	0.3/1.7	0.4/2.7	7.2/48	0/0

Cream, Light Double, Elmlea*, 1 tbsp/15ml

37/248	0.4/2.8	0.6/4.1	3.7/24.5	0/0.3

Cream, Light Single, Elmlea*, 1 tbsp/15ml

19/124	0.5/3.1	1/6.4	1.4/9.5	0/0.3

Cream, Single, Fresh, Sainsbury's*, 1 tbsp/15ml

28/188	0.4/2.6	0.6/3.9	2.7/18	0/0

Cream, Soured, Fresh, Sainsbury's*, 1 tbsp/15ml

28/188	0.4/2.6	0.6/3.9	2.7/18	0/0

Cream, Soured, Tesco*, 1tbsp/15ml

28/188	0.4/2.6	0.6/3.9	2.7/18	0/0

Cream, Swirls Light, Half-Fat, Anchor*, 1 serving/30ml

14/45	0.2/0.6	0.5/1.8	1.2/3.9	0/0

Cream, Whipping, Elmlea*, 1 tbsp/15ml

43/285	0.4/2.4	0.5/3.5	4.4/29	0/0.2

Cream, Whipping, Tesco*, 1 tbsp/15ml

56/374	0.3/1.9	0.5/3.1	5.9/39.3	0/0

Crème Fraîche, BGTY, Sainsbury's*, 1oz/28g

46/164	1/3.5	1.4/5	4.2/15	0/0

Crème Fraîche, Half-Fat, Asda*, 1 serving/50g

87/173	2.5/4.9	2.3/4.6	7.5/15	0/0

Crème Fraîche, Half-Fat, Marks & Spencer*, 1fl oz/30ml

60/200	1.3/4.3	1.1/3.5	5.6/18.7	0/0

kcal serv/100g	prot serv/100g	carb serv/100g	fat serv/100g	fibre serv/100g
Crème Fraîche, Healthy Eating, Tesco*, 1fl oz/30ml				
51/170	1.1/3.5	1.5/5	4.5/15	0/0
Halloumi, Total*, 1oz/28g				
90/320	5.6/20	0.2/0.8	7/25	0/0
Milk, Dried Skimmed, Instant, Powder, Tesco*, 1oz/28g				
100/358	9.8/35	14.6/52	0.3/1.1	0/0
Milk, Evaporated, Light, Carnation*, 1 serving/25g				
28/110	1.9/7.5	2.6/10.5	1/4	0/0
Milk, Full-Fat, Pasteurised Standardised, Sainsbury's*, 1fl oz/30ml				
20/68	1/3.2	1.4/4.7	1.2/4	0/0
Milk, Semi-Skimmed, Asda*, ¼ pint/125ml				
61/49	4.3/3.4	6.3/5	2.1/1.7	0/0
Milk, Semi-Skimmed, Cravendale*, 1 serving/200ml				
98/49	6.8/3.4	10/5	3.4/1.7	0/0
Milk, Semi-Skimmed, Long-Life, Tesco*, 1 serving/20ml				
10/49	0.7/3.4	1/5	0.3/1.7	0/0
Milk, Skimmed, Fresh, Asda*, 1 glass/250ml				
85/34	8.5/3.4	12.5/5	0/0	0/0
Milk, Skimmed, Tesco*, 1 pint/50ml				
17/34	1.7/3.3	2.5/5	0.1/0.1	0/0
Milk, Soya, So Good*, 1fl oz/30ml				
15/50	1/3.4	1.6/5.3	0.5/1.7	0/0
Milk, Soya, Tesco*, 1 serving/100ml				
45/45	3.6/3.6	2.9/2.9	2.1/2.1	1/1
Milk, Whole, Fresh, Asda*, 1 serving/200ml				
128/64	6.4/3.2	9.4/4.7	7.2/3.6	0/0
Milk, Whole, Organic, Marks & Spencer*, 1 bottle/568ml				
386/68	18.2/3.2	26.7/4.7	22.7/4	0/0
Provamel*, Soya Alternative To Milk, Calcium & Vitamins, 1 carton/250ml				
113/45	9/3.6	7.3/2.9	5.3/2.1	2.5/1
Provamel*, Yoghurt, Peach, Alpro Soya, 1 pot/125g				
109/87	4.8/3.8	15.5/12.4	2.8/2.2	0.4/0.3
Yoghurt Drink, Actimel, Orange, Danone*, 1fl oz/30ml				
26/88	0.8/2.7	4.8/16	0.5/1.5	0/0
Yoghurt Drink, Actimel, Original, 0% Fat, Danone*, 1fl oz/30ml				
10/33	0.8/2.8	1.5/4.9	0/0.1	0.6/1.9
Yoghurt Drink, Actimel, Original, Danone*, 1fl oz/30ml				
25/83	0.8/2.8	4.3/14.3	0.5/1.6	0/0

kcal serv/100g	prot serv/100g	carb serv/100g	fat serv/100g	fibre serv/100g
Yoghurt Drink, Light, Yakult*, 1 pot/66ml				
31/47	0.9/1.3	8.1/12.2	0/0	1.2/1.8
Yoghurt Drink, Yakult*, 1 pot/65ml				
51/78	0.9/1.4	11.6/17.8	0.1/0.1	0/0
Yoghurt, Apple & Cinnamon, COU, Marks & Spencer*, 1 pot/150g				
68/45	6.3/4.2	9.2/6.1	0.2/0.1	0.3/0.2
Yoghurt, Apricot, Custard-Style, Shapers, Boots*, 1 pot/146g				
82/56	5.7/3.9	12.1/8.3	1.2/0.8	0.3/0.2
Yoghurt, Apricot, Healthy Living, Tesco*, 1 pot/125g				
68/54	6.4/5.1	9.9/7.9	0.4/0.3	1.4/1.1
Yoghurt, Apricot, Low-Fat, Benecol*, 1 pot/150g				
119/79	5.6/3.7	21.9/14.6	0.9/0.6	0/0
Yoghurt, Apricot, Low-Fat, Tesco*, 1 pot/125g				
111/89	6.1/4.9	16.8/13.4	2.1/1.7	0.3/0.2
Yoghurt, Apricot, Organic, Yeo Valley*, 1 pot/150g				
146/97	6.5/4.3	18.6/12.4	5/3.3	0.2/0.1
Yoghurt, Apricot, Vitality, Muller*, 1 pot/200g				
196/98	9.4/4.7	31.6/15.8	3.6/1.8	0/0
Yoghurt, Banana Choco Flakes Corner, Muller*, 1 pot/150g				
218/145	6.2/4.1	33.8/22.5	6.5/4.3	0/0
Yoghurt, Banana, Light, Muller*, 1 pot/200g				
106/53	8.8/4.4	17.4/8.7	0.2/0.1	0/0
Yoghurt, Bio Activia with Cereals, Danone*, 1 pot/125g				
123/98	5.1/4.1	19.5/15.6	2.6/2.1	0/0
Yoghurt, Bio Activia with Prunes, Danone*, 1 pot/125g				
124/99	4.1/3.3	19/15.2	3.5/2.8	0/0
Yoghurt, Bio Activia with Raspberry, Danone*, 1 pot/125g				
113/90	4.5/3.6	16.3/13	3.5/2.8	0/0
Yoghurt, Bio Fruits with Cherries, 0% Fat, Danone*, 1 pot/125g				
65/52	4.5/3.6	11.4/9.1	0.1/0.1	0/0
Yoghurt, Black Cherry, BGTY, Sainsbury's*, 1 pot/125g				
64/51	5.9/4.7	9.5/7.6	0.3/0.2	0.1/0.1
Yoghurt, Black Cherry, Extra Fruit, Low-Fat, Ski*, 1 pot/125g				
120/96	4.3/3.4	21.5/17.2	1.9/1.5	0.1/0.1
Yoghurt, Black Cherry, Fat-Free, Weight Watchers*, 1 pot/120g				
55/46	5/4.2	8.4/7	0.1/0.1	0.1/0.1
Yoghurt, Black Cherry, Thick & Fruity, Weight Watchers*, 1 pot/120.8g				
58/48	5.1/4.2	9.1/7.5	0.1/0.1	0.1/0.1

	kcal serv/100g	prot serv/100g	carb serv/100g	fat serv/100g	fibre serv/100g
Yoghurt, Blackberry & Raspberry, Fruit Corner, Muller*, 1 pot/175g					
	193/110	6.5/3.7	26.3/15	6.8/3.9	0/0
Yoghurt, Blackberry, Fat-Free, BGTY, Sainsbury's*, 1 pot/150g					
	101/67	5.1/3.4	20.4/13.6	0.2/0.1	2.4/1.6
Yoghurt, Blackberry, Sveltesse 0%, Nestle*, 1 pot/125g					
	63/50	5.4/4.3	9.9/7.9	0.1/0.1	0/0
Yoghurt, Blackcurrant Smooth, Ski*, 1 pot/125g					
	129/103	6.3/5	20.5/16.4	2.4/1.9	0/0
Yoghurt, Blackcurrant, BGTY, Sainsbury's*, 1 pot/200g					
	100/50	9.6/4.8	14.6/7.3	0.4/0.2	0.2/0.1
Yoghurt, Blackcurrant, Low-Fat, Tesco*, 1 pot/125g					
	110/88	6.1/4.9	16.5/13.2	2.1/1.7	0.5/0.4
Yoghurt, Blueberry, Fruit Corner, Muller*, 1 pot/175g					
	196/112	6.5/3.7	27.1/15.5	6.8/3.9	0/0
Yoghurt, Blueberry, Light, Muller*, 1 pot/200g					
	98/49	8.8/4.4	15.4/7.7	0.2/0.1	0/0
Yoghurt, Champagne Rhubarb, Finest, Tesco*, 1 pot/150g					
	213/142	5/3.3	25.2/16.8	10.4/6.9	0.3/0.2
Yoghurt, Citrus Fruit, Fat-Free, Weight Watchers*, 1 pot/120g					
	52/43	4.9/4.1	7.6/6.3	0.1/0.1	0.2/0.2
Yoghurt, Country Berries, Virtually Fat-Free, Light, Muller*, 1 pot/200g					
	104/52	8.8/4.4	16.6/8.3	0.2/0.1	0/0
Yoghurt, Fruit Halo Strawberry & Vanilla, Light, Muller*, 1 pot/145g					
	116/80	5.2/3.6	22.9/15.8	0.4/0.3	0/0
Yoghurt, Fruit Halo, Peach, Pineapple & Passion Fruit, Light, Muller*, 1 pot/145g					
	123/85	5.5/3.8	24.5/16.9	0.4/0.3	0/0
Yoghurt, Greek-Style, Sainsbury's*, 1 serving/200g					
	258/129	9.2/4.6	9.6/4.8	20.4/10.2	0/0
Yoghurt, Greek, 0% Fat, Total*, 1 pot/150g					
	84/56	15/10	6/4	0/0	0/0
Yoghurt, Greek, Light, Total*, 1 pot/150g					
	120/80	9/6	4.5/3	7.5/5	0/0
Yoghurt, Greek, Original, Total*, 1oz/28g					
	36/130	1.7/6	1.1/4	2.8/10	0/0
Yoghurt, Greek, Shape*, 1 serving/100g					
	108/108	7.1/7.1	12.7/12.7	2.7/2.7	0/0

	kcal serv/100g	prot serv/100g	carb serv/100g	fat serv/100g	fibre serv/100g
Yoghurt, Hazelnut, Low-Fat, Tesco*, 1 pot/150g					
	147/98	6.8/4.5	21/14	4.1/2.7	0/0
Yoghurt, Lemon, COU, Marks & Spencer*, 1 pot/200g					
	80/40	8.4/4.2	10.8/5.4	0.2/0.1	0/0
Yoghurt, Lemon, Fat-Free, Weight Watchers*, 1 pot/120g					
	49/41	4.8/4	7/5.8	0.1/0.1	0/0
Yoghurt, Mango, BGTY, Sainsbury's*, 1 pot/125g					
	66/53	6/4.8	10.4/8.3	0.1/0.1	1.5/1.2
Yoghurt, Mango, Weight Watchers*, 1 pot/120g					
	54/45	4.7/3.9	8.5/7.1	0.1/0.1	1.3/1.1
Yoghurt, Natural, Bio, Virtually Fat-Free, Tesco*, 1 serving/100g					
	47/47	5.5/5.5	5.8/5.8	0.2/0.2	0/0
Yoghurt, Natural, Biopot, Set, Onken*, 1 pot/150g					
	101/67	5.9/3.9	7.2/4.8	5.4/3.6	0/0
Yoghurt, Natural, Danone*, 1 pot/125g					
	71/57	4/3.2	4.8/3.8	3.6/2.9	0/0
Yoghurt, Natural, Low-Fat, Asda*, 1oz/28g					
	17/62	1.7/6.1	2/7.1	0.3/1	0/0
Yoghurt, Natural, Low Fat, Tesco*, 1 pot/200g					
	112/56	11.2/5.6	11.6/5.8	2.2/1.1	0/0
Yoghurt, Peach & Apricot, Healthy Living, Tesco*, 1 pot/92g					
	42/46	3.8/4.1	6.5/7.1	0.1/0.1	0/0
Yoghurt, Peach & Apricot, Shape*, 1 pot/120g					
	54/45	5.5/4.6	7/5.8	0.1/0.1	0.1/0.1
Yoghurt, Peach Melba, Sveltesse 0%, Nestle*, 1 pot/125.5g					
	64/51	5.4/4.3	10.3/8.2	0.1/0.1	0/0
Yoghurt, Peach, BGTY, Sainsbury's*, 1 pot/125g					
	61/49	5.9/4.7	9/7.2	0.3/0.2	0.3/0.2
Yoghurt, Peach, Bio Activia 0%, Danone*, 1 pot/125g					
	64/51	4.6/3.7	11.1/8.9	0/0	0/0
Yoghurt, Peach, Bio, Virtually Fat-Free, Shape*, 1 pot/120g					
	55/46	5.6/4.7	7/5.8	0.1/0.1	0.1/0.1
Yoghurt, Peach, Fat-Free, Weight Watchers*, 1 pot/118g					
	53/45	5/4.2	7.9/6.7	0.1/0.1	0.2/0.2
Yoghurt, Peach, Low-Fat, Sainsbury's*, 1 pot/125g					
	114/91	5.4/4.3	18.8/15	1.9/1.5	0.1/0.1
Yoghurt, Peach, Low-Fat, Ski*, 1 pot/125g					
	126/101	6.1/4.9	20.4/16.3	2.3/1.8	0/0

kcal serv/100g	prot serv/100g	carb serv/100g	fat serv/100g	fibre serv/100g
Yoghurt, Raspberry, Fat-Free, Weight Watchers*, 1 pot/120g				
49/41	5/4.2	6.8/5.7	0.1/0.1	0.4/0.3
Yoghurt, Raspberry, Light, Healthy Living, Tesco*, 1 pot/200g				
76/38	7.4/3.7	11.4/5.7	0.2/0.1	0/0
Yoghurt, Raspberry, Low-Fat, Asda*, 1 pot/125g				
121/97	5.9/4.7	21.3/17	1.4/1.1	0/0
Yoghurt, Raspberry, Low-Fat, Muller*, 1 pot/150g				
152/101	7.2/4.8	24.2/16.1	2.9/1.9	0/0
Yoghurt, Raspberry, Low-Fat, Ski*, 1 pot/125g				
125/100	6.1/4.9	19.9/15.9	2.4/1.9	0/0
Yoghurt, Raspberry, Low-Fat, Tesco*, 1 pot/125g				
123/98	6.1/4.9	19.4/15.5	2.3/1.8	0.4/0.3
Yoghurt, Raspberry, Virtually Fat-Free, Tesco*, 1 pot/125g				
51/41	5.1/4.1	7.3/5.8	0.3/0.2	1.4/1.1
Yoghurt, Strawberry, BGTY, Sainsbury's*, 1 pot/123g				
64/52	5.8/4.7	9.5/7.7	0.2/0.2	0.1/0.1
Yoghurt, Strawberry, COU, Marks & Spencer*, 1 pot/125g				
63/50	5.4/4.3	8/6.4	0.1/0.1	0.1/0.1
Yoghurt, Strawberry, Crumble Corner, Muller*, 1 pot/150g				
222/148	5/3.3	32.6/21.7	8/5.3	0/0
Yoghurt, Strawberry, Extra Light, 0.1% Fat, Muller*, 1 pot/200g				
118/59	10/5	17.6/8.8	0.2/0.1	0/0
Yoghurt, Strawberry, Fat-Free, Weight Watchers*, 1 pot/120g				
52/43	4.9/4.1	7.4/6.2	0.1/0.1	0.1/0.1
Yoghurt, Strawberry, Fruit Corner, Muller*, 1 pot/175g				
207/118	6.5/3.7	29.9/17.1	6.8/3.9	0/0
Yoghurt, Strawberry, Healthy Living, Tesco*, 1 pot/175g				
70/40	3.7/2.1	13.5/7.7	0.2/0.1	0.5/0.3
Yoghurt, Strawberry, Light, 99.9% Fat-Free, Ski*, 1 pot/125g				
60/48	5.9/4.7	9.6/7.7	0.1/0.1	1.3/1
Yoghurt, Strawberry, Lite, Onken*, 1 pot/235g				
110/47	12.2/5.2	14.3/6.1	0.5/0.2	0.5/0.2
Yoghurt, Strawberry, Low-Fat, Benecol*, 1 pot/150g				
119/79	5.6/3.7	22.2/14.8	0.9/0.6	0/0
Yoghurt, Strawberry, Low-Fat, Shape*, 1 pot/100g				
56/56	4.9/4.9	5.9/5.9	1.1/1.1	0.1/0.1
Yoghurt, Strawberry, Low-Fat, Ski*, 1 pot/125g				
124/99	6/4.8	19.8/15.8	2.3/1.8	0/0

	kcal serv/100g	prot serv/100g	carb serv/100g	fat serv/100g	fibre serv/100g

CRACKERS, CRISPS, SNACKS AND SNACK BARS

Bites, Bacon Rice, Asda*, 1 pack/30g

136/452	2.1/7	21/70	4.8/16	0.1/0.4

Bites, Bacon, Crispy, Shapers, Boots*, 1 bag/23g

99/431	1.8/8	15.2/66	3.5/15	0.7/3

Bites, Cheese & Ham, Sainsbury's*, 1 pack/21g

65/309	2/9.7	3/14.4	5/23.6	0.2/1

Cheddars, Mini, McVitie's*, 1 bag/30g

161/535	3.3/11	16.3/54.4	9.1/30.3	0.6/2

Cheese Puffs, Shapers, Boots*, 1 bag/16g

84/523	1/6.4	9.4/59	4.6/29	0.3/1.6

Chipsticks, Salt & Vinegar, Smiths, Walkers*, 1 bag/22g

105/476	1.5/6.8	13.1/59.5	5.2/23.5	0/0

Crackerbread, Golden Wheat, Ryvita*, 1 slice/6g

19/317	0.5/8.3	3.9/65	0.2/3.3	0.2/3.3

Crackerbread, Wholemeal, Ryvita*, 1 slice/5.6g

19/319	0.6/10.8	4.3/71.5	0.3/4.2	0.4/6.5

Crackers, 99% Fat-Free, Rakusen's*, 1 cracker/5g

18/366	0.5/10.9	4.4/88.9	0/0.9	0/0

Crackers, Bath Oliver, Jacob's*, 1 cracker/12g

52/432	1.2/9.6	8.1/67.6	1.6/13.7	0.3/2.6

Crackers, Biscuits For Cheese, TTD, Sainsbury's*, 1 cracker/8g

39/493	0.7/8.6	4.9/61	1.9/23.8	0.2/3.1

Crackers, Black Olive, Marks & Spencer*, 1 cracker/4.1g

19/485	0.3/8.3	2.4/59.4	0.9/23.5	0.2/4.3

Crackers, Bran, Jacob's*, 1 cracker/7g

32/454	0.7/9.7	4.4/62.8	1.3/18.2	0.2/3.2

Crackers, Cheddars, McVitie's*, 1 cracker/4g

22/543	0.4/10	2.2/55.1	1.3/31.3	0.1/2.6

Crackers, Cheese Biscuit Thins, Safeway*, 1 cracker/4g

22/545	0.5/11.9	2.1/52.6	1.3/31.9	0.1/2.5

Crackers, Cheese Melts, Carr's*, 1 cracker/4g

19/468	0.4/9.4	2.3/58	0.9/22.1	0.1/3

Crackers, Cheese Thins, Asda*, 1 cracker/4g

21/532	0.5/12	2/49	1.3/32	0/0

Crackers, Choice Grain, Jacob's*, 1 cracker/7g

30/435	0.6/9.2	4.6/65.4	1.1/15.2	0.3/4.7

	kcal serv/100g	prot serv/100g	carb serv/100g	fat serv/100g	fibre serv/100g

Crackers, Cornish Wafer, Jacob's*, 1 cracker/9g

	48/528	0.7/8	4.9/54.4	2.8/31.2	0.2/2.4

Crackers, Cream with Flaked Salt, TTD, Sainsbury's*, 1 cracker/7.4g

	35/500	0.6/8.5	4.5/64.8	1.6/22.9	0.2/2.7

Crackers, Cream, BGTY, Sainsbury's*, 1 cracker/8g

	32/400	0.9/10.9	5.7/71.7	0.6/7.7	0.2/3.1

Crackers, Cream, Half-Fat, Safeway*, 1 cracker/8g

	32/406	6/74.4	0.2/2.4	0.6/7.2	0.2/2.9

Crackers, Cream, Jacob's*, 1 cracker/8g

	35/438	0.8/10.2	5.4/66.9	1.2/14.4	0.2/2.9

Crackers, Cream, Lower Fat, Tesco*, 1 cracker/5g

	20/393	0.6/11	3.6/72.4	0.3/6.6	0.2/3.1

Crackers, Cream, Sainsbury's*, 1 cracker/8.3g

	34/422	0.8/9.5	5.3/66.7	1.2/15.2	0.2/2.8

Crackers, Cream, Tesco*, 1 cracker/5g

	22/444	0.4/8.4	3.5/70	0.7/14.5	0.2/3.1

Crackers, Garlic & Herb, Jacob's*, 1 cracker/100g

	27/27	0.6/0.6	4.1/4.1	1/1	0.2/0.2

Crackers, Herb & Spice, Jacob's*, 1 cracker/6g

	27/457	0.6/9.5	4.1/67.5	1/16.5	0.2/2.7

Crackers, Hovis, Jacob's*, 1 cracker/6g

	27/447	0.6/10.2	3.6/60	1.1/18.5	0.3/4.4

Crackers, Krackawheat, McVitie's*, 1 cracker/7g

	36/515	0.6/9.1	4.4/62.4	1.8/25.4	0.3/4.8

Crackers, Matzo, Rakusen's*, 1 cracker/4g

	15/370	0.4/8.8	3.2/80.2	0.1/1.5	0.2/4

Crackers, Melts, Carr's*, 1 cracker/4g

	18/451	0.4/10.2	2.3/57	0.8/20.2	0.2/5

Crackers, Olive Oil & Oregano, Italian, Jacob's*, 1 cracker/6g

	26/437	0.6/10.3	4/66.3	0.9/14.5	0.2/4

Crackers, Pesto, Jacob's*, 1 cracker/6g

	27/450	0.6/9.7	4/66.5	1/16.1	0.2/2.7

Crackers, Ritz, Original, Jacob's*, 1 cracker/3g

	15/509	0.2/6.9	1.7/55.6	0.9/28.8	0.1/2

Crackers, Sesame & Poppy, Tesco*, 1 cracker/3g

	15/506	0.3/9.4	1.6/53.7	0.8/28.2	0.1/3.4

Crackers, Tuc, Jacob's*, 1 cracker/4g

	21/530	0.3/7.8	2.5/62.2	1.1/27.8	0.1/2.1

kcal serv/100g	prot serv/100g	carb serv/100g	fat serv/100g	fibre serv/100g

Crisps, Bacon Rashers, COU, Marks & Spencer*, 1 bag/20g

| 72/360 | 1.9/9.4 | 15.5/77.5 | 0.6/2.9 | 0.7/3.5 |

Crisps, Bacon, Shapers, Boots*, 1 bag/23g

| 99/431 | 1.8/8 | 15.2/66 | 3.5/15 | 0.7/3 |

Crisps, Bagels, Sour Cream & Chive, Shapers, Boots*, 1 bag/25g

| 94/377 | 2.4/9.7 | 19.5/78 | 0.7/2.9 | 0.5/1.9 |

Crisps, Baked Beans, Walkers*, 1 bag/35g

| 184/525 | 2.3/6.5 | 17.5/50 | 11.6/33 | 1.4/4 |

Crisps, Baked Potato, COU, Marks & Spencer*, 1 bag/25g

| 88/350 | 2.1/8.5 | 19.1/76.4 | 0.6/2.3 | 1.4/5.7 |

Crisps, Barbecue, Hand-Cooked, Tesco*, 1 bag/40g

| 187/468 | 2.6/6.6 | 21.5/53.8 | 10/25.1 | 2.1/5.2 |

Crisps, Barbecue, Walkers*, 1 bag/35g

| 186/530 | 2.3/6.5 | 17.5/50 | 11.6/33 | 1.4/4.1 |

Crisps, BBQ Chilli & Mesquite, Pan-Fried, TTD, Sainsbury's*, 1 sm pack/50g

| 239/478 | 4/8 | 25.7/51.3 | 13.4/26.7 | 2.7/5.4 |

Crisps, Beef & Onion, Walkers*, 1 bag/35g

| 186/530 | 2.3/6.5 | 17.5/50 | 11.6/33 | 1.4/4.1 |

Crisps, Butter & Chive, COU, Marks & Spencer*, 1 bag/26g

| 95/365 | 2/7.7 | 20.1/77.3 | 0.5/1.9 | 1.2/4.6 |

Crisps, Caramelised Onion & Mature Cheddar Cheese, Marks & Spencer*, 1 bag/40.4g

| 208/520 | 2.6/6.6 | 20/50.1 | 13.2/33 | 2/5 |

Crisps, Chargrilled Chicken Crinkles, Shapers, Boots*, 1 bag/20g

| 96/482 | 1.3/6.6 | 12/60 | 4.8/24 | 0.8/4 |

Crisps, Chargrilled Steak, Max, Walkers*, 1 bag/55g

| 289/525 | 3.6/6.5 | 27.5/50 | 18.2/33 | 2.2/4 |

Crisps, Cheddar & Chive, Pret A Manger*, 1 bag/40g

| 187/468 | 2.8/7 | 21.5/53.8 | 9.9/24.8 | 2.4/6 |

Crisps, Cheddar & Onion, Thick & Crunchy, McCoys*, 1 bag/49g

| 250/511 | 3.2/6.6 | 25.7/52.4 | 15/30.6 | 2.3/4.7 |

Crisps, Cheese & Chives, Walkers*, 1 bag/35g

| 186/530 | 2.3/6.5 | 17.5/50 | 11.6/33 | 1.4/4.1 |

Crisps, Cheese & Onion, Flavour Crinkles, Shapers, Boots*, 1 bag/20g

| 96/482 | 1.3/6.6 | 12/60 | 4.8/24 | 0.8/4 |

Crisps, Cheese & Onion, Golden Wonder*, 1 bag/25g

| 131/524 | 1.5/6.1 | 12.3/49.2 | 8.4/33.6 | 0.5/2 |

kcal serv/100g	prot serv/100g	carb serv/100g	fat serv/100g	fibre serv/100g
Crisps, Cheese & Onion, KP*, 1 bag/25g				
134/534	1.7/6.6	12.2/48.7	8.7/34.8	1.2/4.8
Crisps, Cheese & Onion, Lites, Walkers*, 1 bag/28g				
130/465	2.1/7.5	17.1/61	5.9/21	1.1/4
Crisps, Cheese & Onion, McCoys*, 1 bag/35g				
177/506	2.2/6.4	18.8/53.8	10.3/29.5	1.4/4
Crisps, Cheese & Onion, Walkers*, 1 bag/35g				
194/553	2.3/6.5	17.5/50	11.6/33	1.4/4.1
Crisps, Cheese Curls, Shapers, Boots*, 1 bag/13.9g				
74/525	0.6/4.5	8/57	4.3/31	0.4/2.7
Crisps, Chicken & Thyme Flavour, Oven-Roasted, Walkers*, 1 bag/40g				
194/485	2.6/6.5	21.6/54	10.8/27	1.8/4.5
Crisps, Golden Lights, Golden Wonder*, 1 bag/21g				
91/435	1.1/5.4	13.5/64.5	3.6/17.2	0/0
Crisps, Hand-cooked, Marks & Spencer*, 1 bag/40g				
198/495	2.2/5.4	22.8/56.9	10.9/27.2	1.8/4.5
Crisps, Honey Roast Ham, Marks & Spencer*, 1 bag/24.5g				
133/530	1.7/6.6	12.3/49	8.5/34.1	1.2/4.6
Crisps, Lightly Salted, Kettle Chips*, 1 bag/50g				
124/247	3.2/6.4	25.8/51.5	1.5/3	3/6
Crisps, Lightly Salted, Pret A Manger*, 1 bag/40g				
198/495	2.3/5.8	23.2/58	11.4/28.5	1.7/4.3
Crisps, Lightly Salted, Traditional Pan-Fried, TTD, Sainsbury's*, 1 bag/50g				
236/472	3.1/6.2	26.8/53.6	12.9/25.8	2.6/5.1
Crisps, Marmite Flavour, Walkers*, 1 bag/34.5g				
176/510	2.2/6.5	16.9/49	11/32	1.4/4
Crisps, New York Cheddar, Kettle Chips*, 1 bag/50g				
242/483	3.4/6.7	27/53.9	13.4/26.7	2.3/4.5
Crisps, Oven Roasted Chicken & Thyme Sensations, Walkers*, 1 bag/40g				
194/485	2.6/6.5	21.6/54	10.8/27	1.8/4.5
Crisps, Paprika, Mini Hoops, Shapers, Boots*, 1 bag/13.0g				
64/494	1.1/8.7	7/54	3.5/27	0.3/2.2
Crisps, Pickled Onion, Pret A Manger*, 1 bag/40g				
177/443	3/7.5	20.8/52	9.1/22.8	2.9/7.3
Crisps, Pickled Onion, Walkers*, 1 bag/35g				
186/530	2.3/6.5	17.5/50	11.6/33	1.4/4.1
Crisps, Prawn Cocktail, BGTY, Sainsbury's*, 1 bag/25g				
118/473	1.6/6.3	14.7/58.6	5.9/23.7	1.4/5.7

kcal serv/100g	prot serv/100g	carb serv/100g	fat serv/100g	fibre serv/100g
Crisps, Prawn Cocktail, Golden Wonder*, 1 bag/25g				
130/521	1.5/5.8	12.3/49	8.4/33.5	0.5/2
Crisps, Prawn Cocktail, Walkers*, 1 bag/35g				
186/530	2.3/6.5	17.5/50	11.6/33	1.4/4.1
Crisps, Ready Salted, BGTY, Sainsbury's*, 1 bag/25g				
122/486	1.7/6.8	13.9/55.7	6.6/26.2	1.7/6.6
Crisps, Ready Salted, Golden Lights, Golden Wonder*, 1 bag/21g				
92/440	1.1/5.1	13.5/64.3	3.8/18	0/0
Crisps, Ready Salted, Golden Wonder*, 1 bag/25g				
135/539	1.4/5.5	12.5/49.9	8.8/35.3	0.5/2
Crisps, Ready Salted, KP*, 1 bag/24g				
131/545	1.3/5.6	11.5/47.9	8.8/36.8	1.2/4.9
Crisps, Ready Salted, Lites, Walkers*, 1 bag/28g				
132/470	2.1/7.5	16.8/60	6.2/22	1.1/4
Crisps, Ready Salted, Walkers*, 1 bag/35g				
186/530	2.3/6.5	19.3/55	11.9/34	1.4/4.1
Crisps, Roast Beef & Mustard, Thick-Cut, Brannigans*, 1 bag/40g				
203/507	3/7.6	20.7/51.7	12/30	1.5/3.7
Crisps, Roast Chicken Flavour, BGTY, Sainsbury's*, 1 bag/25g				
118/473	1.6/6.2	14.7/58.9	5.9/23.6	1.4/5.7
Crisps, Roast Chicken, Golden Wonder*, 1 bag/25g				
131/522	1.6/6.2	12.2/48.6	8.4/33.6	0.5/2
Crisps, Roast Chicken, Walkers*, 1 bag/35g				
184/525	2.3/6.5	17.5/50	11.6/33	1.4/4
Crisps, Salt & Black Pepper, Hand-cooked, Marks & Spencer*, 1 bag/40g				
180/450	2.3/5.7	22/55	9.2/22.9	2.1/5.2
Crisps, Salt & Vinegar, BGTY, Sainsbury's*, 1 bag/25g				
121/482	1.6/6.5	14.3/57.3	6.3/25.2	1.3/5.2
Crisps, Salt & Vinegar, Big Eat, Walkers*, 1 bag/55.0g				
289/525	3.6/6.5	27.5/50	18.2/33	2.2/4
Crisps, Salt & Vinegar, Golden Lights, Golden Wonder*, 1 bag/21g				
91/435	1/4.9	13.5/64.1	3.7/17.8	0.9/4.3
Crisps, Salt & Vinegar, Golden Wonder*, 1 bag/25g				
131/522	1.4/5.4	12.1/48.5	8.5/34	0.5/2
Crisps, Salt & Vinegar, KP*, 1 bag/25g				
133/532	1.4/5.5	12.2/48.7	8.8/35	1.2/4.7
Crisps, Salt & Vinegar, Lites, Walkers*, 1 bag/28g				
130/465	2.1/7.5	17.1/61	5.9/21	1.1/4

	kcal serv/100g	prot serv/100g	carb serv/100g	fat serv/100g	fibre serv/100g
Crisps, Salt & Vinegar, Max, Walkers*, 1 bag/55g					
	289/525	3.6/6.5	27.5/50	18.2/33	2.2/4
Crisps, Salt & Vinegar, Pret A Manger*, 1 bag/40g					
	186/465	2.7/6.8	22/55	10.1/25.3	2.4/6
Crisps, Salt & Vinegar, Walkers*, 1 bag/35g					
	186/530	2.3/6.5	17.5/50	11.6/33	1.4/4.1
Crisps, Sea Salt with Crushed Black Peppercorns, Kettle Chips*, 1 bag/50g					
	225/449	2.9/5.7	27.5/55	11.5/22.9	2.6/5.2
Crisps, Smoked Ham & Pickle, Thick-Cut, Brannigans*, 1 bag/40g					
	203/507	2.8/7	21.1/52.8	11.9/29.8	1.5/3.8
Crisps, Smoky Bacon, BGTY, Sainsbury's*, 1 bag/25g					
	118/472	1.6/6.5	14.6/58.5	5.9/23.6	1.4/5.7
Crisps, Smoky Bacon, Golden Wonder*, 1 bag/25g					
	131/523	1.5/5.9	12.3/49.1	8.4/33.7	0.5/2
Crisps, Smoky Bacon, Walkers*, 1 bag/35g					
	186/530	2.3/6.5	17.5/50	11.6/33	1.4/4.1
Crisps, Sour Cream & Chive Crinkles, Shapers, Boots*, 1 bag/20g					
	96/482	1.3/6.6	12/60	4.8/24	0.8/4
Crisps, Sour Cream & Chive, Reduced-Fat, Marks & Spencer*, 1 bag/40g					
	192/480	2.6/6.5	24/60	9.6/24	2.6/6.5
Crisps, Sour Cream & Chives, Jordans*, 1 bag/30g					
	125/417	2.2/7.3	21/69.9	3.6/12	0.8/2.7
Crisps, Sour Cream & Onion, Lights, Golden Wonder*, 1 bag/21g					
	91/435	1.1/5.4	13.5/64.5	3.6/17.2	1.2/5.9
Crisps, Spare Rib Flavour, Chinese, Walkers*, 1 bag/34.5g					
	184/525	2.3/6.5	17.5/50	11.6/33	1.4/4
Crisps, Spiced Chilli, McCoys*, 1 bag/50g					
	250/500	3.1/6.1	27.1/54.2	14.4/28.8	2.1/4.2
Crisps, Thai Sweet Chilli, Sensations, Walkers*, 1 bag/35g					
	170/485	2.3/6.5	18.9/54	9.5/27	1.6/4.5
Crisps, Tomato Ketchup, Walkers*, 1 bag/35g					
	186/530	2.3/6.5	17.5/50	11.6/33	1.4/4.1
Crisps, Traditional, Hand-Cooked, Finest, Tesco*, 1 bag/150g					
	708/472	9.6/6.4	79.4/52.9	39.2/26.1	7.7/5.1
Crisps, Vegetable Chips, Pret A Manger*, 1 bag/25g					
	126/504	1.4/5.6	9.3/37.2	9.2/36.8	2.5/10
Crisps, Vegetable, Pan-Fried, Sainsbury's*, ¼ bag/25g					
	102/407	1.2/4.6	9.1/36.5	6.8/27	1.6/6.4

kcal serv/100g	prot serv/100g	carb serv/100g	fat serv/100g	fibre serv/100g
Dairylea Dunkers, Jumbo Munch, Dairylea, Kraft*, 1 serving/50g				
150/300	3.6/7.2	13.3/26.5	9.3/18.5	0.6/1.2
Dairylea Dunkers, Smokey Bacon, Dairylea, Kraft*, 1 pack/45g				
135/300	3.3/7.3	10.8/24	8.8/19.5	0/0
Dairylea Lunchables, Double Cheese, Dairylea, Kraft*, 1 pack/110g				
413/375	19.8/18	18.7/17	28.6/26	0.3/0.3
Dairylea Lunchables, Harvest Ham, Dairylea, Kraft*, 1 pack/110g				
314/285	18.2/16.5	18.2/16.5	18.7/17	0.3/0.3
Discos, Pickled Onion, KP*, 1 bag/31g				
155/500	1.1/3.7	18.2/58.6	8.6/27.8	0.9/2.9
Discos, Salt & Vinegar, KP*, 1 bag/31g				
153/493	1.2/3.8	17.7/57.2	8.6/27.6	0.9/2.8
Doritos, Cool Original, Walkers*, 1 bag/40g				
204/510	3/7.5	24.8/62	10.4/26	1.4/3.5
Doritos, Hint of Lime, Walkers*, 1 bag/35g				
170/485	2.6/7.5	20.3/58	8.8/25	2.6/7.5
Doritos, Mexican Hot, Walkers*, 1 bag/40g				
202/505	3.2/8	22.8/57	10.8/27	1.4/3.5
Doritos, Tangy Cheese, Walkers*, 1 bag/40g				
210/525	2.8/7	25.2/63	10.8/27	1.4/3.5
Frazzles, Bacon, Smiths, Walkers*, 1 bag/23g				
108/470	1.8/8	13.6/59	5.2/22.4	0/0
French Fries, Cheese & Onion, Walkers*, 1 bag/22g				
94/425	1.2/5.4	14.1/64	3.5/16	0.9/4.2
French Fries, Ready Salted, Walkers*, 1 bag/22g				
95/430	1.1/5.1	14.1/64	3.7/17	0.9/4.3
French Fries, Salt & Vinegar, COU, Marks & Spencer*, 1 pack/25g				
88/350	1.3/5.1	20.2/80.9	0.4/1.6	0.6/2.3
French Fries, Salt & Vinegar, Eat Smart, Safeway*, 1 pack/20g				
75/375	1/5.1	16.2/80.9	0.3/1.6	0.5/2.3
French Fries, Salt & Vinegar, Walkers*, 1 bag/22g				
92/420	1.1/5	13.9/63	3.5/16	0.9/4.2
French Fries, Worcester Sauce, Walkers*, 1 bag/22g				
92/420	1.1/5.1	14.1/64	3.5/16	0.9/4.2
Fries, Scampi, Smiths, Walkers*, 1 bag/27g				
134/496	3.5/13	14.2/52.5	7/26	0/0
Frisps, Tasty Cheese & Onion, Frisps*, 1 bag/31g				
162/521	2/6.3	16.2/52.4	9.9/31.8	1.3/4.3

	kcal serv/100g	prot serv/100g	carb serv/100g	fat serv/100g	fibre serv/100g
Hula Hoops, Barbecue Beef Flavour, Hula Hoops*, 1 bag/34g					
	170/500	1.3/3.9	20/58.7	9.4/27.5	0.8/2.4
Hula Hoops, Cheese & Onion, KP*, 1 bag/34g					
	179/525	1.3/3.9	19.3/56.8	10.7/31.4	0.7/2.2
Monster Munch, Flamin' Hot, Walkers*, 1 bag/25g					
	118/470	1.8/7	13.8/55	6.3/25	0.5/1.8
Monster Munch, Pickled Onion, Walkers*, 1 bag/25g					
	120/480	1.5/6	14.3/57	6.3/25	0.4/1.7
Monster Munch, Roast Beef, Walkers*, 1 pack/25g					
	119/475	1.7/6.6	14.5/58	6/24	0.4/1.5
Nik Naks, Cream 'n' Cheesy, Golden Wonder*, 1 bag/34g					
	185/545	1.7/5.1	19.1/56.1	11.4/33.4	0/0
Nik Naks, Nice 'n' Spicy, Golden Wonder*, 1 bag/34g					
	185/545	1.6/4.7	18.9/55.5	11.4/33.4	0.3/1
Nik Naks, Rib 'n' Saucy, Golden Wonder*, 1 bag/34g					
	185/545	1.7/5.1	18.9/55.7	11.4/33.4	0.4/1.1
Nik Naks, Scampi 'n' Lemon, Golden Wonder*, 1 bag/34g					
	195/573	1.7/5	16.9/49.6	13.4/39.4	0.5/1.4
Onion Rings, Pickled, COU, Marks & Spencer*, 1 bag/20g					
	68/340	0.9/4.7	16.1/80.7	0.3/1.5	0.7/3.7
Onion Rings, Pickled, Healthy Eating, Tesco*, 1 pack/15g					
	51/340	0.9/6.2	11.2/74.7	0.3/1.8	1/6.5
Popcorn, Butter Toffee, Tesco*, 1 pack/350g					
	1418/405	7.7/2.2	286/81.7	27/7.7	15.1/4.3
Popcorn, Ready Salted, Microwave, Popz*, 1 serving/20g					
	101/504	1.4/7	10.3/51.5	6/30	1.8/9.2
Popcorn, Salted, Blockbuster*, 1 bowl/25g					
	121/482	2.1/8.2	14.5/57.8	6.1/24.3	1.4/5.5
Popcorn, Sweet, Blockbuster*, 1 serving/100g					
	470/470	6.2/6.2	67.2/67.2	17.9/17.9	6/6
Popcorn, Toffee, 90% Fat-Free, Butterkist*, 1 pack/35g					
	142/406	1/2.8	27.2/77.7	3.3/9.3	0/0
Pork Scratchings, KP*, 1 pack/20g					
	125/624	9.5/47.3	0.1/0.5	9.6/48.1	0.1/0.5
Pork Scratchings, Tavern Snacks*, 1 pack/30g					
	187/624	14.2/47.3	0.2/0.5	14.4/48.1	0.2/0.5
Pot Noodle*, Beef & Tomato, 1 pot/90g					
	382/424	9.6/10.7	54.3/60.3	14/15.5	3.3/3.7

kcal serv/100g	prot serv/100g	carb serv/100g	fat serv/100g	fibre serv/100g
Pot Noodle*, Chow Mein, 1 pot/89g				
385/433	10.3/11.6	53.8/60.5	14.2/16	2.4/2.7
Pot Noodle*, Nice 'n' Spicy, 1 pot/87g				
380/437	8.4/9.7	53.5/61.5	14.7/16.9	2.3/2.7
Pot Noodle*, Spicy Curry, 1 pot/89g				
379/426	8.7/9.8	54.7/61.5	13.9/15.6	2.7/3
Pot Noodle*, Sweet & Sour, 1 pot/86g				
376/437	8.1/9.4	54.4/63.2	13.9/16.2	2.3/2.7
Prawn Crackers, Asda*, 1 serving/25g				
134/535	0.5/2	13.3/53	8.8/35	0/0
Prawn Crackers, Marks & Spencer*, 1 pack/15g				
83/550	0.5/3	9.3/62.3	4.8/32	0/0
Prawn Crackers, Sainsbury's*, 1 cracker/3g				
16/537	0.1/2.4	1.8/60.4	1/31.7	0/0.8
Prawn Crackers, Tesco*, ⅓ pack/20g				
114/568	0.7/3.7	8.8/44	8.4/41.9	0.1/0.5
Pringles, Barbecue, Pringles*, 1 serving/50g				
267/533	2.5/4.9	24/48	18/36	2.6/5.1
Pringles, Cheese & Onion, Pringles*, 1 serving/50g				
266/532	2.3/4.5	23.5/47	18/36	2.5/4.9
Pringles, Original, Pringles*, 1 serving/50g				
274/547	2.4/4.7	23.5/47	19/38	2.6/5.1
Pringles, Paprika, Pringles*, 1 serving/50g				
268/535	2.9/5.7	23/46	18/36	2.5/5
Pringles, Salt & Vinegar, Pringles*, 1 serving/50g				
265/530	2.3/4.5	23.5/47	18/36	2.4/4.8
Pringles, Sour Cream & Onion, Pringles*, 1 serving/50g				
270/539	2.7/5.3	23/46	18.5/37	2.5/4.9
Pringles, Sour Cream & Onion, Right, Pringles*, 1 serving/50g				
233/466	2.7/5.4	28/56	12.5/25	2.3/4.6
Quavers, Cheese, Walkers*, 1 bag/16g				
82/515	0.5/3	9.8/61	4.6/29	0.2/1.2
Quavers, Prawn Cocktail, Walkers*, 1 bag/16g				
82/510	0.4/2.6	9.8/61	4.5/28	0.2/1.2
Quavers, Salt & Vinegar, Walkers*, 1 bag/16g				
80/500	0.4/2.3	9.3/58	4.6/29	0.2/1.1
Rice Crackers, Japanese, Mini, Sunrise*, 1 serving/50g				
180/360	3.5/7	41.5/83	0/0	3.5/7

kcal serv/100g	prot serv/100g	carb serv/100g	fat serv/100g	fibre serv/100g
Rice Crackers, Thin, Blue Dragon*, 3 crackers/5g				
20/395	0.3/6.1	4.2/84.4	0.2/3.7	0/0
Skips, Bacon, KP*, 1 pack/17.1g				
81/474	1.1/6.5	10.6/62.1	3.8/22.2	0.4/2.3
Skips, Prawn Cocktail, KP*, 1 bag/17g				
88/516	0.6/3.4	10.2/59.9	5/29.2	0.2/1.4
Snack-a-Jacks, Barbecue Flavour, Jumbo, Quaker*, 1 serving/10g				
38/376	0.7/7	8/80	0.3/2.5	0.1/1
Snack-a-Jacks, Barbecue Flavour, Quaker*, 1 pack/30g				
126/421	2/6.5	23.1/77	3/10	0.3/1
Snack-a-Jacks, Caramel Flavour, Jumbo, Quaker*, 1 cake/13g				
52/397	0.7/5	11.3/87	0.3/2.5	0.1/1
Snack-a-Jacks, Caramel, Quaker*, 1 bag/35g				
140/401	1.9/5.5	30.1/86	1.2/3.5	0.2/0.5
Snack-a-Jacks, Cheddar Cheese Flavour, Jumbo, Quaker*, 1 cake/10g				
40/399	0.9/8.5	8.1/81	0.4/4	0.1/1
Snack-a-Jacks, Cheddar Cheese Flavour, Quaker*, 1 bag/30g				
128/427	2.4/8	21.9/73	3/10	0.3/1
Snack-a-Jacks, Chocolate, Jumbo, Quaker*, 1 cake/12g				
49/406	0.7/5.5	10.2/85	0.5/4.5	0.1/1
Snack-a-Jacks, Creamy Lemon Flavour, Quaker*, 1 pack/35g				
137/390	1.8/5	30.5/87	0.9/2.5	0.4/1
Snack-a-Jacks, Crispy Cheese, Quaker*, 1 pack/30g				
122/407	2.4/8	23.4/78	2/6.5	0.3/1
Snack-a-Jacks, Salt & Vinegar, Quaker*, 1 bag/30g				
123/410	2/6.5	23.3/77.5	2.4/8	0.3/1
Snack-a-Jacks, Savoury Salted, Quaker*, 1 bag/30g				
124/414	2.3/7.5	23.1/77	2.4/8	0.3/1
Snack-a-Jacks, Sour Cream & Chive, Quakers*, 1 pack/30g				
123/410	2.3/7.5	23.1/77	2.4/8	0.3/1
Snack Bars, All-Day Breakfast, Weight Watchers*, 1 bar/50g				
179/358	3.4/6.8	36.1/72.2	2.3/4.6	1.6/3.2
Snack Bars, Alpen* Apple & Blackberry with Yoghurt, Weetabix*, 1 bar/29g				
122/421	1.7/5.7	21.2/73	3.4/11.8	0/0
Snack Bars, Alpen*, Fruit & Nut with Milk Chocolate, Weetabix*, 1 bar/29g				
125/431	2/7	19.7/68	4.2/14.5	0/0
Snack Bars, Alpen*, Fruit & Nut, Weetabix*, 1 bar/28g				
110/394	1.8/6.5	19.9/71.2	2.6/9.2	0/0

kcal serv/100g	prot serv/100g	carb serv/100g	fat serv/100g	fibre serv/100g
Snack Bars, Alpen*, Strawberry with Yoghurt, Weetabix, 1 bar/29g				
123/425	1.6/5.6	21.3/73.5	3.5/12.1	0/0
Snack Bars, AM, Cereal, Apple, McVitie's*, 1 bar/40g				
160/400	1.7/4.3	26.2/65.5	5.4/13.5	1.2/3
Snack Bars, AM, Cereal, Berry, McVitie's*, 1 bar/30g				
146/486	2/6.5	20.6/68.8	6.2/20.5	0.2/0.5
Snack Bars, AM, Cereal, Fruit & Nut, McVitie's*, 1 bar/35g				
167/477	2.3/6.6	22.7/64.9	7.5/21.4	1.2/3.4
Snack Bars, AM, Cereal, Grapefruit, McVitie's*, 1 bar/35g				
136/389	1.8/5.1	24.8/70.9	3.3/9.4	1.1/3.1
Snack Bars, AM, Cereal, Orange Marmalade, McVitie's*, 1 bar/40g				
151/378	1.8/4.5	21.3/53.3	7.2/18	0.7/1.8
Snack Bars, AM, Cereal, Raisin & Nut, McVitie's*, 1 bar/35.1g				
148/422	2.2/6.4	21.7/62.1	5.7/16.4	0.8/2.4
Snack Bars, AM, Cereal, Strawberry, McVitie's*, 1 bar/34.9g				
138/395	2/5.7	24.7/70.5	3.5/10.1	0.9/2.7
Snack Bars, AM, Muesli Fingers, McVitie's*, 1 bar/35g				
154/440	2.1/6	20.9/59.8	6.9/19.6	1.1/3.1
Snack Bars, Apple & Cinnamon, Chewy, GFY, Asda*, 1 bar/27g				
95/351	1.6/6	20/74	0.9/3.4	2.2/8
Snack Bars, Apricot & Almond, Chewy & Crisp, Tesco*, 1 bar/27g				
122/452	1.7/6.2	16.2/60	5.6/20.8	0.7/2.6
Snack Bars, Blue Riband, Double Choc, Nestle*, 1 bar/22g				
113/513	1.1/5.1	13.9/63.1	5.9/26.7	0.2/1.1
Snack Bars, Brunch, Cranberry & Orange, Cadbury's*, 1 bar/35g				
154/440	2.2/6.2	23.8/67.9	5.6/15.9	0/0
Snack Bars, Brunch, Hazelnut, Cadbury's*, 1 bar/35g				
163/465	2.5/7.1	21.4/61	7.6/21.6	0/0
Snack Bars, Cappuccino Coll, Marks & Spencer*, 1 bar/35g				
185/529	2.1/6	17.5/50	12.3/35	0.4/1
Snack Bars, Caramel Crisp, Go Ahead, McVitie's*, 1 bar/33g				
141/428	1.6/4.8	24.8/75.1	4/12	0.3/0.8
Snack Bars, Cereal, Apple & Raisin, Harvest, Quaker*, 1 bar/22g				
87/396	1.1/5	15.4/70	2.5/11.5	0.9/4
Snack Bars, Cereal, Apple & Sultana, Go Ahead, McVitie's*, 1 bar/35g				
137/392	1.4/4.1	27.2/77.6	2.5/7.2	0.6/1.8
Snack Bars, Cereal, Apple, Chewy, BGTY, Sainsbury's*, 1 bar/25g				
85/340	1.2/4.8	19/76	0.5/2	0.5/2

kcal serv/100g	prot serv/100g	carb serv/100g	fat serv/100g	fibre serv/100g
Snack Bars, Cereal, Apricot & Yoghurt, Shapers, Boots*, 1 bar/27g				
99/366	1/3.7	20.3/75	1.5/5.7	0.9/3.3
Snack Bars, Cereal, Apricot Yoghurt, COU, Marks & Spencer*, 1 bar/25g				
90/360	1.5/6.1	19.2/76.6	0.6/2.5	0.7/2.9
Snack Bars, Cereal, Apricot, Perfectly Balanced, Waitrose*, 1 bar/25g				
89/356	1.2/4.9	19.2/76.9	0.8/3.2	1/3.8
Snack Bars, Cereal, Berry & Cream, COU, Marks & Spencer*, 1 bar/20g				
72/360	1.1/5.3	15.9/79.7	0.5/2.3	0.6/3.1
Snack Bars, Cereal, Chewy & Crisp with Choc Chips, Tesco*, 1 bar/27g				
125/463	2.5/9.2	14.6/54	6.3/23.4	1/3.8
Snack Bars, Cereal, Chewy & Crisp with Roasted Nuts, Tesco*, 1 bar/27g				
127/471	2.5/9.3	15.4/57	6.2/22.9	0.7/2.5
Snack Bars, Cereal, Coconut Muesli, Kellogg's*, 1 bar/25g				
108/430	1.3/5	16.3/65	4.3/17	1.3/5
Snack Bars, Cereal, Cranberrry & Blackcurrant, Healthy Living, Tesco*, 1 bar/25g				
79/316	1.4/5.5	17.1/68.2	0.6/2.3	2.2/8.6
Snack Bars, Cereal, Cranberry & Orange, Weight Watchers*, 1 bar/28g				
102/365	1.3/4.5	21.7/77.6	1.1/4.1	0.6/2.3
Snack Bars, Cereal, Cranberry, Eat Smart, Safeway*, 1 bar/25g				
86/345	1.2/4.7	18.9/75.7	0.6/2.3	1/3.9
Snack Bars, Cereal, Frosties & Milk, Kellogg's*, 1 bar/27g				
122/450	2.7/10	18.4/68	4.3/16	0.3/1
Snack Bars, Cereal, Fruit & Nut Break, Jordans*, 1 bar/37g				
135/374	2.5/7	22.8/63.2	3.7/10.4	2.9/8.1
Snack Bars, Cereal, Golden Grahams, Nestle*, 1 bar/25g				
106/425	1.6/6.5	17.2/68.8	3.4/13.7	0/0
Snack Bars, Cereal, Granola, Starbucks*, 1 bar/90g				
324/360	7.2/8	34.7/38.6	19.2/21.3	4.3/4.8
Snack Bars, Cereal, Hazelnut & Pistachio, Go Ahead, McVitie's*, 1 bar/35g				
147/419	1.9/5.4	23.9/68.3	4.8/13.8	0.8/2.3
Snack Bars, Cereal, Honey, Sultana & Sesame, COU, Marks & Spencer*, 1 bar/20g				
70/350	1/4.8	16.3/81.7	0.4/2.1	0.7/3.4
Snack Bars, Cereal, Lemon & Sultana, Eat Smart, Safeway*, 1 bar/25g				
89/355	1.1/4.2	19.6/78.4	0.6/2.2	0.7/2.6
Snack Bars, Cereal, Maple, Healthy Living, Tesco*, 1 bar/25g				
93/372	1.4/5.5	19.2/76.6	1.2/4.9	0.5/2

kcal serv/100g	prot serv/100g	carb serv/100g	fat serv/100g	fibre serv/100g

Snack Bars, Cereal, Muesli Break, Breakfast in a Bar, Jordans*, 1 bar/46g

| 178/387 | 2.7/5.9 | 30.6/66.6 | 5/10.8 | 2/4.3 |

Snack Bars, Cereal, Raisin & Nut Snack Bar, Benecol*, 1 bar/25g

| 98/390 | 1/3.9 | 17.1/68.5 | 2.8/11.1 | 0.5/2 |

Snack Bars, Cereal, Rice Krispies & Milk, Kellogg's*, 1 bar/20g

| 84/421 | 1.4/7 | 14/70 | 2.6/13 | 0.1/0.3 |

Snack Bars, Cereal, Roast Hazelnut, Organic, Jordans*, 1 bar/33g

| 150/455 | 2.6/8 | 18.7/56.7 | 7.2/21.8 | 2.6/7.8 |

Snack Bars, Cereal, Roasted Peanut, Weight Watchers*, 1 bar/26g

| 104/400 | 2.5/9.5 | 17.2/66.1 | 2.8/10.8 | 0.7/2.8 |

Snack Bars, Cereal, Sultana & Honey, Jordans*, 1 bar/36g

| 130/361 | 2.2/6 | 23.7/65.9 | 3/8.2 | 3.3/9.2 |

Snack Bars, Cereal, Toffee Apple, Eat Smart, Safeway*, 1 bar/25g

| 23/90 | 0.3/1 | 4.9/19.6 | 0.2/0.7 | 0.2/0.7 |

Snack Bars, Cereal, White Chocolate Muesli, Kellogg's*, 1 bar/25g

| 110/440 | 1.3/5 | 17.5/70 | 4/16 | 0.5/2 |

Snack Bars, Cheerios Cereal & Milk Bar, Nestle*, 1 bar/24g

| 98/407 | 1.8/7.6 | 15.5/64.5 | 3.2/13.2 | 0/0 |

Snack Bars, Chocolate & Orange, Shapers, Boots*, 1 bar/26g

| 98/378 | 1.1/4.2 | 19/73 | 3.4/13 | 0.4/1.5 |

Snack Bars, Chocolate & Raisin, Shapers, Boots*, 1 bar/27g

| 95/353 | 1.3/4.7 | 20.5/76 | 2.5/9.1 | 0.7/2.7 |

Snack Bars, Chocolate Brownie, Big Softies, To Go, Fox's*, 1 bar/25g

| 87/348 | 1.4/5.5 | 18.7/74.9 | 0.7/2.9 | 0/0 |

Snack Bars, Chocolate, Crisp, Weight Watchers*, 1 bar/25g

| 92/369 | 1.4/5.4 | 18.8/75.1 | 2.6/10.2 | 0.2/0.8 |

Snack Bars, Coco Pops & Milk Bar, Kellogg's*, 1 bar/20g

| 90/450 | 1.6/8 | 13.8/69 | 3.2/16 | 0.2/1 |

Snack Bars, Coconut Chocolate Crisp, Weight Watchers*, 1 bar/25g

| 89/356 | 0.9/3.6 | 17.8/71.2 | 2.6/10.4 | 0.8/3.2 |

Snack Bars, Crispy Caramel, Shapers, Boots*, 1 bar/24g

| 96/400 | 0.9/3.9 | 16.1/67 | 4.1/17 | 0.1/0.4 |

Snack Bars, Crunchy, Honey & Almond, Jordans*, 1 bar/33g

| 153/465 | 2.9/8.8 | 18.5/56.1 | 7.5/22.8 | 1.9/5.8 |

Snack Bars, Crunchy, Maple & Pecan, Jordans*, 1 bar/33g

| 153/464 | 2.5/7.7 | 18.7/56.8 | 7.6/22.9 | 2.1/6.5 |

Snack Bars, Fruit & Nut Crisp, Go Ahead, McVitie's*, 1 bar/23.0g

| 99/430 | 1.2/5.3 | 16.4/71.3 | 3.2/13.7 | 0.4/1.7 |

kcal serv/100g	prot serv/100g	carb serv/100g	fat serv/100g	fibre serv/100g
Snack Bars, Frusli, Absolutely Apricot, Jordans*, 1 bar/33g				
120/365	1.7/5	21.1/63.8	3.3/10	2.1/6.3
Snack Bars, Frusli, Blueberry Burst, Jordans*, 1 bar/33g				
133/402	1.6/4.8	22.7/68.8	3.9/11.9	1.5/4.6
Snack Bars, Frusli, Cranberry & Apple, Jordans*, 1 bar/34g				
131/385	1.7/5.1	23.4/68.9	3.4/9.9	2/5.8
Snack Bars, Frusli, Raisin & Hazelnut, Jordans*, 1 bar/34g				
145/426	2.1/6.3	20.8/61.3	5.9/17.3	1.3/3.9
Snack Bars, Frusli, Tangy Citrus, Jordans*, 1 bar/33g				
130/393	1.4/4.1	23.2/70.4	3.5/10.5	1.4/4.3
Snack Bars, Frusli, Wild Berries, Jordans*, 1 bar/33g				
128/387	1.5/4.6	24.8/75.2	2.5/7.5	1.1/3.3
Snack Bars, Harvest Cheweee, Choc Chip, Quaker*, 1 bar/22g				
94/426	1.3/6	14.1/64	3.5/16	0.7/3
Snack Bars, Harvest Cheweee, Toffee, Quaker*, 1 bar/22g				
94/427	1.1/5	15/68.2	3.3/15	0.7/3.2
Snack Bars, Harvest Cheweee, White Chocolate Chip, Quaker*, 1 bar/22g				
94/425	1.3/6	14.7/67	3.4/15.5	0.8/3.5
Snack Bars, Milk Chocolate Chip & Hazelnut, Snack, Benecol*, 1 bar/25g				
99/395	1.2/4.7	16.1/64.5	3.3/13.1	0.6/2.5
Snack Bars, Nutri-Grain, Apple, Kellogg's*, 1 bar/37g				
130/350	1.5/4	25.2/68	3/8	1.1/3
Snack Bars, Nutri-Grain, Blueberry, Kellogg's*, 1 bar/37g				
130/350	1.5/4	25.2/68	3/8	1.1/3
Snack Bars, Nutri-Grain, Cherry, Kellogg's*, 1 bar/37g				
133/360	1.5/4	25.2/68	3/8	1.1/3
Snack Bars, Nutri-Grain, Chocolate, Kellogg's*, 1 bar/37g				
137/370	1.7/4.5	24.8/67	3.7/10	1.1/3
Snack Bars, Nutri-Grain, Elevenses Ginger, Kellogg's*, 1 bar/45g				
170/378	2.5/5.6	30/66.7	4/8.9	1.5/3.3
Snack Bars, Nutri-Grain, Elevenses, Kellogg's*, 1 bar/45g				
162/360	2.3/5	30.2/67	3.6/8	1.6/3.5
Snack Bars, Nutri-Grain, Strawberry, Kellogg's*, 1 bar/37g				
133/360	1.5/4	25.5/69	3/8	1.1/3
Snack Bars, Orange Crunch, Go Ahead, McVitie's*, 1 bar/23g				
99/430	0.9/4.1	17.9/78	2.9/12.8	0.2/0.8
Snack Bars, Raisin & Hazelnut, Weight Watchers*, 1 bar/24g				
95/396	1.2/5	17.1/71.3	2.4/10	0.7/2.9

kcal serv/100g	prot serv/100g	carb serv/100g	fat serv/100g	fibre serv/100g
Snack Bars, Tracker, Breakfast Banana, Mars*, 1 bar/37g				
176/476	1.7/4.7	23.4/63.3	8.4/22.6	3.5/9.4
Snack Bars, Tracker, Chocolate Chip, Mars*, 1 bar/37g				
188/509	3.2/8.6	20.6/55.8	10.3/27.9	0/0
Snack Bars, Tracker, Roasted Nut, Mars*, 1 bar/27g				
139/515	2.6/9.8	14.4/53.5	7.9/29.1	0/0
Snack Bars, Tracker, Strawberry, Mars*, 1 bar/27g				
129/479	1.3/4.7	17.2/63.6	6.2/22.8	0/0
Space Raiders, Pickled Onion, Space Raiders*, 1 bag/16g				
74/461	1.1/7	9.8/61.4	3.3/20.8	0.5/3.4
Space Raiders, Salt & Vinegar, Space Raiders*, 1 bag/16.9g				
81/478	1.2/6.9	10.5/61.7	3.8/22.6	0.4/2.2
Squares, Rice Krispies, Chocolate Caramel, Kellogg's*, 1 bar/21g				
90/430	0.9/4.5	15.5/74	2.7/13	0.1/0.5
Squares, Rice Krispies, Chocolate, Kellogg's*, 1 bar/18g				
74/410	0.8/4.5	13.7/76	1.8/10	0.3/1.5
Thai Bites, Lightly Salted, Jacob's*, 1 pack/25g				
94/375	1.7/6.9	19.9/79.7	0.8/3.2	0/0.1
Thai Bites, Oriental Spice, Jacob's*, 1 pack/25g				
93/373	1.8/7.1	19.5/78	0.9/3.6	0.1/0.2
Thai Bites, Seaweed Flavour, Jacob's*, 1 pack/25g				
94/377	1.8/7.1	20/80	0.8/3.2	0.1/0.5
Thai Bites, Sweet Herb, Jacob's*, 1 pack/25g				
93/372	1.8/7.1	19.7/78.8	0.8/3.2	0.1/0.2
Tortilla Chips, Chilli Flavour, Somerfield*, 1 serving/50g				
242/484	3.4/6.8	30.1/60.1	12.1/24.1	2.7/5.3
Tortilla Chips, Cool, Salted, Sainsbury's*, 1 serving/50g				
253/506	3.3/6.5	29.3/58.6	13.7/27.3	2.2/4.3
Tortilla Chips, Cool, Tesco*, 1 serving/50g				
246/492	3.7/7.4	29.5/58.9	12.6/25.2	2.3/4.6
Tortilla Chips, Lightly Salted, Marks & Spencer*, 1 serving/20g				
99/495	1.4/7	12.4/62.2	5/25	0.8/4
Tortilla Chips, Lightly Salted, Waitrose*, 1 bag/40g				
188/471	2.6/6.5	23.4/58.6	9.4/23.4	1.7/4.3
Tortilla Chips, Waitrose*, 1 serving/25g				
128/510	2/7.9	16.4/65.5	6/24	1.1/4.5
Twiglets, Original, Jacob's*, 1 bag/30g				
117/390	3.6/12	18.4/61.3	3.2/10.8	2/6.8

kcal serv/100g	prot serv/100g	carb serv/100g	fat serv/100g	fibre serv/100g

Twiglets, Tangy, Jacob's*, 1 bag/30g

| 136/454 | 2.4/8.1 | 16.8/55.9 | 6.6/22 | 1.6/5.4 |

Waffles, Barbecue Flavour, American-Style, Shapers, Boots*, 1 pack/20g

| 95/476 | 0.9/4.5 | 13/65 | 4.4/22 | 0.7/3.7 |

Waffles, Ready Salted, Marks & Spencer*, 1 bag/40g

| 194/485 | 0.8/2.1 | 26.2/65.6 | 9.4/23.6 | 0.6/1.6 |

Waffles, Smokey Bacon, BGTY, Sainsbury's*, 1 bag/12g

| 41/344 | 0.7/5.6 | 9.2/76.3 | 0.2/1.8 | 0.2/1.5 |

Wheat Crunchies, Bacon, Crispy, Golden Wonder*, 1 bag/35g

| 172/491 | 3.9/11.1 | 19.6/55.9 | 8.7/24.9 | 1/2.8 |

Wheat Crunchies, Spicy Tomato, Golden Wonder*, 1 bag/35g

| 171/488 | 3.7/10.7 | 19.4/55.5 | 8.7/24.8 | 1.1/3 |

Wheat Crunchies, Worcester Sauce, Golden Wonder*, 1 bag/35g

| 170/487 | 3.7/10.7 | 19.2/54.9 | 8.7/24.9 | 1.1/3 |

Winders, Real Fruit, Kellogg's*, 1 serving/18g

| 67/370 | 0.1/0.5 | 13.9/77 | 1.3/7 | 0.5/3 |

Wotsits, BBQ, Walkers*, 1 bag/21g

| 109/521 | 1.5/7.2 | 11.7/55.8 | 6.3/29.9 | 0.3/1.2 |

Wotsits, Cheesy, Walkers*, 1 pack/19g

| 104/545 | 1.5/8 | 10.3/54 | 6.3/33 | 0.2/1 |

Wotsits, Prawn Cocktail, Walkers*, 1 pack/21g

| 109/520 | 1.2/5.5 | 11.6/55 | 6.5/31 | 0.2/1.1 |

DESSERTS AND ICE CREAM

Angel Delight, Butterscotch Flavour, Kraft*, 1 sachet/59g

| 280/475 | 1.4/2.4 | 43.4/73.5 | 11.2/19 | 0/0 |

Angel Delight, Raspberry Flavour, Kraft*, 1 sachet/59g

| 289/490 | 1.5/2.5 | 42.5/72 | 12.4/21 | 0/0 |

Angel Delight, Strawberry Flavour, Kraft*, 1 sachet/59g

| 286/485 | 1.5/2.5 | 41.9/71 | 12.4/21 | 0/0 |

Brandy Snap, Baskets, Askeys*, 1 basket/20g

| 98/490 | 0.4/1.9 | 14.5/72.7 | 4.3/21.3 | 0/0 |

Bread & Butter Pudding, BGTY, Sainsbury's*, 1 serving/120g

| 161/134 | 6.7/5.6 | 27.6/23 | 2.6/2.2 | 1/0.8 |

Bread & Butter Pudding, Finest, Tesco*, 1 serving/153g

| 379/248 | 7.5/4.9 | 37.6/24.6 | 22/14.4 | 1.4/0.9 |

	kcal serv/100g	prot serv/100g	carb serv/100g	fat serv/100g	fibre serv/100g

Bread & Butter Pudding, Individual, Waitrose*, 1 pudding/116g

| 247/213 | 6.3/5.4 | 28.3/24.4 | 12.1/10.4 | 0.3/0.3 |

Bread & Butter Pudding, Marks & Spencer*, 1 serving/125g

| 359/287 | 6.6/5.3 | 30.1/24.1 | 24.3/19.4 | 1/0.8 |

Bread & Butter Pudding, Sainsbury's*, 1 pudding/230g

| 446/194 | 11/4.8 | 50.4/21.9 | 22.3/9.7 | 0.9/0.4 |

Cheesecake, Blackcurrant Devonshire, McVitie's*, ⅙ cheesecake/67g

| 190/288 | 2.5/3.8 | 19.6/29.7 | 11.3/17.1 | 1.1/1.7 |

Cheesecake, Blackcurrant Swirl, Heinz*, ⅓ portion/87g

| 241/277 | 3.6/4.1 | 26.4/30.3 | 13.4/15.4 | 3.1/3.6 |

Cheesecake, Chocolate & Hazelnut, Gold, Sara Lee*, 1 slice/65g

| 205/316 | 3.8/5.9 | 18.7/28.7 | 12.8/19.7 | 0.7/1.1 |

Cheesecake, Chocolate Brownie, Tesco*, 1 serving/101g

| 400/396 | 4.8/4.8 | 32.1/31.8 | 28/27.7 | 0.8/0.8 |

Cheesecake, Chocolate, American-Style, Asda*, 1 cheesecake/390g

| 1486/381 | 19.5/5 | 167.7/43 | 81.9/21 | 23.4/6 |

Cheesecake, Double Chocolate Wedge, Sainsbury's*, 1 portion/75g

| 327/436 | 4.3/5.7 | 21.8/29 | 24.8/33 | 1.3/1.7 |

Cheesecake, Lemon Creamy & Light, Marks & Spencer*, ⅙ cake/67.5g

| 238/350 | 2.4/3.5 | 22/32.3 | 13.9/20.4 | 0.3/0.4 |

Cheesecake, Lemon, Pret A Manger*, 1 pot/150g

| 382/255 | 2.7/1.8 | 21.9/14.6 | 31.4/20.9 | 0.3/0.2 |

Cheesecake, Mandarin, Co-Op*, 1 slice/99g

| 297/300 | 4/4 | 31.7/32 | 16.8/17 | 0.3/0.3 |

Cheesecake, Mandarin, GFY, Asda*, 1 serving/97g

| 194/200 | 3.9/4 | 34.9/36 | 4.3/4.4 | 0.8/0.8 |

Cheesecake, Mandarin, Low-Fat, Tesco*, 1 serving/70g

| 145/207 | 2.3/3.3 | 25.9/37 | 3.3/4.7 | 1/1.4 |

Cheesecake, Raspberry Rapture, Tesco*, 1 serving/109.5g

| 332/302 | 4.2/3.8 | 27.9/25.4 | 22.7/20.6 | 0.7/0.6 |

Cheesecake, Sticky Toffee, Iceland*, 1 cheesecake/116g

| 331/285 | 4.4/3.8 | 39.3/33.9 | 17.3/14.9 | 0.1/0.1 |

Cheesecake, Sticky Toffee, Tesco*, 1 slice/66g

| 248/375 | 2.6/4 | 23.3/35.3 | 16/24.2 | 0.3/0.5 |

Cheesecake, Strawberry, 95% Fat-Free, Marks & Spencer*, 1 slice/98g

| 187/191 | 5/5.1 | 33.1/33.8 | 3.9/4 | 0.3/0.3 |

Cheesecake, Strawberry, Individual, Weight Watchers*, 1 cheesecake/103g

| 199/193 | 5.7/5.5 | 34.9/33.9 | 3.3/3.2 | 1.9/1.8 |

kcal serv/100g	prot serv/100g	carb serv/100g	fat serv/100g	fibre serv/100g
Cheesecake, Strawberry, SmartPrice, Asda*, 1 cheesecake/90g				
239/265	4.5/5	28.8/32	11.7/13	1/1.1
Cheesecake, Toffee, Marks & Spencer*, 1 serving/105g				
357/340	5.5/5.2	39.1/37.2	22.6/21.5	0.9/0.9
Cheesecake, Triple Chocolate, Waitrose*, ⅙ cheesecake/76g				
262/349	4.1/5.4	28.7/38.3	14.5/19.3	0.9/1.2
Cheesecake, Vanilla, Tesco*, 1 serving/115g				
417/363	6.6/5.7	33.8/29.4	28.4/24.7	0.7/0.6
Choc Ices, Dark, Somerfield*, 1 ice/62ml				
186/300	1.9/3	15.5/25	13/21	0/0
Choc Ices, Dark, Tesco*, 1 ice/43.4g				
136/316	1.3/3	11.8/27.4	9.2/21.4	0.3/0.7
Choc Ices, Light, Tesco*, 1 ice/43g				
138/322	1.5/3.4	11.7/27.1	9.5/22.1	0.2/0.5
Choc Ices, Mini Mix, Magnum-Style, Eis Stern, Lidl*, 1 ice/38.6g				
130/334	1.6/4.2	11.3/29	9/23	0/0
Choc Ices, Value, Tesco*, 1 ice/31g				
87/281	0.8/2.6	7.7/24.8	5.9/19	0.2/0.6
Christmas Pudding, Luxury, Safeway*, ⅛ pudding/114g				
316/277	3.5/3.1	54.6/47.9	9.2/8.1	1.5/1.3
Christmas Pudding, Sticky Toffee, Tesco*, ¼ pudding/114g				
372/326	2.9/2.5	73.5/64.5	7.3/6.4	0.9/0.8
Christmas Pudding, Tesco*, 1 serving/113g				
305/270	2.7/2.4	62.2/55	6.7/5.9	1.7/1.5
Crème Brulee, Marks & Spencer*, 1 pot/100g				
360/360	3.3/3.3	13/13	32.6/32.6	0/0
Crème Caramel, Sainsbury's*, 1 pot/100g				
102/102	2.5/2.5	21.1/21.1	0.9/0.9	0/0
Crème Caramel, Tesco*, 1 pot/100g				
113/113	2.4/2.4	20/20	2.6/2.6	0/0
Crumble, Apple & Blackberry, Asda*, 1 serving/175g				
427/244	4.7/2.7	66.5/38	15.8/9	2.1/1.2
Crumble, Apple & Blackberry, Marks & Spencer*, 1 serving/135g				
398/295	4.7/3.5	60.6/44.9	15.1/11.2	2.2/1.6
Crumble, Apple & Blackberry, Sainsbury's*, 1 serving/110g				
232/211	3.3/3	40.8/37.1	6.2/5.6	2.3/2.1
Crumble, Apple & Blackberry, Tesco*, 1 crumble/335g				
667/199	8.7/2.6	134.3/40.1	10.4/3.1	6.4/1.9

kcal serv/100g	prot serv/100g	carb serv/100g	fat serv/100g	fibre serv/100g
Crumble, Apple & Custard, Asda*, 1 serving/125g				
250/200	2.9/2.3	40/32	8.8/7	0/0
Crumble, Apple & Toffee, Weight Watchers*, 1 pot/98g				
206/210	2.1/2.1	36.8/37.6	5.6/5.7	1.6/1.6
Crumble, Apple with Custard, Individual, Sainsbury's*, 1 pudding/120g				
286/238	2.4/2	37.7/31.4	13.9/11.6	2.9/2.4
Crumble, Apple, Somerfield*, 1 serving/195g				
454/233	4.9/2.5	71.8/36.8	16.4/8.4	2.1/1.1
Crumble, Apple, Tesco*, 1 serving/150g				
342/228	3/2	50.4/33.6	14.3/9.5	1.8/1.2
Crumble, Bramley Apple, Marks & Spencer*, 1 serving/149g				
387/260	6.6/4.4	60/40.3	13.7/9.2	1.6/1.1
Crumble, Bramley Apple, Sainsbury's*, 1 serving/100g				
248/248	2/2	35.4/35.4	10.9/10.9	2.3/2.3
Crumble, Rhubarb, Marks & Spencer*, 1 serving/133g				
366/275	4.5/3.4	56.7/42.6	13.2/9.9	1.9/1.4
Crumble, Rhubarb, Sainsbury's*, 1 serving/50g				
112/224	1.6/3.1	20.2/40.4	2.8/5.6	0.9/1.8
Crumble, Topping, Sainsbury's*, 1 serving/47g				
188/401	2.8/5.9	23.6/50.3	9.2/19.6	2.5/5.3
Custard, Devon, Low-Fat, Ambrosia*, ⅓ pot/141g				
102/72	4.1/2.9	17.9/12.7	1.6/1.1	0.1/0.1
Custard, Fresh, Co-Op*, 1 serving/125g				
150/120	6.3/5	17.5/14	6.3/5	0.6/0.5
Custard, Fresh, Healthy Eating, Tesco*, 1 serving/100g				
103/103	2.3/2.3	17.3/17.3	2.7/2.7	0.2/0.2
Custard, Fresh, Sainsbury's*, 1 serving/125g				
158/126	3.3/2.6	19.3/15.4	7.5/6	0.1/0.1
Custard, Half-Fat, Safeway*, 1 serving/100ml				
105/105	2.3/2.3	17.3/17.3	2.7/2.7	0.7/0.7
Custard, Low-Fat, Ready-To-Serve, Bird's*, 1oz/28g				
24/87	0.8/2.8	4.3/15.5	0.4/1.4	0/0
Custard, Original, Ready-To-Serve, Bird's*, 1oz/28g				
29/102	0.8/2.8	4.3/15.5	0.8/3	0/0
Custard, Powder, Original Flavour, Bird's*, 1oz/28g				
99/355	0.1/0.4	24.4/87	0.1/0.5	0/0
Custard, Ready-To-Eat, Low-Fat, Tesco*, 1 pot/150g				
132/88	4.4/2.9	24.3/16.2	2/1.3	0.3/0.2

kcal serv/100g	prot serv/100g	carb serv/100g	fat serv/100g	fibre serv/100g
Custard, Ready-To Serve, Low-Fat, Co-Op*, 1 can/425g				
319/75	12.8/3	59.5/14	3/0.7	0/0
Custard, Ready-To-Serve, BGTY, Sainsbury's*, ⅓ pot/166g				
163/98	4.3/2.6	25.9/15.6	4.6/2.8	0.2/0.1
Custard, Ready-To-Serve, Healthy Eating, Tesco*, 1oz/28g				
22/77	0.8/2.9	3.6/13	0.4/1.5	0/0
Custard, Ready-To-Serve, Somerfield*, 1oz/28g				
29/103	0.8/3	4.8/17	0.8/3	0/0
Custard, Smooth & Creamy, Fresh, Tesco*, 1 serving/100g				
123/123	2.5/2.5	15/15	5.9/5.9	0.3/0.3
Custard, Vanilla, COU, Marks & Spencer*, 1 pot/140g				
147/105	6/4.3	23.2/16.6	3.5/2.5	0.8/0.6
Dessert, Banoffee, Frozen, Healthy Living, Tesco*, 1 serving/60g				
92/153	1.5/2.5	17.9/29.9	1.6/2.6	0.4/0.6
Dessert, Banoffee, Weight Watchers*, 1 pot/80g				
154/192	3.6/4.5	28.2/35.3	3/3.7	0.6/0.8
Dessert, Black Cherry & Chocolate, COU, Marks & Spencer*, 1 pack/115g				
132/115	4.1/3.6	26/22.6	1.6/1.4	1.4/1.2
Dessert, Cafe Latte, COU, Marks & Spencer*, 1 pot/120g				
162/135	6/5	28.8/24	2.6/2.2	1.1/0.9
Dessert, Cafe Mocha, COU, Marks & Spencer*, 1 dessert/115g				
155/135	6.3/5.5	25.1/21.8	3.1/2.7	1.2/1
Dessert, Chocolate & Cherry, COU, Marks & Spencer*, 1 pot/130g				
156/120	3.4/2.6	31.9/24.5	2.1/1.6	1.2/0.9
Dessert, Chocolate & Coconut, COU, Marks & Spencer*, 1 pot/125g				
169/135	4.5/3.6	32/25.6	2.8/2.2	0.9/0.7
Dessert, Chocolate & Honeycomb Iced, Weight Watchers*, 1 pot/58g				
92/159	1.8/3.1	15.3/26.3	2.5/4.3	0.5/0.8
Dessert, Chocolate & Mallow Iced, GFY, Asda*, 1 pot/150ml				
140/93	3/2	28/18.7	1.8/1.2	3.4/2.3
Dessert, Chocolate & Mallow, Iced, Weight Watchers*, 1 pot/150ml				
140/93	3/2	28/18.7	1.8/1.2	3.4/2.3
Dessert, Chocolate & Vanilla Caramel, Dairy, Yoplait Petits Filous*, 1 pot/60g				
101/169	2.9/4.8	14.2/23.6	3.7/6.2	0/0
Dessert, Chocolate & Vanilla, Heavenly Swirls, Healthy Living, Tesco*, 1 pot/73g				
104/143	2.2/3	19.6/26.9	1.9/2.6	0.5/0.7

	kcal serv/100g	prot serv/100g	carb serv/100g	fat serv/100g	fibre serv/100g

Dessert, Chocolate Brownie, Asda*, ⅙ brownie/63.5g

171/271	3.2/5	23.9/38	6.9/11	2.8/4.4

Dessert, Chocolate Brownie, Marks & Spencer*, ¼ pack/143.5g

612/425	6.8/4.7	57/39.6	39.6/27.5	1.4/1

Dessert, Chocolate Chip Sponge & Chocolate Custard, COU,
Marks & Spencer*, 1 pot/125g

181/145	5.4/4.3	33.6/26.9	2.5/2	1.6/1.3

Dessert, Chocolate Fudge Brownie, Tesco*, 1 pot/125g

374/299	5.8/4.6	50.3/40.2	16.6/13.3	1.6/1.3

Dessert, Chocolate Muffin, COU, Marks & Spencer*, 1 serving/110g

149/135	5.1/4.6	29.2/26.5	2.1/1.9	1/0.9

Dessert, Chocolate Profiterole, Sainsbury's*, ⅙ pot/95.0g

192/202	5.1/5.4	23.8/25.1	8.5/8.9	0.8/0.8

Dessert, Chocolate Profiterole, Tesco*, 1 serving/76g

281/370	3.3/4.3	21.2/27.9	20.3/26.7	0.3/0.4

Dessert, Chocolate Toffee, Weight Watchers*, 1 pot/90.1g

164/182	4.4/4.9	31.5/35	3.2/3.5	1.6/1.8

Dessert, Chocolate, Campina*, 1 pot/125g

186/149	4/3.2	23.1/18.5	8.6/6.9	0/0

Dessert, Chocolate, COU Marks & Spencers*, 1 serving/120g

168/140	6.7/5.6	31.7/26.4	2.5/2.1	1.3/1.1

Dessert, Chocolate, Value, Tesco*, 1 pot/115g

112/97	3.2/2.8	18.1/15.7	3/2.6	0/0

Dessert, Double Chocolate Brownie, Weight Watchers*, 1 serving/82g

151/184	3.7/4.5	27.3/33.3	3/3.6	1.8/2.2

Dessert, Irish Cream Caffe Latte, Marks & Spencer*, 1 pot/118.5g

161/135	6/5	28.6/24	2.6/2.2	1.1/0.9

Dessert, Lemon Meringue, Weight Watchers*, 1 pot/170g

321/189	4.1/2.4	73.3/43.1	0.9/0.5	1/0.6

Dessert, Profiterole, Marks & Spencer*, 1 pot/61g

209/342	3.4/5.5	17.8/29.1	13.5/22.1	0.3/0.5

Dessert, Raspberry & Chardonnay, COU, Marks & Spencer*, 1 serving/135g

155/115	2.2/1.6	34.4/25.5	0.7/0.5	3.6/2.7

Dessert, Rice, Lite, Muller*, 1 pot/150g

116/77	5.3/3.5	20.4/13.6	1.4/0.9	0/0

Dessert, Rolo, Nestle*, 1 pot/78g

191/245	2.4/3.1	23.6/30.3	9.5/12.2	0.2/0.3

kcal serv/100g	prot serv/100g	carb serv/100g	fat serv/100g	fibre serv/100g

Dessert, Summer Fruits, Yoghurt, Iced, BGTY, Sainsbury's*, ¼ pot/85g

105/124	2.8/3.3	21.8/25.6	0.8/0.9	0.4/0.5

Dessert, Vanilla & Toffee, Heavenly Swirls, Healthy Living. Tesco*, 1 pot/73g

106/145	1.8/2.5	20.5/28.1	1.8/2.5	0.4/0.5

Dessert, Vanilla Flavour, Iced, Healthy Eating, Tesco*, 1 serving/50g

67/134	2/3.9	12.1/24.1	1.2/2.4	2.3/4.6

Dessert, Vanilla Sponge & Custard with Raspberry Conserve, COU, Marks & Spencer*, 1 serving/140g

189/135	3.4/2.4	39.6/28.3	1.7/1.2	2.4/1.7

Dessert, Vanilla with Strawberries Swirl, Weight Watchers*, 1 pot/57g

81/142	1.4/2.5	13.3/23.4	2.2/3.9	0.1/0.2

Dessert, Vanilla, Frozen, GFY, Asda*, 1 serving/52g

72/139	1.4/2.7	11.4/22	2.3/4.5	0/0

Dessert, Vanilla, Too Good To Be True, Frozen, Wall's*, 1 serving/50ml

35/70	1/2	7.5/14.9	0.2/0.4	0.1/0.1

Fool, Apricot, BGTY, Sainsbury's*, 1 pot/113g

87/77	4/3.5	9/8	3.8/3.4	0.3/0.3

Fool, Blackcurrant, BGTY, Sainsbury's*, 1 pot/113g

89/79	4/3.5	11.8/10.4	2.9/2.6	0.7/0.6

Fool, Rhubarb, Fruit, BGTY, Sainsbury's*, 1 pot/120g

90/75	3.5/2.9	11.4/9.5	3.4/2.8	0.4/0.3

Fool, Strawberry, Fruit, BGTY, Sainsbury's*, 1 pot/120g

100/83	3.6/3	13.8/11.5	3.4/2.8	1.2/1

Fool, Strawberry, Fruit, Somerfield*, 1 pot/114g

201/176	3.4/3	18.2/16	12.5/11	0/0

Fromage Frais, 0% Fat, Vitalinea*, 1 tbsp/28g

14/50	2.1/7.4	1.3/4.7	0/0.1	0/0

Fromage Frais, Apricot, Tesco*, 1 pot/100g

77/77	6.5/6.5	6/6	3/3	1.3/1.3

Fromage Frais, Apricot, Weight Watchers*, 1 pot/100g

47/47	6.2/6.2	5.4/5.4	0.1/0.1	0.2/0.2

Fromage Frais, Banoffee Toffee, Weight Watchers*, 1 pot/100g

64/64	5.7/5.7	10/10	0.1/0.1	1.1/1.1

Fromage Frais, Blackcurrant, Eat Smart, Safeway*, 1 pot/100g

60/60	7.9/7.9	6.1/6.1	0.2/0.2	0.5/0.5

Fromage Frais, Blackcurrant, Healthy Eating, Tesco*, 1 pot/100g

59/59	7.7/7.7	6.5/6.5	0.2/0.2	0.6/0.6

	kcal serv/100g	prot serv/100g	carb serv/100g	fat serv/100g	fibre serv/100g

Fromage Frais, Chocolate & Orange, Weight Watchers*, 1 pot/100g

64/64	5.7/5.7	10/10	0.1/0.1	1.1/1.1

Fromage Frais, COU, Marks & Spencer*, 1 pot/100g

48/48	7.8/7.8	4.5/4.5	0.1/0.1	0.5/0.5

Fromage Frais, Fruit On The Bottom, Better For You, Morrisons*, 1 pot/100g

66/66	5.6/5.6	10.6/10.6	0.2/0.2	0/0

Fromage Frais, Fruit, Weight Watchers*, 1 pot/100g

48/48	5.4/5.4	6.3/6.3	0.1/0.1	0.3/0.3

Fromage Frais, Lemon Pie, Low-Fat, Sainsbury's*, 1 pot/90g

108/120	6/6.7	15.6/17.3	2.4/2.7	0.2/0.2

Fromage Frais, Munch Bunch, Nestle*, 1 pot/42g

50/119	3.2/7.6	6.2/14.8	1.2/2.9	0/0

Fromage Frais, Natural, Healthy Eating, Tesco*, 1 serving/65g

30/46	5.1/7.8	2.1/3.3	0.1/0.2	0/0

Fromage Frais, Peach, BGTY, Sainsbury's*, 1 pot/100g

53/53	7.2/7.2	5.5/5.5	0.2/0.2	0.5/0.5

Fromage Frais, Peach, Weight Watchers*, 1 pot/100g

48/48	5.4/5.4	6.4/6.4	0.1/0.1	0.2/0.2

Fromage Frais, Petits Filous, Yoplait*, 1 pot/60g

76/127	3.9/6.5	8.7/14.5	2.8/4.7	0/0

Fromage Frais, Raspberry & Redcurrant, BGTY, Sainsbury's*, 1 pot/100g

49/49	7.2/7.2	4.5/4.5	0.2/0.2	1.9/1.9

Fromage Frais, Raspberry & Strawberry, Weight Watchers*, 1 pot/100g

48/48	5.4/5.4	6.2/6.2	0.1/0.1	0.3/0.3

Fromage Frais, Raspberry, COU, Marks & Spencer*, 1 pot/100g

49/49	7.8/7.8	4.9/4.9	0.1/0.1	0.4/0.4

Fromage Frais, Raspberry, Healthy Eating, Tesco*, 1 pot/100g

53/53	6.2/6.2	6.6/6.6	0.2/0.2	0.3/0.3

Fromage Frais, Raspberry, Low-Fat, Sainsbury's*, 1 pot/90g

96/107	5.2/5.8	13.6/15.1	2.3/2.6	0.1/0.1

Fromage Frais, Raspberry, Muller*, 1 pot/50g

68/135	3.1/6.1	6.8/13.5	3.2/6.3	0/0

Fromage Frais, Raspberry, Weight Watchers*, 1 pot/100g

49/49	5.3/5.3	6.9/6.9	0.1/0.1	1.2/1.2

Fromage Frais, Red Cherry, Healthy Eating, Tesco*, 1 pot/100g

55/55	6.2/6.2	7.2/7.2	0.2/0.2	0.1/0.1

kcal serv/100g	prot serv/100g	carb serv/100g	fat serv/100g	fibre serv/100g
Fromage Frais, Rhubarb & Crumble, Low-Fat, Sainsbury's*, 1 pot/90g				
96/107	6/6.7	12.7/14.1	2.3/2.6	0.4/0.4
Fromage Frais, Strawberry, BGTY, Sainsbury's*, 1 pot/100g				
48/48	7.2/7.2	4.3/4.3	0.2/0.2	1.4/1.4
Fromage Frais, Strawberry, Healthy Eating, Tesco*, 1 pot/100g				
54/54	6.2/6.2	6.8/6.8	0.2/0.2	0.1/0.1
Fromage Frais, Strawberry, Weight Watchers*, 1 pot/100g				
47/47	5.4/5.4	6.2/6.2	0.1/0.1	0.2/0.2
Fromage Frais, with Cereal, Shape Rise, Danone*, 1 serving/165g				
205/124	10.7/6.5	39.5/23.9	2.1/1.3	0.9/0.5
Ice Cream Bar, Caramel, Cadbury's*, 1 bar/64g				
188/294	2.4/3.7	20.7/32.4	10.6/16.6	0/0
Ice Cream Cone, Carousel Wafer Company*, 1 cone/2g				
7/342	0.3/12.6	1.3/65	0.1/3.7	0/0
Ice Cream Cone, Chocolate & Vanilla, Good Choice, Iceland*, 1 cone/110ml				
161/146	3/2.7	25.2/22.9	7.2/6.5	0.9/0.8
Ice Cream Cone, Chocolate, Vanilla & Hazelnut, Sainsbury's*, 1 cone/62g				
190/306	2.8/4.5	21/33.9	10.5/16.9	0.4/0.6
Ice Cream Cone, Cornetto, GFY, Asda*, 1 cone/67.2g				
161/241	2/3	24.8/37	6/9	0.1/0.1
Ice Cream Cone, Cornetto, Wall's*, 1 cone/75g				
195/260	2.8/3.7	25.9/34.5	9.7/12.9	0/0
Ice Cream Cone, Flake 99 Cadbury's*, 1 cone/125ml				
204/163	3/2.4	24.5/19.6	11/8.8	0/0
Ice Cream Cone, Strawberry & Vanilla, Asda*, 1 cone/115ml				
193/168	2.1/1.8	26/22.6	9/7.8	0.1/0.1
Ice Cream, Baileys, Haagen-Dazs*, 1oz/28g				
73/260	1.3/4.5	6.2/22.2	4.8/17.1	0/0
Ice Cream, Belgian Chocolate, Haagen-Dazs*, 1oz/28g				
89/318	1.3/4.6	8/28.4	5.8/20.7	0/0
Ice Cream, Bournville, Cadbury's*, 1 bar/120g				
258/215	4.2/3.5	31.2/26	13.9/11.6	0/0
Ice Cream, Caramel, Carte d'Or*, 2 boules/50g				
106/212	1.3/2.6	15.4/30.8	4.4/8.7	0/0
Ice Cream, Cherrylicious, Tesco*, 1 serving/57.7g				
122/210	1.6/2.8	21.5/37	3.2/5.6	0.1/0.2
Ice Cream, Choc Chip Cookie Dough, Ben & Jerry's*, 1 serving/100g				
230/230	3/3	23/23	14/14	0/0

kcal serv/100g	prot serv/100g	carb serv/100g	fat serv/100g	fibre serv/100g
Ice Cream, Choc Chip, Haagen-Dazs*, 1oz/28g				
80/286	1.3/4.7	6.9/24.8	5.2/18.7	0/0
Ice Cream, Chocolate Flavour, Soft Scoop, Sainsbury's*, 1 serving/70g				
122/174	2.2/3.1	16.5/23.6	5.3/7.5	0.2/0.3
Ice Cream, Chocolate Fudge Brownie, Ben & Jerry's*, 1 serving/100g				
260/260	0/0	31/31	13/13	2/2
Ice Cream, Chocolate Fudge Swirl, Haagen-Dazs*, 1oz/28g				
77/276	1.3/4.6	7.2/25.6	4.8/17.2	0/0
Ice Cream, Chocolate Honeycomb, COU, Marks & Spencer*, 1 serving/100ml				
150/150	3.5/3.5	31.5/31.5	2.6/2.6	0.7/0.7
Ice Cream, Chocolate Midnight Cookies, Haagen-Dazs*, 1oz/28g				
81/289	1.4/4.9	8/28.7	4.8/17.2	0/0
Ice Cream, Chocolate, Weight Watchers*, 1 serving/100ml				
92/92	1.8/1.8	15.2/15.2	2.5/2.5	0.5/0.5
Ice Cream, Chocolatino, Tesco*, 1 serving/100g				
243/243	4.4/4.4	32.2/32.2	10.8/10.8	0.6/0.6
Ice Cream, Chunky Monkey, Ben & Jerry's*, 1 serving/100g				
280/280	4/4	28/28	17/17	1/1
Ice Cream, Coconut, Carte d'Or*, 1 serving/100ml				
125/125	1.8/1.8	14/14	7.1/7.1	0.5/0.5
Ice Cream, Cookies & Cream, Haagen-Dazs*, 1oz/28g				
73/262	1.3/4.6	6.3/22.6	4.8/17	0/0
Ice Cream, Cornish Clotted, Marks & Spencer*, 1 pot/90g				
207/230	2.5/2.8	19.6/21.8	13.1/14.5	0.1/0.1
Ice Cream, Cream of Cornish Vanilla, Wall's*, 1 serving/111ml				
100/90	1.9/1.7	12.2/11	4.8/4.3	0.1/0.1
Ice Cream, Dairy Milk, Cadbury's*, 1 stick/120ml				
286/238	4.2/3.5	31.1/25.9	16.8/14	0/0
Ice Cream, Double Chocolate, Nestle*, 1 serving/77.5g				
250/320	3.7/4.8	26.3/33.7	14.4/18.4	0/0
Ice Cream, Galaxy, Mars*, 1 bar/60ml				
203/339	2.8/4.7	17.8/29.7	13.4/22.4	0/0
Ice Cream, Honey, I'm Home, Ben & Jerry's*, 1 serving/100g				
260/260	0/0	28/28	15/15	0/0
Ice Cream, Lemon Pie, Haagen-Dazs*, 1oz/28g				
73/262	1.1/3.9	6.9/24.5	4.6/16.3	0/0
Ice Cream, Magnum Moments, Wall's*, 1 serving/18ml				
58/323	0.7/4	5.4/30	3.7/20.8	0/0

	kcal serv/100g	prot serv/100g	carb serv/100g	fat serv/100g	fibre serv/100g
Ice Cream, Maple & Walnut, American, Sainsbury's*, ⅛ pot/68g					
	121/179	2.1/3.1	17.3/25.6	4.9/7.2	0.1/0.2
Ice Cream, Mars, Mars*, 1 bar/75g					
	260/346	3.8/5.1	27.9/37.2	14.8/19.7	0/0
Ice Cream, Mocha Coffee Indulgence, Sainsbury's*, ¼ pot/82g					
	178/217	2.6/3.2	18.1/22.1	10.6/12.9	0.1/0.1
Ice Cream, Neapolitan, Soft Scoop, Asda*, 1 scoop/47g					
	83/176	1.5/3.1	10.8/23	3.8/8	0/0
Ice Cream, Pralines & Cream, Haagen-Dazs*, 1oz/28g					
	77/276	1.2/4.2	7.3/26.2	4.8/17.2	0/0
Ice Cream, Raspberry Pavlova, Sainsbury's*, 1 serving/100g					
	202/202	2.7/2.7	26.6/26.6	9.4/9.4	3.3/3.3
Ice Cream, Raspberry Ripple, Soft Scoop, Asda*, 1 scoop/46g					
	75/164	1.2/2.5	11.5/25	2.8/6	0/0
Ice Cream, Raspberry Ripple, Soft Scoop, Sainsbury's*, 1 serving/75g					
	128/170	2/2.6	18.2/24.2	5.3/7	0.2/0.3
Ice Cream, Raspberry Ripple, Soft Scoop, Tesco*, 2 scoops/50g					
	79/157	1.3/2.5	11.5/23	3.1/6.1	0.1/0.2
Ice Cream, Rum & Raisin, Organic, Iceland*, 1oz/28g					
	55/195	1.3/4.5	7.9/28.1	2/7.2	0/0
Ice Cream, Screwball, Tesco*, 1 screwball/61g					
	116/190	1.8/2.9	15.4/25.2	5.2/8.6	0.2/0.3
Ice Cream, Strawberry & Cream, Mivvi, Nestle*, 1 serving/60g					
	118/196	1.6/2.6	17.6/29.4	4.6/7.6	0.1/0.2
Ice Cream, Strawberry Cheesecake, Haagen-Dazs*, 1oz/28g					
	74/266	1.1/3.9	7.4/26.5	4.5/16.1	0/0
Ice Cream, Strawberry, Haagen-Dazs*, 1oz/28g					
	67/241	1.1/4	6/21.5	4.3/15.5	0/0
Ice Cream, The Full Vermonty, Ben & Jerry's*, 1 serving/100g					
	280/280	0/0	27/27	18/18	1/1
Ice Cream, Toffee Crème, Haagen-Dazs*, 1oz/28g					
	74/265	1.3/4.5	7.5/26.7	4.4/15.6	0/0
Ice Cream, Toffee Ripple, Tesco*, 1 serving/100g					
	173/173	2.7/2.7	24.4/24.4	7.2/7.2	0.1/0.1
Ice Cream, Tropical Fruit Sorbet, Waitrose*, 1 lolly/109.8g					
	90/82	1.7/1.5	16/14.5	2.2/2	0.2/0.2
Ice Cream, Vanilla Caramel Fudge, Ben & Jerry's*, 1 serving/100g					
	260/260	4/4	28/28	14/14	0/0

	kcal serv/100g	prot serv/100g	carb serv/100g	fat serv/100g	fibre serv/100g
Ice Cream, Vanilla Choc Fudge, Tofutti*, 1 tub/500ml					
	825/165	8/1.6	100/20	45/9	2/0.4
Ice Cream, Vanilla Dairy, Finest, Tesco*, 1 serving/92g					
	227/247	4.1/4.5	16.6/18	16/17.4	0.3/0.3
Ice Cream, Vanilla with Strawberry Swirl, Mini Tub, Weight Watchers*, 1 mini tub/57.0g					
	81/142	1.4/2.5	13.3/23.4	2.2/3.9	0.1/0.2
Ice Cream, Vanilla, COU, Marks & Spencer*, ¼ pot/79g					
	111/140	1.3/1.7	20.5/25.9	2.2/2.8	0.6/0.8
Ice Cream, Vanilla, Dairy, Organic, Yeo Valley*, 1 serving/100g					
	206/206	4.9/4.9	21.3/21.3	11.2/11.2	0/0
Ice Cream, Vanilla, Haagen-Dazs*, 1oz/28g					
	70/250	1.3/4.5	5.5/19.7	4.8/17.1	0/0
Ice Cream, Vanilla, Organic, Sainsbury's*, 1 serving/85g					
	176/207	3.7/4.3	17.4/20.5	10.2/12	0.1/0.1
Ice Cream, Vanilla, Organic, Waitrose*, 1 serving/125g					
	178/142	3.4/2.7	15.5/12.4	11.3/9	0/0
Ice Cream, Vanilla, Really Creamy, Asda*, 1 serving/50g					
	98/196	1.8/3.5	11.5/23	5/10	0.1/0.1
Ice Cream, Vanilla, SmartPrice, Asda*, 1 scoop/40g					
	55/137	1.1/2.8	7.6/19	2.4/6	0.1/0.2
Ice Cream, Vanilla, Soft Scoop, 25% Less Fat, Asda*, 1oz/28g					
	42/149	0.8/2.9	6.4/23	1.4/5	0/0
Ice Cream, Vanilla, Soft Scoop, BGTY, Sainsbury's*, 1 serving/75g					
	104/139	2/2.7	16.2/21.6	3.5/4.6	0.2/0.2
Ice Cream, Vanilla, Soft Scoop, Light, 94% Fat-Free, Wall's*, 1 serving/100ml					
	80/80	1.4/1.4	12.4/12.4	2.9/2.9	0.1/0.1
Ice Cream, Vanilla, Soft Scoop, Marks & Spencer*, 1 scoop/125ml					
	225/180	3.6/2.9	29.8/23.8	10.1/8.1	0.1/0.1
Ice Cream, Vanilla, Thorntons*, 1oz/28g					
	63/225	1.4/4.9	5.7/20.5	3.8/13.6	0/0
Ice Cream, Vanilla, Too Good to be True, Walls*, 1 serving/50ml					
	35/70	1/2	7.5/14.9	0.2/0.4	0.1/0.1
Ice Cream, Vanilla, with Vanilla Pods, Sainsbury's*, 1 serving/100g					
	195/195	3.5/3.5	22.5/22.5	10.1/10.1	0.1/0.1
Ice Cream, Viennetta, Chocolate, Wall's*, ¼ pot/80g					
	200/250	3.3/4.1	19.2/24	12.2/15.2	0/0

kcal serv/100g	prot serv/100g	carb serv/100g	fat serv/100g	fibre serv/100g
Ice Cream, Viennetta, Forest Fruit, Wall's*, 1 serving/98g				
265/270	3.3/3.4	26.7/27.2	15.9/16.2	0/0
Ice Cream, Viennetta, Mint, Wall's*, 1 serving/80g				
204/255	2.7/3.4	18.4/23	13.3/16.6	0/0
Ice Cream, Viennetta, Vanilla, Wall's*, ¼ bar/80gg				
204/255	2.6/3.3	18.4/23	13.4/16.7	0/0
Ice Lolly, Blackcurrant, Ribena*, 1 lolly/52ml				
41/79	0/0	10/19.2	0/0	0/0
Ice Lolly, Fab, Nestle*, 1 lolly/57g				
82/144	0.5/0.8	13.5/23.7	2.8/4.9	0/0
Ice Lolly, Orange, Real Juice, Sainsbury's*, 1 lolly/72ml				
63/88	0.5/0.7	15.1/21	0.1/0.1	0.1/0.1
Ice Lolly, Rocket, Co-Op*, 1 lolly/60g				
42/70	0/0	10.2/17	0/0	0/0
Ice Lolly, Vanilla Cream, Covered in White Chocolate, Mmmm, Tesco*, 1 ice cream/85g				
258/303	2.7/3.2	25.2/29.6	16.2/19.1	0.7/0.8
Mousse, Aero Chocolate, Nestle*, 1 pot/59g				
109/185	3/5.1	12.4/21	5.3/8.9	0.3/0.5
Mousse, Black Cherry, Lite, Onken*, 1 pot/150g				
156/104	6.9/4.6	26.9/17.9	2.3/1.5	0.4/0.3
Mousse, Cadbury's Light Chocolate, St Ivel*, 1 pot/64g				
79/123	4/6.2	11.1/17.3	2/3.2	0/0
Mousse, Chocolate & Hazelnut, Onken*, 1 pot/125g				
173/138	4.1/3.3	22.3/17.8	7.5/6	0/0
Mousse, Chocolate & Mint, COU, Marks & Spencer*, 1 pot/90g				
108/120	4.9/5.4	16/17.8	2.3/2.6	0.5/0.5
Mousse, Chocolate & Vanilla, Weight Watchers*, 1 pot/80g				
106/132	3.5/4.4	17.8/22.2	2.2/2.8	0.7/0.9
Mousse, Chocolate, Asda*, 1 pot/60.9g				
127/209	2.3/3.8	16/26.3	6/9.9	0.7/1.1
Mousse, Chocolate, BGTY, Sainsbury's*, 1 pot/62.5g				
78/126	2.5/4	13.3/21.5	1.7/2.7	0.7/1.1
Mousse, Chocolate, COU, Marks & Spencer*, 1 pot/70g				
81/115	4.1/5.8	11.6/16.6	1.9/2.7	0.7/1
Mousse, Chocolate, Eat Smart, Safeway*, 1 pot/62g				
81/130	2.5/4.1	13.3/21.5	1.7/2.7	0.7/1.1

kcal serv/100g	prot serv/100g	carb serv/100g	fat serv/100g	fibre serv/100g
Mousse, Chocolate, GFY, Asda*, 1 pot/62.5g				
85/136	2.4/3.8	15/24	1.7/2.7	0/0
Mousse, Chocolate, Healthy Eating, Tesco*, 1 pot/60g				
80/134	2.6/4.4	13.9/23.2	1.6/2.6	0.6/1
Mousse, Chocolate, Italian-Style, Tesco*, 1 pot/90g				
243/270	4.5/5	29.5/32.8	11.9/13.2	2.2/2.4
Mousse, Chocolate, Light, Cadbury's*, 1 pot/55g				
69/125	3.4/6.2	9.6/17.5	1.8/3.2	0/0
Mousse, Chocolate, Pret A Manger*, 1 pot/110g				
314/285	3/2.7	18.6/16.9	25.2/22.9	1.4/1.3
Mousse, Chocolate, Sainsbury's*, 1 pot/62g				
122/197	2.5/4	15.7/25.4	5.5/8.8	0.7/1.1
Mousse, Fruit Juice, Shape*, 1 pot/100g				
115/115	3.5/3.5	18.5/18.5	2.8/2.8	0/0
Mousse, Lemon, COU, Marks & Spencer*, 1 pot/70g				
81/115	2/2.9	13.6/19.4	1.7/2.4	2.5/3.5
Mousse, Lemon, Dessert, Sainsbury's*, 1 pot/62.5g				
114/182	2.3/3.6	12.9/20.7	5.9/9.4	0.4/0.6
Mousse, Lemon, GFY, Asda*, 1 pot/62.5g				
72/114	2.1/3.4	12/19	1.7/2.7	0/0
Mousse, Lemon, Healthy Eating, Tesco*, 1 pot/60g				
57/95	2/3.4	8.6/14.3	1.6/2.7	0.4/0.7
Mousse, Lemon, Lite, Onken*, 1 pot/150g				
156/104	6.9/4.6	27/18	2.4/1.6	0/0
Mousse, Lemon, Onken*, 1 pot/150g				
219/146	7.7/5.1	23.7/15.8	10.4/6.9	0.1/0.1
Mousse, Lemon, Tesco*, 1 pot/60g				
67/111	2/3.4	10.9/18.2	1.6/2.7	0/0
Mousse, Orange & Lemon, Light, Muller*, 1 pot/150g				
147/98	6.5/4.3	29/19.3	0.6/0.4	0/0
Mousse, Orange Fruit Juice, Shape*, 1 pot/100g				
116/116	3.5/3.5	18.5/18.5	2.8/2.8	0/0
Mousse, Peach, Onken*, 1 pot/150g				
200/133	7.2/4.8	20.3/13.5	9.9/6.6	0/0
Mousse, Raspberry Ripple, Economy, Sainsbury's*, 1 serving/50g				
39/78	0.7/1.3	4.9/9.7	1.9/3.7	0.2/0.3
Mousse, Raspberry, COU, Marks & Spencer*, 1 pot/70g				
81/115	2.1/3	13.7/19.6	1.7/2.4	2.7/3.9

kcal serv/100g	prot serv/100g	carb serv/100g	fat serv/100g	fibre serv/100g
Mousse, Raspberry, Lite, Onken*, 1 pot/150g				
152/101	6.9/4.6	26/17.3	2.3/1.5	1.6/1
Mousse, Rhubarb & Vanilla, Onken*, 1 pot/150g				
210/140	7.5/5	23.7/15.8	9.5/6.3	0.3/0.2
Mousse, Rhubarb, COU, Marks & Spencer*, 1 pot/70g				
88/125	2/2.9	18/25.7	1.5/2.1	2.9/4.2
Mousse, Rhubarb, Lite, Onken*, 1 pot/150g				
155/103	6.9/4.6	26.7/17.8	2.3/1.5	0.5/0.3
Mousse, Strawberry, Asda*, 1 pot/64g				
107/167	2.2/3.5	11.5/18	5.8/9	0.1/0.2
Mousse, Strawberry, Light, Muller*, 1 pot/150g				
147/98	6.5/4.3	29.1/19.4	0.6/0.4	0/0
Mousse, Strawberry, Lite, Onken*, 1 pot/150g				
153/102	6.9/4.6	26/17.3	2.4/1.6	1.7/1.1
Mousse, Strawberry, Onken*, 1 pot/150g				
200/133	7.2/4.8	20.3/13.5	9.9/6.6	0/0
Mousse, Strawberry, Weight Watchers*, 1 pot/90g				
124/138	2.7/3	23/25.5	2.4/2.7	0.5/0.5
Mousse, Summer Fruits, Light, Muller*, 1 pot/149g				
143/96	6.4/4.3	27.9/18.7	0.6/0.4	0/0
Mousse, Tropical Fruits, Light, Muller*, 1 pot/150g				
150/101	6.4/4.3	29.8/20	0.6/0.4	0/0
Pavlova, Raspberry, Marks & Spencer*, 1 serving/84g				
193/230	1.9/2.3	28/33.3	8.1/9.6	0.3/0.3
Pavlova, Raspberry, Tesco*, 1 serving/65g				
191/294	1.8/2.7	27.2/41.8	8.4/12.9	0.7/1.1
Pavlova, Sticky Toffee, Sainsbury's*, ⅙ pack/61g				
249/415	2.2/3.7	37.9/63.1	9.8/16.4	0.5/0.9
Pavlova, Strawberry, COU, Marks & Spencer*, 1 pot/95g				
147/155	2.3/2.4	29/30.5	2.3/2.4	0.8/0.8
Pie, Apple & Blackberry, Shortcrust, Marks & Spencer*, 1 serving/142g				
469/330	6.1/4.3	71.3/50.2	17.8/12.5	1.6/1.1
Pie, Apple & Blackberry, Tesco*, 1 serving/106g				
287/271	4.5/4.2	40.7/38.4	11.9/11.2	1.8/1.7
Pie, Apple & Blackcurrant, Mr Kipling*, 1 pie/66g				
220/334	2.2/3.4	33.7/51	8.5/12.9	0/0
Pie, Apple, Deep-Filled, Farmfoods*, 1oz/28g				
74/266	1/3.6	9.6/34.3	3.6/12.7	0.6/2.2

kcal serv/100g	prot serv/100g	carb serv/100g	fat serv/100g	fibre serv/100g
Pie, Apple, Deep-Filled, Sainsbury's*, ¼ pie/137g				
374/273	5.2/3.8	48.8/35.6	17.5/12.8	2.2/1.6
Pie, Apple, Individual, Somerfield*, 1 pie/47.2g				
178/379	1.6/3.5	25/53.2	7.9/16.9	0.6/1.3
Pie, Apple, Puff Pastry, Marks & Spencer*, 1 pie/135g				
338/250	3.2/2.4	42.3/31.3	17.1/12.7	1.4/1
Pie, Apple, SmartPrice, Asda*, 1 serving/47g				
178/379	1.6/3.5	24.9/53	8/17	0.6/1.3
Pie, Apple, Tesco*, 1 pie/47g				
191/406	1.6/3.3	27.9/59.4	8.1/17.2	0.7/1.5
Pie, Banoffee Cream, American Dream, McVitie's*, 1 portion/70g				
277/396	3/4.3	25.7/36.7	17.9/25.5	0.6/0.8
Pie, Banoffee, Shape*, 1 serving/120g				
175/146	4/3.3	33.6/28	2.8/2.3	0.6/0.5
Pie, Banoffee, Tesco*, 1 pie/112g				
381/340	4.1/3.7	50.8/45.4	17.8/15.9	1.3/1.2
Pie, Cherry, Shortcrust, Marks & Spencer*, 1 pie/142g				
412/290	5.1/3.6	61.6/43.4	15.5/10.9	1.1/0.8
Pie, Key Lime, Sainsbury's*, ¼ pie/80g				
280/350	3.4/4.2	41.4/51.8	11.2/14	0.6/0.7
Pie, Lemon Meringue, Marks & Spencer*, ⅙ pie/78g				
215/275	3/3.9	31.5/40.4	8.6/11	0.6/0.8
Pie, Lemon Meringue, Weight Watchers*, 1 serving/85g				
161/189	2/2.4	36.6/43.1	0.4/0.5	0.5/0.6
Pie, Mince, Deep-Filled, Sainsbury's*, 1 pie/67g				
240/358	2.3/3.5	36.9/55	9.2/13.8	0.9/1.4
Pie, Mince, Deep-Filled, Tesco*, 1 pie/57g				
215/376	2.2/3.9	33.1/57.8	8.2/14.3	0.9/1.6
Pie, Mince, Finest, Tesco*, 1 pie/61g				
234/384	2.6/4.3	36.5/59.9	8.6/14.1	1.6/2.7
Pie, Mince, Lattice, Marks & Spencer*, 1 pie/51g				
204/400	2.2/4.4	29.6/58	8.6/16.8	2.1/4.1
Pie, Mince, Mini, Waitrose*, 1 pie/30g				
150/501	1.7/5.7	15.4/51.3	9.1/30.3	0.5/1.7
Pie, Mince, Mr Kipling*, 1 pie/62g				
231/372	2.4/3.8	35.2/56.8	8.9/14.4	0.9/1.5
Pie, Mississippi Mud, Tesco*, 1 serving/104g				
399/384	5.5/5.3	34.4/33.1	26.6/25.6	1.9/1.8

kcal serv/100g	prot serv/100g	carb serv/100g	fat serv/100g	fibre serv/100g
Pie, Rhubarb, Sara Lee*, 1 serving/89.6g				
225/250	2.6/2.9	25.8/28.7	12.4/13.8	1.2/1.3
Provamel*, Alpro Soya, Caramel Flavoured Soya Dessert, 1 pot/125g				
103/82	3.8/3	17.1/13.7	2.1/1.7	0.4/0.3
Provamel*, Alpro Soya, Chocolate-Flavoured Soya Dessert, 1 pot/125g				
110/88	3.8/3	17.3/13.8	2.9/2.3	1.1/0.9
Provamel*, Alpro Soya, Vanilla-Flavoured Dessert, 1 pot/125g				
100/80	3.8/3	16.3/13	2.3/1.8	0/0
Provamel*, Black Cherry Yofu, 1 pot/125g				
106/85	4.6/3.7	16.1/12.9	2.6/2.1	1.5/1.2
Pudding, Chocolate Marks & Spencer*, 1 serving/105g				
401/382	6.5/6.2	42.7/40.7	22.7/21.6	1.2/1.1
Pudding, Chocolate Sponge, Healthy Eating, Tesco*, 1 pudding/102.5g				
197/191	4.5/4.4	35.7/34.7	3.9/3.8	0.9/0.9
Pudding, Chocolate with Chocolate Sauce, BGTY, Sainsbury's*, 1 pudding/110.3g				
161/146	3.9/3.5	31.5/28.6	2.1/1.9	2.5/2.3
Pudding, Chocolate with Chocolate Sauce, Heinz*, ¼ can/77g				
213/277	1.6/2.1	36.3/47.2	6.8/8.8	0.6/0.8
Pudding, Chocolate, BGTY, Sainsbury's*, 1 pudding/110g				
293/266	5.2/4.7	56.7/51.5	5.2/4.7	0.7/0.6
Pudding, Chocolate, Perfectly Balanced, Waitrose*, 1 pot/105g				
196/187	4/3.8	37.8/36	3.3/3.1	0.8/0.8
Pudding, Eve's, BGTY, Sainsbury's*, 1 pudding/145g				
164/113	3.2/2.2	33.9/23.4	1.7/1.2	1/0.7
Pudding, Forest Fruit Sponge, Eat Smart, Safeway*, 1 pot/88.2g				
150/170	3.7/4.2	29.5/33.5	1.6/1.8	2.3/2.6
Pudding, Jam Roly Poly & Custard, Co-Op*, 1 serving/105g				
263/250	3.2/3	46.2/44	7.4/7	0.8/0.8
Pudding, Lemon, BGTY, Sainsbury's*, 1 serving/100g				
151/151	2.9/2.9	31/31	1.9/1.9	0.5/0.5
Pudding, Lemon, Perfectly Balanced, Waitrose*, 1 serving/105g				
212/202	3.6/3.4	43.8/41.7	2.5/2.4	0.6/0.6
Pudding, Macaroni, Creamed, Ambrosia*, 1 can/425g				
374/88	15.3/3.6	62.1/14.6	7.2/1.7	1.3/0.3
Pudding, Spotted Dick, Asda*, 1 serving/105g				
282/269	3/2.9	36/34.3	14/13.3	1.4/1.3

kcal serv/100g	prot serv/100g	carb serv/100g	fat serv/100g	fibre serv/100g
Pudding, Sticky Toffee, Marks & Spencer*, 1 pudding/105g				
337/321	3.7/3.5	54.5/51.9	11.6/11	1.2/1.1
Pudding, Sticky Toffee, Tesco*, 1 serving/110g				
287/261	3.6/3.3	35/31.8	14.7/13.4	0.8/0.7
Pudding, Summer Pudding, Waitrose*, 1 pot/120g				
125/104	2.4/2	27.7/23.1	0.5/0.4	1.7/1.4
Pudding, Treacle Sponge, Heinz*, 1 serving/160g				
445/278	4/2.5	78.2/48.9	13/8.1	1/0.6
Rice Pudding, 50% Less Fat, Asda*, ½ can/212g				
170/85	6.6/3.3	32.4/16.2	1.6/0.8	0.4/0.2
Rice Pudding, Apple, 99% Fat-Free, Mullerice, Muller*, 1 pot/150g				
125/83	5.3/3.5	23/15.3	1.4/0.9	0/0
Rice Pudding, BGTY, Sainsbury's*, ½ can/212g				
180/85	7/3.3	34.3/16.2	1.7/0.8	0.4/0.2
Rice Pudding, Caramel, Mullerice, Muller*, 1 pot/200g				
210/105	7/3.5	34.8/17.4	4.8/2.4	0/0
Rice Pudding, Creamed with Sultanas & Nutmeg, Ambrosia*, ½ can/200g				
210/105	6.4/3.2	33.2/16.6	5.8/2.9	0.2/0.1
Rice Pudding, Creamed, Asda*, 1 serving/215.4g				
196/91	6.9/3.2	34.4/16	3.4/1.6	0/0
Rice Pudding, Creamed, Canned, Ambrosia*, 1 can/425g				
383/90	13.2/3.1	64.6/15.2	8.1/1.9	0/0
Rice Pudding, Creamed, Healthy Eating, New, Tesco*, 1 can/215g				
146/68	7.7/3.6	24.5/11.4	1.9/0.9	0/0
Rice Pudding, Creamed, Healthy Eating, Tesco*, 1oz/28g				
19/68	1/3.6	3.2/11.4	0.2/0.6	0/0
Rice Pudding, Light, Mullerice, Muller*, 1 pot/100g				
72/72	3.5/3.5	12.2/12.2	0.9/0.9	0/0
Rice Pudding, Low-Fat, Canned, Ambrosia*, ½ can/200g				
162/81	6.4/3.2	30.4/15.2	1.6/0.8	0/0
Rice Pudding, Low-Fat, No Added Sugar, Weight Watchers*, ½ can/212g				
155/73	7.8/3.7	24.2/11.4	3.2/1.5	0/0
Rice Pudding, Low-Fat, Pot, Ambrosia*, 1 pot/150g				
129/86	5/3.3	24.2/16.1	1.4/0.9	0/0
Rice Pudding, Original, 99% Fat-Free, Mullerice, Muller*, 1 pot/150g				
108/72	5.9/3.9	17.7/11.8	1.5/1	0/0
Rice Pudding, Raisin & Nutmeg, Muller*, 1 pot/200g				
244/122	6.6/3.3	44/22	4.6/2.3	0/0

	kcal serv/100g	prot serv/100g	carb serv/100g	fat serv/100g	fibre serv/100g
Rice Pudding, Raspberry, Muller*, 1 pot/200g					
	228/114	6.8/3.4	40/20	4.6/2.3	0/0
Rice Pudding, Strawberry, 99% Fat-Free, Muller*, 1 serving/150g					
	116/77	5.3/3.5	20.4/13.6	1.4/0.9	0/0
Rice Pudding, Strawberry, Muller*, 1 pot/150g					
	173/115	5.1/3.4	30/20	3.6/2.4	0/0
Rice Pudding, Toffee, 99% Fat-Free, Muller*, 1 tub/150g					
	119/79	5/3.3	21.5/14.3	1.5/1	0/0
Rice Pudding, Vanilla Custard, Mullerice, Muller*, 1 pot/200g					
	250/125	6.6/3.3	44.2/22.1	5.2/2.6	0/0
Semolina Pudding, Creamed, Ambrosia*, 1 can/425g					
	344/81	14/3.3	55.7/13.1	7.2/1.7	0.9/0.2
Sorbet, Lemon, Tesco*, 1 serving/75g					
	80/106	0/0	19.7/26.2	0/0	0.3/0.4
Sorbet, Mango, Tropical, Haagen-Dazs*, 1oz/28g					
	32/116	0.1/0.2	8/28.6	0/0.1	0/0
Sorbet, Mango, Waitrose*, 1 pot/100g					
	90/90	0.1/0.1	22.1/22.1	0/0	0.6/0.6
Sorbet, Orange, Del Monte*, 1 sorbet/500g					
	625/125	1/0.2	160.5/32.1	0.5/0.1	0/0
Sorbet, Peach & Vanilla Fruit Swirl, Healthy Living, Tesco*, 1 pot/73g					
	93/127	0.8/1.1	21.1/28.9	0.6/0.8	0.4/0.5
Sorbet, Raspberry & Blackberry, Fat-Free, Marks & Spencer*, 1 sorbet/125g					
	140/112	0.5/0.4	34.4/27.5	0/0	0.8/0.6
Sorbet, Raspberry, Tesco*, 1 serving/70ml					
	97/138	0.4/0.5	23.8/34	0/0	0/0
Sponge Fingers, Boudoir, Sainsbury's*, 1 biscuit/5g					
	20/396	0.4/8.1	4.1/82.8	0.2/3.6	0/0.4
Strudel, Apple, Sainsbury's*, ⅙ portion/90g					
	269/299	3.2/3.6	32.7/36.4	13.9/15.4	1.7/1.9
Strudel, Apple, Tesco*, 1 serving/150g					
	432/288	5/3.3	54.6/36.4	21.6/14.4	4.2/2.8
Sundae, Chocolate & Orange, Weight Watchers*, 1 pot/102g					
	137/134	1.2/1.2	25.8/25.2	2.2/2.2	0.2/0.2
Sundae, Chocolate & Vanilla Ice Cream, Tesco*, 1 sundae/70.2g					
	139/199	2/2.8	19.3/27.5	6/8.6	0.4/0.5
Sundae, Chocolate Brownie, Finest, Tesco*, 1 serving/215g					
	808/376	6.7/3.1	64.7/30.1	58.1/27	0.9/0.4

kcal serv/100g	prot serv/100g	carb serv/100g	fat serv/100g	fibre serv/100g
Sundae, Chocolate, Eat Smart, Safeway*, 1 serving/97g				
150/155	3.4/3.5	28.1/29	2.6/2.7	4.2/4.3
Sundae, Chocolate, Healthy Eating, Tesco*, 1 serving/130g				
199/153	5.9/4.5	32.4/24.9	5.1/3.9	0.8/0.6
Sundae, Strawberry & Vanilla, Weight Watchers*, 1 pot/105g				
148/141	1.3/1.2	30.6/29.1	2.2/2.1	0.3/0.3
Tart, Bakewell, Marks & Spencer*, ¼ tart/75g				
345/460	5.6/7.5	36.1/48.1	20/26.7	1.6/2.1
Tart, Bakewell, Somerfield*, ¼ tart/80g				
296/370	4/5	36/45	15.2/19	0/0
Tart, Egg Custard, Marks & Spencer*, 1 tart/85g				
243/286	5.4/6.3	29.5/34.7	12.3/14.5	0.6/0.7
Tart, Egg Custard, Safeway*, 1 tart/85g				
225/265	4.5/5.3	28.3/33.3	10.7/12.6	0.7/0.8
Tart, Egg Custard, Sainsbury's*, 1 tart/85g				
230/270	5.2/6.1	25.6/30.1	12/14.1	0.6/0.7
Tart, Egg Custard, Tesco*, 1 cake/82g				
214/261	5.1/6.2	25.8/31.5	10/12.2	0.9/1.1
Tart, Fruit, Safeway*, 1 tart/180g				
425/236	4.9/2.7	55.1/30.6	20.5/11.4	0/0
Tart, Italian Lemon & Almond, Sainsbury's*, 1 slice/49g				
182/371	3.6/7.4	15.6/31.9	11.6/23.7	2/4.1
Tart, Jam, Assorted, Tesco*, 1 tart/35g				
123/351	1.2/3.4	18.2/51.9	5/14.4	0.4/1.2
Tart, Jam, Real Fruit, Mr Kipling*, 1 tart/35g				
136/389	1.2/3.5	21.4/61	5.1/14.5	0/0
Tart, Lemon & Raspberry, Finest, Tesco*, 1 tart/120g				
360/300	6.2/5.2	46.1/38.4	16.8/14	3.5/2.9
Tart, Lemon Curd, Lyons*, 1 tart/30g				
122/406	1.1/3.7	17.8/59.3	5.1/17	0/0
Tart, Lemon, Marks & Spencer*, ⅙ tart/50g				
208/415	2.5/5	16.4/32.7	14.7/29.3	0.5/0.9
Tart, Pear & Chocolate with Brandy, TTD, Sainsbury's*, ⅙ tart/90g				
261/290	3.2/3.5	28.8/32	14.8/16.4	1.3/1.4
Tart, Strawberry & Fresh Cream, Finest, Tesco*, 1 tart/129g				
350/271	4.3/3.3	40.1/31.1	19.1/14.8	1.5/1.2
Tart, Toffee Pecan, Marks & Spencer*, 1 tart/91g				
414/455	5.5/6	44.1/48.5	24.1/26.5	1.8/2

kcal serv/100g	prot serv/100g	carb serv/100g	fat serv/100g	fibre serv/100g
Tiramisu, BGTY, Sainsbury's*, 1 pot/90g				
140/156	4.1/4.5	25.5/28.3	2.4/2.7	0.3/0.3
Tiramisu, COU, Marks & Spencer*, 1 serving/95g				
138/145	3.5/3.7	25.6/26.9	2.6/2.7	0.6/0.6
Tiramisu, Italian, Co-Op*, 1 pack/90g				
230/255	4.5/5	33.3/37	9/10	0.4/0.4
Tiramisu, Italian, Safeway*, 1 serving/125g				
353/282	5.5/4.4	43/34.4	17.5/14	2/1.6
Tiramisu, Morrisons*, 1 pot/90g				
248/276	3.6/4	34.2/38	9.9/11	0/0
Tiramisu, Trifle, Sainsbury's*, 1 serving/100g				
243/243	2.3/2.3	23.2/23.2	15.7/15.7	0.6/0.6
Tiramisu, Waitrose*, 1 pot/90g				
221/246	5.8/6.4	24.5/27.2	11.2/12.4	0/0
Trifle, Chocolate, Healthy Living, Tesco*, 1 serving/150g				
189/126	6/4	32.1/21.4	4.1/2.7	6.9/4.6
Trifle, Chocolate, Light Milk, Cadbury's*, 1 pot/90g				
171/190	5/5.6	23/25.5	6.6/7.3	0/0
Trifle, Chocolate, Tesco*, 1 serving/125g				
313/250	5.4/4.3	30/24	19/15.2	0.9/0.7
Trifle, Fruit Cocktail, Individual, Shape*, 1 trifle/115g				
136/118	3.7/3.2	22.5/19.6	3.1/2.7	1.8/1.6
Trifle, Fruit Cocktail, Individual, Tesco*, 1 pot/113g				
175/155	1.9/1.7	22.1/19.6	8.8/7.8	0.7/0.6
Trifle, Sherry, Sainsbury's*, 1 serving/132g				
215/162	3.2/2.4	26.7/20.1	10/7.5	0.4/0.3
Trifle, Strawberry, COU, Marks & Spencer*, 1 serving/142g				
170/120	4.3/3	31/21.8	3.3/2.3	0.4/0.3
Trifle, Strawberry, Healthy Eating, Tesco*, 1 serving/113g				
114/101	1.9/1.7	20.9/18.5	2.5/2.2	0.7/0.6
Trifle, Strawberry, Healthy Living, Tesco*, 1 pot/150g				
161/107	3.4/2.3	29/19.3	3.5/2.3	4/2.7
Trifle, Strawberry, Individual, Shape*, 1 pot/115g				
137/119	3.8/3.3	22.8/19.8	3.1/2.7	1.8/1.6
Trifle, Strawberry, Individual, Somerfield*, 1 trifle/125g				
208/166	2.5/2	27.5/22	10/8	0/0
Trifle, Strawberry, Marks & Spencer*, 1 trifle/50g				
81/161	1/2	8.9/17.7	4.6/9.2	0.3/0.6

kcal serv/100g	prot serv/100g	carb serv/100g	fat serv/100g	fibre serv/100g
Trifle, Strawberry, Sainsbury's*, ¼ trifle/125g				
232/186	2.7/2.2	27.1/21.7	12.5/10	0.2/0.2
Trifle, Strawberry, Tesco*, 1 serving/83g				
140/169	1.3/1.6	14.7/17.7	8.5/10.2	0.6/0.7
Trifle, Summerfruit, BGTY, Sainsbury's*, 1 trifle/125g				
151/121	1.5/1.2	24/19.2	5.5/4.4	0.6/0.5
Wafers, Cafe Curls, Rolled, Askeys*, 1 curl/5g				
21/422	0.3/5.8	4/80.3	0.4/8.6	0/0
Wafers, Ice Cream, Askeys*, 2 wafers/3g				
11/380	0.3/11	2.4/79	0.1/2.5	0/0

DRINKS

kcal serv/100g	prot serv/100g	carb serv/100g	fat serv/100g	fibre serv/100g
Apple Juice Drink, No-Added-Sugar, Asda*, 1 glass/200ml				
10/5	0/0	2/1	0/0	0/0
Apple Juice, Chilled, Asda*, 1 glass/200ml				
98/49	0.2/0.1	24/12	0/0	0/0
Appletise, Schweppes*, 1 glass/200ml				
98/49	0/0	23.6/11.8	0/0	0/0
Baileys*, Irish Cream, Original, 1 glass/37g				
130/350	1.2/3.2	7.4/20	5.8/15.7	0/0
Beer, Extra Light, Sleeman Breweries*, 1 bottle/341ml				
90/26	0/0	2.5/0.7	0/0	0/0
Beer, Ginger, Classic, Schweppes*, 1 can/330ml				
115/35	0/0	27.7/8.4	0/0	0/0
Beer, Ginger, Diet, Sainsbury's*, 1 glass/200ml				
2/1	0/0	0.2/0.1	0/0	0/0
Beer, Ginger, Light, Waitrose*, 1 glass/250ml				
3/1	0/0	0/0	0.3/0.1	0.3/0.1
Beer, Ginger, Sainsbury's*, 1 can/330ml				
178/54	0/0	42.9/13	0/0	0/0
Beer, Ginger, Traditional-Style, Tesco*, 1 can/330ml				
218/66	0/0	53.1/16.1	0/0	0/0
Beer, Ultra, Michelob*, 1 bottle/275ml				
88/32	0/0	2.5/0.9	0/0	0/0
Beer, Weissbier, Alcohol-Free, Erdinger*, 1 bottle/500ml				
125/25	2/0.4	26.5/5.3	0/0	0/0

kcal serv/100g	prot serv/100g	carb serv/100g	fat serv/100g	fibre serv/100g
Beer, Wheat, Tesco*, 1 bottle/500ml				
155/31	2.5/0.5	2/0.4	0/0	0/0
Bitter Lemon, Diet, Asda*, 1 glass/200ml				
4/2	0/0	0.6/0.3	0/0	0/0
Bitter Lemon, Low-Calorie, Tesco*, 1 glass/200ml				
6/3	0/0	1.5/0.8	0/0	0/0
Bitter Lemon, Sainsbury's*, 1 glass/250ml				
45/18	0.3/0.1	11/4.4	0.3/0.1	0.3/0.1
Caro, Instant Beverage, No Caffeine, Nestle Uk Ltd*, 1 pot/50g				
133/265	2.8/5.5	30/60	0.2/0.3	0/0
Cherryade, Sugar-Free, Tesco*, 1 glass/250ml				
3/1	0/0	0/0	0/0	0/0
Chocolate Drink, Instant Break, Milk, Cadbury's*, 4 rounded tsp/28g				
119/425	3.1/10.9	18/64.2	3.9/14	0/0
Cider, Medium Sweet, Somerfield*, 1 pint/568ml				
233/41	0/0	28.4/5	0/0	0/0
Cider, Value, Tesco*, 1 pint/568ml				
153/27	0/0	4.5/0.8	0/0	0/0
Cocoa Powder, Cadbury's*, 1 tbsp/16g				
52/322	3.7/23.1	1.7/10.5	3.3/20.8	0/0
Coffee Mate, Lite, Nestle*, 2 tsps/5g				
20/398	0.1/2.5	4.2/83.9	0.3/6.9	0/0
Coffee Mate, Nestle*, 2 tsp/7g				
36/520	0.1/1.2	4.2/60.5	2.1/30.3	0/0
Coffee, Cafe Vanilla, Nescafe*, 1 sachet/18.5g				
82/432	1.8/9.7	13.9/73	2.2/11.4	0/0
Coffee, Caffe Mocha, Starbucks*, 1 tall/200ml				
278/139	9.8/4.9	30/15	15.8/7.9	1.4/0.7
Coffee, Cappuccino, Cafe Mocha, Dry, Maxwell House*, 1 serving/23g				
100/434	1/4.3	18/78.2	2.5/10.8	0/0
Coffee, Cappuccino, Cafe Specials, Dry, Marks & Spencer*, 1 serving/14g				
55/395	2/14	8.3/59	1.6/11.5	0.1/0.7
Coffee, Cappuccino, Chocolate, Tall, Pret A Manger*, 1 serving/355ml				
106/30	5.9/1.7	7.6/2.1	5.8/1.6	0/0
Coffee, Cappuccino, Dry, Maxwell House*, 1 mug/15g				
53/350	1.8/12	9.6/64	1.4/9.6	0.1/0.4
Coffee, Cappuccino, For Filter Systems, Kenco*, 1 sachet/6g				
23/375	1.1/19	2.6/44	0.8/13.5	0/0

	kcal serv/100g	prot serv/100g	carb serv/100g	fat serv/100g	fibre serv/100g

Coffee, Cappuccino, Instant, Kenco*, 1 sachet/20g

80/401	2.7/13.5	11.1/55.7	2.8/13.8	0/0

Coffee, Cappuccino, Instant, Made Up, Maxwell House*, 1 serving/280g

123/44	1.7/0.6	16.2/5.8	5.3/1.9	0/0

Coffee, Cappuccino, Instant, Unsweetened, Douwe Egberts*, 1 serving/12g

48/400	1.3/11	6.4/53	1.9/16	0/0

Coffee, Cappuccino, Low-Sugar, Tesco*, 1 serving/13g

55/425	2.4/18.4	5.6/43.3	2.6/19.8	0.1/0.4

Coffee, Cappuccino, Marks & Spencer*, 1 serving/164g

66/40	2.5/1.5	7.2/4.4	2.6/1.6	0.1/0.1

Coffee, Cappuccino, Nescafe*, 1 sachet/13g

52/398	1.5/11.5	8.7/66.6	1.2/9.5	0/0

Coffee, Cappuccino, Original Mugsticks, Maxwell House*, 1 serving/18g

73/406	2.6/14.4	9.5/52.8	2.8/15.6	0/0

Coffee, Cappuccino, Sainsbury's*, 1 serving/12g

49/411	1.8/14.9	6.3/52.9	1.9/15.5	0/0.4

Coffee, Cappuccino, Swiss Chocolate, Nescafe*, 1 sachet/20g

81/404	2.1/10.5	13.1/65.3	2.3/11.5	0.6/2.9

Coffee, Cappuccino, Unsweetened Taste, Maxwell House*, 1 serving/15g

65/434	2.6/17.4	7.1/47.6	2.9/19.3	0/0.3

Coffee, Cappuccino, Unsweetened, Dry, Nescafe*, 1 sachet/12g

51/427	1.8/14.9	6.6/54.7	2/16.6	0/0

Coffee, Frappe Iced, Nestle*, 1 serving/25g

96/384	3.8/15	18/72	1/4	0.1/0.5

Coffee, Frappuccino, Blended Coffee, Starbucks*, 1 serving/454ml

260/57	5/1.1	52/11.5	3.5/0.8	0/0

Coffee, Frappuccino, Caramel, Coffee-Based, Starbucks*,
1 grande size/473ml

279/59	4.7/1	54.9/11.6	3.3/0.7	0/0

Coffee, Frappuccino, Mango Citrus Tea, Starbucks*, 1 tall/220ml

180/82	1/0.5	40/18.2	0/0	0/0

Coffee, Frappuccino, Starbucks*, 1 drink/281ml

190/68	6/2.1	39/13.9	3/1.1	0/0

Coffee, Frappuccino, Strawberries & Cream, Starbucks*,
1 serving/Grande/473ml

581/123	15/3.2	92/19.5	17/3.6	0/0

Coffee, Ice Mocha Drink, Nescafe, Nestle*, 1 bottle/280ml

160/57	3.1/1.1	29.4/10.5	3.4/1.2	0/0

kcal serv/100g	prot serv/100g	carb serv/100g	fat serv/100g	fibre serv/100g
Coffee, Latte, 'a' Mocha, Cafe Met*, 1 bottle/290ml				
174/60	9.3/3.2	26.1/9	4.1/1.4	0/0
Coffee, Latte, Cafe, Marks & Spencer*, 1 serving/190g				
143/75	8.2/4.3	15.8/8.3	5.3/2.8	0/0
Coffee, Latte, Nescafe*, 1 sachet/21g				
98/469	3/14.5	11/52.4	4.7/22.5	0/0
Coffee, Latte, Pret A Manger*, 1 serving/336g				
194/58	10.5/3.1	13.2/3.9	11.2/3.3	7/2.1
Coffee, Latte, Skimmed Milk, Starbucks*, 1 serving/260ml				
88/34	8.8/3.4	13/5	0.3/0.1	0/0
Coffee, Latte, Whole Milk, Starbucks*, 1 tall/355.2ml				
180/51	10/2.8	14/3.9	10/2.8	0/0
Coffee, Moch 'a' Latte, CafeMet*, 1 bottle/290ml				
174/60	9.3/3.2	26.1/9	4.1/1.4	0/0
Cranberry & Raspberry Juice Drink, Asda*, 1 glass/250ml				
135/54	0.5/0.2	32.5/13	0/0	0/0
Cream Soda, Traditional-Style, Tesco*, 1 can/330ml				
139/42	0/0	34.3/10.4	0/0	0/0
Crush, Morello Cherry, Finest, Tesco*, 1 bottle/250ml				
115/46	0/0	28/11.2	0/0	0/0
Crush, Orange & Raspberry, Freshly-Squeezed, Finest, Tesco*, 1fl oz/30ml				
17/56	0.2/0.5	3.8/12.6	0/0.1	0.1/0.2
Crush, Orange & Raspberry, Safeway*, 1 serving/100ml				
57/57	0.5/0.5	13.6/13.6	0.1/0.1	0.2/0.2
Crush, Orange, Cool, Diet, Sainsbury's*, 1 can/330ml				
10/3	0.2/0.1	2/0.6	0.2/0.1	0.2/0.1
Dandelion & Burdock, Drink, Ben Shaws Original*, 1 lge can/440ml				
128/29	0/0	30.8/7	0/0	0/0
Diamond White, Cider, 1fl oz/30ml				
11/36	0/0	0.8/2.6	0/0	0/0
Dr Pepper*, Coca-Cola*, 1 bottle/500ml				
210/42	0/0	54.5/10.9	0/0	0/0
Dr Pepper*, Soda, Diet, 1fl oz/30ml				
0/1	0/0	0/0.1	0/0	0/0
Energy Drink, Red Rooster, Hi Energy Mixer, Cott Beverages Ltd*, 1 can/250ml				
113/45	1.5/0.6	25.8/10.3	0/0	0/0

	kcal serv/100g	prot serv/100g	carb serv/100g	fat serv/100g	fibre serv/100g
Fanta, Lemon, The Coca Cola Co*, 1 can/330ml					
	165/50	0/0	39.6/12	0/0	0/0
Fanta, Light, The Coca-Cola Co*, 1 glass/250ml					
	5/2	0/0	1.3/0.5	0/0	0/0
Fanta, Orange, The Coca-Cola Co*, 1 can/330ml					
	142/43	0/0	34.3/10.4	0/0	0/0
Fruit Drink, Alive Tropical Torrent, The Coca Cola Co*, 1 glass/200ml					
	88/44	0/0	22/11	0/0	0/0
Fruit Drink, Apple & Blackcurrant, No Added Sugar, Safeway*, 1fl oz/30ml					
	2/8	0/0.1	0.3/1	0/0	0/0
Fruit Drink, Blackcurrant & Apple, Shapers, Boots*, 1 bottle/500ml					
	10/2	0/0	1/0.2	0/0	0/0
Fruit Drink, Five Fruits, Five Alive*, 1 carton/250ml					
	125/50	0/0	30/12	0/0	0/0
Fruit Infusion, Peach, Lime & Ginger, Marks & Spencer*, 1 serving/250ml					
	88/35	0/0	21.3/8.5	0/0	0/0
High Lights, Cadbury's*, 1 cup/200ml					
	40/20	2/1	5/2.5	1.4/0.7	0.6/0.3
High Lights, Caffe Latte, Cadbury's*, 1 serving/200g					
	40/20	2/1	5/2.5	1.4/0.7	0/0
High Lights, Choc Malt Hot Chocolate, Cadbury's*, 1 serving/200ml					
	44/22	2/1	5/2.5	1.4/0.7	0.6/0.3
High Lights, Choc Mint, Cadbury's*, 1 serving/200ml					
	40/20	2/1	5/2.5	1.4/0.7	0.6/0.3
High Lights, Dairy Fudge, Cadbury's*, 1 serving/200ml					
	40/20	2/1	5.6/2.8	1/0.5	0.4/0.2
High Lights, Espresso, Cadbury's*, 1 serving/200ml					
	35/18	2.5/1.3	3.9/2	0.9/0.5	0/0
High Lights, Orange, Cadbury's*, 1 serving/200ml					
	40/20	2/1	4.6/2.3	1.4/0.7	0/0
High Lights, Toffee Flavour, Chocolate Drink, Cadbury's*, 1 serving/200ml					
	40/20	2/1	5.2/2.6	1.4/0.7	0/0
Hot Chocolate, Chocolate Break, Tesco*, 1 serving/21g					
	110/524	1.7/7.9	12.4/58.9	6/28.5	0.4/1.7
Hot Chocolate, Chocolate Time, Safeway*, 1 serving/30g					
	123/411	2.8/9.4	20.3/67.8	3.4/11.4	0.5/1.8
Hot Chocolate, Galaxy, Mars*, 1 mug/28g					
	115/411	2/7	19.2/68.7	3.4/12.1	0/0

kcal serv/100g	prot serv/100g	carb serv/100g	fat serv/100g	fibre serv/100g
Hot Chocolate, Instant, BGTY, Sainsbury's*, 1 sachet/28g				
16/56	0.6/2.1	3/10.6	0.2/0.6	0.1/0.3
Hot Chocolate, Instant, Cadbury's*, 1 sachet/28g				
119/426	3.1/10.9	18/64.2	3.9/14	0.6/2.3
Hot Chocolate, Instant, GFY, Asda*, 1 mug/200ml				
106/53	3.6/1.8	20/10	1.2/0.6	0.8/0.4
Hot Chocolate, Instant, Tesco*, 1 serving/32g				
132/414	2.6/8	21.9/68.3	3.9/12.1	0.2/0.7
Hot Chocolate, Maltesers, Malt Drink, Instant, Mars*, 1 serving/220ml				
104/47	1.9/0.9	17/7.7	3/1.4	0/0
Hot Chocolate, Velvet, Cadbury's*, 1 serving/28g				
136/487	2.4/8.6	16.2/57.8	6.9/24.6	0.6/2
Hot Chocolate, with Whipped Cream Grande, Starbucks*, **1 grande mug/473ml**				
440/93	15/3.2	44/9.3	24/5.1	2/0.4
Iron Bru, Diet, Barr's*, 1 can/330ml				
2/1	0.3/0.1	0.3/0.1	0/0	0/0
Lager, Amstel, Heineken N V*, 1 pint/568ml				
227/40	2.8/0.5	17/3	0/0	0/0
Lager, Becks*, 1 can/275ml				
113/41	0/0	8.3/3	0/0	0/0
Lager, Budweiser, Anheuser-Busch*, 1 bottle/330ml				
133/40	1/0.3	9.6/2.9	0/0	0/0
Lager, Export, Foster's*, 1 pint/568ml				
210/37	0/0	12.5/2.2	0/0	0/0
Lager, Foster's*, 1 pint/568ml				
227/40	0/0	17.6/3.1	0/0	0/0
Lager, French Premier, Somerfield*, 1 bottle/250ml				
108/43	0/0	10/4	0/0	0/0
Lager, Heineken, Heineken N V*, 1 pint/568ml				
256/45	2.8/0.5	17/3	0/0	0/0
Lager, Miller Pilsner*, 1 bottle/500ml				
150/30	1.5/0.3	12/2.4	0/0	0/0
Lager, Pils, Holsten*, 1 can/440ml				
167/38	1.3/0.3	10.6/2.4	0/0	0/0
Lager, Premium, Tesco*, 1 can/440ml				
229/52	1.8/0.4	17.6/4	0/0	0/0

kcal serv/100g	prot serv/100g	carb serv/100g	fat serv/100g	fibre serv/100g
Lager, Stella Artois*, 1 can/550ml				
222/40	1.7/0.3	16/2.9	0/0	0/0
Lemonade, 7-Up, Light, Britvic*, 1 can/330ml				
4/1	0.3/0.1	0.7/0.2	0/0	0/0
Lemonade, Asda*, 1 glass/250ml				
83/33	0/0	20/8	0/0	0/0
Lemonade, Cloudy, Diet, Safeway*, 1 can/330ml				
7/2	0/0	0.7/0.2	0/0	0/0
Lemonade, Cloudy, Diet, Sainsbury's*, 1 can/330ml				
7/2	0.3/0.1	0.7/0.2	0.3/0.1	1/0.3
Lemonade, Cloudy, Sainsbury's*, 1 glass/250ml				
118/47	0.3/0.1	30/12	0.3/0.1	0.3/0.1
Lemonade, Diet, Asda*, 1 glass/250ml				
3/1	0/0	0.3/0.1	0.3/0.1	0/0
Lemonade, Shapers, Boots*, 1 bottle/500ml				
13/3	0/0	0/0	0/0	0/0
Lemonade, Sprite, Light, Sprite*, 1fl oz/30ml				
0/2	0/0	0/0	0/0	0/0
Lemonade, Still, Marks & Spencer*, 1 glass/250ml				
5/49	0/0.1	1.3/12.9	0/0	0/0
Lemonade, Still, Tesco*, 1 glass/200ml				
100/50	0/0	24/12	0/0	0/0
Lucozade, Hydro Active, Smithkline Beecham*, 1fl oz/30ml				
3/10	0/0	0.6/2	0/0	0/0
Lucozade, Orange Energy Drink, Smithkline Beecham*, 1 bottle/500ml				
350/70	0/0	86/17.2	0/0	0/0
Lucozade, Original, Smithkline Beecham*, 1 sm bottle/345ml				
252/73	0/0	61.8/17.9	0/0	0/0
Lucozade, Sport Isotonic Lemon Body Fuel, Smithkline Beecham*, 1 bottle/500ml				
140/28	0/0	32/6.4	0/0	0/0
Lucozade, Sport, Orange, SmithKline Beecham*, 1 bottle/500ml				
140/28	0/0	32/6.4	0/0	0.5/0.1
Lucozade, Tropical, SmithKline Beecham*, 1 bottle/380ml				
266/70	0/0	65.4/17.2	0/0	0/0
Milk Drink, Mars Extra Milk Chocolate Caramel, Mars*, 1 bottle/330g				
224/68	11.6/3.5	39.9/12.1	1/0.3	0/0

	kcal serv/100g	prot serv/100g	carb serv/100g	fat serv/100g	fibre serv/100g
Milk Shake, Banana Flavour, Frijj*, 1 bottle/500ml					
	310/62	17/3.4	50.5/10.1	4/0.8	0/0
Milk Shake, Banana Flavour, Shapers, Boots*, 1 bottle/250ml					
	201/80	14/5.6	32/12.8	1.9/0.8	4.8/1.9
Milk Shake, Banana, Yazoo*, 1 bottle/500ml					
	325/65	15.5/3.1	51.5/10.3	6.5/1.3	0/0
Milk Shake, Chocolate Flavour, BGTY, Sainsbury's*, 1 bottle/500ml					
	290/58	26.5/5.3	40/8	2.5/0.5	4.5/0.9
Milk Shake, Chocolate Flavoured, Fresh, Thick, Frijj*, 1 bottle/500ml					
	345/69	17.5/3.5	58/11.6	5/1	0/0
Milk Shake, Chocolate, Extreme, Frijj*, 1 bottle/500g					
	425/85	19.5/3.9	63.5/12.7	10.5/2.1	0/0
Milk Shake, Strawberry Flavour, Thick, Low-Fat, Frijj*, 1 bottle/250ml					
	155/62	8.5/3.4	25.3/10.1	2/0.8	0/0
Milk Shake, Strawberry, Thick, Somerfield*, 1 milkshake/250ml					
	275/110	10/4	37.5/15	10/4	0/0
Milk Shake, Vanilla Flavour, BGTY, Sainsbury's*, 1 bottle/500ml					
	230/46	26.5/5.3	29.5/5.9	0.5/0.1	2/0.4
Milk Shake, Vanilla, Frijj*, 1 bottle/500ml					
	320/64	17/3.4	53.5/10.7	4/0.8	0/0
Multivitamins Drink, Tropicana*, 1fl oz/30ml					
	16/52	0.2/0.5	3.2/10.5	0/0	0/0.1
Options*, Choca Mocha Drink, 1 sachet/10g					
	36/359	1.4/14.1	5/50.1	1.1/11.4	0.7/7
Options*, Chocolate Au Lait Drink, 1 sachet/10g					
	36/355	1.2/11.8	5.5/54.5	1/10	0.7/7.3
Options*, Hot Chocolate, Belgian Chocolate, Instant, 1 serving/11g					
	40/363	1.4/12.4	6/54.9	1.1/10.4	0.8/7.5
Options*, Hot Chocolate, Diet Friendly, 1 sachet/11ml					
	40/364	1.6/14.3	5.6/50.6	1.3/11.6	0.8/7.1
Options*, Hot Chocolate, Irish Cream, 1 sachet/10.9g					
	39/357	1.5/13.9	5.5/50	1.2/11.3	0.9/8.1
Options*, Hot Chocolate, Orange Flavour, 1 serving/11ml					
	40/364	1.6/14.2	5.6/50.8	1.3/11.6	0.8/7.1
Orange Drink, Sparkling, Shapers, Boots*, 1 bottle/500ml					
	15/3	0.5/0.1	2/0.4	0.5/0.1	0/0
Orange Juice, Freshly Squeezed, Asda*, 1 glass/200ml					
	88/44	1.2/0.6	20/10	0/0	0.2/0.1

kcal serv/100g	prot serv/100g	carb serv/100g	fat serv/100g	fibre serv/100g

Provamel*, Soya Alternative To Milk, ½ pint/284ml

| 102/36 | 10.2/3.6 | 1.7/0.6 | 6/2.1 | 3.4/1.2 |

Provamel*, Strawberry Flavour Soya Alternative To Milk, 1 carton/250ml

| 160/64 | 9/3.6 | 19.3/7.7 | 5.3/2.1 | 3/1.2 |

Red Bull, 1 can/250ml

| 113/45 | 0/0 | 28.3/11.3 | 0/0 | 0/0 |

Red Bull, Sugar-Free*, 1 can/250ml

| 8/3 | 0/0 | 2.5/1 | 0/0 | 0/0 |

Ribena*, Blackcurrant, Diluted with Water, 1 serving/180ml

| 81/45 | 0/0 | 19.8/11 | 0/0 | 0/0 |

Ribena*, Light, 1 bottle/288ml

| 63/22 | 0/0 | 15/5.2 | 0/0 | 0/0 |

Shandy, Bitter, Original, Ben Shaws*, 1 can/330ml

| 89/27 | 0/0 | 19.8/6 | 0/0 | 0/0 |

Shandy, Lemonade, Traditional-Style, Tesco*, 1 can/330ml

| 63/19 | 0/0 | 15.5/4.7 | 0/0 | 0/0 |

SlimFast, Banana Deluxe Meal Replacement Drink, SlimFast*, 1 serving/325ml

| 215/66 | 13.5/4.2 | 36.6/11.3 | 2.5/0.8 | 4.7/1.4 |

SlimFast, Coffee Mocha, Ready-to-Drink, SlimFast*, 1 shake/325ml

| 215/66 | 13.7/4.2 | 34.5/10.6 | 2.6/0.8 | 4.9/1.5 |

SlimFast, French Vanilla, Ready-To-Drink, SlimFast*, 1 can/325ml

| 215/66 | 13.7/4.2 | 34.5/10.6 | 2.6/0.8 | 4.9/1.5 |

SlimFast, Peach Shake, SlimFast*, 1 can/325ml

| 215/66 | 13.7/4.2 | 34.5/10.6 | 2.6/0.8 | 4.9/1.5 |

SlimFast, Strawberry Supreme, Ready-To-Drink, SlimFast*, 1 can/325ml

| 215/66 | 13.7/4.2 | 34.5/10.6 | 2.6/0.8 | 4.9/1.5 |

SlimFast, Vanilla Shake, Ready-To-Drink, SlimFast*, 1 can/325ml

| 215/66 | 13.7/4.2 | 34.5/10.6 | 2.6/0.8 | 4.9/1.5 |

Smoothie, Apple, Raspberries & Banana, P & J*, 1 bottle/330ml

| 188/57 | 2.3/0.7 | 40.3/12.2 | 1/0.3 | 0/0 |

Smoothie, Apricot & Peach, COU, Marks & Spencer*, 1 serving/250ml

| 100/40 | 2.3/0.9 | 20.8/8.3 | 0.9/0.4 | 1/0.4 |

Smoothie, Banana, Marks & Spencer*, 1 bottle/500ml

| 270/54 | 8.5/1.7 | 61/12.2 | 0.5/0.1 | 4/0.8 |

Smoothie, Blackberry & Blueberry, Innocent*, 1 bottle/250ml

| 120/48 | 1.5/0.6 | 28.8/11.5 | 0.3/0.1 | 0/0 |

kcal serv/100g	prot serv/100g	carb serv/100g	fat serv/100g	fibre serv/100g
Smoothie, Blackcurrants & Gooseberries, For Autumn, Innocent*, 1 bottle/250ml				
118/47	1.3/0.5	31.3/12.5	0.3/0.1	0/0
Smoothie, Boysenberry & Raspberry, Fruit, Sainsbury's*, 1 bottle/250ml				
108/43	1.8/0.7	25/10	0.3/0.1	4/1.6
Smoothie, Cranberries & Rasperries, Pure Fruit, Innocent*, 1 serving/250ml				
103/41	1.3/0.5	23.8/9.5	0.5/0.2	0/0
Smoothie, Cranberries & Strawberries, Innocent*, 1 serving/250ml				
103/41	1.3/0.5	23.8/9.5	0.5/0.2	0/0
Smoothie, Daily Detox, P & J*, 1 bottle/250ml				
143/57	2/0.8	32.8/13.1	0.5/0.2	0/0
Smoothie, Ginseng & Ace Vitamins, Marks & Spencer*, 1 bottle/250ml				
138/55	1.8/0.7	32.5/13	0.5/0.2	2.3/0.9
Smoothie, It's Alive, P & J*, 1 bottle/250ml				
150/60	1.8/0.7	34/13.6	0.8/0.3	0/0
Smoothie, Mango & Passion Fruit, Innocent*, 1 bottle/250ml				
138/55	1/0.4	32/12.8	0.5/0.2	0/0
Smoothie, Mango & West Indian Cherry, Plus, Tesco*, 1 serving/250ml				
133/53	1.6/0.6	30.6/12.2	0.6/0.2	1.3/0.5
Smoothie, Mango, Pineapple & Passion Fruit, Eat Smart, Safeway*, 1 bottle/250ml				
135/54	1.3/0.5	31.5/12.6	0/0	2.8/1.1
Smoothie, Mango, Pineapple & Passionfruit, Marks & Spencer*, 1 bottle/500ml				
290/58	3.5/0.7	60.5/12.1	2.5/0.5	4.5/0.9
Smoothie, Orange & Mango, Safeway*, 1 bottle/250ml				
130/52	1.3/0.5	30.3/12.1	0.5/0.2	1.8/0.7
Smoothie, Orange, Mango & Apricot, COU, Marks & Spencer*, 1 bottle/250ml				
130/52	1.5/0.6	27.5/11	1.5/0.6	1.5/0.6
Smoothie, Orange, Strawberry & Guava, Sainsbury's*, 1 serving/300ml				
159/53	0.9/0.3	36/12	0.6/0.2	2.4/0.8
Smoothie, Oranges & Mangoes, Get Your Vits, P & J*, 1 bottle/250ml				
128/51	1.5/0.6	29/11.6	0.5/0.2	0/0
Smoothie, Oranges Mangoes & Bananas, P & J*, 1 bottle/330ml				
195/59	3/0.9	44.9/13.6	0.7/0.2	2.3/0.7

kcal serv/100g	prot serv/100g	carb serv/100g	fat serv/100g	fibre serv/100g
Smoothie, Peach, Mild & Fruity, Campina*, 1 bottle/330ml				
211/64	8.9/2.7	43.2/13.1	0/0	0/0
Smoothie, Peaches & Bananas, P & J*, 1 bottle/330ml				
188/57	2.3/0.7	44.9/13.6	1/0.3	0/0
Smoothie, Pineapple, Banana & Coconut, P & J*, 1 bottle/330ml				
234/71	2.6/0.8	40.6/12.3	4.6/1.4	0/0
Smoothie, Pineapple, Banana & Mango Fruit, Finest, Tesco*, 1 glass/200ml				
94/47	0.2/0.1	22.4/11.2	0.4/0.2	0/0
Smoothie, Pineapple, Banana & Pear, Asda*, 1 bottle/250ml				
147/59	1.2/0.5	34/13.6	0.3/0.1	0.8/0.3
Smoothie, Pineapple, Banana & Pear, Princes*, 1 bottle/250ml				
153/61	1.3/0.5	34.8/13.9	0.5/0.2	1.3/0.5
Smoothie, Pineapple, Mango & Lime, Way To Five, Sainsbury's*, 1 bottle/250g				
120/48	1/0.4	28.3/11.3	0.3/0.1	0.8/0.3
Smoothie, Raspberry, Marks & Spencer*, 1 serving/250ml				
138/55	4.3/1.7	30.5/12.2	1.5/0.6	4.8/1.9
Smoothie, Strawberries & Bananas, Innocent*, 1 bottle/250ml				
118/47	1/0.4	26.8/10.7	0.5/0.2	0/0
Smoothie, Strawberries & Bananas, P & J*, 1 bottle/330ml				
172/52	3/0.9	38/11.5	1/0.3	0/0
Smoothie, Strawberry & Banana Fruit, Finest, Tesco*, 1 bottle/250ml				
135/54	0.8/0.3	31.3/12.5	0.8/0.3	1.3/0.5
Smoothie, Strawberry & Cherry, Organic, Marks & Spencer*, 1 bottle/250ml				
138/55	2/0.8	30.8/12.3	0.8/0.3	1/0.4
Smoothie, Strawberry & Raspberry, Shapers, Boots*, 1 bottle/250ml				
110/44	1.5/0.6	25/10	0.5/0.2	1.5/0.6
Smoothie, Strawberry & White Chocolate, Marks & Spencer*, 1 serving/250ml				
100/40	6.3/2.5	13.8/5.5	2.5/1	0.3/0.1
Smoothie, Strawberry Dairy, Shapers, Boots*, 1 bottle/250ml				
120/48	4.3/1.7	24.3/9.7	0.8/0.3	1.3/0.5
Smoothie, Vanilla & Honey, Sainsbury's*, 1 bottle/250ml				
238/95	8/3.2	37/14.8	6/2.4	0.8/0.3
Smoothie, Vanilla Bean, Marks & Spencer*, 1 bottle/500ml				
450/90	16.5/3.3	69.5/13.9	13/2.6	0/0
Squash, Blackcurrant, High Juice, Marks & Spencer*, 1 glass/250ml				
50/20	0.3/0.1	13/5.2	0/0	0.3/0.1

	kcal serv/100g	prot serv/100g	carb serv/100g	fat serv/100g	fibre serv/100g
Squash, Fruit & Barley Orange, Robinson's*, 1 av serving/50ml					
	8/16	0.2/0.3	1.3/2.6	0/0	0/0
Squash, Lemon, High Juice, Sainsbury's*, 1 glass diluted/250ml					
	98/39	0.3/0.1	22.8/9.1	0.3/0.1	0.3/0.1
Squash, Lemon, Whole, Low-Sugar, Sainsbury's*, 1 glass/250ml					
	5/2	0.3/0.1	0.5/0.2	0.3/0.1	0.3/0.1
Squash, Mixed Fruit, Low-Sugar, Sainsbury's*, 1 glass/250ml					
	5/2	0.3/0.1	0.5/0.2	0.3/0.1	0.3/0.1
Squash, Orange & Pineapple, Original, Robinson's*, 1 serving/250ml					
	138/55	2.5/1	32.5/13	0/0	0/0
Squash, Orange, Sainsbury's*, 1 glass/250ml					
	8/3	0.3/0.1	1.3/0.5	0.3/0.1	0.3/0.1
Squash, Pink Grapefruit, High Juice, Sainsbury's*, 1 serving/250ml					
	103/41	0.3/0.1	24.8/9.9	0.3/0.1	0.3/0.1
Squash, Tropical Fruits, High Juice Sainsbury's*, 1 serving/250ml					
	95/38	0.3/0.1	23.3/9.3	0.3/0.1	0.3/0.1
Summer Fruits, Light, Oasis*, 1 bottle/500ml					
	16/3	0/0	2/0.4	0/0	0/0
Summer Fruits, Oasis*, 1 bottle/500ml					
	185/37	0/0	45/9	0/0	0/0
Sunny Delight*, 1 glass/200ml					
	88/44	0.2/0.1	20/10	0.4/0.2	0/0
Sunny Delight*, Light, 1 glass/200ml					
	16/8	0.2/0.1	2/1	0.4/0.2	0/0
Tea, Lemon Iced, Costa*, 1 bottle/275ml					
	91/33	0/0	22/8	0/0	0/0
Tea, Lemon, Original, Instant Drink, Lift*, 1 serving/15g					
	53/352	0/0	13.1/87	0/0	0/0
Tea, Peach Flavour, Lift*, 1 cup/15g					
	58/384	0/0.3	14.3/95.6	0/0	0/0
Tea, Peach, Iced, Twinings*, 1 serving/200ml					
	60/30	0.2/0.1	14.6/7.3	0.2/0.1	0/0
Tonic Water, Indian, Slimline, Schweppes*, 1 pub measure/188ml					
	3/2	0.8/0.4	0.1/0.1	0/0	0/0
Tonic Water, Marks & Spencer*, 1 bottle/500ml					
	100/20	0/0	24/4.8	0/0	0/0
Vimto*, 1 can/330ml					
	147/45	0/0	36.3/11	0/0	0/0

kcal serv/100g	prot serv/100g	carb serv/100g	fat serv/100g	fibre serv/100g

Vimto*, Grape Blackcurrant & Raspberry Juice Drink, 1 bottle/500ml

| 223/45 | 0/0 | 55/11 | 0/0 | 0/0 |

Vimto*, Light, 1 can/330ml

| 17/5 | 0/0 | 4/1.2 | 0/0 | 0/0 |

Water, Lemon & Elderflower, Slightly Sparkling, Tesco*, 1 glass/200ml

| 2/1 | 0/0 | 0.2/0.1 | 0/0 | 0/0 |

Water, Lemon & Lime Flavoured, Marks & Spencer*, 1 glass/250ml

| 13/5 | 0/0 | 2.5/1 | 0/0 | 0/0 |

Water, Mandarin & Cranberry, Still, Marks & Spencer*, 1 bottle/500ml

| 100/20 | 0/0 | 25/5 | 0/0 | 0/0 |

Water, Orange & Peach, Touch of Fruit, Volvic*, 1 bottle/400ml

| 93/23 | 0/0 | 22/5.5 | 0/0 | 0/0 |

Water, Peach & Lemon, Still, Marks & Spencer*, 1 bottle/500ml

| 100/20 | 0/0 | 25/5 | 0/0 | 0/0 |

Water, Peach, Perfectly Clear, Silver Spring Mineral Water Co*, 1 bottle/500ml

| 4/1 | 0/0 | 0/0 | 0/0 | 0/0 |

Water, Spring, Apple & Cherry Flavoured, Sparkling, Sainsbury's*, 1 glass/250ml

| 5/2 | 0.3/0.1 | 0.5/0.2 | 0.3/0.1 | 0.3/0.1 |

Water, Spring, Apple & Raspberry Flavoured, Sainsbury's*, 1fl oz/30ml

| 1/2 | 0/0.1 | 0/0.1 | 0/0.1 | 0/0.1 |

Water, Spring, Boysenberry, Shapers, Boots*, 1 bottle/700ml

| 7/1 | 0/0 | 0.7/0.1 | 0/0 | 0/0 |

Water, Spring, Peach Flavour, Shapers, Boots*, 1 bottle/500ml

| 5/1 | 0/0 | 0/0 | 0/0 | 0/0 |

Water, Spring, Peach Flavoured, No Added Sugar, Asda*, 1 glass/200ml

| 4/2 | 0/0 | 0.4/0.2 | 0/0 | 0/0 |

EATING OUT AND FAST FOOD

Bread, Garlic Pizza, Domino's Pizza*, 1 slice/40g

| 115/295 | 4.7/12 | 16.1/41.4 | 3.5/9 | 0.9/2.3 |

Bread, Garlic, Pizza Hut*, 1 slice/24g

| 101/419 | 2.1/8.7 | 11.5/48.1 | 5.1/21.3 | 0.6/2.7 |

Breakfast, Big Breakfast, McDonald's*, 1 breakfast/256g

| 591/231 | 26.1/10.2 | 39.9/15.6 | 36.4/14.2 | 4.1/1.6 |

	kcal serv/100g	prot serv/100g	carb serv/100g	fat serv/100g	fibre serv/100g
Burgers, Bacon & Cheese, McDonald's*, 1 burger/141g					
	358/254	19.9/14.1	33.7/23.9	15.9/11.3	2.7/1.9
Burgers, Bacon Double Cheeseburger, Bunless, Burger King*, **1 burger/138g**					
	607/440	41.4/30	5.5/4	42.8/31	0/0
Burgers, Big Mac, McDonald's*, 1 Big Mac/215g					
	492/229	26.7/12.4	44.1/20.5	23/10.7	5.4/2.5
Burgers, Big Tasty, McDonald's*, 1 pack/348g					
	804/231	40.7/11.7	50.8/14.6	50.5/14.5	5.6/1.6
Burgers, Cheeseburger, Bacon Double, Burger King*, 1 pack/191g					
	510/267	36.3/19	30.6/16	26.7/14	1.9/1
Burgers, Cheeseburger, Burger King*, 1 burger/141g					
	379/269	22/15.6	42.3/30	18.9/13.4	2/1.4
Burgers, Cheeseburger, Double, McDonalds*, 1 burger/171g					
	438/256	26.5/15.5	33.2/19.4	20/11.7	3.1/1.8
Burgers, Cheeseburger, McDonald's*, 1 burger/122g					
	300/246	15.9/13	33.2/27.2	11.6/9.5	2.6/2.1
Burgers, Chicken Fillet, Kentucky Fried Chicken*, 1 burger/213g					
	469/220	32/15	40.5/19	19.6/9.2	3.4/1.6
Burgers, Chicken Flamer, Burger King*, 1 sandwich/162g					
	308/190	20.4/12.6	30.1/18.6	11.8/7.3	3.1/1.9
Burgers, Chicken Sandwich, Burger King*, 1 sandwich/224g					
	659/294	25/11.2	52.9/23.6	39/17.4	2.9/1.3
Burgers, Chicken Whopper, Lite, Burger King*, 1 Whopper/159g					
	339/213	24.3/15.3	29.3/18.4	13.8/8.7	0/0
Burgers, Double Whopper with Cheese, Burger King*, 1 pack/378g					
	934/247	52.9/14	49.1/13	60.5/16	3.8/1
Burgers, Double Whopper, Burger King*, 1 sandwich/353g					
	918/260	47.7/13.5	53/15	56.8/16.1	3.9/1.1
Burgers, Filet-O-Fish, McDonald's*, 1 pack/161g					
	388/241	16.1/10	40.3/25	17.7/11	1.1/0.7
Burgers, Fillet Towermeal, Kentucky Fried Chicken*, 1 pack/283g					
	656/232	36.6/13	55.9/19.8	31.8/11.2	4.1/1.5
Burgers, Hamburger, Burger King*, 1 burger/128g					
	339/265	18.9/14.8	30/23.4	16/12.5	1.9/1.5
Burgers, Hamburger, McDonald's*, 1 burger/108g					
	254/235	13.2/12.2	33/30.6	7.7/7.1	2.5/2.3

kcal serv/100g	prot serv/100g	carb serv/100g	fat serv/100g	fibre serv/100g

Burgers, McChicken Grill with BBQ Sauce, McDonald's*, 1 pack/215g

| 309/144 | 26/12.1 | 39/18.1 | 5.5/2.6 | 4.7/2.2 |

Burgers, McChicken Premiere, McDonald's*, 1 burger/244g

| 547/224 | 26.8/11 | 38.8/15.9 | 28.1/11.5 | 3.2/1.3 |

Burgers, McChicken Sandwich, McDonald's*, 1 pack/167g

| 376/225 | 16.5/9.9 | 38.6/23.1 | 17.2/10.3 | 3.7/2.2 |

Burgers, Quarter Pounder with Cheese, McDonald's*, 1 burger/206g

| 515/250 | 31.1/15.1 | 37.5/18.2 | 26.8/13 | 3.7/1.8 |

Burgers, Quarter Pounders, Deluxe, McDonald's*, 1 burger/253g

| 521/206 | 28.8/11.4 | 40.7/16.1 | 26.8/10.6 | 4.3/1.7 |

Burgers, Quarter Pounders, McDonald's*, 1 burger/178g

| 424/238 | 25.8/14.5 | 37.2/20.9 | 19/10.7 | 3.7/2.1 |

Burgers, Quarter Pounders, Wimpy*, 1 serving/100g

| 540/540 | 28.1/28.1 | 42.3/42.3 | 29.9/29.9 | 6.7/6.7 |

Burgers, Spicy Bean, Burger King*, 1 burger/239g

| 504/211 | 18.9/7.9 | 62.6/26.2 | 19.8/8.3 | 9.3/3.9 |

Burgers, Steak Premiere, McDonald's*, 1 burger/229g

| 453/198 | 34.1/14.9 | 44.4/19.4 | 14.2/6.2 | 3.7/1.6 |

Burgers, Vegetable, Deluxe, McDonald's*, 1 burger/210g

| 422/201 | 9.7/4.6 | 54.2/25.8 | 18.7/8.9 | 5.9/2.8 |

Burgers, Veggie, Burger King*, 1 burger/223g

| 433/194 | 14.7/6.6 | 55.5/24.9 | 16.9/7.6 | 7.6/3.4 |

Burgers, Whopper Junior with Cheese, Burger King*, 1 burger/167g

| 421/252 | 20/12 | 30.1/18 | 23.4/14 | 1.7/1 |

Burgers, Whopper with Cheese, Burger King*, 1 pack/299g

| 724/242 | 32.9/11 | 47.8/16 | 44.9/15 | 3/1 |

Burgers, Whopper with Mayo, Burger King*, 1 Whopper/278g

| 678/244 | 28.9/10.4 | 52.8/19 | 38.9/14 | 3.9/1.4 |

Burgers, Whopper, Burger King*, 1 Whopper/274g

| 641/234 | 30.1/11 | 46.6/17 | 38.4/14 | 2.7/1 |

Burgers, Zinger Fillet, Kentucky Fried Chicken*, 1 serving/185g

| 445/241 | 25.8/13.9 | 41.5/22.4 | 19.6/10.6 | 2.6/1.4 |

Burgers, Zinger Tower, Kentucky Fried Chicken*, 1 serving/256g

| 620/242 | 31.7/12.4 | 51.7/20.2 | 31.9/12.5 | 3.3/1.3 |

Burgers, Zinger, Meal, Kentucky Fried Chicken*, 1 meal/305g

| 735/241 | 68.3/22.4 | 32.3/10.6 | 42.7/14 | 4.3/1.4 |

Cadbury's Byte, McDonald's*, 1 Byte/14g

| 67/478 | 0.9/6.5 | 9.1/64.7 | 2.9/20.7 | 0.2/1.7 |

kcal serv/100g	prot serv/100g	carb serv/100g	fat serv/100g	fibre serv/100g
Cake, Birthday, McDonald's*, 1 portion/158g				
406/257	2.5/1.6	62.6/39.6	15/9.5	0.5/0.3
Cake, Chocolate Chip Brownie, McDonald's*, 1 brownie/19g				
68/360	0.9/4.9	11.2/58.8	2.4/12.7	0.4/1.9
Cannelloni, Pizza Express*, 1 serving/100g				
631/631	22.8/22.8	50.5/50.5	37.8/37.8	0/0
Cheesecake, Domino's Pizza*, 1 serving/132g				
396/300	6.6/5	37.6/28.5	24.6/18.6	0/0
Cheesecake, Pizza Express*, 1 slice/100g				
347/347	5.9/5.9	24.8/24.8	24.8/24.8	0/0
Chicken, Drumsticks, Extra Crispy, Kentucky Fried Chicken*, 1 drumstick/67g				
195/291	14.9/22.3	7/10.4	12/17.9	0.9/1.4
Chicken, Dunkers, Domino's Pizza*, 1oz/28g				
62/220	6.6/23.5	0.4/1.5	3.7/13.3	0.1/0.5
Chicken, Popcorn, Large, Kentucky Fried Chicken*, 1 serving/170g				
1054/620	51/30	61.2/36	68/40	0/0
Chicken, Popcorn, Small, Kentucky Fried Chicken*, 1 serving Sm/99g				
358/362	16.8/17	20.8/21	22.8/23	0.2/0.2
Chicken, Strippers, Domino's Pizza*, 1oz/28g				
61/219	6.5/23.3	3.8/13.4	2.2/8	0.3/1
Chicken, Strips, Crispy, Kentucky Fried Chicken*, 1 strip/50g				
134/268	9.3/18.6	7.3/14.5	7.6/15.1	0.7/1.5
Chicken, Wings, Take-Away, Pizza Hut*, 1 pack/178g				
466/262	40.1/22.5	3/1.7	32.8/18.4	2.3/1.3
Chicken, Wings, with Sour Cream & Chive Dip, Pizza Hut*, 1 pack/178g				
680/382	40.6/22.8	3.4/1.9	56.1/31.5	2.3/1.3
Chicken McNuggets, McDonald's*, 6 pieces/109g				
254/233	18.6/17.1	11.6/10.6	14.8/13.6	2.1/1.9
Chicken Select, McDonald's*, 2 Selects/82.1g				
184/224	11.2/13.7	12.1/14.8	9.6/11.7	1.1/1.3
Chicken, Breast, Kentucky Fried Chicken*, 1 breast/161g				
370/230	40/24.8	11/6.8	19/11.8	0/0
Chicken, Breast, Original Recipe, Kentucky Fried Chicken*, 1 breast/161g				
596/370	64.4/40	17.7/11	30.6/19	0/0
Chicken, Fillets, Burger King*, 1 serving/72g				
101/140	20.1/27.9	0.3/0.4	2.2/3.1	0/0

kcal serv/100g	prot serv/100g	carb serv/100g	fat serv/100g	fibre serv/100g

Chicken, Hot Wing, Kentucky Fried Chicken*, 1 wing/22g

| 75/341 | 4/18.2 | 4/18.2 | 5/22.7 | 0.2/0.8 |

Coffee, Cappuccino, Regular, Burger King*, 1 serving/200ml

| 36/18 | 2/1 | 6/3 | 0.2/0.1 | 0.2/0.1 |

Coffee, UHT Creamer, McDonald's*, 1 cup/14ml

| 17/123 | 0.6/4.2 | 0.6/4.2 | 1.4/10 | 0/0 |

Coke, Burger King*, 1 med/400ml

| 172/43 | 0/0 | 42.4/10.6 | 0/0 | 0/0 |

Coke, Coca Cola, McDonald's*, 1 med/400ml

| 172/43 | 0/0 | 42/10.5 | 0/0 | 0/0 |

Coleslaw, Kentucky Fried Chicken*, 1 portion/142g

| 231/163 | 2/1.4 | 26/18.3 | 13.5/9.5 | 3/2.1 |

Corn, On The Cob, Kentucky Fried Chicken*, 1 cob/162g

| 150/93 | 4.9/3 | 35/21.6 | 1.5/0.9 | 1.9/1.2 |

Dip Pot, Barbeque Sauce, Burger King*, 1 serving/25g

| 31/125 | 0.2/0.6 | 7.2/28.7 | 0.1/0.3 | 0.1/0.4 |

Dip, Garlic & Herb, Domino's*, 1 pot/28g

| 194/693 | 0.4/1.4 | 0.7/2.5 | 21.1/75.4 | 0.1/0.4 |

Dip, Garlic, Olive Oil & Butter, Pizza Express*, ½ pot/17g

| 106/621 | 0.3/1.5 | 0.5/2.8 | 11.5/67.4 | 0.1/0.5 |

Dough Balls, Pizza Express*, 8 dough balls/50g

| 200/400 | 7.1/14.3 | 42.5/85 | 1.6/3.2 | 0/0 |

Doughnuts, Chocolate Donut, McDonald's*, 1 Donut/79g

| 329/417 | 3.9/4.9 | 36.3/45.9 | 18.8/23.8 | 1.9/2.4 |

Doughnuts, Chocolate Donut, Mini, McDonald's*, 1 Donut/17g

| 64/375 | 1.2/6.8 | 8/46.9 | 3/17.8 | 0.3/1.6 |

Doughnuts, Cinnamon Donut, McDonald's*, 1 Donut/72g

| 302/419 | 3.7/5.1 | 31/43.1 | 18.1/25.1 | 2.7/3.8 |

Doughnuts, Sugared Donut, McDonald's*, 1 Donut/72g

| 303/421 | 3.6/5 | 30.7/42.6 | 18.4/25.6 | 2.7/3.7 |

Dressing, Balsamic with Olive Oil, Pizza Express*, 1 serving/10g

| 42/421 | 0/0.3 | 1/10.3 | 4.1/41.2 | 0/0 |

Dressing, Honey & Mustard, Burger King*, 1 sachet/40g

| 32/80 | 0.6/1.5 | 5.8/14.5 | 0.8/2 | 0.3/0.8 |

Dressing, Olive Oil, Pizza Express*, 2 tsp/5g

| 29/573 | 0.1/1.4 | 0.2/3.4 | 3.2/63 | 0/0 |

Dressing, Salad, Pizza Express*, 1 serving/5g

| 29/573 | 0.1/1.4 | 0.2/3.4 | 3.2/63 | 0/0 |

	kcal serv/100g	prot serv/100g	carb serv/100g	fat serv/100g	fibre serv/100g
Fanta, Orange, McDonald's*, 1 regular/251ml					
	108/43	0/0	26.1/10.4	0/0	0/0
Filet-O-Fish, McDonald's*, 1 pack/161g					
	388/241	16.1/10	40.3/25	17.7/11	1.1/0.7
Fish Fingers, McDonald's*, 3 fingers/74g					
	164/221	10/13.5	14.9/20.2	7.1/9.6	2.3/3.1
Flatbread, Chicken Salsa, McDonald's*, 1 serving/100g					
	480/480	27.3/27.3	57.6/57.6	15.5/15.5	0/0
Flatbread, Greek, McDonald's*, 1 flatbread/100g					
	433/433	21.2/21.2	47.3/47.3	20.7/20.7	3.8/3.8
French Fries, King Size, Salted, Burger King*, 1 bag/170g					
	539/317	6/3.5	71.9/42.3	25/14.7	4.9/2.9
French Fries, Medium, Salted, Burger King*, 1 bag/116g					
	369/318	3.9/3.4	49/42.2	16.9/14.6	3.9/3.4
French Fries, Small, Salted, Burger King*, 1 bag/74g					
	229/310	2/2.7	30.9/41.8	11/14.8	2/2.7
Fries, McDonald's *, 1 reg portion/78g					
	207/265	3/3.8	28.3/36.3	9/11.5	2.8/3.6
Fries, Medium, Kentucky Fried Chicken*, 1 serving/100g					
	294/294	3.8/3.8	36.4/36.4	14.8/14.8	3.1/3.1
Fries, Wimpy*, 1 serving/100g					
	295/295	3.7/3.7	42.4/42.4	12.1/12.1	3.5/3.5
Fruit Bag, Happy Meal, McDonald's*, 1 bag/80g					
	34/43	0.2/0.2	8/10	0.1/0.1	1.4/1.8
Fruit, A Croquer, McDonald's*, 1 serving/80g					
	47/59	0.3/0.4	10.8/13.5	0.3/0.4	1.8/2.3
Hash Browns, Burger King*, 1 hash brown/102g					
	318/312	7.3/7.2	32.9/32.3	19.8/19.4	3.9/3.8
Hash Browns, McDonald's*, 1 portion/56g					
	127/227	1.2/2.2	14.2/25.3	7.3/13	2.1/3.8
Hot Chocolate, McDonald's*, 1fl oz/30ml					
	101/336	1/3.4	18.3/60.9	2.6/8.7	0.6/2
Hot Chocolate, Regular, McDonald's*, 1 regular/32.4ml					
	122/380	2.2/7	25.3/79	1.3/4	0/0
Hot Dog, & Ketchup, McDonald's*, 1 serving/116g					
	296/255	11.1/9.6	29.9/25.8	14.6/12.6	1.5/1.3
Hot Dog, American-Style, Tesco*, 1 sausage/75g					
	164/218	9.5/12.7	2.6/3.4	12.8/17.1	0/0

kcal serv/100g	prot serv/100g	carb serv/100g	fat serv/100g	fibre serv/100g
Hot Dog, Farmfoods*, 1 sausage/50g				
84/168	5/10	2.5/5	6/12	0.5/1
Ice Cream Cone, McDonald's*, 1 cone/98g				
157/160	4.4/4.5	23.9/24.4	4.9/5	0/0
Ice Cream Cone, with Flake, McDonald's*, 1 cone/107g				
204/191	5.1/4.8	28.9/27	7.7/7.2	0/0
Ice Cream, Dairy, Pizza Hut*, 1 portion/141.7g				
273/192	6.5/4.6	33.1/23.3	12.6/8.9	0.3/0.2
Ice Cream, Vanilla, Pizza Express*, 1 serving/100g				
119/119	0.9/0.9	13.8/13.8	6.8/6.8	0/0
Jacket Skins, Pizza Hut*, 1 portion/ 223.5g				
571/255	7.6/3.4	51.5/23	37.2/16.6	4.7/2.1
Jacket Skins, with Sour Cream & Chive Dip, Pizza Hut*, 1 portion/223.5g				
311/139	3.1/1.4	20.8/9.3	24.2/10.8	1.8/0.8
Ketchup, Dip Pot, Burger King*, 1 pot/25g				
27/107	0.3/1	6.2/24.7	0/0.1	0.2/0.6
Ketchup, Sachet, Burger King*, 1 sachet/15g				
16/107	0.2/1	3.7/24.7	0/0.1	0.1/0.6
Ketchup, Tomato, McDonald's*, 1 portion/20g				
26/131	0.3/1.4	6.2/31.2	0/0.1	0/0
Lasagne, Pizza Hut*, 1 serving/350g				
669/191	39.4/11.3	62.4/17.8	29.2/8.3	9.3/2.7
Lemonade, Sprite, McDonald's*, 1 regular/251ml				
108/43	0/0	26.4/10.5	0/0	0/0
McFlurry, Creme Egg, Cadbury, McDonald's*, 1 pack/203g				
390/192	8.3/4.1	60.7/29.9	13.2/6.5	0/0
McFlurry, Crunchie, McDonald's*, 1 portion/183g				
321/175	7.7/4.2	47.9/26.1	11.4/6.2	0/0
McFlurry, Dairy Milk, McDonalds's*, 1 portion/181g				
280/154	8.2/4.5	44.2/24.3	13.1/7.2	0/0
McFlurry, Jammie Dodger, McDonald's*, 1 serving/128g				
256/200	5/3.9	43/33.6	8.2/6.4	0.4/0.3
McFlurry, Smarties, McDonald's*, 1 serving/185g				
327/177	7.8/4.2	48.5/26.2	11.5/6.2	0.4/0.2
McMuffin, Bacon & Egg, Double, McDonald's*, 1 pack/226g				
573/253	33.3/14.7	25.8/11.4	37.1/16.4	1.8/0.8
McMuffin, Bacon & Egg, McDonald's*, 1 McMuffin/141g				
345/245	20/14.2	26.1/18.5	18/12.8	1.8/1.3

	kcal serv/100g	prot serv/100g	carb serv/100g	fat serv/100g	fibre serv/100g
McMuffin, Egg, McDonald's*, 1 McMuffin/127g					
	281/221	15.5/12.2	25.9/20.4	12.8/10.1	1.9/1.5
McMuffin, Sausage & Egg, McDonald's*, 1 McMuffin/176g					
	426/242	24.3/13.8	25.9/14.7	24.8/14.1	1.8/1
McMuffin, Scrambled Egg, McDonald's*, 1 McMuffin/147g					
	294/200	16/10.9	25.7/17.5	14.1/9.6	1.9/1.3
Melt, Toasted Ham & Cheese, McDonald's*, 1 serving/100g					
	239/239	11.2/11.2	30.6/30.6	8/8	1.8/1.8
Milk Shake, Banana, McDonald's*, 1 regular/336g					
	396/118	10.8/3.2	66.5/19.8	10.1/3	0/0
Milk Shake, Chocolate, McDonald's*, 1 regular/336g					
	403/120	11.4/3.4	66.9/19.9	10.1/3	0/0
Milk Shake, Strawberry, McDonald's*, 1 regular/336g					
	400/119	10.8/3.2	67.2/20	10.1/3	0/0
Milk Shake, Vanilla, McDonald's*, 1 regular/336g					
	383/114	10.8/3.2	63.2/18.8	10.1/3	0/0
Milk, Semi-Skimmed, Organic, McDonald's*, 1 bottle/250ml					
	123/49	8.5/3.4	12.5/5	4.3/1.7	0/0
Muffin, Buttered with Preserve, McDonald's*, 1 muffin/93g					
	234/252	5.5/5.9	44.7/48.1	3.7/4	1.9/2
Muffin, Buttered, McDonald's*, 1 muffin/63g					
	158/250	5.4/8.6	25.6/40.7	3.7/5.9	1.8/2.9
Mushrooms, Garlic, Pizza Hut*, 1 pack/112.2g					
	217/192	6.7/5.9	22.3/19.7	11.2/9.9	3.8/3.4
Mushrooms, Garlic, with BBQ Dip, Pizza Hut*, 1 pack/112.2g					
	264/234	7/6.2	34.5/30.5	11.3/10	3.8/3.4
Mushrooms, Garlic, with Sour Cream & Chive Dip, Pizza Hut*,					
1 pack/112.2g					
	429/380	7.2/6.4	22.6/20	34.8/30.8	3.8/3.4
Onion Rings, Large, Burger King*, 1 serving/120g					
	348/290	5.8/4.8	43.7/36.4	16.7/13.9	4.6/3.8
Onion Rings, Regular, Burger King*, 1 serving/90g					
	261/290	4.3/4.8	32.8/36.4	12.5/13.9	3.4/3.8
Orange Juice, Pure, McDonald's*, 1 regular/200ml					
	94/47	1.4/0.7	20.6/10.3	0/0	0.2/0.1
Pancake, & Sausage, McDonald's*, 1 portion/262g					
	671/256	16/6.1	89.9/34.3	27/10.3	2.9/1.1

kcal serv/100g	prot serv/100g	carb serv/100g	fat serv/100g	fibre serv/100g

Pancake, & Syrup, McDonald's*, 1 pack/209g

| 531/254 | 5/2.4 | 87.6/41.9 | 15.9/7.6 | 1.3/0.6 |

Pasta Salad, with Chicken, McDonald's*, 1 serving/190g

| 266/140 | 12.5/6.6 | 37.2/19.6 | 6.7/3.5 | 0.4/0.2 |

Pie, Apple Slice, Colonels Pies, Kentucky Fried Chicken*, 1 slice/113g

| 310/274 | 1.9/1.7 | 44/38.9 | 13.9/12.3 | 0/0 |

Pie, Apple, McDonald's*, 1 pie/78g

| 225/289 | 2.2/2.8 | 25.9/33.2 | 12.6/16.1 | 1.1/1.4 |

Pie, Dutch Apple, Burger King*, 1 pie/113g

| 339/300 | 1.9/1.7 | 52/46 | 13.9/12.3 | 0.9/0.8 |

Pie, Strawberry Creme, Slice, Kentucky Fried Chicken*, 1 slice/78g

| 279/358 | 4.2/5.4 | 32/41 | 15/19.2 | 2/2.5 |

Pizza, American Hot, Pizza Express*, 1 pizza/521.9g

| 788/151 | 33.4/6.4 | 98.1/18.8 | 32.4/6.2 | 10.4/2 |

Pizza, Cheese & Tomato, 9.5", Domino's Pizza*, 1 slice/52g

| 125/241 | 6.7/12.8 | 18.1/34.9 | 2.9/5.6 | 1.7/3.2 |

Pizza, Chicken Supreme, Medium Pan, Pizza Hut*, ½ med pizza/300g

| 810/270 | 39/13 | 87/29 | 36/12 | 6/2 |

Pizza, Deluxe, 9.5", Domino's Pizza*, 1 slice/66g

| 171/259 | 8.4/12.8 | 19.2/29.1 | 6.7/10.1 | 1.6/2.4 |

Pizza, Full House, 9.5", Domino's Pizza*, 1 slice/74g

| 183/247 | 9.3/12.5 | 18.9/25.5 | 7.8/10.5 | 1.3/1.8 |

Pizza, Ham & Mushroom, The Italian, Medium 12", Pizza Hut*, 1 slice/96g

| 270/281 | 13.1/13.6 | 34/35.4 | 10.2/10.6 | 2.5/2.6 |

Pizza, Hawaiian, Medium Pan, Pizza Hut*, 1 slice/96g

| 241/251 | 12.1/12.6 | 28/29.2 | 8.9/9.3 | 1.3/1.4 |

Pizza, Margherita, Medium Pan, Pizza Hut*, 1 slice/85g

| 239/281 | 10.8/12.7 | 26.4/31.1 | 10/11.8 | 1.8/2.1 |

Pizza, Margherita, Pizza Express*, 1 pizza/269.7g

| 527/195 | 27.5/10.2 | 82.4/30.5 | 9.7/3.6 | 3.8/1.4 |

Pizza, Margherita, Stuffed Crust Original, Pizza Hut*, 1 slice/125.3g

| 330/262 | 18.8/14.9 | 35.9/28.5 | 12.3/9.8 | 1.3/1 |

Pizza, Margherita, The Italian, Medium, Pizza Hut*, 1 slice/95g

| 292/307 | 14.4/15.2 | 37.5/39.5 | 10.3/10.8 | 2.2/2.3 |

Pizza, Meat Feast, Medium Pan, Pizza Hut*, 1 slice/114g

| 324/284 | 16.6/14.6 | 27.8/24.4 | 16.2/14.2 | 1/0.9 |

Pizza, Meat Feast, The Italian, 12", Pizza Hut*, 1 slice/113g

| 341/302 | 17.4/15.4 | 34.2/30.3 | 16.2/14.3 | 2.6/2.3 |

kcal serv/100g	prot serv/100g	carb serv/100g	fat serv/100g	fibre serv/100g
Pizza, Meaty, The Edge, Pizza Hut*, 1 slice/64g				
207/323	10.6/16.6	14.9/23.3	11.6/18.2	0/0
Pizza, Mighty Meaty, 9.5", Domino's Pizza*, ⅙ pizza/71g				
177/249	9.9/13.9	18.1/25.5	7.2/10.2	2/2.8
Pizza, Mixed Grill, 9.5", Domino's Pizza*, 1 slice/75g				
178/237	9/12	19.7/26.2	7/9.3	1.7/2.3
Pizza, Pepperoni Passion, 9.5", Domino's Pizza*, 1 slice/65g				
186/286	8.8/13.6	20.5/31.5	7.5/11.6	0.9/1.4
Pizza, Pepperoni, The Insider, Pizza Hut*, 1 slice/137g				
360/263	17/12.4	34.9/25.5	17/12.4	2.1/1.5
Pizza, Quattro Formaggi, Pizza Express*, 1 pizza/528g				
723/137	32.4/6.1	101/19.1	22.1/4.2	0/0
Pizza, Supreme, Medium Pan, Pizza Hut*, 1 slice/105.7g				
292/275	13.4/12.6	26.6/25.1	14.6/13.8	1.3/1.2
Pizza, Supreme, The Italian, Medium, Pizza Hut*, 1 slice/106g				
297/280	13.8/13	35.4/33.4	12.1/11.4	2.2/2.1
Pizza, Tandoori Hot, 9.5", Domino's Pizza*, 1 slice/67g				
137/205	8.2/12.2	18.6/27.8	3.5/5.2	1.9/2.8
Pizza, The Works, The Edge, Pizza Hut*, 1 slice/64g				
161/252	8.3/12.9	14.1/22	8/12.5	0/0
Pizza, Tomato & Cheese, Thin & Crispy, Marks & Spencer*, 1 pizza/300g				
705/235	33/11	83.1/27.7	28.2/9.4	3.6/1.2
Pizza, Veg-a-Roma without Cheese, Domino's Pizza*, 1 sm pizza/354g				
712/201	29.7/8.4	118.2/33.4	13.5/3.8	9.6/2.7
Pizza, Vegetarian, Original Medium, Pizza Hut*, 1 slice/93.5g				
227/241	10.5/11.2	26.3/28	8.8/9.4	1.8/1.9
Pizza, Vegetarian, Supreme, 9.5", Domino's Pizza*, 1 slice/71g				
137/193	7.7/10.8	19.2/27	3.3/4.6	1.7/2.4
Pizza, Veggie, The Edge, Pizza Hut*, 1 slice/60g				
137/228	6.8/11.4	14.8/24.6	5.6/9.3	0/0
Pizza, Veneziana, Pizza Express*, 1 pizza/300g				
614/205	26.3/8.8	92.7/30.9	18.7/6.2	0/0
Potato, Wedges, Domino's Pizza*, 1 serving/198g				
428/216	8.1/4.1	60/30.3	17.2/8.7	0/0
Potato, Wedges, McDonald's, 1 portion/176g				
368/208	5.8/3.3	46.2/26.1	17.9/10.1	3.9/2.2
Roll, Bacon with Brown Sauce, McDonald's*, 1 roll/118g				
289/245	15.1/12.8	36.8/31.2	9.9/8.4	1.7/1.4

kcal serv/100g	prot serv/100g	carb serv/100g	fat serv/100g	fibre serv/100g
Salad, Burger King*, 1 serving/165g				
34/21	2/1.2	5.8/3.5	0.3/0.2	4.3/2.6
Salad, Chicken Caesar, Pizza Express*, 1 serving/100g				
519/519	32/32	39/39	29/29	0/0
Salad, Feta Cheese & Pasta, McDonald's*, 1 pack/250g				
240/96	9.5/3.8	28/11.2	9.8/3.9	2.3/0.9
Salad, Pasta & Tuna, McDonald's*, 1 pack/244g				
217/89	11/4.5	30.5/12.5	5.4/2.2	2.2/0.9
Salad, Potato, Kentucky Fried Chicken*, 1 portion/160g				
229/143	4/2.5	22.9/14.3	13.9/8.7	2.9/1.8
Salad, Tomato & Mozzarella, Starter, Pizza Express*, 1 serving/100g				
288/288	15.6/15.6	5.9/5.9	22.4/22.4	0/0
Salad, Warm Chicken, No Dressing, Kentucky Fried Chicken*, 1 salad/100g				
302/302	28.4/28.4	22/22	11.1/11.1	1.9/1.9
Sandwich, Chicken Club, Burger King*, 1 pack/242g				
620/256	29.8/12.3	54/22.3	31.9/13.2	3.9/1.6
Sandwich, Chicken, Burger King*, 1 pack/224g				
659/294	25/11.2	52.9/23.6	39/17.4	2.9/1.3
Sandwich, Egg & Bacon, Burger King*, 1 pack/139g				
296/213	15.4/11.1	30.2/21.7	12.6/9.1	2.6/1.9
Sandwich, McChicken Sandwich, New, McDonald's*, 1 sandwich/100g				
375/375	16.5/16.5	38.6/38.6	17.2/17.2	3.8/3.8
Sandwich, Sausage, Bacon & Egg, Burger King*, 1 pack/182g				
430/236	24/13.2	31.9/17.5	23.1/12.7	3.1/1.7
Sauce, Barbeque, McDonald's*, 1 portion/32g				
55/173	0.7/2.2	12.3/38.3	0.4/1.2	0/0
Sauce, Curry, Sweet, McDonald's*, 1 portion/32g				
61/192	0.4/1.2	13.2/41.1	0.8/2.5	0/0
Sauce, Mustard, Mild, McDonald's*, 1 portion/30g				
64/212	0.3/1	7.4/24.8	3.6/12.1	0/0
Sauce, Sweet & Sour, McDonald's*, 1 portion/32g				
59/183	0.1/0.4	13.9/43.5	0.3/0.8	0/0
Saveloy, Unbattered, Takeaway, 1 saveloy/65g				
192/296	9/13.8	7/10.8	14.5/22.3	0.5/0.8
Sundae, Hot Caramel, McDonald's*, 1 sundae/189g				
357/189	7.2/3.8	64.1/33.9	8.3/4.4	0/0
Sundae, Hot Fudge, McDonald's*, 1 sundae/187g				
352/188	8.4/4.5	56.1/30	10.7/5.7	0/0

	kcal serv/100g	prot serv/100g	carb serv/100g	fat serv/100g	fibre serv/100g

Sundae, No Topping, McDonald's*, 1 sundae/149g

219/147	6.3/4.2	32.2/21.6	7.6/5.1	0/0

Sundae, Strawberry, McDonald's*, 1 sundae/186g

296/159	6.3/3.4	51.2/27.5	7.6/4.1	0/0

Tea, UHT Skimmed Milk, McDonald's*, 1 cup/14ml

10/74	0.5/3.7	0.8/5.4	0.6/4.1	0/0

Topping, Bruschetta, Pizza Express*, 1 serving/99.9g

452/452	8.7/8.7	49.9/49.9	24.6/24.6	0/0

Twister, Kentucky Fried Chicken*, 1 Twister/240g

600/250	21.8/9.1	51.8/21.6	33.8/14.1	3.8/1.6

Wrap, Twister, Kentucky Fried Chicken*, 1 Twister/252g

670/266	27/10.7	54.9/21.8	38/15.1	3/1.2

Yoghurt, Berry Crunch, McDonald's*, 1 serving/194.8g

224/115	6.8/3.5	36.9/18.9	5.1/2.6	2.3/1.2

FISH AND SEAFOOD

Calamari, Battered with Tartar Sauce Dip, Tesco*, 1 pack/210g

573/273	18.7/8.9	32.3/15.4	41/19.5	1.3/0.6

Calamari, Battered, Marks & Spencer*, 1 pack/160g

424/265	22.9/14.3	25.3/15.8	25.8/16.1	1.1/0.7

Calamari, Battered, Young's*, 1 serving/150g

266/177	11.7/7.8	19.5/13	15.6/10.4	2.3/1.5

Calamari, Marks & Spencer*, 1oz/28g

65/231	3.9/13.9	3.2/11.5	4/14.4	0.1/0.5

Calamari, Rings in Batter, Waitrose*, ½ pack/85g

227/267	11.8/13.9	12.1/14.2	14.6/17.2	0.5/0.6

Caviar, Lumpfish, John West*, 1oz/28g

26/92	3.6/13	0.3/1	1.1/4	0/0

Cod, & Salmon, Steam Cuisine, COU, Marks & Spencer*, 1 pack/400g

340/85	27.2/6.8	35.6/8.9	7.2/1.8	4.8/1.2

Cod, Battered, Chip Shop-Style, Aldi*, 1 serving/150g

293/195	20/13.3	11.6/7.7	18.5/12.3	2.1/1.4

Cod, Battered, Chip Shop, Youngs*, 1 portion/113g

237/210	13/11.5	16.2/14.3	13.7/12.1	0.7/0.6

Cod, Breaded, In Oven Crisp Crumb, Morrisons*, 1 serving/100g

201/201	12.4/12.4	17.5/17.5	9/9	1/1

	kcal serv/100g	prot serv/100g	carb serv/100g	fat serv/100g	fibre serv/100g

Cod, Breaded, Portions, GFY, Asda*, 1 portion/125g

| | 169/135 | 17.5/14 | 18.8/15 | 2.6/2.1 | 1.3/1 |

Cod, Cakes, Big Time, Bird's Eye*, 1 cake/114g

| | 185/162 | 8.7/7.6 | 19/16.7 | 8.2/7.2 | 1.1/1 |

Cod, Fillets, Breaded, Chunky, Prime, Tesco*, 1 fillet/135g

| | 246/182 | 17.4/12.9 | 16.7/12.4 | 12.2/9 | 2.3/1.7 |

Cod, Fillets, Breaded, Chunky, Reduced-Fat, Tesco*, 1 fillet/135g

| | 201/149 | 19/14.1 | 14/10.4 | 7.7/5.7 | 2.7/2 |

Cod, Fillets, Breaded, GFY, Asda*, 1 fillet/123g

| | 185/150 | 17.2/14 | 20.9/17 | 3.6/2.9 | 1.8/1.5 |

Cod, Fillets, Chunky in Breadcrumbs, Better for You, Morrisons*, 1 fillet/124g

| | 166/134 | 15.3/12.3 | 20.1/16.2 | 2.6/2.1 | 1.7/1.4 |

Cod, Fillets, Chunky, BGTY, Sainsbury's*, 1 fillet/139g

| | 228/165 | 22.2/16.1 | 17.8/12.9 | 7.5/5.4 | 1.8/1.3 |

Cod, Fillets, Extra Large, Harry Ramsdens*, 1 fillet/190g

| | 433/228 | 19.6/10.3 | 35.5/18.7 | 24.3/12.8 | 1.5/0.8 |

Cod, Fillets, In a Sweet Red Pepper Sauce, GFY, Asda*, ½ pack/170g

| | 143/84 | 25.5/15 | 3.9/2.3 | 2.7/1.6 | 0.2/0.1 |

Cod, Fillets, in Breadcrumbs, Bird's Eye*, 1 serving/112g

| | 190/170 | 14.3/12.8 | 15.9/14.2 | 7.7/6.9 | 0.6/0.5 |

Cod, Fillets, in Chip Shop Batter, Marks & Spencer*, 1 serving/135g

| | 285/211 | 16.9/12.5 | 15.2/11.3 | 17/12.6 | 1.4/1 |

Cod, Fillets, in Ovencrisp Batter, Tesco*, 1 portion/142g

| | 240/169 | 17.2/12.1 | 23.1/16.3 | 8.7/6.1 | 0.4/0.3 |

Cod, Fillets, in Parsley Sauce, BGTY, Sainsbury's*, 1 pack/351g

| | 316/90 | 40.7/11.6 | 4.6/1.3 | 15.1/4.3 | 2.5/0.7 |

Cod, Fillets, Mornay, Sainsbury's*, 1 serving/153g

| | 236/154 | 23.3/15.2 | 3.4/2.2 | 14.4/9.4 | 1.4/0.9 |

Cod, Fish & Chips, Waitrose*, 1 pack/283g

| | 849/300 | 40.8/14.4 | 95.4/33.7 | 34/12 | 13.6/4.8 |

Cod, in Bubble Batter, Youngs*, 1 fish/135g

| | 315/233 | 14.9/11 | 20.4/15.1 | 19.7/14.6 | 0.8/0.6 |

Cod, in Butter Sauce, Ross*, 1 serving/150g

| | 126/84 | 13.7/9.1 | 4.8/3.2 | 5.9/3.9 | 0.2/0.1 |

Cod, in Butter Sauce, Sainsbury's*, 1 serving/170g

| | 184/108 | 17.9/10.5 | 5.3/3.1 | 10/5.9 | 0.5/0.3 |

	kcal serv/100g	prot serv/100g	carb serv/100g	fat serv/100g	fibre serv/100g
Cod, Mediterranean, COU, Marks & Spencer*, 1 pack/400g					
	320/80	26/6.5	44.8/11.2	2.8/0.7	9.2/2.3
Cod, Steaks, in Butter Sauce, Bird's Eye*, 1 pack/170g					
	165/97	17/10	6.6/3.9	7.8/4.6	0.2/0.1
Cod, Steaks, in Crispy Batter, Bird's Eye*, 1 steak/124g					
	241/194	12.9/10.4	13.6/11	14.9/12	1.4/1.1
Cod, Steaks, in Parsley Sauce, Bird's Eye*, 1 pack/176g					
	150/85	18.3/10.4	8.8/5	4.6/2.6	0.2/0.1
Cod, Steaks, in Parsley Sauce, Frozen, Bird's Eye*, 1 pack/172.2g					
	155/90	18.1/10.5	9.6/5.6	4.8/2.8	0.2/0.1
Cod, with Sunblush Tomato Sauce, GFY, Asda*, ½ pack/177.3g					
	117/66	23/13	0.2/0.1	2.7/1.5	1.8/1
Crab, Cocktail, Waitrose*, 1 serving/100g					
	217/217	10.8/10.8	3.8/3.8	17.6/17.6	0.4/0.4
Crab, Dressed, in Shell, Asda*, 1 crab/142g					
	64/45	9.7/6.8	0/0	2.7/1.9	0/0
Crab, Dressed, John West*, 1 can/43g					
	61/143	7.7/18	0.9/2	3/7	0/0
Crab, Sticks, Sainsbury's*, 1 stick/16g					
	18/113	1.1/7	3.4/21	0/0.1	0/0.1
Crepes, Lobster, Finest, Tesco*, 1 serving/160g					
	250/156	17.1/10.7	22.4/14	10.2/6.4	1.9/1.2
Crumble, Fish & Prawn, Youngs*, 1 pie/375g					
	476/127	21.8/5.8	36.4/9.7	27/7.2	4.9/1.3
Crumble, Ocean, Good Choice, Iceland*, 1 pack/340g					
	377/111	24.5/7.2	49/14.4	9.2/2.7	3.7/1.1
Crumble, Salmon, Youngs*, 1 pie/339g					
	380/112	15.6/4.6	44.1/13	15.6/4.6	2.4/0.7
Fish & Chips, Safeway*, 1 pack/249g					
	518/208	19.9/8	62.3/25	20.9/8.4	8.7/3.5
Fish Bake, Haddock & Prawn, COU, Marks & Spencer*, 1 bake/340g					
	289/85	24.8/7.3	24.8/7.3	9.5/2.8	1.4/0.4
Fish Bake, Italiano, Bird's Eye*, ½ pack/205g					
	180/88	23.6/11.5	7.4/3.6	6.4/3.1	0.6/0.3
Fish Bake, Vegetable Tuscany, Bird's Eye*, ½ pack/201g					
	195/97	23.7/11.8	4.4/2.2	9.2/4.6	1.2/0.6
Fish Balls, Gefilte, Marks & Spencer*, 1 pack/200g					
	280/140	28.2/14.1	23.8/11.9	7.8/3.9	2/1

kcal serv/100g	prot serv/100g	carb serv/100g	fat serv/100g	fibre serv/100g
Fish Cakes, Bubbly Batter, Youngs*, 1 fish cake/44.1g				
109/247	3.1/7.1	9/20.5	6.6/15.1	0.6/1.4
Fish Cakes, Cod & Pancetta, Cafe Culture, Marks & Spencer*, 1 fish cake/85g				
166/195	7.8/9.2	6.1/7.2	13.2/15.5	1.7/2
Fish Cakes, Cod, Asda*, 1 fish cake/72.2g				
163/227	5/7	18/25	7.9/11	1.7/2.3
Fish Cakes, Cod, in Crunch Crumb, Bird's Eye*, 1 fish cake/52g				
85/163	4.6/8.8	8.4/16.2	3.6/7	0.4/0.7
Fish Cakes, Cod, Sainsbury's*, 1 fish cake/90g				
176/195	8.6/9.5	15.8/17.5	8.1/9	0.7/0.8
Fish Cakes, Cod, Tesco*, 1 fish cake/49g				
94/192	4.2/8.6	9.2/18.8	4.5/9.1	0.4/0.8
Fish Cakes, Haddock, Asda*, 1 fish cake/88g				
181/206	7/8	18.5/21	8.8/10	1.3/1.5
Fish Cakes, Haddock, Smoked, Tesco*, 1 fish cake/90g				
171/190	7.7/8.6	20.3/22.5	6.6/7.3	1/1.1
Fish Cakes, Marks & Spencer*, 1 fish cake/80g				
180/225	6.4/8	14.4/18	10.6/13.3	0/0
Fish Cakes, Prawn, Tesco*, 1 fish cake/90g				
209/232	7.4/8.2	26.3/29.2	8.2/9.1	1.6/1.8
Fish Cakes, Salmon & Dill, Waitrose*, 1 fish cake/85g				
179/211	7.7/9.1	15/17.6	9.9/11.6	1.9/2.2
Fish Cakes, Salmon, Asda*, 1 fish cake/86g				
215/250	6.9/8	19.8/23	12/14	1.2/1.4
Fish Cakes, Salmon, Bird's Eye*, 1 fish cake/50g				
84/168	4.8/9.5	6.1/12.2	4.5/9	0.7/1.4
Fish Cakes, Salmon, Marks & Spencer*, 1 fish cake/86g				
181/210	7.8/9.1	13/15.1	10.9/12.7	1.5/1.7
Fish Cakes, Salmon, Sainsbury's*, 1 fish cake/90g				
167/186	11.9/13.2	15.7/17.4	6.4/7.1	1.1/1.2
Fish Cakes, Salmon, Tesco*, 1 fish cake/50g				
110/219	5.1/10.1	6.9/13.7	6.9/13.7	0.5/0.9
Fish Cakes, Smoked Haddock, Sainsbury's*, 1 fish cake/63.2g				
127/201	6.9/11	11.2/17.8	6/9.5	1.3/2.1
Fish Cakes, Thai Crab & Prawn, Tesco*, 1 fish cake/115g				
269/234	10.1/8.8	20/17.4	16.6/14.4	1.4/1.2

kcal serv/100g	prot serv/100g	carb serv/100g	fat serv/100g	fibre serv/100g
Fish Cakes, Tuna, Marks & Spencer*, 1 fish cake/85g				
170/200	8.5/10	12.7/14.9	9.4/11	1.4/1.6
Fish Cakes, Tuna, Tesco*, 1 fish cake/90g				
182/202	8.3/9.2	22.5/25	6.6/7.3	1.2/1.3
Fish Fingers, 100% Cod Fillet, Bird's Eye*, 1 finger/30g				
56/186	3.9/13	4.7/15.6	2.4/7.9	0.2/0.7
Fish Fingers, Chip Shop, Youngs*, 1 finger/30g				
75/251	2.8/9.3	5/16.6	4.9/16.4	0.4/1.2
Fish Fingers, Cod Fillet, Asda*, 1 finger/31g				
66/214	4/13	5.6/18	3.1/10	0/0
Fish Fingers, Cod Fillet, Bird's Eye*, 1 finger/30g				
53/177	3.8/12.7	4.2/14.1	2.3/7.7	0.3/1
Fish Fingers, Cod Fillet, Waitrose*, 1 finger/30g				
55/183	3.6/11.9	5.1/16.9	2.3/7.5	0.2/0.7
Fish Fingers, Cod, Tesco*, 1 finger/30g				
56/188	3.7/12.3	5/16.8	2.4/7.9	0.5/1.6
Fish Fingers, Haddock Fillet, Bird's Eye*, 1 finger/29g				
48/167	3.6/12.4	3.8/13.2	2.1/7.2	0.3/0.9
Fish Fingers, Hoki Fillet, Bird's Eye*, 1 finger/30g				
58/193	3.8/12.6	4.7/15.6	2.7/8.9	0.2/0.7
Fish Fingers, in Crispy Batter, Bird's Eye*, 1 finger/29g				
63/218	3/10.4	4.6/15.8	3.7/12.6	0.1/0.4
Fish Fingers, Ross*, 1 finger/26g				
48/186	3.1/12.1	4.6/17.6	2/7.5	0.2/0.8
Fish Fingers, Sainsbury's*, 1 finger/27g				
52/194	3.6/13.4	4.3/16	2.3/8.5	0.2/0.7
Haddock, & Chips, Marks & Spencer*, 1oz/28g				
52/187	2/7	6.3/22.6	2.1/7.6	0.6/2.1
Haddock, Cheese & Chive Sauce, Healthy Eating, Tesco*, 1 pack/360g				
284/79	45.7/12.7	9.4/2.6	7.2/2	0.4/0.1
Haddock, Fillets, Battered, Asda*, 1 fillet/100g				
241/241	13/13	18/18	13/13	2.5/2.5
Haddock, Fillets, Battered, Marks & Spencer*, 1 fillet/125g				
306/245	15.8/12.6	20/16	18.3/14.6	0.9/0.7
Haddock, Fillets, Breadcrumbs, Scottish, Sainsbury's*, 1 fillet/170g				
345/203	22.8/13.4	27.9/16.4	15.8/9.3	1.5/0.9
Haddock, Fillets, Breaded, Tesco*, 1 fillet/142g				
251/177	20.3/14.3	21.3/15	9.7/6.8	1.3/0.9

kcal serv/100g	prot serv/100g	carb serv/100g	fat serv/100g	fibre serv/100g
Haddock, Fillets, in Cheese Mornay Sauce, Marks & Spencer*, ½ pack/190g				
219/115	25.7/13.5	3.4/1.8	11.6/6.1	0.1/0.1
Haddock, Fillets, in Tomato Herb Sauce, BGTY, Sainsbury's*, ½ pack/165g				
150/91	21.3/12.9	5.9/3.6	4.6/2.8	0.2/0.1
Haddock, Smoked, with Cheese & Chive, GFY, Asda, ½ pack/185.7g				
195/105	27.9/15	5.8/3.1	6.7/3.6	0.6/0.3
Herring, Rollmop, with Onion, Asda*, 1 rollmop/65g				
89/137	8.6/13.2	6.7/10.3	3.1/4.8	0.5/0.8
Hoki, in Breadcrumbs, Youngs*, 1 piece/156g				
275/176	22.3/14.3	18.3/11.7	13.6/8.7	1.2/0.8
Hoki, Steaks, in Crunch Crumb, Bird's Eye*, 1 steak/115.2g				
250/217	15.1/13.1	19.8/17.2	12.2/10.6	0.9/0.8
Lemon Sole, & Butter, Marks & Spencer*, 1oz/28g				
49/174	4.2/15.1	0/0.1	3.5/12.6	0/0
Lemon Sole, Breadcrumbs, Marks & Spencer*, 1oz/28g				
63/225	3.1/11.2	4.8/17.1	3.6/12.7	0.2/0.7
Lemon Sole, Fillets, Chunky Breaded, Tesco*, 1 portion/160g				
366/229	17/10.6	33.8/21.1	18.1/11.3	1.4/0.9
Lemon Sole, Fillets, Lightly Dusted, Marks & Spencer*, 1 fillet/112.5g				
181/160	15.7/13.9	11.3/10	8.7/7.7	1.1/1
Mackerel, Fillets, in Spicy Tomato Sauce, Princes*, 1 can/125g				
250/200	17/13.6	5.9/4.7	17.6/14.1	0/0
Mackerel, Fillets, in Tomato Sauce, Princes*, 1 can/125g				
254/203	17/13.6	4.1/3.3	18.8/15	0/0
Mackerel, Fillets, in Tomato Sauce, Sainsbury's*, 1 can/125g				
204/163	17.5/14	2.5/2	13.8/11	0.1/0.1
Mackerel, Fillets, Peppered, Asda*, ½ pack/130g				
430/331	28.6/22	0/0	35.1/27	0/0
Mackerel, Fillets, Peppered, Smoked, Safeway*, 1 fillet/135g				
478/354	25.5/18.9	0/0	41.7/30.9	0/0
Mackerel, Fillets, Peppered, Smoked, Sainsbury's*, 1 serving/106g				
388/366	22/20.8	0.6/0.6	33/31.1	0.1/0.1
Marlin, Steaks, Chargrilled, Sainsbury's*, 1 serving/240g				
367/153	56.6/23.6	1.9/0.8	14.6/6.1	1.4/0.6
Parcels, Smoked Salmon, Marks & Spencer*, 1 parcel/55g				
151/275	8.5/15.4	0.4/0.7	13/23.6	0/0
Parcels, Smoked Salmon, Tesco*, 1 serving/50g				
147/293	8.2/16.4	0/0	12.7/25.3	0.1/0.2

	kcal serv/100g	prot serv/100g	carb serv/100g	fat serv/100g	fibre serv/100g
Pie, Admiral, Youngs*, 1 serving/250g					
	263/105	12/4.8	26.5/10.6	11.5/4.6	1.8/0.7
Pie, Admiral's, Ross*, 1 pie/340g					
	357/105	16.3/4.8	37.1/10.9	15.6/4.6	2.4/0.7
Pie, Fish, Better for You, Morrisons*, 1 pack/350g					
	301/86	17.5/5	35/10	10.2/2.9	3.2/0.9
Pie, Fish, Creamy, Finest, Tesco*, 1 serving/300g					
	438/146	30.9/10.3	17.1/5.7	27.3/9.1	2.4/0.8
Pie, Fish, GFY, Asda*, 1 pack/356.4g					
	360/101	21.4/6	49.8/14	8.2/2.3	3.2/0.9
Pie, Fish, Luxury with Mature Cheddar Mashed Potato, Sainsbury's*, ½ pack/301g					
	394/131	21.1/7	27.7/9.2	22.3/7.4	2.1/0.7
Pie, Fish, Topped with Potato, GFY, Asda*, 1 pack/450g					
	414/92	27/6	40.5/9	16.2/3.6	5/1.1
Pie, Fisherman's, Sainsbury's*, 1 pack/300g					
	195/65	11.7/3.9	29.1/9.7	3.6/1.2	3.6/1.2
Pie, Fisherman's, Youngs*, 1 pack/375g					
	499/133	23.3/6.2	42/11.2	26.3/7	3/0.8
Pie, Haddock Cumberland, Marks & Spencer*, 1 pie/300g					
	390/130	24.6/8.2	31.8/10.6	18/6	1.2/0.4
Pie, Mariner's, Ross*, 1 pie/340g					
	435/128	17/5	47.3/13.9	20.1/5.9	3.4/1
Pie, Ocean, BGTY, Sainsbury's*, 1 pack/350g					
	270/77	18.9/5.4	36.8/10.5	5.3/1.5	3.9/1.1
Pie, Ocean, Youngs*, 1 serving/187.5g					
	250/133	11.7/6.2	21.1/11.2	13.2/7	1.5/0.8
Pie, Smoked Haddock, Eat Smart, Safeway*, 1 pack/400g					
	376/94	32.4/8.1	40.4/10.1	9.6/2.4	4.8/1.2
Plaice, Fillets, Baked, Sainsbury's*, 1 serving/100g					
	234/234	13/13	19.2/19.2	11.7/11.7	1.1/1.1
Plaice, Fillets, Breaded, Asda*, 1 serving/150g					
	389/259	13.5/9	33/22	22.5/15	2.1/1.4
Plaice, Fillets, Breaded, Chunky, Boneless, Tesco*, 1 fillet/160g					
	318/199	18.6/11.6	27.2/17	15/9.4	1.4/0.9
Prawn Creole, Spicy, BGTY, Sainsbury's*, 1 pack/400g					
	436/109	16.8/4.2	83.6/20.9	3.6/0.9	1.6/0.4

	kcal serv/100g	prot serv/100g	carb serv/100g	fat serv/100g	fibre serv/100g

Prawn Toast, Chinese Snack Selection, Mini, Tesco*, 1 toast/11g

36/330	1/9.4	2.1/18.8	2.7/24.2	0.2/1.9

Prawn Toast, Sesame, Occasions, Sainsbury's*, 1 toast/12.0g

34/283	1.2/9.9	2.3/19.2	2.2/18.5	0.2/2

**Prawns &, Noodles in Sweet Chilli Sauce, COU, Marks & Spencer*,
1 pack/400g**

240/60	18/4.5	37.2/9.3	1.6/0.4	5.2/1.3

**Prawns, Sweet & Sour, Cantonese, Microwave Easy Steam, Sainsbury's*,
1 pack/400g**

424/106	17.2/4.3	67.2/16.8	9.6/2.4	12/3

Prawn Cocktail, Sainsbury's*, 1 serving/200g

706/353	15.8/7.9	5.4/2.7	69/34.5	1/0.5

Prawns, Batter Crisp, Lyons*, 1 pack/160g

350/219	12.8/8	29.1/18.2	20.3/12.7	1.8/1.1

Prawns, Chilli & Coriander, Marks & Spencer*, 1 serving/70g

67/95	12.5/17.9	0.4/0.6	1.5/2.2	0.4/0.6

Prawns, Chilli, Battered, Marks & Spencer*, 1oz/28g

63/225	2/7.2	6.7/23.8	3.2/11.5	0.1/0.5

Prawns, Chinese, Oriental Express*, 1 serving/320g

218/68	10.2/3.2	44.2/13.8	1.9/0.6	6.1/1.9

Prawns, Filo & Breaded Wrapped, Marks & Spencer*, 1 serving/19g

45/235	1.8/9.5	3.9/20.4	2.5/13	0.3/1.4

Prawns, in Creamy Garlic Sauce, Youngs*, 1 serving/158g

261/165	13.4/8.5	0.5/0.3	22.9/14.5	0/0

Prawns, in Red Thai Curry Sauce, Youngs*, 1 pack/255g

197/77	12.2/4.8	16.6/6.5	8.7/3.4	2/0.8

Prawns, King, in Filo, Finest, Tesco*, 1 prawn/20g

38/189	2.6/13	5.6/27.8	0.6/2.9	0.3/1.6

Salmon, Blinis, Smoked, Marks & Spencer*, 1oz/28g

67/240	3.3/11.9	5.3/18.9	3.6/13	0.5/1.8

Salmon, En Croute, Sainsbury's*, 1 serving/179g

533/298	17.4/9.7	32.9/18.4	35.8/20	2.1/1.2

Salmon, Fillets, & Butter, Marks & Spencer*, 1oz/28g

64/230	4.7/16.7	0/0	5/18	0/0

Salmon, Fillets, Foil Baked, Tesco*, 1 fillet/130g

234/180	26.3/20.2	0/0	14.3/11	0/0

Salmon, Fillets, in Creamy Dill Sauce, Bird's Eye*, 1 pack/340g

333/98	19/5.6	29.6/8.7	15.3/4.5	4.4/1.3

kcal serv/100g	prot serv/100g	carb serv/100g	fat serv/100g	fibre serv/100g
Salmon, Fillets, in White Wine & Parsley Dressing, Tesco*, 1 fillet/150g				
291/194	26.3/17.5	0.5/0.3	20.4/13.6	0.9/0.6
Salmon, Fillets, Poached, Marks & Spencer*, 1oz/28g				
56/200	6.1/21.7	0/0.1	3.6/12.7	0/0
Salmon, Fillets, Scottish Poached, Tesco*, 1 serving/112g				
216/193	23/20.5	0.7/0.6	13.6/12.1	0.7/0.6
Salmon, Fillets, with a Cream Sauce, Scottish, Marks & Spencer*, 1 serving/200g				
360/180	27.6/13.8	2/1	26/13	0.2/0.1
Salmon, Fillets, with Lemon & Herb Butter, Asda*, 1 fillet/125g				
305/244	25/20	0.5/0.4	22.5/18	0/0
Salmon, Flakes, Honey Roast, Marks & Spencer*, 1oz/28g				
56/200	7.7/27.6	0.9/3.2	2.5/8.8	0/0
Salmon, Flakes, Honey Roast, Sainsbury's*, 1 serving/100g				
169/169	23.8/23.8	0.5/0.5	8/8	0.1/0.1
Salmon, Flakes, Honey Roast, Scottish, Asda*, ½ pack/68.1g				
145/213	15.6/23	1.1/1.6	8.8/13	0.5/0.7
Salmon, Flakes, Honey Roasted, Tesco*, 1 serving/100g				
211/211	21.5/21.5	2.3/2.3	12.9/12.9	0/0
Salmon, Flakes, Poached, Marks & Spencer*, 1oz/28g				
53/190	6.7/24	0/0	2.9/10.5	0/0
Salmon, Florentine, Asda*, 1 serving/190g				
306/161	30.4/16	3.4/1.8	19/10	0/0
Salmon, in a Watercress Sauce, Marks & Spencer*, 1 pack/400g				
480/120	28.4/7.1	32.4/8.1	27.2/6.8	6.8/1.7
Salmon, Minted Potatoes & Vegetables, Steam Cuisine, Marks & Spencer*, 1 pack/400g				
470/118	30.8/7.7	24.8/6.2	29.6/7.4	5.2/1.3
Salmon, with Herb Vegetables, Healthy Eating, Tesco*, 1 pack/350g				
228/65	23.1/6.6	13.3/3.8	9.1/2.6	3.2/0.9
Sardines, in Brine, Tesco*, ½ can/42g				
79/189	9.6/22.8	0/0	4.6/10.9	0/0
Sardines, in Tomato Sauce, Asda*, 1 can/120g				
218/182	21.6/18	0.6/0.5	14.4/12	0/0
Sardines, in Tomato Sauce, Princes*, 1 can/120g				
228/190	22.8/19	1.9/1.6	14.3/11.9	0/0
Sardines, in Tomato Sauce, Skinless & Boneless, Sainsbury's*, 1 can/120g				
143/119	26.5/22.1	1.2/1	3.6/3	0.1/0.1

	kcal serv/100g	prot serv/100g	carb serv/100g	fat serv/100g	fibre serv/100g

Scampi, & Chips, Tesco*, 1 serving/450g

689/153	23/5.1	100.8/22.4	21.6/4.8	7.2/1.6

Scampi, Breaded, Asda*, 1 serving/70g

181/258	9.8/14	13.3/19	9.8/14	0.9/1.3

Scampi, Breaded, Safeway*, 1 pack/340g

755/222	35.4/10.4	74.1/21.8	35.4/10.4	5.4/1.6

Scampi, Breaded, Scottish, Sainsbury's*, 1oz/28g

61/219	3.1/11	4.9/17.4	3.3/11.7	0.4/1.4

Scampi, Breaded, Wholetail, Tesco*, ½ pack/85g

193/227	8.2/9.7	20.1/23.6	8.8/10.4	0.9/1.1

Seafood Cocktail, Asda*, 1oz/28g

26/92	3.9/14	1.6/5.7	0.4/1.5	0/0.1

Seafood Medley, Steam Cuisine, Marks & Spencer*, 1 pack/400g

320/80	34/8.5	18/4.5	12.4/3.1	5.2/1.3

Sushi, Californian, Fish Roll, Nigiri & Maki Selection, Marks & Spencer*, 1 serving/200g

300/150	13/6.5	51.6/25.8	4.6/2.3	2/1

Sushi, Californian, Yakatori, Marks & Spencer*, 1 serving/200g

340/170	12.8/6.4	50/25	9.4/4.7	2/1

Sushi, Deluxe, Pret A Manger*, 1 pack/350g

522/149	20.2/5.8	91.7/26.2	8.5/2.4	3.2/0.9

Sushi, Fish Nigiri, Adventurous, Tesco*, 1 med pack/200g

270/135	14.2/7.1	43.4/21.7	4.4/2.2	1/0.5

Sushi, Fish Selection Box, Marks & Spencer*, 1 serving/220g

396/180	14.5/6.6	59.6/27.1	9.9/4.5	2/0.9

Sushi, Fish Selection, Marks & Spencer*, 1 serving/210g

315/150	13.7/6.5	54.2/25.8	4.8/2.3	2.1/1

Sushi, Fish, Large Box, Tesco*, 1 box/290g

423/146	14.2/4.9	74.8/25.8	7.5/2.6	2.3/0.8

Sushi, Fish, Medium Box, Tesco*, 1 box/195g

281/144	9.9/5.1	50.1/25.7	4.5/2.3	1.4/0.7

Sushi, Fish, Small, Tesco*, 1 serving/105g

148/141	6.2/5.9	25.1/23.9	2.5/2.4	0.6/0.6

Sushi, Komachi Set, Waitrose*, 1 box/235g

425/181	14.3/6.1	73.6/31.3	8.2/3.5	3.3/1.4

Sushi, Medium Box, Marks & Spencer*, 1 serving/215g

366/170	20.9/9.7	52.2/24.3	6/2.8	1.9/0.9

kcal serv/100g	prot serv/100g	carb serv/100g	fat serv/100g	fibre serv/100g

Sushi, Nigiri, Marks & Spencer*, 1 serving/190g

| 285/150 | 9.9/5.2 | 48.8/25.7 | 4.8/2.5 | 1.7/0.9 |

Sushi, Prawn & Salmon Selection, Marks & Spencer*, 1 serving/150g

| 218/145 | 8.3/5.5 | 41.1/27.4 | 2.6/1.7 | 0.9/0.6 |

Sushi, Salmon & Roll Set, Small, Sainsbury's*, 1 serving/101g

| 167/165 | 4.9/4.9 | 30.7/30.4 | 2.6/2.6 | 0.8/0.8 |

Sushi, Salmon Feast Box, Marks & Spencer*, 1 pack/200g

| 330/165 | 11.2/5.6 | 54/27 | 5.8/2.9 | 2/1 |

Sushi, Selection, Shapers, Boots*, 1 pack/189g

| 293/155 | 9.6/5.1 | 52.9/28 | 4.7/2.5 | 4.2/2.2 |

Sushi, Taiko Vegetable Set, Waitrose*, 1 serving/135g

| 254/188 | 5.9/4.4 | 50.1/37.1 | 3.2/2.4 | 1.9/1.4 |

Sushi, Tesco*, 1 pack/195g

| 285/146 | 9.9/5.1 | 50.5/25.9 | 4.5/2.3 | 1.4/0.7 |

Sushi, Tokyo Set, Marks & Spencer*, 1 pack/150g

| 240/160 | 11/7.3 | 38/25.3 | 4.7/3.1 | 0.9/0.6 |

Sushi, Vegetarian, Marks & Spencer*, 1 pack/223g

| 290/130 | 9.1/4.1 | 56.9/25.5 | 3.3/1.5 | 2.9/1.3 |

Sushi, Vegetarian, Tesco*, 1 pack/132g

| 185/140 | 4.1/3.1 | 35.9/27.2 | 2.8/2.1 | 1.2/0.9 |

Sushi, Yo!, Salmon Lunch Set, Sainsbury's*, 1 pack/150g

| 242/161 | 8.9/5.9 | 42.2/28.1 | 4.2/2.8 | 1.2/0.8 |

Trout, Rainbow, Fillets, with Lemon & Rosemary Butter, Marks & Spencer*, 1 serving/230g

| 460/200 | 40.3/17.5 | 3.2/1.4 | 32/13.9 | 1.2/0.5 |

Trout, Rosemary-Crusted, Finest, Tesco*, 1 trout/150g

| 264/176 | 24.3/16.2 | 18.3/12.2 | 10.4/6.9 | 1.5/1 |

Tuna Snack Pot, Italian, Weight Watchers*, 1 pot/240g

| 245/102 | 21.8/9.1 | 20.4/8.5 | 8.6/3.6 | 1.2/0.5 |

Tuna Snack Pot, Oriental, Weight Watchers*, 1 pot/240g

| 269/112 | 21.6/9 | 30.2/12.6 | 7/2.9 | 0.7/0.3 |

Tuna Snack Pot, Provencale, Weight Watchers*, 1 pot/240g

| 266/111 | 23.5/9.8 | 24.5/10.2 | 8.2/3.4 | 1.2/0.5 |

Tuna, All-Day Light Meal, Italian, John West*, 1 serving/100g

| 141/141 | 11/11 | 13/13 | 5/5 | 0/0 |

Tuna, in a Red Chilli & Lime Dressing, Princes*, 1 sachet/85g

| 102/120 | 18.3/21.5 | 0.9/1 | 2.8/3.3 | 0/0 |

kcal serv/100g	prot serv/100g	carb serv/100g	fat serv/100g	fibre serv/100g
Tuna, in a Tikka Dressing, Princes*, 1 sachet/85g				
116/137	15.8/18.6	4.7/5.5	3.8/4.5	0/0
Tuna, in Garlic & Herb Mayonnaise, John West*, ½ can/92g				
243/264	11/12	3.7/4	20.4/22.2	0.2/0.2
Tuna, in Light Lemon Mayonnaise, Princes*, 1 can/80g				
99/124	13.4/16.8	2.8/3.5	3.8/4.8	0/0
Tuna, in Thousand Island Dressing, John West*, 1 can/185g				
287/155	33.3/18	9.4/5.1	13/7	0.4/0.2
Tuna, Light Lunch, French-Style, John West*, 1 pack/250g				
208/83	19.5/7.8	19/7.6	6/2.4	2.5/1
Tuna, Light Lunch, Mediterranean, John West*, 1 pack/250g				
180/72	20/8	18.8/7.5	2.8/1.1	2.8/1.1
Tuna, Light Lunch, Nicoise-Style, John West*, 1 pack/250g				
241/96	26/10.4	22.3/8.9	5.3/2.1	7.1/2.8
Tuna, Mayonnaise with Sweetcorn, John West*, ½ can/92g				
231/251	11/12	4.1/4.5	19/20.6	0.2/0.2
Tuna, Mayonnaise, Weight Watchers*, 1 can/80g				
114/142	9.2/11.5	5/6.2	6.3/7.9	0.1/0.1
Tuna, Steaks, Chargrilled, Italian, Sainsbury's*, 1 serving/125g				
199/159	31.4/25.1	0.3/0.2	8/6.4	0.6/0.5
Tuna, Steaks, Finest, Tesco*, 1 serving/120g				
138/115	31.2/26	0.7/0.6	1.1/0.9	0/0
Tuna, Steaks, in Oriental Sauce, Good Choice, Iceland*, 1 pack/260g				
333/128	58/22.3	21.1/8.1	1.8/0.7	1/0.4
Tuna, Tomato & Herb, Weight Watchers*, 1 can/80g				
79/99	9.3/11.6	4.1/5.1	2.9/3.6	0.4/0.5
Tuna, with a Twist, French Dressing, John West*, 1 pack/85g				
135/159	12.9/15.2	2.4/2.8	8.2/9.7	0.1/0.1
Tuna, with a Twist, Lime & Black Pepper Dressing, John West*, 1 pack/85g				
133/156	13.3/15.6	2.4/2.8	7.8/9.2	0/0
Tuna, with Light Mayonnaise, Princes*, 1 sachet/100g				
112/112	20.5/20.5	3/3	2/2	0/0

MEAT PRODUCTS

Bacon Bits, Smoked, Sainsbury's*, 1 pack/250g				
585/234	46/18.4	0.3/0.1	44.5/17.8	0.3/0.1

kcal serv/100g	prot serv/100g	carb serv/100g	fat serv/100g	fibre serv/100g
Bacon Bits, Smoked, Somerfield*, 1oz/28g				
75/269	6.7/24	0/0	5.3/19	0/0
Bacon, Chops, BBQ, Sainsbury's*, 1 chop/78g				
184/236	16.5/21.2	3.6/4.6	11.5/14.8	0.1/0.1
Bacon, Chops, in Cheese Sauce, Tesco*, 1 serving/185g				
311/168	30.2/16.3	10.4/5.6	16.5/8.9	2.8/1.5
Bacon, Chops, Marks & Spencer*, 1 chop/103g				
232/225	16.4/15.9	0/0	18.5/18	0/0
Bacon, Chops, Reduced-Salt, Somerfield*, 1 chop/68g				
165/243	15.1/22.2	0/0	11.6/17.1	0/0
Bacon, Crispy Strips, Unsmoked, Marks & Spencer*, 1 serving/25g				
121/485	13.9/55.6	0.1/0.4	7.3/29.2	0/0
Bacon, Diced, Below 5% Fat, Healthy Choice, Asda*, 1oz/28g				
28/101	5.3/19	0.3/1	0.6/2.3	0.3/0.9
Bacon, Extra Lean, Marks & Spencer*, 1 rasher/30g				
33/110	6.1/20.2	0/0	1/3.4	0/0
Bacon, Half-Fat, Marks & Spencer*, 1 pack/40g				
162/405	3.4/8.4	27.6/69	4.2/10.5	0.9/2.3
Bacon, Lean & Low, Danepak*, 1 serving/26g				
44/171	4.8/18.3	0/0	2.8/10.9	0/0
Bacon, Maple Cure, Medallions, So Good, Somerfield*, 1 slice/25g				
42/168	7.7/30.7	0.6/2.5	1/3.9	0/0
Bacon, Rashers, COU, Marks & Spencer*, 1 pack/20g				
72/360	1.9/9.4	15.5/77.5	0.6/2.9	0.7/3.5
Bacon, Rashers, Smoked Rindless, Healthy Eating, Tesco*, 1 rasher/20g				
21/106	4/19.8	0/0	0.6/3	0/0
Bacon, Rashers, Unsmoked, Rindless, Healthy Eating, Tesco*, 1 rasher/20g				
21/106	4/19.8	0/0	0.6/3	0/0
Bacon, Rindless, Smoked, Danish, Healthy Eating, Tesco*, 1 rasher/20g				
21/106	4/19.8	0/0	0.6/3	0/0
Bacon, Smoked Medallions, BGTY, Sainsbury's*, 1 rasher/18g				
26/143	5.4/29.9	0.1/0.8	0.4/2.2	0/0.1
Beef Grill Steak, Bird's Eye*, 1 steak/66g				
205/310	10.7/16.2	2.4/3.6	16.9/25.6	0.1/0.1
Beef Grill Steak, Black Pepper, Tesco*, 1 serving/87g				
261/300	14.1/16.2	7.5/8.6	19.4/22.3	0/0
Beef Grill Steak, Iceland*, 1 grillsteak/93g				
322/346	23/24.7	0.7/0.8	25.2/27.1	0/0

kcal serv/100g	prot serv/100g	carb serv/100g	fat serv/100g	fibre serv/100g
Beef Grill Steak, Mighty, Bird's Eye*, 1 serving/134g				
420/313	28/20.9	6.7/5	31/23.1	0.2/0.1
Beef Grill Steak, Peppered, Asda*, 1 serving/170g				
386/227	37.7/22.2	9.7/5.7	21.8/12.8	1/0.6
Beef Grill Steak, Peppered, Sainsbury's*, 1 serving/172g				
378/220	36.5/21.2	8.8/5.1	21.8/12.7	0.3/0.2
Beef Grill Steak, Ross*, 1 grillsteak/61g				
182/298	9.3/15.2	1.2/2	15.6/25.5	0.2/0.3
Beef, Casserole, Steak, BGTY, Sainsbury's*, 1 serving/100g				
122/122	22.6/22.6	0.1/0.1	3.5/3.5	0.1/0.1
Beef, Mince, 5% Fat, GFY, Asda*, 1 serving/227g				
279/123	54.5/24	0/0	6.8/3	0/0
Beef, Mince, 90% Lean, Marks & Spencer*, 1 serving/100g				
175/175	21.9/21.9	0/0	9.6/9.6	0/0
Beef, Mince, British, Tesco*, ½ pack/120g				
278/232	22.7/18.9	0/0	20.9/17.4	0/0
Beef, Mince, British, Value, Tesco*, 1 serving/125g				
396/317	20.4/16.3	0/0	34.3/27.4	0/0
Beef, Mince, Extra-Lean, Sainsbury's*, 1oz/28g				
49/174	6.1/21.9	0/0.1	2.7/9.6	0/0.1
Beef, Mince, Steak, 95% Fat-Free, BGTY, Sainsbury's*, 1oz/28g				
35/124	6/21.3	0/0.1	1.2/4.3	0/0.1
Beef, Patties, Oriental, Perfectly Balanced, Waitrose*, ½ pack/200g				
238/119	19.2/9.6	27.6/13.8	5.6/2.8	2.4/1.2
Beef, Potted, Yorkshire, Sutherland*, 1 serving/10g				
20/199	1.7/17.2	0.1/1.1	1.4/14	0/0
Beef, Stewed Steak, & Onions with Gravy, John West*, ½ can/205g				
269/131	28.7/14	6.2/3	14.4/7	0/0
Beef, Stewed Steak, SmartPrice, Asda*, 1 serving/205g				
230/112	28.7/14	5.7/2.8	10.3/5	0/0
Burgers, Beef with Onion, Bird's Eye*, 1 burger/41g				
114/278	6.3/15.3	1.4/3.5	9.2/22.5	0.1/0.2
Burgers, Beef, 100%, Sainsbury's*, 1 burger/44g				
133/302	9.4/21.4	0.4/0.9	10.4/23.6	0.4/0.9
Burgers, Beef, Quarter Pounders, 100% Prime, Asda*, 1 burger/86g				
254/299	22.1/26	1.4/1.6	17.9/21	0/0

kcal serv/100g	prot serv/100g	carb serv/100g	fat serv/100g	fibre serv/100g

Burgers, Beef, Quarter Pounders, Aberdeen Angus, Marks & Spencer*, 1 burger/113g

| 254/225 | 22.4/19.8 | 1.8/1.6 | 17.5/15.5 | 0/0 |

Burgers, Beef, Quarter Pounders, Bird's Eye*, 1 burger/139g

| 386/278 | 21.3/15.3 | 4.9/3.5 | 31.3/22.5 | 0.3/0.2 |

Burgers, Beef, Quarter Pounders, Farmfoods*, 1 burger/113g

| 289/256 | 16.3/14.4 | 6.1/5.4 | 22.1/19.6 | 0.1/0.1 |

Burgers, Beef, Quarterpounders, Flame-Grilled, Rustlers*, 1 burger/190g

| 557/293 | 28.3/14.9 | 46.2/24.3 | 28.7/15.1 | 0/0 |

Burgers, Beef, Tesco*, 1 burger/47g

| 110/234 | 10.5/22.3 | 4.1/8.7 | 5.7/12.1 | 0.5/1.1 |

Burgers, BGTY, Sainsbury's*, 1 burger/110g

| 177/161 | 22.9/20.8 | 7.8/7.1 | 6.1/5.5 | 1.2/1.1 |

Burgers, Cheeseburger, with Relish, American-Style, Tesco*, 1 burger/61.4g

| 131/215 | 8.7/14.2 | 10.7/17.5 | 6/9.8 | 2.6/4.2 |

Burgers, Chicken, Bird's Eye*, 1 burger/57g

| 147/258 | 7.8/13.6 | 9.6/16.8 | 8.7/15.2 | 0.2/0.4 |

Burgers, Quarter Pounder with Cheese & Buns, Sainsbury's*, 1 burger/198g

| 471/238 | 30.9/15.6 | 37.8/19.1 | 22.8/11.5 | 2.8/1.4 |

Faggots, Pork, Mr Brains*, 1 serving/189g

| 242/128 | 10/5.3 | 22.5/11.9 | 12.5/6.6 | 1.1/0.6 |

Frankfurters, Herta*, 1 frankfurter/35g

| 117/335 | 4.2/12 | 0.7/2 | 10.9/31 | 0/0 |

Frankfurters, Jumbo, Herta*, 1 frankfurter/80g

| 236/295 | 9.4/11.7 | 0.3/0.4 | 22/27.5 | 0/0 |

Frankfurters, Jumbo, Marks & Spencer*, 1 frankfurter/94g

| 277/295 | 11/11.7 | 0.4/0.4 | 25.9/27.5 | 0/0 |

Frankfurters, Real German, Meica*, 1 frankfurter/42g

| 100/239 | 5/12 | 0.2/0.5 | 8.8/21 | 0/0 |

Gammon Joint, Irish, with Honey & Mustard Glaze, Tesco*, 1 serving/100g

| 161/161 | 18.1/18.1 | 3.2/3.2 | 8.5/8.5 | 0.2/0.2 |

Gammon Joint, with Honey & Mustard Glaze, Tesco*, 1 pack/450g

| 725/161 | 81.5/18.1 | 14.4/3.2 | 38.3/8.5 | 0.9/0.2 |

Gammon Steaks, Below 5% Fat, Asda*, 1 pack/250g

| 253/101 | 47.5/19 | 2.5/1 | 5.8/2.3 | 2.3/0.9 |

	kcal serv/100g	prot serv/100g	carb serv/100g	fat serv/100g	fibre serv/100g

Gammon Steaks, Unsmoked, Healthy Eating, Tesco*, 1 serving/110g

100/91	20.5/18.6	1.1/1	1.5/1.4	0/0

Gammon Steaks, Unsmoked, Prime, Asda*, 1 steak/250g

280/112	45/18	0.5/0.2	11/4.4	0/0

Gammon Steaks, with Honey & Mustard, GFY, Asda*, ½ pack/190g

270/142	39.9/21	8.6/4.5	8.4/4.4	0/0

Gammon, Breaded British, Marks & Spencer*, 1oz/28g

28/100	6/21.4	0.1/0.4	0.4/1.4	0/0

Gammon, Breaded, Wiltshire, Marks & Spencer*, 1oz/28g

39/140	6.6/23.6	0.4/1.6	1.3/4.7	0/0

Gammon, Dry Cured, Ready-to-Roast, Marks & Spencer*, ½ joint/255g

255/100	52.3/20.5	1.3/0.5	3.8/1.5	1.3/0.5

Gammon, Honey Roast, Dry Cured, British Gammon, TTD, Sainsbury's*, 1 slice/35g

50/142	8.4/24	1.2/3.3	1.3/3.6	0/0.1

Gammon, Unsmoked, British Steaks, Marks & Spencer*, 1 steak/140g

273/195	40.7/29.1	0.4/0.3	11.8/8.4	0/0

Ham, Turkey, Smoked, Wafer-Thin, Bernard Matthews*, 1 serving/10g

11/112	1.4/14.4	0.4/3.8	0.4/4.4	0/0

Hot Dog, American-Style, Sainsbury's*, 1 sausage/50g

144/288	6.5/13	0.3/0.5	13/26	0/0

Hot Dog, Big American-Style, Princes*, 1 sausage/27g

53/197	2.3/8.5	1.9/7	4.1/15	0/0

Hot Dog, Canned, Ye Olde Oak*, 1 hot dog/33g

54/165	3.8/11.5	1.7/5	4/12	0/0

Hot Dog, in Brine, Premium, Ye Olde Oak*, 1 sausage/23g

39/168	2.5/11	0.9/4	2.8/12	0.2/1

Hot Dog, Jumbo, Co-Op*, 1 sausage/75g

169/225	9.8/13	3/4	13.5/18	0/0

Hot Dog, Lancaster*, 4 sausages/92g

138/150	9.2/10	3.7/4	9.7/10.5	0/0

Hot Dog, Mini, Tesco*, 1 hot dog/10g

22/218	1.3/12.7	0.3/3.4	1.7/17.1	0/0

Hot Dog, Princes*, 1 sausage/23g

42/183	1.8/8	1.2/5	3.3/14.5	0/0

Hot Dog, SmartPrice Asda*, 1 sausage/23g

31/135	2.3/10	0.8/3.5	2.1/9	0/0

	kcal serv/100g	prot serv/100g	carb serv/100g	fat serv/100g	fibre serv/100g
Hot Dog, Value, Tesco*, 1 sausage/27g					
	59/218	3.4/12.7	0.9/3.4	4.6/17.1	0/0
Kebab, BBQ Pork, Sainsbury's*, 1 serving/90g					
	65/72	9.9/11	1.3/1.4	2.2/2.4	0.8/0.9
Lamb, Grill Steak, Bird's Eye*, 1 grillsteak/71g					
	170/239	11.7/16.5	1.3/1.9	13.1/18.4	0.5/0.7
Lamb, Grill Steak, Minted, Asda*, 1 grillsteak/100g					
	298/298	28/28	6/6	18/18	0/0
Lamb, Grill Steak, Prime, Asda*, 1 steak/63g					
	192/304	13.9/22	1.4/2.2	14.5/23	0/0
Lamb, Steak, Bernard Matthews*, 1 steak/140g					
	151/108	25.5/18.2	1/0.7	5/3.6	0/0
Lamb, Steak, BGTY, Sainsbury's*, 1 serving/125g					
	185/148	30.1/24.1	0.1/0.1	7.3/5.8	0.1/0.1
Lamb, Steak, Leg, Grilled, Bernard Matthews*, 1 steak/140g					
	209/149	33/23.6	0.4/0.3	8.3/5.9	0/0
Lamb, Steak, Leg, Healthy Eating, Tesco*, 1 steak/150g					
	165/110	30.2/20.1	0/0	5/3.3	0/0
Lamb, Steak, with Redcurrant & Mint Sauce, Asda*, 1 steak/142.8g					
	327/229	22.9/16	11.4/8	18.6/13	0/0
Liver, Calves, with Fresh Sage Butter, Marks & Spencer*, 1 serving/116.7g					
	211/180	15/12.8	11.8/10.1	12.5/10.7	1.8/1.5
Pasty, Bite-Size Pasties, Food To Go, Sainsbury's*, 1 serving/60g					
	226/377	4.9/8.2	18.7/31.2	14.6/24.4	0.9/1.5
Pasty, Cornish Roaster, Ginsters*, 1 pasty/130g					
	417/321	11.1/8.5	38.9/29.9	24.2/18.6	1.7/1.3
Pasty, Cornish, BGTY, Sainsbury's*, 1 pasty/135g					
	308/228	10.4/7.7	38.1/28.2	12.7/9.4	2.2/1.6
Pasty, Cornish, Cheese & Onion, Ginsters*, 1 pasty/130g					
	511/393	13.5/10.4	39.9/30.7	33/25.4	3/2.3
Pasty, Cornish, Chicken & Bacon, Ginsters*, 1 pasty/227g					
	579/255	12.3/5.4	58.3/25.7	32.9/14.5	2/0.9
Pasty, Cornish, Marks & Spencer*, 1 pasty/150g					
	480/320	9.8/6.5	41/27.3	30.5/20.3	2.3/1.5
Pasty, Cornish, Mini, Marks & Spencer*, 1 pasty/72g					
	227/315	4.8/6.7	15.1/21	16.3/22.6	0.7/1
Pasty, Cornish, Mini, Sainsbury's*, 1 pasty/70g					
	280/400	5.1/7.3	19.7/28.1	20.1/28.7	1.1/1.5

kcal serv/100g	prot serv/100g	carb serv/100g	fat serv/100g	fibre serv/100g
Pasty, Cornish, Original, Ginsters*, 1 pasty/227g				
568/250	13.6/6	43.1/19	35.9/15.8	2.5/1.1
Pasty, Cornish, Pork Farms*, 1 pasty/250g				
673/269	19.3/7.7	57/22.8	40.8/16.3	0/0
Pasty, Cornish, Safeway*, 1 pasty/170g				
490/288	12.8/7.5	38.4/22.6	31.6/18.6	2.6/1.5
Pasty, Cornish, SmartPrice, Asda*, 1 pasty/94g				
286/304	7.5/8	30.1/32	15/16	1.6/1.7
Pasty, Cornish, Tesco*, 1 pasty/150g				
467/311	10.2/6.8	32.9/21.9	32.7/21.8	2.4/1.6
Pasty, Cornish, Traditional-Style, Geo Adams*, 1 pasty/165g				
488/296	11.7/7.1	41.9/25.4	30.4/18.4	2.1/1.3
Pasty, Steak & Onion, Marks & Spencer*, 1 pasty/164g				
459/280	14.3/8.7	31.5/19.2	30.8/18.8	2.3/1.4
Pasty, Tandoori & Vegetable, Holland & Barrett*, 1 pack/110g				
232/211	4.7/4.3	32.3/29.4	9.4/8.5	2/1.8
Pâté, Ardennes, Asda*, 1 serving/50g				
143/286	7/13.9	1.8/3.6	12/24	0.7/1.3
Pâté, Brussels with Garlic, Asda*, 1 serving/50g				
170/340	5.4/10.7	2/4	15.7/31.3	1.3/2.5
Pâté, Brussels, Asda*, 1 serving/50g				
175/350	5.4/10.7	2.2/4.4	16.1/32.2	0.9/1.7
Pie, Buffet Pork, Farmfoods*, 1 pie/65g				
252/388	5.7/8.8	18.3/28.2	17.4/26.7	0.7/1
Pie, Chicken & Mushroom, Farmfoods*, 1 pie/110g				
271/246	6.2/5.6	24.6/22.4	16.4/14.9	1/0.9
Pie, Chicken & Vegetable, Farmfoods*, 1 pie/128g				
384/300	9.2/7.2	32.5/25.4	24.1/18.8	1.8/1.4
Pie, Cottage, Classic British, Sainsbury's*, 1 pack/450g				
500/111	28.4/6.3	50/11.1	20.7/4.6	2.7/0.6
Pie, Minced Beef & Onion, Bird's Eye*, 1 pie/145g				
419/289	10.3/7.1	38.1/26.3	25.1/17.3	1/0.7
Pie, Minced Beef & Onion, Farmfoods*, 1 pie/128g				
378/295	9.3/7.3	31.2/24.4	23.9/18.7	1.3/1
Pie, Minced Beef & Onion, Sainsbury's*, 1 pie/150g				
410/273	10.2/6.8	41.7/27.8	22.5/15	1.4/0.9
Pie, Minced Beef & Onion, Tesco*, 1 pie/150g				
455/303	8.6/5.7	41.1/27.4	28.5/19	2.6/1.7

	kcal serv/100g	prot serv/100g	carb serv/100g	fat serv/100g	fibre serv/100g
Pie, Pork & Egg, Marks & Spencer*, ¼ pie/108g					
	379/351	10.5/9.7	21.4/19.8	28/25.9	0.9/0.8
Pie, Pork & Pickle, Bowyers*, 1 pie/150g					
	576/384	15/10	39.5/26.3	41/27.3	0/0
Pie, Pork & Pickle, Pork Farms*, 1 pie/50g					
	185/370	4.3/8.5	15.1/30.1	12/24	0/0
Pie, Pork, Buffet, Bowyers*, 1 pie/60g					
	217/362	6.2/10.4	14.9/24.9	14.7/24.5	0/0
Pie, Pork, Melton Mowbray, Cured, Marks & Spencer*, 1 pie/290g					
	1044/360	29.3/10.1	75.1/25.9	71.1/24.5	2.9/1
Pie, Pork, Melton Mowbray, Medium, Somerfield*, ¼ pie/70g					
	275/393	7.7/11	18.9/27	18.9/27	0/0
Pie, Pork, Melton Mowbray, Mini, Tesco*, 1 pie/50g					
	196/392	6.3/12.6	10.4/20.8	14.4/28.7	1.5/2.9
Pie, Pork, Melton Mowbray, Safeway*, 1 pie/50g					
	197/393	5.5/10.9	15.7/31.3	12.5/24.9	0.5/0.9
Pie, Pork, Melton Mowbray, Tesco*, 1 sm pie/148g					
	679/459	14.8/10	42.9/29	49.9/33.7	1.9/1.3
Pie, Pork, Melton, Mini, Marks & Spencer*, 1oz/28g					
	112/400	3/10.8	8/28.4	7.6/27.3	0.3/1.2
Pie, Pork, Melton, Mini, Pork Farms*, 1 pie/50g					
	200/399	4.5/8.9	13.1/26.2	14.6/29.2	0/0
Pie, Pork, Mini, Tesco*, 1 pie/45g					
	162/359	4.6/10.2	11.7/25.9	10.7/23.8	0.5/1
Pie, Pork, Somerfield*, 1 pie/110g					
	442/402	12.1/11	26.4/24	31.9/29	0/0
Pie, Potato & Meat, Farmfoods*, 1 pie/158g					
	416/263	8.5/5.4	34.8/22	26.9/17	1.6/1
Pie, Scotch, Co-Op*, 1 pie/132g					
	408/309	9.6/7.3	36/27.3	24.9/18.9	2/1.5
Pie, Scotch, Farmfoods*, 1 pie/151g					
	430/285	11.8/7.8	40.5/26.8	24.6/16.3	1.8/1.2
Pie, Steak & Ale, Fray Bentos*, 1 pie/425g					
	697/164	32.3/7.6	55.3/13	38.7/9.1	0/0
Pie, Steak & Kidney, Bird's Eye*, 1 pie/146g					
	419/287	11/7.5	35.6/24.4	25.8/17.7	2.5/1.7
Pie, Steak & Mushroom, Bird's Eye*, 1 pie/142g					
	389/274	10.7/7.5	32.2/22.7	24.1/17	2.8/2

	kcal serv/100g	prot serv/100g	carb serv/100g	fat serv/100g	fibre serv/100g
Pie, Steak & Mushroom, Co-Op*, 1 pie/454g					
	1158/255	40.9/9	90.8/20	68.1/15	4.5/1
Pie, Steak & Onion, Farmfoods*, 1 pie/127g					
	382/301	7.6/6	33.5/26.4	24.3/19.1	1.3/1
Pie, Steak, Tesco*, 1 serving/205g					
	556/271	14.8/7.2	47.8/23.3	33.8/16.5	2.9/1.4
Pie, Turkey & Ham, Farmfoods*, 1 pie/147g					
	404/275	12.6/8.6	39/26.5	21.9/14.9	2.1/1.4
Pork, Chinese, Steak, Asda*, 1 serving/250g					
	508/203	55/22	10/4	27.5/11	3.3/1.3
Pork, Escalope, BGTY, Sainsbury's*, ½ pack/200g					
	274/137	62.2/31.1	0/0	2.8/1.4	0/0
Pork, Escalope, British, Healthy Eating, Tesco*, 1 escalope/125g					
	138/110	26.6/21.3	0/0	3.4/2.7	0/0
Pork, Escalope, GFY, Asda*, 1 escalope/120g					
	182/152	37.2/31	0/0	3.7/3.1	0/0
Pork, Honey Roast, Loin, Sainsbury's*, 1 slice/12g					
	20/165	2.8/23.6	0.3/2.7	0.8/6.6	0/0.1
Pork, Hot & Spicy, Steak, Shoulder, Waitrose*, 1 steak/100g					
	207/207	19.5/19.5	1.3/1.3	13.7/13.7	0/0
Pork, Medallions, Loin, BGTY, Sainsbury's*, 1 pack/220g					
	142/129	29.9/27.2	0/0	2.4/2.2	0.9/0.8
Pork &, Chestnut Stuffing, Marks & Spencer*, 1oz/28g					
	64/230	1.5/5.3	3.5/12.6	4.8/17.1	1/3.7
Pork, BBQ, Chunky, Tesco*, 1 pack/170g					
	226/133	39.6/23.3	7.8/4.6	4.1/2.4	0.3/0.2
Pork, Chinese, Steaks, Shoulder, Sainsbury's*, 1 steak/100g					
	243/243	28.6/28.6	1.6/1.6	13.6/13.6	1.1/1.1
Pork, Diced, Healthy Eating, Tesco*, 1 serving/75g					
	83/110	16/21.3	0/0	2/2.7	0/0
Pork, Fillet, BGTY, Sainsbury's*, ½ pack/175g					
	256/146	54.1/30.9	0.2/0.1	4.4/2.5	0.2/0.1
Pork, Lunch Tongue, Tesco*, 1 serving/125g					
	228/182	25.5/20.4	1/0.8	13.5/10.8	0/0
Pork, Medallions, Healthy Eating, Tesco*, 1 serving/113.5g					
	125/110	24.3/21.3	0/0	3.1/2.7	0/0
Pork, Mince, Extra Lean, BGTY, Sainsbury's*, 1 serving/227g					
	320/141	43.8/19.3	0.2/0.1	16.1/7.1	1.4/0.6

kcal serv/100g	prot serv/100g	carb serv/100g	fat serv/100g	fibre serv/100g
Pork, Mince, Healthy Eating, Tesco*, 1 pack/400g				
444/111	80.8/20.2	2.8/0.7	12/3	0/0
Ribs, Barbecue, American-Style, Tesco*, 1 serving/250g				
595/238	62.5/25	28.8/11.5	25.5/10.2	0.8/0.3
Ribs, Pork, Chinese-Style, Grilled, Safeway*, 1 serving/100g				
309/309	24.8/24.8	6.2/6.2	20.5/20.5	0/0
Ribs, Pork, Chinese-Style, Jumbo, Sainsbury's*, 1oz/28g				
82/293	7.6/27.3	1.2/4.2	5.2/18.6	0/0.1
Sausage, Aberdeen Angus Beef, Asda*, 1 sausage/77g				
203/263	12.3/16	5.4/7	14.6/19	0.4/0.5
Sausage, Aberdeen Angus, Safeway*, 1 sausage/55.9g				
142/254	10.1/18.1	3.4/6.1	9.8/17.5	0.7/1.2
Sausage, Beef, Premium, Morrisons*, 1 sausage/67g				
164/245	10.4/15.5	3.1/4.6	12.3/18.3	0.7/1
Sausage, Beef, Thick, Butcher's Choice, Tesco*, 1 sausage/57g				
171/300	6.1/10.7	3.6/6.3	14.7/25.8	0.6/1
Sausage, Best Olde English, Safeway*, 1 sausage/53g				
164/310	8.4/15.8	4.4/8.3	12.6/23.8	0.7/1.3
Sausage, BGTY, Sainsbury's*, 1 sausage/50g				
95/189	8.5/16.9	5.5/10.9	4.3/8.6	0.3/0.5
Sausage, Bockwurst German, Princes*, 1 sausage/45g				
113/251	4.7/10.5	0.2/0.5	10.4/23	0/0
Sausage, Bockwurst, in Brine, Ye Olde Oak*, 1 sausage/40.5g				
105/255	4.5/11	0.4/1	9.4/23	0/0
Sausage, Cambridge Gluten-Free, Waitrose*, 1 sausage/121g				
258/213	17.7/14.6	2.3/1.9	19.7/16.3	1.6/1.3
Sausage, Chicken & Tarragon, Butcher's Choice, Sainsbury's*, 1 sausage/47g				
106/225	8.5/18.1	2.7/5.8	6.8/14.4	0.1/0.2
Sausage, Chipolata, Cumberland, Asda*, 1 sausage/33g				
84/255	4.3/13	5.6/17	5/15	0.5/1.5
Sausage, Chipolata, Cumberland, Finest, Tesco*, 1 chipolata/28g				
66/235	4.4/15.6	0.9/3.1	5/17.8	0.2/0.7
Sausage, Chipolata, Cumberland, TTD, Sainsbury's*, 1 sausage grilled/46g				
138/299	9/19.5	2.2/4.8	10.2/22.1	0.6/1.2
Sausage, Chipolata, Finest Cumberland, Tesco*, 1 sausage/37g				
99/267	4.8/12.9	1.5/4	8.2/22.2	0.1/0.3

	kcal serv/100g	prot serv/100g	carb serv/100g	fat serv/100g	fibre serv/100g
Sausage, Chipolata, Lamb & Rosemary, Tesco*, 1 sausage/31.6g					
	69/218	3.6/11.3	2.6/8.3	4.9/15.5	0/0
Sausage, Chipolata, Pork & Tomato, Organic, Tesco*, 1 chipolata/28g					
	79/283	3.4/12.2	1.2/4.3	6.7/24.1	0.3/0.9
Sausage, Chipolata, Pork, Finest, Tesco*, 1 sausage/28g					
	78/280	3.8/13.7	1.1/3.9	6.5/23.3	0.1/0.2
Sausage, Chipolata, Pork, Premium, Waitrose*, 1 chipolata/28.5g					
	70/242	4.2/14.6	0.4/1.4	5.7/19.8	0.4/1.5
Sausage, Chipolata, Pork, Safeway*, 1 sausage/25.2g					
	61/242	3.2/12.8	2.5/10	4.2/16.8	0.3/1.2
Sausage, Chipolata, Pork, Somerfield*, 1 chipolata/28g					
	80/286	3.4/12	2.8/10	6.2/22	0/0
Sausage, Chipolata, Pork, Ultimate, TTD, Sainsbury's*, 1 sausage/45g					
	112/248	7.9/17.6	2.4/5.3	7.8/17.4	0.5/1.2
Sausage, Chipolata, Value, Tesco*, 1 sausage/28.3g					
	82/292	2.4/8.4	3.2/11.6	6.6/23.6	0.7/2.4
Sausage, Choice Pork, Co-Op*, 1 sausage/57g					
	200/350	5.7/10	5.1/9	17.7/31	1.1/2
Sausage, Chorizo, Bites, Mini, Sainsbury's*, ½ pack/32.6g					
	141/426	8.4/25.5	0.8/2.3	11.6/35	0.2/0.7
Sausage, Chorizo, Marks & Spencer*, 1 sausage/57g					
	140/245	8.2/14.4	4/7	10.4/18.3	1/1.7
Sausage, Chorizo, Sliced, Tesco*, 1 serving/80g					
	234/292	21/26.3	1.1/1.4	16.1/20.1	0/0
Sausage, Chorizo, Spanish Slices, Tesco*, 1 slice/20g					
	59/297	5.4/26.8	0.5/2.6	4/19.9	0/0
Sausage, Chorizo, Spicy, Marks & Spencer*, 1 sausage/67g					
	154/230	8.7/13	6.9/10.3	10.5/15.6	0.6/0.9
Sausage, Chorizo, Tesco*, 1 sausage/53g					
	161/303	6.2/11.7	2.3/4.4	14/26.5	0.5/0.9
Sausage, Classic Sicilian-Style, TTD, Sainsbury's*, 1 sausage/49g					
	135/275	8.2/16.8	0.2/0.5	11/22.5	0.4/0.9
Sausage, Classic Toulouse, TTD, Sainsbury's*, 1 sausage/44.5g					
	138/310	10.3/23.2	0.9/2.1	10.4/23.3	0.4/0.9
Sausage, Cocktail, Garnish Selection, Marks & Spencer*, 2 sausages/31g					
	110/355	3.3/10.6	1.7/5.4	10.1/32.5	0.5/1.5
Sausage, Cocktail, Occasions, Sainsbury's*, 1 sausage/9g					
	31/353	1.1/12.1	0.9/9.8	2.6/29.5	0/0.3

	kcal serv/100g	prot serv/100g	carb serv/100g	fat serv/100g	fibre serv/100g

Sausage, Cumberland Pork, Butcher's Choice, Sainsbury's*, 1 sausage/57g

148/260	11.3/19.8	2.5/4.3	10.4/18.2	0.1/0.1

Sausage, Cumberland Pork, Safeway*, 1 sausage/57g

156/273	8.1/14.2	5.7/10	11.2/19.6	0.6/1

Sausage, Cumberland Pork, Waitrose*, 1 sausage/112g

317/283	14.9/13.3	6.5/5.8	25.8/23	2.2/2

Sausage, Cumberland Ring, Finest, Tesco*, 1 ring/227g

606/267	29.3/12.9	9.1/4	50.4/22.2	0.7/0.3

Sausage, Cumberland Ring, TTD, Sainsbury's*, 1 sausage/142g

410/289	25.1/17.7	8.8/6.2	30.5/21.5	1.1/0.8

Sausage, Cumberland, Butcher's Choice, Tesco*, 1 sausage/56g

180/321	6.2/11.1	4.3/7.6	15.3/27.4	1/1.8

Sausage, Cumberland, GFY, Asda*, 1 sausage/49g

72/147	8.3/17	4.9/10	2.1/4.3	0.3/0.7

Sausage, Cumberland. Less Than 5% Fat, Safeway*, 1 sausage/57g

78/137	10.1/17.8	4.6/8	2.2/3.8	0.6/1.1

Sausage, Extra Lean, Grilled, BGTY, Sainsbury's*, 1 sausage/49g

96/196	8.2/16.7	6.8/13.9	4/8.2	0.3/0.6

Sausage, Extra Lean, Marks & Spencer*, 1 sausage/55g

61/110	8.4/15.3	4/7.2	1.8/3.3	1.6/2.9

Sausage, Extra Special Toulouse, Asda*, 1 sausage/65g

212/326	9.8/15	5.2/8	16.9/26	0.4/0.6

Sausage, Frozen, SmartPrice, Asda*, 1 sausage/40g

116/291	3.2/8	5.2/13	9.2/23	0.4/0.9

Sausage, Frozen, Value, Tesco*, 1 sausage/38g

110/290	3.4/8.9	4.2/11.1	8.9/23.3	0.4/1.1

Sausage, Garlic, Strong, Asda*, 1 slice/11g

24/217	1.7/15	0.1/1	1.9/17	0/0

Sausage, Garlic, Tesco*, 1 slice/12g

22/183	2.1/17.7	0.4/3	1.3/11.1	0/0

Sausage, German Extrawurst, Waitrose*, 1 slice/12.5g

39/303	1.8/13.8	0.1/0.8	3.5/27.2	0/0

Sausage, Glamorgan with Cheese & Leek, TTD, Sainsbury's*, 1 sausage/53g

171/323	10/18.9	1.7/3.3	13.8/26	0.3/0.6

Sausage, Glamorgan, Organic, Waitrose*, 1 sausage/41.8g

81/194	6.1/14.5	4.7/11.2	4.2/10.1	0.7/1.7

Sausage, Great British Banger Lincolnshire, 5% Fat, Asda*, 1 sausage/42g

96/229	6.3/15	5.5/13	5.5/13	0.5/1.2

	kcal serv/100g	prot serv/100g	carb serv/100g	fat serv/100g	fibre serv/100g

Sausage, Grilled, Healthy Eating, Tesco*, 1 sausage/46g

| 82/178 | 6.9/15 | 6/13 | 3.2/7 | 0.5/1 |

Sausage, Hot Mustard Porker, Tesco*, 1 sausage/52g

| 143/275 | 8.4/16.1 | 4.2/8.1 | 10.3/19.8 | 1.6/3.1 |

Sausage, Irish Recipe, Morrisons*, 1 serving/50g

| 176/351 | 4.4/8.7 | 14.1/28.1 | 11.3/22.6 | 0.5/1 |

Sausage, Irish Recipe, Sainsbury's*, 1 sausage/40g

| 111/277 | 4.9/12.2 | 7.5/18.8 | 6.9/17.2 | 0.2/0.6 |

Sausage, Irish Recipe, Tesco*, 1 sausage/52g

| 146/281 | 5.7/10.9 | 5.7/11 | 11.2/21.5 | 0.1/0.2 |

Sausage, Irish, Frozen, Tesco*, 1 sausage/46g

| 129/281 | 5/10.9 | 5.1/11 | 9.9/21.5 | 0.5/1.1 |

Sausage, Lincolnshire Pork, Butcher's Choice, Sainsbury's*, 1 sausage/47g

| 146/310 | 8.6/18.3 | 2.6/5.5 | 11.2/23.9 | 0.1/0.2 |

Sausage, Lincolnshire Pork, Tesco*, 1 sausage/46g

| 161/349 | 4.5/9.7 | 4.9/10.6 | 13.7/29.8 | 0.2/0.5 |

Sausage, Lincolnshire, BGTY, Sainsbury's*, 1 sausage/48.0g

| 94/196 | 8.2/17.1 | 5.3/11.1 | 4.4/9.2 | 0.2/0.4 |

Sausage, Lincolnshire, GFY, Asda*, 1 sausage/50g

| 74/147 | 8.5/17 | 5/10 | 2.2/4.3 | 0.5/1 |

Sausage, Lincolnshire, Somerfield*, 1 sausage/28.5g

| 79/281 | 3.6/13 | 2.2/8 | 6.2/22 | 0/0 |

Sausage, Lincolnshire, Tesco*, 1 sausage/60g

| 177/295 | 6.8/11.4 | 3.2/5.3 | 15.2/25.4 | 0/0 |

Sausage, Lincolnshire, Thick, Asda*, 1 sausage/41.6g

| 90/214 | 6.7/16 | 6.3/15 | 4.2/10 | 0.7/1.6 |

Sausage, Lincolnshire, Thick, Premium, Sainsbury's*, 1 sausage/48g

| 147/306 | 6.8/14.1 | 5.9/12.3 | 10.7/22.3 | 0.1/0.3 |

Sausage, Lincolnshire, TTD, Sainsbury's*, 1 sausage/59g

| 150/258 | 11.5/19.8 | 3.5/6.1 | 9.9/17.1 | 0.5/0.8 |

Sausage, Lincolnshire, Waitrose*, 1 sausage/48g

| 91/189 | 6.4/13.3 | 2.9/6 | 6/12.4 | 0.4/0.9 |

Sausage, Lorne, Marks & Spencer*, 1 sausage/75g

| 240/320 | 8.4/11.2 | 10.7/14.3 | 18.9/25.2 | 1.4/1.8 |

Sausage, Mediterranean Style Paprika, Waitrose*, 1 sausage/67g

| 190/283 | 8.1/12.1 | 3.1/4.6 | 16.1/24 | 1.3/1.9 |

Sausage, Mediterranean-Style, 95% Fat-Free, Bowyers*, 1 sausage/50g

| 60/120 | 7/13.9 | 4.5/8.9 | 1.6/3.2 | 0/0 |

kcal serv/100g	prot serv/100g	carb serv/100g	fat serv/100g	fibre serv/100g
Sausage, Micro, Wall's*, 1 sausage/45g				
149/330	5.5/12.2	6/13.4	11.4/25.3	1/2.3
Sausage, Mini, Skinless, Asda*, 1 sausage/8g				
22/279	0.8/10	1.4/17	1.5/19	0/0.3
Sausage, Pistachio, Waitrose*, 1 slice/12g				
32/267	1.7/14	0.1/1	2.8/23	0/0.1
Sausage, Pork & Apple, Finest, Tesco*, 1 sausage/75g				
180/240	9.3/12.4	5.5/7.3	13.4/17.9	1.4/1.9
Sausage, Pork & Apple, Lean Recipe, Wall's*, 1 sausage/57g				
79/139	8.3/14.5	5.4/9.4	2.6/4.5	1.3/2.3
Sausage, Pork & Apple, Marks & Spencer*, 1 sausage/57g				
125/220	6.9/12.1	5/8.8	9.1/15.9	1.3/2.2
Sausage, Pork & Apple, Sainsbury's*, 1 sausage/67g				
184/275	12.3/18.4	5.2/7.8	12.7/18.9	1.1/1.7
Sausage, Pork & Beef, Farmfoods*, 1 sausage/45g				
125/277	4.2/9.3	3.6/7.9	10.4/23.1	0.4/0.9
Sausage, Pork & Beef, Freshbake*, 1 sausage/45g				
114/253	3.9/8.7	6.4/14.3	8.1/17.9	0.9/1.9
Sausage, Pork & Beef, Somerfield*, 1 sausage/57g				
164/288	4.6/8	8/14	12.5/22	0/0
Sausage, Pork & Beef, Thick, Iceland*, 1 sausage/53g				
165/312	5.5/10.4	6.4/12.1	13.1/24.7	0.3/0.6
Sausage, Pork & Beef, Thick, Tesco*, 1 sausage/46g				
139/302	3.1/6.7	8.6/18.7	10.3/22.3	0.2/0.5
Sausage, Pork & Herb, BGTY, Sainsbury's*, 1 sausage/50.3g				
72/143	8.5/16.9	6.3/12.6	1.4/2.8	0.7/1.3
Sausage, Pork & Herb, COU, Marks & Spencer*, 1 sausage/59g				
65/110	9/15.2	5.3/8.9	1.2/2	0.5/0.9
Sausage, Pork & Herb, Finest, Tesco*, 1 sausage/75g				
224/298	10.1/13.4	2.2/2.9	19.4/25.9	0.2/0.2
Sausage, Pork & Leek, Extra Special, Asda*, 1 sausage/70g				
179/255	5.6/8	9.1/13	13.3/19	1.7/2.4
Sausage, Pork & Leek, Finest, Tesco*, 1 sausage/75.6g				
194/255	8.9/11.8	5.7/7.5	15.1/19.8	0.5/0.7
Sausage, Pork & Leek, Tesco*, 1 sausage/75g				
226/301	7.5/10	5.1/6.8	19.5/26	0.3/0.4
Sausage, Pork & Leek, The Best, Safeway*, 1 sausage/52g				
133/256	7.5/14.4	2.8/5.4	10.2/19.7	0.6/1.1

kcal serv/100g	prot serv/100g	carb serv/100g	fat serv/100g	fibre serv/100g
Sausage, Pork & Leek, TTD, Sainsbury's*, 1 sausage/44g				
125/284	10.1/23	1/2.2	9/20.4	0.5/1.2
Sausage, Pork & Onion, Asda*, 1 sausage/42g				
108/257	8.4/20	2.5/6	7.1/17	0.8/1.8
Sausage, Pork & Stilton Cheese, Budgens*, 1 sausage/57g				
175/308	7.4/13.1	4/7	14.4/25.3	0/0
Sausage, Pork & Stilton, Finest, Tesco*, 1 sausage/75g				
244/325	10/13.3	3.5/4.7	21.1/28.1	0.5/0.6
Sausage, Pork & Sun-Dried Tomato, Shire*, 1 sausage/67g				
183/273	8.6/12.8	5.1/7.6	14.3/21.3	0.1/0.2
Sausage, Pork & Tomato, Somerfield*, 1 sausage/57g				
157/275	7.4/13	3.4/6	12.5/22	0/0
Sausage, Pork Cocktail , Tesco*, 1 sausage/14g				
39/279	1.7/12.1	1.3/9.2	3/21.5	0.2/1.1
Sausage, Pork Cocktail, Marks & Spencer*, 1 sausage/50g				
170/340	6.3/12.6	5.4/10.7	13.8/27.5	0.5/0.9
Sausage, Pork with Mozzarella, Italian-Style, Tesco*, 1 sausage/75.6g				
206/271	9.1/12	7.7/10.1	15.4/20.3	0.8/1
Sausage, Pork, 95% Fat-Free, Bowyers*, 1 sausage/52g				
55/105	8/15.3	3.6/7	1.2/2.4	0/0
Sausage, Pork, Apricot & Lovage, Waitrose*, 1 sausage/67g				
165/246	7.5/11.2	8.6/12.9	11.1/16.6	0.9/1.3
Sausage, Pork, Butcher's Choice, Tesco*, 1 sausage/57g				
166/292	6.7/11.7	3.6/6.3	14/24.5	1.2/2.1
Sausage, Pork, Chilli & Coriander, Grilled, Sainsbury's*, 1 sausage/54g				
123/228	10.2/18.9	1.9/3.5	8.3/15.4	1/1.8
Sausage, Pork, Cocktail, Cooked, Geo Adams*, 1 sausage/8.9g				
30/336	1.2/13.2	1/10.6	2.4/26.8	0/0.3
Sausage, Pork, COU, Marks & Spencer*, 1 sausage/57g				
66/115	8.9/15.6	5.4/9.5	1.2/2.1	0.8/1.4
Sausage, Pork, Eat Smart, Grilled, Safeway*, 2 sausages/91g				
120/132	20.7/22.7	6.6/7.3	1.2/1.3	1.1/1.2
Sausage, Pork, Economy, Sainsbury's*, 1 sausage/40g				
116/289	5/12.6	6.7/16.8	7.6/19	0.2/0.5
Sausage, Pork, Extra Lean Premium, Waitrose*, 1 serving/57g				
89/156	9.8/17.2	1.5/2.7	4.8/8.5	1/1.8
Sausage, Pork, Extra Lean, Better For You, Morrisons*, 1 sausage/54g				
63/116	8.6/16	2.7/5	1.9/3.6	0.1/0.2

kcal serv/100g	prot serv/100g	carb serv/100g	fat serv/100g	fibre serv/100g

Sausage, Pork, Extra Lean, BGTY, Grilled, Sainsbury's*, 1 sausage/50g

| 95/189 | 8.5/16.9 | 5.5/10.9 | 4.3/8.6 | 0.3/0.5 |

Sausage, Pork, Extra Lean, Butcher's Choice, Sainsbury's*, 1 sausage/50g

| 91/181 | 10.4/20.7 | 2.1/4.1 | 4.6/9.1 | 0.1/0.1 |

Sausage, Pork, Extra Lean, GFY, Asda*, 1 sausage/57g

| 89/156 | 10/17.5 | 3/5.2 | 4.1/7.2 | 0.2/0.4 |

Sausage, Pork, Farmfoods*, 1 sausage/45g

| 151/336 | 5.2/11.5 | 4/8.8 | 12.7/28.3 | 0.5/1 |

Sausage, Pork, Finest, Tesco*, 1 sausage/76g

| 214/282 | 10/13.2 | 2.3/3 | 18.3/24.1 | 0.7/0.9 |

Sausage, Pork, Free-Range, Waitrose*, 1 sausage/57g

| 144/252 | 9.2/16.2 | 1.4/2.4 | 11.2/19.7 | 0.2/0.3 |

Sausage, Pork, Frozen, Tesco*, 2 sausages/85g

| 244/287 | 9.4/11.1 | 7.6/8.9 | 19.6/23 | 0.5/0.6 |

Sausage, Pork, Garlic & Herb, Speciality, Waitrose*, 1 sausage/67g

| 185/276 | 8.5/12.7 | 1.5/2.2 | 16.1/24 | 0.7/1.1 |

Sausage, Pork, Garlic & Herb, Tesco*, 1 sausage/75.6g

| 198/261 | 8.6/11.3 | 7.4/9.7 | 15/19.7 | 0.9/1.2 |

Sausage, Pork, Good Intentions, Somerfield*, 1 sausage/57g

| 116/203 | 9.9/17.3 | 5.5/9.7 | 6/10.6 | 0.4/0.7 |

Sausage, Pork, Ham & Asparagus, Tesco*, 1 sausage/75.7g

| 173/228 | 11.3/14.9 | 2.9/3.8 | 12.9/17 | 0.8/1.1 |

Sausage, Pork, Healthy Eating, Tesco*, 1 sausage/46g

| 117/254 | 5.4/11.7 | 11.1/24.1 | 5.7/12.3 | 0.2/0.5 |

Sausage, Pork, Honey Roast, Westaways*, 1 sausage/75g

| 183/244 | 9.8/13.1 | 9.6/12.8 | 11.7/15.6 | 0/0 |

Sausage, Pork, Jumbo, Asda*, 1 sausage/74g

| 155/209 | 12.6/17 | 11.1/15 | 6.7/9 | 0.7/1 |

Sausage, Pork, Jumbo, Budgens*, 1 sausage/113g

| 351/309 | 11.9/10.5 | 10.2/9 | 29.2/25.7 | 0/0 |

Sausage, Pork, Less Than 5% Fat, Safeway*, 2 sausages/106.4g

| 149/141 | 18.2/17.2 | 9.1/8.6 | 4.5/4.2 | 1.2/1.1 |

Sausage, Pork, Low-Fat, 95% Fat-Free, Asda*, 1 sausage/50g

| 73/145 | 8.7/17.3 | 5.3/10.5 | 2.2/4.3 | 0.5/1 |

Sausage, Pork, Marks & Spencer*, 1oz/28g

| 98/350 | 3.2/11.4 | 2.5/8.8 | 8.5/30.3 | 0.3/1 |

Sausage, Pork, Olde English-Style, Safeway*, 1 sausage/53g

| 155/293 | 7.4/13.9 | 5.5/10.4 | 11.5/21.7 | 0.8/1.5 |

kcal serv/100g	prot serv/100g	carb serv/100g	fat serv/100g	fibre serv/100g
Sausage, Pork, Organic, Sainsbury's*, 1 sausage/40g				
127/312	7.5/18.5	0.4/0.9	10.6/26	0.4/1.1
Sausage, Pork, Organic, Tesco*, 1 sausage/50g				
116/231	7.4/14.8	3.3/6.5	8.1/16.2	0.4/0.7
Sausage, Pork, Roasted Pepper & Chilli, COU, Marks & Spencer*,				
1 sausage/57g				
57/100	8.7/15.2	4/7.1	1.1/2	1.2/2.1
Sausage, Pork, Thick, Good Choice, Iceland*, 1 sausage/50g				
94/188	8.1/16.2	6.1/12.2	4.1/8.2	0.3/0.6
Sausage, Pork, Thick, Half-Fat, Butcher's Choice, Tesco*, 1 sausage/57g				
112/196	7.7/13.5	5.2/9.1	6.6/11.5	0.9/1.6
Sausage, Pork, Thick, Healthy Eating, Tesco*, 1 sausage/52g				
61/117	7.4/14.2	4.4/8.5	1.5/2.9	0.5/0.9
Sausage, Pork, Thick, Lean Recipe, Wall's*, 1 sausage/57g				
75/132	8.8/15.4	4.8/8.5	2.3/4.1	1.2/2.1
Sausage, Pork, Thick, Low-Fat, Iceland*, 1 sausage/50g				
95/189	6.2/12.3	9.7/19.4	3.5/6.9	0/0
Sausage, Pork, Thick, Premium, Sainsbury's, 1 sausage/49g				
147/301	7.4/15.1	3.8/7.7	11.4/23.3	0.1/0.2
Sausage, Pork, Thick, Somerfield*, 1 sausage/44.9g				
123/274	6.9/15.3	3.7/8.3	9/20	0.8/1.8
Sausage, Pork, Thick, Wall's*, 1 sausage/45g				
154/343	5.4/11.9	5.1/11.4	12.3/27.4	0.4/0.9
Sausage, Pork, Thin-Link, Tesco*, 1 sausage/25g				
68/272	3.7/14.8	4.8/19.2	3.8/15.2	0.3/1.2
Sausage, Pork, Traditionally-Made, Finest, Tesco*, 1 sausage/75g				
210/280	10.3/13.7	2.9/3.9	17.5/23.3	0.2/0.2
Sausage, Pork, Ultimate, TTD, Sainsbury's*, 1 sausage/54g				
136/252	9.2/17.1	2.8/5.2	9.8/18.1	0.5/1
Sausage, Pork, Value, Sainsbury's*, 1 sausage/37g				
109/294	4.3/11.6	6.4/17.3	7.3/19.8	0.3/0.7
Sausage, Tuna & Herb, Sainsbury's*, 1 sausage/47g				
109/231	9.2/19.6	4.7/10	5.9/12.5	0.7/1.5
Sausage, Tuna & Smoked Salmon, Healthy Living, Tesco*, 1 sausage/67g				
90/134	12/17.9	1.9/2.8	3.8/5.7	1.3/2
Sausage, Tuna, Mediterranean-Style, Sainsbury's*, 1 serving/50g				
102/204	7.6/15.1	7.4/14.7	4.8/9.5	0.6/1.2

	kcal serv/100g	prot serv/100g	carb serv/100g	fat serv/100g	fibre serv/100g
Sausage, Turkey & Chicken, Butcher's Choice, Tesco*, 1 sausage/56.7g					
	110/193	7.9/13.8	4.7/8.3	6.6/11.6	0.6/1
Sausage, Turkey & Pork, Bernard Matthews*, 1 sausage/55g					
	137/249	5.6/10.2	7.2/13.1	9.5/17.3	0/0
Sausage, Turkey, Asda*, 1 serving/56g					
	98/175	7.8/14	2.8/5	6.2/11	0/0
Sausage, Turkey, Premium, Somerfield*, 1 sausage/57g					
	76/134	10.3/18	4/7	2.3/4	0/0
Sausage, Turkey, Somerfield*, 1 sausage/114g					
	186/163	17.1/15	8/7	10.3/9	0/0
Sausage, Tuscan, Marks & Spencer*, 1 sausage/66g					
	145/220	9.8/14.9	3/4.6	10.6/16	0.4/0.6
Sausage Meat, Marks & Spencer*, 1oz/28g					
	98/350	2.7/9.8	3.2/11.3	8.4/29.9	0.4/1.3
Sausage Roll, Asda*, 1 roll/64g					
	248/388	5.1/8	16.6/26	17.9/28	0.6/1
Sausage Roll, Basics, Party-Size, Somerfield*, 1 roll/13g					
	45/343	0.9/7	3.8/29	2.9/22	0/0
Sausage Roll, BGTY, Sainsbury's*, 1 roll/65g					
	200/308	6.2/9.6	18.1/27.9	11.4/17.6	0.9/1.4
Sausage Roll, Buffet, Healthy Eating, Tesco*, 1 roll/30g					
	83/278	2.9/9.6	9.4/31.2	3.8/12.8	0.5/1.5
Sausage Roll, Cocktail, Sainsbury's*, 1 roll/15g					
	57/381	1.2/8.2	4/26.4	4.1/27	0.2/1
Sausage Roll, Co-Op*, 1 roll/66g					
	244/370	5.3/8	16.5/25	17.8/27	1.3/2
Sausage Roll, Ginsters*, 1 roll/140g					
	753/538	18.2/13	47.2/33.7	54.7/39.1	3.1/2.2
Sausage Roll, Healthy Eating, Tesco*, 1 roll/70g					
	195/278	6.7/9.6	21.8/31.2	9/12.8	1.1/1.5
Sausage Roll, Large, Sainsbury's*, 1 roll/43g					
	164/382	3.1/7.3	12.1/28.1	11.5/26.7	0.5/1.2
Sausage Roll, Marks & Spencer*, 1 roll/32g					
	130/405	2.9/9.2	6.8/21.4	10/31.2	0.3/0.9
Sausage Roll, Mini, Tesco*, 1 roll/15g					
	53/356	1.4/9	3.6/23.9	3.7/24.9	0.2/1.5
Sausage Roll, Party-Size, Tesco*, 1 roll/12g					
	39/327	0.7/6.2	3.1/26.2	2.6/21.9	0.2/1.3

kcal serv/100g	prot serv/100g	carb serv/100g	fat serv/100g	fibre serv/100g
Sausage Roll, Party, Sainsbury's*, 1 roll/12g				
54/422	1.1/8.7	3.4/26.7	4/31.1	0.2/1.2
Sausage Roll, Pork Farms*, 1 roll/54g				
213/395	5.2/9.6	11.7/21.6	16.2/30	0/0
Sausage Roll, Pork, Large, Marks & Spencer*, 1 roll/63g				
236/375	5.7/9	14.2/22.5	17.6/27.9	0.4/0.7
Sausage Roll, Snack, GFY, Asda*, 1 roll/34g				
112/329	3.2/9.4	9/26.5	7/20.6	0.3/0.9
Savoury Eggs, Mini, Asda*, 1 egg/19g				
58/303	2/10.3	3.4/17.7	4/21.2	0.3/1.5
Savoury Eggs, Mini, Tesco*, 1 egg/20g				
68/342	2.2/11.2	4.6/23	4.6/22.8	0.2/0.9
Scotch Eggs, Asda*, 1 egg/114g				
286/251	12.8/11.2	15.6/13.7	19.2/16.8	1.6/1.4
Scotch Eggs, Mini, Sainsbury's*, 1 egg/12.2g				
39/329	1.3/10.9	2.3/18.9	2.8/23.3	0.1/1
Scotch Eggs, Sainsbury's*, 1 egg/116g				
287/247	13.2/11.4	15.3/13.2	19.1/16.5	0.7/0.6
Scotch Eggs, Tesco*, 1 egg/114g				
309/271	13.1/11.5	19.4/17	19.8/17.4	1/0.9
Spare Ribs, American-Style, Somerfield*, ½ pack/125g				
303/242	23.5/18.8	19.5/15.6	14.5/11.6	2.3/1.8
Spare Ribs, Cantonese, Sainsbury's*, 1 serving/300g				
633/211	54.3/18.1	30.9/10.3	32.4/10.8	1.2/0.4
Spare Ribs, Chinese-Style, Asda*, 1 serving/300g				
642/214	60/20	33/11	30/10	2.4/0.8
Spare Ribs, Chinese-Style, Meal Solutions, Co-Op*, 1 serving/165g				
215/130	13.2/8	6.6/4	14.9/9	0.3/0.2
Spare Ribs, Chinese-Style, Safeway*, ½ pack/285g				
633/222	47/16.5	45.9/16.1	29.1/10.2	6/2.1

POULTRY PRODUCTS

kcal	prot	carb	fat	fibre
Chicken, Balls, Chinese, Marks & Spencer*, 1 ball/16g				
45/280	1.7/10.8	4.7/29.2	2.2/13.6	0.3/2.1
Chicken, Balls, Crispy, Marks & Spencer*, 1 ball/16g				
35/220	2.1/13.3	3.8/23.7	1.3/8.1	0.1/0.5

kcal serv/100g	prot serv/100g	carb serv/100g	fat serv/100g	fibre serv/100g

Chicken, Barbecue Breast Steaks, Spicy, Marks & Spencer*, 1 serving/100g

| 135/135 | 17.7/17.7 | 2/2 | 6.3/6.3 | 0.9/0.9 |

Chicken, Barbecue, Fillets, Mini, Marks & Spencer*, 1oz/28g

| 36/130 | 7.1/25.3 | 1.7/5.9 | 0.2/0.6 | 0.2/0.8 |

Chicken, Barbecue, Southern-Style, GFY, Asda*, 1 serving/165g

| 213/129 | 31.4/19 | 8.3/5 | 6.1/3.7 | 1.7/1 |

Chicken, Battered, Breast, Steaks, Iceland*, 1 breast steak/95g

| 224/236 | 14.6/15.4 | 13.5/14.2 | 12.4/13.1 | 0.9/0.9 |

Chicken, Battered, Crispy, Asda*, 1 piece/95g

| 225/237 | 13.3/14 | 15.2/16 | 12.4/13 | 0/0 |

Chicken, Breaded, Breast, Steaks, Iceland*, 1 breast steak/84g

| 206/245 | 15.9/18.9 | 10.8/12.9 | 11/13.1 | 1.2/1.4 |

Chicken, Breaded, Fillet, Asda*, 1 piece/98g

| 196/200 | 20.6/21 | 10.8/11 | 7.8/8 | 0/0 |

Chicken, Breaded, Portions, Crunchy, Asda*, 1 piece/92g

| 199/216 | 12.9/14 | 12/13 | 11/12 | 0/0 |

Chicken, Breaded, Steaks, Tesco*, 1 steak/95g

| 213/224 | 12.4/13 | 16.1/16.9 | 11/11.6 | 0.4/0.4 |

Chicken, Cajun, Breast, Fillets, Marinated, Sainsbury's*, 1 fillet/93g

| 113/122 | 23/24.7 | 2.4/2.6 | 1.3/1.4 | 0.5/0.5 |

Chicken, Cajun, Breast, Pieces, Sainsbury's*, 1 serving/100g

| 142/142 | 22/22 | 6.3/6.3 | 3.2/3.2 | 0.9/0.9 |

Chicken, Chargrilled, Asda*, 1 slice/25g

| 27/109 | 6/23.9 | 0.1/0.5 | 0.3/1.3 | 0/0 |

Chicken, Chargrilled, Breast, Cured, Marks & Spencer*, 1 slice/19g

| 19/100 | 4/20.9 | 0.1/0.3 | 0.3/1.7 | 0/0 |

Chicken, Chargrilled, Chunky, Tesco*, 1oz/28g

| 32/116 | 7.1/25.5 | 0.3/0.9 | 0.3/1.1 | 0/0 |

Chicken, Chargrilled Fillets, GFY, Asda*, 1 fillet/64g

| 90/140 | 19.2/30 | 0.3/0.4 | 1.3/2 | 0.7/1.1 |

Chicken, Chargrilled Fillets, Sainsbury's*, 1 serving/119g

| 214/180 | 26.3/22.1 | 1.7/1.4 | 11.3/9.5 | 0.8/0.7 |

Chicken, Chargrilled Fillets, Sliced, Marks & Spencer*, 1 serving/140g

| 182/130 | 41.7/29.8 | 0.8/0.6 | 1.4/1 | 0.7/0.5 |

Chicken, Chargrills, Garlic, Bird's Eye*, 1 piece/76g

| 169/222 | 14.6/19.2 | 0.9/1.2 | 11.9/15.6 | 0/0 |

Chicken, Chargrills, Original, Birds Eye*, 1 serving/79g

| 179/227 | 14.6/18.5 | 0.9/1.1 | 13/16.5 | 0/0 |

kcal serv/100g	prot serv/100g	carb serv/100g	fat serv/100g	fibre serv/100g
Chicken, Chilli, Chunks, Breast, Safeway*, 1 serving/100g				
142/142	22.2/22.2	6.3/6.3	3.2/3.2	0/0
Chicken, Chinese, Sliced, Breast, Fillets, Marks & Spencer*, 1 pack/140g				
182/130	31.9/22.8	11.9/8.5	0.4/0.3	1.1/0.8
Chicken, Chinese-Style, Breast Fillets, Asda*, 1oz/28g				
41/148	8.7/31.2	0.3/1.1	0.6/2.1	0.2/0.7
Chicken, Chinese-Style, Mini Breast Fillets, Tesco*, ½ pack/100g				
121/121	24.9/24.9	2.9/2.9	1.1/1.1	0.2/0.2
Chicken, Chinese-Style, Mini Fillets, Marks & Spencer*, 1 pack/190g				
228/120	41.8/22	14.3/7.5	1.3/0.7	2.3/1.2
Chicken, Drumsticks, American-Style, Frozen, Sainsbury's*, 1 drumstick/84g				
195/232	18.4/21.9	6.1/7.3	10.8/12.8	0.7/0.8
Chicken, Drumsticks, BBQ, Asda*, 1oz/28g				
53/189	7/25	0.6/2	2.5/9	0.1/0.3
Chicken, Drumsticks, BBQ, Safeway*, 1 serving/48g				
84/176	11.4/23.8	1.6/3.4	3.8/7.9	0/0
Chicken, Drumsticks, BBQ, Sainsbury's*, 1 drumstick/100g				
195/195	22.4/22.4	6.5/6.5	8.7/8.7	0.1/0.1
Chicken, Drumsticks, Chinese-Style, Asda*, 1oz/28g				
52/184	6.8/24.2	0.5/1.9	2.5/8.8	0.2/0.6
Chicken, Drumsticks, Chinese, Sainsbury's*, 1 drumstick/100g				
171/171	20.9/20.9	5.2/5.2	7.4/7.4	0.8/0.8
Chicken, Drumsticks, Hot & Spicy, Asda*, 1oz/28g				
49/176	7/25	0.3/1	2.2/8	0.1/0.4
Chicken, Drumsticks, Jumbo-Size, Marks & Spencer*, 1oz/28g				
53/190	7.3/26	0.2/0.6	2.7/9.5	0/0
Chicken, Drumsticks, Roast, Asda*, 1oz/28g				
50/180	7/24.9	0.3/1	2.4/8.5	0/0
Chicken, Drumsticks, Roast, Safeway*, 1 serving/85.2g				
150/176	21.2/24.9	0.3/0.3	7.1/8.3	0/0
Chicken, Drumsticks, Roasted, Tesco*, 1 drumstick/70g				
125/179	18.3/26.1	0.2/0.3	5.7/8.1	0/0
Chicken, Drumsticks, Sainsbury's*, 1 drumstick/100g				
183/183	25.3/25.3	0.1/0.1	9.1/9.1	0.1/0.1
Chicken, Drumsticks, Tesco*, 1 serving/100g				
230/230	17.6/17.6	0/0	17.7/17.7	0/0

	kcal serv/100g	prot serv/100g	carb serv/100g	fat serv/100g	fibre serv/100g
Chicken, Drumsticks, with Skin, Asda*, 1 drumstick/125g					
	231/185	32.5/26	0/0	11.3/9	0/0
Chicken, Drumsticks, without Skin, Tesco*, 1 drumstick/121g					
	152/126	23/19	0/0	6.7/5.5	0/0
Chicken, Escalope, Bernard Matthews*, 1 escalope/143g					
	390/273	13.6/9.5	26.2/18.3	25.7/18	0/0
Chicken, Escalope, Breast, Marks & Spencer*, 1 pack/310g					
	372/120	62.6/20.2	4.7/1.5	13.3/4.3	1.9/0.6
Chicken, Escalope, Breast, Quick-Cook, Healthy Living, Tesco*, 1 serving/100g					
	106/106	23.7/23.7	0/0	1.2/1.2	0/0
Chicken, Escalope, Breast, Tesco*, 1 serving/100g					
	103/103	23/23	0.6/0.6	1/1	0.8/0.8
Chicken, Escalope, Crispy Crumb, Sainsbury's*, 1 escalope/121.3g					
	381/315	19.1/15.8	25.4/21	22.5/18.6	2.1/1.7
Chicken, Escalope, GFY, Asda*, 1 escalope/128g					
	330/258	19.2/15	23/18	17.9/14	0.5/0.4
Chicken, Escalope, Tomato & Basil, Safeway*, 1 escalope/150g					
	242/161	31.8/21.2	3.3/2.2	11.3/7.5	1.8/1.2
Chicken, Fillets, Baked, Breast, Farmfoods*, 1 serving/100g					
	79/79	17.4/17.4	0.2/0.2	1/1	0.8/0.8
Chicken, Fillets, Coronation, BGTY, Sainsbury's*, 1 fillet/100g					
	136/136	27.1/27.1	2.4/2.4	2.6/2.6	1/1
Chicken, Fillets, Crumbed, Breast, Sainsbury's*, 1 fillet/107g					
	230/215	17.5/16.4	16.7/15.6	10.4/9.7	1.2/1.1
Chicken, Fillets, Hickory Barbecue & Chilli, BGTY, Sainsbury's*, 1 fillet/100g					
	133/133	26.9/26.9	3.6/3.6	1.2/1.2	0.9/0.9
Chicken, Fillets, Honey & Mustard, Mini, Marks & Spencer*, 1 serving/105g					
	142/135	26.1/24.9	4.1/3.9	2.1/2	1.4/1.3
Chicken, Fillets, Hot & Spicy, Breast, Sainsbury's*, 1 fillet/108g					
	211/195	20/18.5	15.8/14.6	7.6/7	1.3/1.2
Chicken, Fillets, Hot & Spicy, Iceland*, 1 serving/92g					
	171/186	16.7/18.2	10/10.9	7.2/7.8	0.8/0.9
Chicken, Fillets, Lime & Coriander, Mini, Breast, Tesco*, ½ pack/100g					
	122/122	25/25	2.5/2.5	1.3/1.3	0.2/0.2
Chicken, Fillets, Lime & Coriander, Mini, Marks & Spencer*, 1 fillet/42g					
	44/105	9.4/22.4	0.9/2.1	0.5/1.2	0.1/0.3

kcal serv/100g	prot serv/100g	carb serv/100g	fat serv/100g	fibre serv/100g
Chicken, Fillets, Mini, Marks & Spencer*, 1oz/28g				
35/125	7.4/26.6	0/0	0.6/2.1	0/0
Chicken, Fillets, Roast, Boneless, Breast, Sainsbury's*, 1 breast/120g				
221/184	30.1/25.1	0.2/0.2	11/9.2	0.1/0.1
Chicken, Fillets, Roast, Breast, Morrisons*, 1 fillet/120g				
221/184	30.1/25.1	0.2/0.2	11/9.2	0.1/0.1
Chicken, Fillets, Roast, Sliced, Skinless, Breast, Marks & Spencer*, 1 serving/240g				
312/130	71.5/29.8	1.4/0.6	2.4/1	1.2/0.5
Chicken, Fillets, Skinless, Cooked, Breast, Marks & Spencer*, 1 serving/100g				
130/130	29.8/29.8	0.6/0.6	1/1	0.5/0.5
Chicken, Fillets, Skinless, Cooked, Breast, Waitrose*, 1 breast/85g				
201/236	44.5/52.4	1/1.2	2.6/3	1/1.2
Chicken, Fillets, Sweet Chilli & Lime, Mini, Marks & Spencer*, 1 serving/210g				
284/135	51.5/24.5	11.8/5.6	3.8/1.8	2.3/1.1
Chicken, Fillets, Tandoori, Mini, Eat Smart, Safeway*, 1 serving/50g				
65/130	13.1/26.2	0.7/1.4	1/2	0.3/0.5
Chicken, Fillets, Tandoori, Mini, Marks & Spencer*, 1 serving/100g				
125/125	23.2/23.2	3.7/3.7	2.1/2.1	0.2/0.2
Chicken, Fillets, Tomato & Basil, Mini, Breast, Tesco*, 1 pack/200g				
262/131	50.4/25.2	4.2/2.1	4.8/2.4	0.4/0.2
Chicken, Fillets, Tomato & Basil, Mini, Marks & Spencer*, 1oz/28g				
32/115	6.1/21.7	0.8/2.9	0.5/1.8	0.1/0.5
Chicken, Fried, Spicy, Sainsbury's*, 1 serving/150g				
414/276	43.2/28.8	4.4/2.9	24.9/16.6	3.2/2.1
Chicken, Garlic, Crunchy, Bird's Eye*, 1 piece/99g				
259/262	14.3/14.4	16.7/16.9	15/15.2	0.9/0.9
Chicken, Goujons, Breast, Fresh, Asda*, 1oz/28g				
30/106	6.7/24	0/0	0.3/1.1	0/0
Chicken, Honey Roast, Asda*, 1 slice/25g				
30/118	6/24	0.3/1.1	0.5/1.9	0/0.1
Chicken, Honey Roast, Thin Sliced, Asda*, 1 slice/13g				
15/116	2.5/19.1	0.4/3.2	0.4/3	0/0.1
Chicken, Mexican, Spicy, Bird's Eye*, 1 piece/103g				
254/247	15/14.6	17/16.5	14/13.6	0.6/0.6
Chicken, Mexican-Style, BGTY, Sainsbury's*, 1 serving/260g				
255/98	17.9/6.9	31.5/12.1	6.5/2.5	5.7/2.2

	kcal serv/100g	prot serv/100g	carb serv/100g	fat serv/100g	fibre serv/100g
Chicken, Mexican-Style, GFY, Asda*, ½ pack/200g					
	256/128	34/17	7.4/3.7	10/5	0.6/0.3
Chicken, Nuggets, Battered, Somerfield*, 1oz/28g					
	69/248	3.9/14	4.5/16	3.9/14	0/0
Chicken, Nuggets, Breaded, Crunchy, Asda*, 1 nugget/14g					
	35/253	2.2/16	2.5/18	1.8/13	0.3/1.9
Chicken, Nuggets, Breaded, Iceland*, 1 nugget/13g					
	35/270	2.5/19.4	2.1/15.8	1.9/14.3	0.1/1.1
Chicken, Nuggets, Breaded, SmartPrice, Asda*, 1 nugget/16g					
	51/320	2.4/15	4.6/29	2.6/16	0.2/1.2
Chicken, Nuggets, Breast, Maitre Choice, Lidl*, 1 serving/100g					
	184/184	16.4/16.4	12.9/12.9	7.4/7.4	0/0
Chicken, Nuggets, Crispy, Premium, Sun Valley*, 5 nuggets/108g					
	295/273	14/13	18.4/17	18.4/17	0/0
Chicken, Nuggets, Crunchy Crumb, Tesco*, 1 serving/100g					
	257/257	13.1/13.1	18.6/18.6	14.5/14.5	0.7/0.7
Chicken, Nuggets, Iceland*, 1 nugget/15g					
	44/290	2.2/14.5	2.8/18.9	2.6/17.4	0.3/2.3
Chicken, Nuggets, in Crispy Breadcrumbs, Sainsbury's*, 4 nuggets/54g					
	137/253	7/12.9	9.8/18.1	7.7/14.3	0.6/1.2
Chicken, Nuggets, Organic, Tesco*, 1 nugget/20g					
	52/258	2.7/13.5	4.5/22.3	2.5/12.7	0.2/1.1
Chicken, Nuggets, Southern-Fried, Bird's Eye*, 1 nugget/17g					
	42/248	2.2/12.9	3/17.8	2.4/14	0.2/1.2
Chicken, Nuggets, Tesco*, 1oz/28g					
	68/243	3.7/13.3	4.5/16.2	3.9/13.9	0.2/0.7
Chicken, Roast, Drumsticks, with Brown Sugar, Sainsbury's*, 1 drumstick/78g					
	144/185	17.9/22.9	1.6/2	7.4/9.5	0.9/1.1
Chicken, Roast, Healthy Living, Tesco*, 1 slice/25g					
	30/118	5.8/23	0.6/2.2	0.5/1.9	0.1/0.2
Chicken, Roast, in Sugar Marinade, Marks & Spencer*, 1 portion/200g					
	370/185	52.8/26.4	0.8/0.4	17.2/8.6	0.2/0.1
Chicken, Roast, Leg Quarter, Waitrose*, 1 quarter/120g					
	230/192	24.4/20.3	0.8/0.7	14.5/12.1	0.6/0.5
Chicken, Roast, Tesco*, 1 slice/20g					
	27/133	4.8/24	0.6/2.8	0.6/2.8	0.1/0.3

kcal serv/100g	prot serv/100g	carb serv/100g	fat serv/100g	fibre serv/100g
Chicken, Roll, Asda*, 1 slice/10g				
17/174	1.5/15	0.4/3.8	1.1/11	0/0
Chicken, Roll, Breast, Sainsbury's, 1 slice/10g				
15/153	1.8/18.4	0.2/1.9	0.8/8	0.1/0.7
Chicken, Roll, SmartPrice, Asda*, 1 slice/14g				
24/174	2.1/15	0.5/3.8	1.5/11	0/0
Chicken, Slices, Breast, Bernard Matthews*, 1 slice/20g				
24/122	3.9/19.3	0.6/3	0.7/3.6	0/0
Chicken, Slices, Cooked, Sainsbury's*, 1 slice/19g				
20/106	4.1/21.4	0.4/2.1	0.2/1.3	0.1/0.3
Chicken, Slices, Roast, Mattessons*, 1 slice/25g				
33/131	6.2/24.8	0.6/2.2	0.9/3.4	0.1/0.5
Chicken, Slices, Roast, Premium, Somerfield*, 1 slice/20g				
23/114	5/25	0.2/1	0.2/1	0/0
Chicken, Southern-Fried, Bird's Eye*, 1 steak/98g				
272/278	14.3/14.6	13.1/13.4	18/18.4	0.9/0.9
Chicken, Southern-Fried, Drumsticks, Tesco*, 1oz/28g				
57/202	4.9/17.6	2.5/8.8	3/10.7	0.1/0.5
Chicken, Southern-Fried, Fillets, Asda*, 1 fillet/86g				
175/203	18.1/21	12/14	6/7	0.4/0.5
Chicken, Southern-Fried, Fillets, Fresh, Sainsbury's*, 1 fillet/104g				
220/212	18.9/18.2	12.9/12.4	10.3/9.9	1/1
Chicken, Southern Fried, Fillets, Frozen, Morrisons*, 1 piece/100g				
181/181	15.1/15.1	9.7/9.7	9.1/9.1	2.3/2.3
Chicken, Southern-Fried, Fillets, Mini, Breast, Tesco*, 1 piece/43.7g				
87/199	7.2/16.5	5.7/13	3.9/9	1/2.3
Chicken, Southern-Fried, Portions, Asda*, 1 portion/95g				
210/221	13.3/14	11.4/12	12.4/13	0/0
Chicken, Southern-Fried, Steaks, Tesco*, 1 steak/137g				
293/214	21.1/15.4	15.2/11.1	16.4/12	1.2/0.9
Chicken, Southern-Fried, Strips, Tesco*, 1 pack/300g				
699/233	56.1/18.7	54.9/18.3	28.2/9.4	4.2/1.4
Chicken, Southern-Fried, Thigh, Tesco*, 1oz/28g				
68/242	4.1/14.7	2.8/10.1	4.5/15.9	0.1/0.5
Chicken, Southern-Fried, Wing, Tesco*, 1 serving/100g				
238/238	15/15	11.7/11.7	14.6/14.6	0.5/0.5
Chicken, Steaks, Hot & Spicy, Tesco*, 1 steak/95g				
200/211	12.8/13.5	10.8/11.4	11.8/12.4	0.8/0.8

	kcal serv/100g	prot serv/100g	carb serv/100g	fat serv/100g	fibre serv/100g
Chicken, Thai, Red, Fillets, Mini, BGTY, Sainsbury's*, 1 serving/100g					
	125/125	20.9/20.9	6.8/6.8	1.6/1.6	0.8/0.8
Chicken, Thai, Red, Fillets, Mini, Marks & Spencer*, 1 serving/210g					
	273/130	47.3/22.5	8.6/4.1	5.3/2.5	0.8/0.4
Chicken, Thai-Style, Red, Fillets, Mini, Breast, Tesco*, ½ pack/100g					
	135/135	26.8/26.8	2.8/2.8	1.8/1.8	0.5/0.5
Chicken, Tikka, Breast Chunks, Safeway*, 1 pack/200g					
	356/178	64.4/32.2	8.2/4.1	7.4/3.7	0/0
Chicken, Tikka, Breast Fillets, Mini, Asda*, 1oz/28g					
	34/123	7.3/26	0.4/1.5	0.5/1.7	0.3/1
Chicken, Tikka, Breast Fillets, Sliced, Marks & Spencer*, 1 pack/140g					
	154/110	30.7/21.9	4.5/3.2	2.4/1.7	1.1/0.8
Chicken, Tikka, Breast Pieces, Sainsbury's*, 1 serving/150g					
	233/155	39.2/26.1	4.8/3.2	6.2/4.1	0.8/0.5
Chicken, Tikka, Breast, Ready-Cooked, Frozen, Fullers Foods, Aldi*, 1 serving/100g					
	127/127	24/24	2.4/2.4	2.4/2.4	2/2
Chicken, Tikka, Fillets, Mini, Marks & Spencer*, 1 serving/100g					
	125/125	24.2/24.2	1.1/1.1	2.6/2.6	1.3/1.3
Chicken, Tikka, Fillets, Roast, Asda*, 1oz/28g					
	36/127	7.3/26	0.6/2.3	0.4/1.5	0.1/0.3
Chicken, Tikka, Pieces, Ready-Cooked, Iceland*, 1 serving/100g					
	135/135	26.8/26.8	1.6/1.6	2.5/2.5	0/0
Chicken, Tikka, Portions, Asda*, 1oz/28g					
	47/169	4.8/17.2	0.1/0.5	3.1/11	0.3/1
Chicken, Wafer-Thin, American-Fried, Bernard Matthews*, 1oz/28g					
	31/111	5/18	0.9/3.1	0.8/3	0/0
Chicken, Wafer-Thin, Roast, Asda*, 1oz/28g					
	31/110	5.9/21	1/3.6	0.4/1.3	0/0
Chicken, Wafer-Thin, Roast, Safeway*, 1 serving/25g					
	28/112	5.2/20.6	0.6/2.4	0.6/2.2	0/0
Chicken, Wafer-Thin, Roast, Sainsbury's*, 1oz/28g					
	34/121	5.1/18.3	1/3.7	1/3.6	0.4/1.6
Chicken, Wafer-Thin, Roast, Tesco*, 1oz/28g					
	36/129	5.4/19.3	1/3.6	1.1/4.1	0/0
Chicken, Wafer-Thin, Sage & Onion, Breast, Bernard Matthews*, 1 serving/25g					
	30/120	5/19.8	0.9/3.5	0.8/3	0/0

	kcal serv/100g	prot serv/100g	carb serv/100g	fat serv/100g	fibre serv/100g
Chicken, Wafer-Thin, Sainsbury's*, 1 pack/100g					
	114/114	20.4/20.4	1.9/1.9	2.7/2.7	0.1/0.1
Chicken, Wings, Chinese-Style, Asda*, 1oz/28g					
	70/250	7.8/28	0.8/3	3.9/14	0.1/0.5
Chicken, Wings, Chinese-Style, Marks & Spencer*, 1 serving/100g					
	260/260	20.5/20.5	7.3/7.3	17/17	0.6/0.6
Chicken, Wings, Hot & Spicy, Asda*, 1 pack/450g					
	1076/239	94.5/21	22.1/4.9	67.5/15	5.9/1.3
Chicken, Wings, Hot & Spicy, Tesco*, ½ pack/325g					
	725/223	73.8/22.7	17.6/5.4	40/12.3	1.3/0.4
Chicken, Wings, Microwave, Tesco*, 1oz/28g					
	72/256	6.4/22.7	2.2/7.8	4.2/14.9	0.1/0.4
Chicken in, Barbeque Sauce, Healthy Eating, Tesco*, 1 breast/170g					
	177/104	31.1/18.3	7.7/4.5	2.4/1.4	1.5/0.9
Chicken in, Leek & Bacon Sauce, Chilled, Co-Op*, 1 pack/400g					
	460/115	60/15	8/2	20/5	0.8/0.2
Chicken in, Mild & Fruity Curry, Breasts, Healthy Eating, Tesco*, **2 breasts/345g**					
	321/93	54.5/15.8	14.1/4.1	5.2/1.5	1.7/0.5
Chicken with, Cranberry & Orange Stuffing, Sainsbury's*, 1 serving/100g					
	201/201	23/23	4.1/4.1	10.3/10.3	0.8/0.8
Chicken with, Garlic & Herbs, Asda*, 1 slice/25g					
	29/114	6/23.9	0.3/1.1	0.4/1.5	0/0
Chicken with, Stuffing, Breast, TTD, Sainsbury's*, 1oz/28g					
	50/180	6/21.5	1.5/5.2	2.3/8.1	0.3/0.9
Curry, Chicken, Mild, Sainsbury's*, 1 can/400g					
	472/118	42/10.5	14/3.5	27.6/6.9	5.2/1.3
Dippers, Chicken, Chinese, Tesco*, ½ pack/150g					
	255/170	26/17.3	12.6/8.4	11.3/7.5	1.4/0.9
Dippers, Chicken, Crispy, Bird's Eye*, 1 dipper/17g					
	48/280	2.1/12.5	2.2/12.9	3.4/19.8	0/0.2
Dippers, Chicken, Crispy, Farmfoods*, 1 dipper/17g					
	42/247	2.4/14.2	2.8/16.4	2.4/13.9	0.1/0.4
Dippers, Chicken, Tikka, Tesco*, 1oz/28g					
	54/193	6/21.5	1.4/5	2.7/9.7	0.3/1
Duck, Breast Fillet, Skinless, Gressingham, TTD, Sainsbury's, **1 serving/160g**					
	192/120	40.6/25.4	0.2/0.1	3.2/2	0.6/0.4

	kcal serv/100g	prot serv/100g	carb serv/100g	fat serv/100g	fibre serv/100g

Duck, Breast Fillets, Sliced, Marks & Spencer*, 1 pack/100g

| 150/150 | 25.3/25.3 | 3.6/3.6 | 3.7/3.7 | 0/0 |

Duck, Crispy in a Plum Sauce, Marks & Spencer*, 1 pack/325g

| 569/175 | 34.8/10.7 | 36.4/11.2 | 31.2/9.6 | 2.9/0.9 |

Duck, Fillets, Free-Range with Red Wine Sauce, Waitrose*, ½ pack/250g

| 378/151 | 41/16.4 | 10.3/4.1 | 19.3/7.7 | 5.5/2.2 |

Duck, in Orange Sauce, Iceland*, 1 serving/200g

| 336/168 | 22.6/11.3 | 14.8/7.4 | 20.8/10.4 | 2.4/1.2 |

Duck, in Oriental Sauce, Iceland*, 1 pack/201.1g

| 352/175 | 24.1/12 | 12.7/6.3 | 22.7/11.3 | 3/1.5 |

Duck, Leg, Crispy, Sainsbury's*, 1 pack/230g

| 598/260 | 35.4/15.4 | 65.1/28.3 | 21.9/9.5 | 0/0 |

Duck, Legs, Meat & Skin, Finest, Tesco*, 1 serving/150g

| 431/287 | 22.5/15 | 0.2/0.1 | 37.8/25.2 | 1.5/1 |

Duck, Roast Cantonese-Style, Tesco*, 1 pack/300g

| 375/125 | 24.6/8.2 | 53.7/17.9 | 6.9/2.3 | 1./0.5 |

Pastrami, Turkey, Wafer-Thin, Marks & Spencer*, 1 serving/100g

| 113/113 | 23.6/23.6 | 1.4/1.4 | 1.6/1.6 | 0/0 |

Pastrami, Turkey, Wafer-Thin, Sainsbury's*, 1 serving/100g

| 108/108 | 19.3/19.3 | 3/3 | 2.1/2.1 | 0.5/0.5 |

Turkey, Escalope, Breaded, Tesco*, 1 escalope/138g

| 298/216 | 18.9/13.7 | 18.5/13.4 | 16.4/11.9 | 2.2/1.6 |

Turkey, Escalope, Lemon & Pepper, Bernard Matthews*, 1 escalope/143g

| 362/253 | 16/11.2 | 24.6/17.2 | 22.2/15.5 | 0/0 |

Turkey, Escalope, Southern-Fried, Somerfield*, 1 pack/280g

| 700/250 | 44.8/16 | 36.4/13 | 42/15 | 0/0 |

Turkey, Escalope, Spicy Mango, Bernard Matthews*, 1 escalope/136g

| 354/260 | 15.8/11.6 | 33.5/24.6 | 17.4/12.8 | 0/0 |

Turkey, Goujons, Bernard Matthews*, 1 goujon/32g

| 78/245 | 3.6/11.3 | 5.8/18.1 | 4.5/14.1 | 0/0 |

Turkey, Breast, Golden Roasted, Bernard Matthews*, 1 piece/38g

| 43/113 | 9.2/24.3 | 0.2/0.4 | 0.6/1.6 | 0/0 |

Turkey, Breast, Hand-Carved, Butter-Basted, TTD, Sainsbury's*, 1oz/28g

| 40/142 | 6.9/24.7 | 0.3/1.2 | 1.1/4.1 | 0.1/0.3 |

Turkey, Breast Steaks, Thai, Bernard Matthews*, 1 serving/175g

| 280/160 | 51.5/29.4 | 8.1/4.6 | 4.7/2.7 | 0/0 |

	kcal serv/100g	prot serv/100g	carb serv/100g	fat serv/100g	fibre serv/100g

Turkey, Breast, Wafer-Thin, Chinese-Style, Bernard Matthews*,
1 pack/100g

110/110	18/18	6.1/6.1	1.5/1.5	0/0

Turkey, Chargrilled, Finely Sliced, No Added Water, Sainsbury's*,
1 slice/16g

17/106	4/24.8	0.1/0.9	0.1/0.4	0.1/0.5

Turkey, Cooked Roll, Dinosaur, Bernard Matthews*, 1 slice/10g

17/170	1.4/13.6	0.6/6	1/10.2	0.1/1.1

Turkey, Fillets, Tikka Marinated, Bernard Matthews*, 1 pack/200g

310/155	43.6/21.8	10.4/5.2	10.4/5.2	3.2/1.6

Turkey, Golden Drummers, Bernard Matthews*, 1 drummer/57g

146/256	7/12.2	5.8/10.1	10.6/18.6	0.5/0.9

Turkey, Honey Roast, Slices, Tesco*, 1 slice/20g

24/122	4.9/24.5	0.4/2.1	0.3/1.7	0.1/0.5

Turkey, Honey Roast, Wafer-Thin, Asda*, 1oz/28g

33/119	5.5/19.6	1.3/4.7	0.7/2.4	0/0

Turkey, Mince, Asda*, 1 serving/120g

173/144	21.6/18	0/0	9.6/8	0/0

Turkey, Mince, BGTY, Sainsbury's*, 1 serving/100g

113/113	21.9/21.9	0.1/0.1	2.8/2.8	0/0

Turkey, Mince, Extra Lean, Iceland*, 1 serving/100g

122/122	19/19	0/0	5.1/5.1	0/0

Turkey, Mince, Frozen, Asda*, 1 serving/100g

147/147	21/21	0/0	7/7	0/0

Turkey, Mince, Healthy Eating, Tesco*, 1 serving/175g

217/124	31.5/18	0/0	10.2/5.8	0/0

Turkey, Mince, Safeway*, 1 serving/150g

264/176	42.8/28.5	0/0	10.2/6.8	0/0

Turkey, Mince, Sainsbury's*, ½ pack/250g

495/198	71.5/28.6	0/0	24/9.6	0/0

Turkey, Rashers Lightly Smoked, Healthy Eating, Tesco*, 1 serving/75g

76/101	14.9/19.8	1.1/1.5	1.4/1.8	0/0

Turkey, Rashers, Bernard Matthews*, 1 slice/25g

26/105	4.5/18	0.9/3.7	0.5/2	0/0

Turkey, Rashers, Healthy Choice, Safeway*, 1 rasher/27g

27/99	5.4/20	0.6/2.4	0.3/1	0/0

Turkey, Rashers, Lightly Smoked, Tesco*, 1 serving/75g

76/101	14.9/19.8	1.1/1.5	1.4/1.8	0/0

	kcal serv/100g	prot serv/100g	carb serv/100g	fat serv/100g	fibre serv/100g

Turkey, Rashers, Original, Unsmoked, Mattesons*, 1 rasher/26g

26/99	5/19.3	0.5/1.8	0.4/1.6	0/0

Turkey, Rashers, Smoked, Mattessons*, 1 rasher/26g

26/99	5/19.3	0.5/1.8	0.4/1.6	0/0

Turkey, Rashers, Unsmoked, Co-Op*, 1 rasher/25g

26/105	4.8/19	0.5/2	0.5/2	0/0

READY MEALS AND SIDE DISHES

Alphabites, Bird's Eye*, 9 bites/56g

75/134	1.1/2	10.9/19.5	3/5.3	0.8/1.4

Bake, Chicken & Mushroom, COU, Marks & Spencer*, 1 serving/360g

324/90	26.3/7.3	37.1/10.3	8.3/2.3	4/1.1

Balti, Chicken & Potato Wedges, Healthy Living, Tesco*, 1 pack/450g

387/86	27/6	48.6/10.8	9.5/2.1	5/1.1

Balti, Chicken Rice, COU, Marks & Spencer*, 1 pack/400g

360/90	30/7.5	50/12.5	3.6/0.9	4/1

Balti, Chicken Tikka, Finest, Tesco*, ½ pack/200g

280/140	31.6/15.8	2.2/1.1	17.2/8.6	6.4/3.2

Balti, Chicken Tikka, Tesco*, 1 pack/350g

466/133	38.9/11.1	22.4/6.4	24.5/7	2.5/0.7

Balti, Chicken, BGTY, Sainsbury's*, 1 pack/400g

356/89	20.4/5.1	63.2/15.8	2.4/0.6	2.8/0.7

Balti, Chicken, Takeaway, Sainsbury's*, 1 pack/400g

404/101	41.6/10.4	19.2/4.8	18/4.5	5.6/1.4

Beans, Baked, Heinz*, 1 serving/415g

303/73	19.1/4.6	54.4/13.1	0.8/0.2	14.9/3.6

Beans, Baked, & Jumbo Sausages, Asda*, 1 serving/210g

317/151	14.7/7	31.5/15	14.7/7	5.5/2.6

Beans, Baked, & Sausage, Asda*, ½ can/205g

252/123	12.3/6	32.8/16	8/3.9	6.2/3

Beans, Baked, & Sausage, GFY, Asda*, 1 serving/217g

178/82	10.2/4.7	21.7/10	5.6/2.6	3.9/1.8

Beans, Baked, & Vegetarian Sausages, in Tomato Sauce, Tesco*, 1 can/420g

538/128	28.1/6.7	57.1/13.6	14.3/3.4	11.3/2.7

	kcal serv/100g	prot serv/100g	carb serv/100g	fat serv/100g	fibre serv/100g

Beans, Baked, American, Heinz*, 1 serving/130g

140/108	6/4.6	27/20.8	0.5/0.4	5/3.8

Beans, Baked, Barbecue, Heinz*, ½ can/100g

82/82	4.9/4.9	14.9/14.9	0.3/0.3	4/4

Beans, Baked, Cheezy, Heinz*, 1oz/28g

53/189	3.2/11.6	6.9/24.5	1.4/4.9	1.7/6.2

Beans, Baked, Healthy Choice, Asda*, 1oz/28g

16/58	0.8/2.9	3.1/11	0.1/0.2	0.7/2.6

Beans, Baked, Healthy Choice, Safeway*, 1 can/220g

205/93	10.3/4.7	38.1/17.3	1.1/0.5	8.1/3.7

Beans, Baked, Healthy Living, Tesco*, 1 sm can/220g

84/38	5.1/2.3	15.1/6.9	0.3/0.1	3.6/1.6

Beans, Baked, in Tomato Sauce, Asda*, 1 serving/100g

77/77	4.6/4.6	14/14	0.3/0.3	3.7/3.7

Beans, Baked, in Tomato Sauce, Healthy Balance, Heinz*, ½ can/207g

139/67	9.5/4.6	24.2/11.7	0.4/0.2	7.7/3.7

Beans, Baked, in Tomato Sauce, Healthy Eating, Tesco*, 1 can/420g

353/84	21.4/5.1	63.4/15.1	1.3/0.3	15.1/3.6

Beans, Baked, in Tomato Sauce, Healthy Selection, Somerfield*, 1 can/220g

125/57	6.6/3	24.2/11	0/0	0/0

Beans, Baked, in Tomato Sauce, Heinz*, ½ can/207g

155/75	9.7/4.7	28.2/13.6	0.4/0.2	7.7/3.7

Beans, Baked, in Tomato Sauce, Makes Sense, Safeway*, 1 can/210.3g

164/78	8.8/4.2	30.9/14.7	0.6/0.3	6.7/3.2

Beans, Baked, in Tomato Sauce, Organic, Sainsbury's*, ½ can/210g

204/97	10.7/5.1	37.8/18	1.1/0.5	7.4/3.5

Beans, Baked, in Tomato Sauce, Tesco*, 1 can/210g

179/85	9.7/4.6	33.4/15.9	0.6/0.3	7.4/3.5

Beans, Baked, in Tomato Sauce, Waitrose*, ½ can/210g

170/81	8.8/4.2	31.1/14.8	1.3/0.6	6.9/3.3

Beans, Baked, in Tomato Sauce, Weight Watchers*, ½ can/207g

137/66	9.7/4.7	23.4/11.3	0.4/0.2	7.7/3.7

Beans, Baked, Marks & Spencer*, 1oz/28g

23/81	1.4/5	5.4/19.2	0.1/0.4	1/3.7

Beans, Baked, Reduced Salt & Sugar, Safeway*, ½ can/210g

195/93	9.9/4.7	36.3/17.3	1.1/0.5	7.8/3.7

	kcal serv/100g	prot serv/100g	carb serv/100g	fat serv/100g	fibre serv/100g
Beans, Baked, Reduced Sugar & Salt, Tesco*, 1 can/420g					
	353/84	21.4/5.1	63.4/15.1	1.3/0.3	15.1/3.6
Beans, Baked, Reduced Sugar & Salt, Waitrose*, ½ can/220g					
	150/68	11/5	25.3/11.5	0.4/0.2	8.1/3.7
Beans, Baked, Sainsbury's*, ½ can/210g					
	179/85	10.3/4.9	32.6/15.5	0.8/0.4	10.9/5.2
Beans, Baked, with Pork Sausages, Heinz*, ½ can/207g					
	184/89	11.4/5.5	23.2/11.2	5.2/2.5	5.4/2.6
Beans, Baked, with Pork Sausages, Tesco*, 1 can/220g					
	279/127	12.5/5.7	32.8/14.9	6.8/3.1	6.4/2.9
Beans, Baked, with Vegetable Sausages, Heinz*, 1 can/200g					
	212/106	12.2/6.1	24.4/12.2	7.2/3.6	5.8/2.9
Beans, Curried, Heinz*, ½ can/100g					
	103/103	4.9/4.9	17.9/17.9	1.3/1.3	4/4
Beans, Mixed, Hot & Spicy, Tesco*, 1 serving/78g					
	61/78	3.9/5	10.4/13.3	0.4/0.5	3/3.9
Beans, Mixed, in a Mild Chilli Sauce, Sainsbury's*, ½ can/208g					
	162/78	10.8/5.2	28.1/13.5	0.6/0.3	10.8/5.2
Beans, Mixed, in Spicy Pepper Sauce, Sainsbury's*, ½ can/210g					
	187/89	9.9/4.7	32.1/15.3	2.1/1	6.7/3.2
Beans, Mixed, Italian-Style, Tesco*, 1 can/300g					
	237/79	18/6	36.3/12.1	2.1/0.7	11.7/3.9
Beans, Refried, Old El Paso*, 1 serving/100g					
	83/83	5/5	13.5/13.5	1/1	0/0
Beef & Gravy, Lean Roast, Bird's Eye*, 1 portion/114g					
	111/97	15.2/13.3	3.4/3	4/3.5	0.1/0.1
Beef Braised Steak, & Mustard Mash, Healthy Eating, Tesco*, 1 pack/450g					
	392/87	33.3/7.4	42.8/9.5	9.5/2.1	3.2/0.7
Beef Braised Steak, & Red Wine with Vegetable Mash, Healthy Living, Tesco*, 1 pack/500g					
	360/72	25.5/5.1	34.5/6.9	13.5/2.7	6/1.2
Beef Braised Steak, COU, Marks & Spencer*, ½ pack/225g					
	180/80	26.8/11.9	8.1/3.6	5/2.2	1.6/0.7
Beef Braised, & Vegetables with Mashed Potato, BGTY, Sainsbury's*, 1 pack/453g					
	331/73	29.4/6.5	40.3/8.9	5.9/1.3	5.4/1.2
Beef Chasseur, & Potato Mash, BGTY, Sainsbury's*, 1 pack/450g					
	468/104	39.6/8.8	49.5/11	12.6/2.8	3.2/0.7

	kcal serv/100g	prot serv/100g	carb serv/100g	fat serv/100g	fibre serv/100g

Beef in, Red Wine with Mashed Potato, Healthy Living, Tesco*, 1 pack/400g

288/72   13.6/3.4   40.8/10.2   7.6/1.9   6.8/1.7

Beef with, Oyster Sauce, Ooodles of Noodles, Oriental Express*, 1 pack/425g

378/89   20.8/4.9   60.4/14.2   5.5/1.3   6.4/1.5

Beef with, Vegetable Rice, Hot & Sour, COU, Marks & Spencer*, 1 pack/400g

360/90   22/5.5   57.6/14.4   5.6/1.4   2.4/0.6

Beef, Strips, Stir-Fry, Fresh, Healthy Living, Tesco*, 1 serving/125g

138/110   28.9/23.1   0/0   2.5/2   0.8/0.6

Bhaji, Onion, Asda*, 1 mini bhaji/49g

96/196   2.9/6   9.8/20   4.9/10   1/2

Bhaji, Onion, Indian Starter Selection, Marks & Spencer*, 1 bhaji/22g

65/295   1.3/5.7   3.5/15.8   5.1/23.3   0.6/2.8

Bhaji, Onion, Mini, Indian Snack Selection, Occasions, Sainsbury's*, 1 bhaji/21.8g

46/211   1.1/4.8   4.3/19.7   2.8/12.6   0.7/3.2

Bhaji, Onion, Mini, Tesco*, 1 serving/23g

48/210   1.7/7.3   6.1/26.7   1.9/8.2   0.3/1.3

Bhaji, Onion, Safeway*, 1 bhaji/23g

40/175   1.3/5.7   4.7/20.3   1.7/7.5   0.8/3.5

Biryani, Chicken, Marks & Spencer*, 1 pack/400g

800/200   31.2/7.8   79.2/19.8   40.4/10.1   4.8/1.2

Biryani, Chicken, Weight Watchers*, 1 pack/330g

300/91   19.8/6   46.9/14.2   3.6/1.1   2/0.6

Bolognese Shells, Italiana, Weight Watchers*, 1 can/395g

284/72   20.9/5.3   38.7/9.8   5.1/1.3   3.2/0.8

Cannelloni, Ricotta & Spinach, COU, Marks & Spencer*, 1 pack/360g

288/80   20.9/5.8   34.9/9.7   6.8/1.9   5.4/1.5

Cannelloni, Spinach & Ricotta, BGTY, Sainsbury's*, 1 serving/300g

297/99   14.7/4.9   47.7/15.9   5.1/1.7   3/1

Cannelloni, Spinach & Ricotta, Healthy Eating, Tesco*, 1 pack/340g

326/96   15.3/4.5   46.6/13.7   8.8/2.6   4.4/1.3

Cannelloni, Spinach & Ricotta, Italiano, Tesco*, 1 pack/425g

510/120   20/4.7   52.7/12.4   24.2/5.7   3.8/0.9

Casserole, Beef & Ale, Finest, Tesco*, ½ pack/300g

222/74   36.6/12.2   11.7/3.9   3.3/1.1   1.2/0.4

kcal serv/100g	prot serv/100g	carb serv/100g	fat serv/100g	fibre serv/100g
Casserole, Beef & Red Wine, BGTY, Sainsbury's*, 1 pack/300g				
192/64	24/8	20.1/6.7	1.8/0.6	2.7/0.9
Casserole, Beef with Dumplings, COU, Marks & Spencer*, ½ pack/226g				
215/95	20.3/9	20.6/9.1	5.4/2.4	1.4/0.6
Casserole, Chicken & Dumplings, Healthy Living, Tesco*, 1 pack/450g				
441/98	33.3/7.4	50/11.1	12.2/2.7	2.7/0.6
Casserole, Chicken & White Wine, BGTY, Sainsbury's*, 1 serving/300g				
216/72	21.6/7.2	17.7/5.9	6.6/2.2	3.9/1.3
Casserole, Chicken with Herb Dumplings, COU, Marks & Spencer*, ½ pack/227.8g				
205/90	24.2/10.6	16.4/7.2	4.3/1.9	1.4/0.6
Casserole, Chicken, GFY, Asda*, 1 pack/400g				
280/70	20/5	32/8	8/2	6/1.5
Casserole, Chicken, Marks & Spencer*, 1 pack/200g				
230/115	14.8/7.4	21.8/10.9	8.8/4.4	1.8/0.9
Casserole, Lamb & Rosemary, BGTY, Sainsbury's*, 1 serving/300g				
192/64	21.3/7.1	20.4/6.8	2.7/0.9	1.8/0.6
Casserole, Lamb & Rosemary, Marks & Spencer*, 1 pack/454g				
409/90	44/9.7	25/5.5	15/3.3	4.5/1
Casserole, Vegetable with Herb Dumplings, COU, Marks & Spencer*, 1 pack/450g				
270/60	7.2/1.6	45.5/10.1	5.4/1.2	4.5/1
Chicken, Arrabiata, GFY, Asda*, 1 pack/340g				
228/67	16/4.7	30.6/9	4.4/1.3	0/0
Chicken, Cajun, & Potato Hash, Healthy Eating, Tesco*, 1 pack/450g				
428/95	29.7/6.6	52.7/11.7	10.8/2.4	4.1/0.9
Chicken, Cajun, Breast Fillet, Good Choice, Iceland*, 1 fillet/80.3g				
106/132	20.9/26.1	2.8/3.5	1.2/1.5	0/0
Chicken, Chargrilled, & Vegetable Medley, Healthy Eating, Tesco*, 1 pack/450g				
270/60	29.3/6.5	26.1/5.8	5.4/1.2	4.1/0.9
Chicken, Chargrilled, Breast, in Creamy Mushroom & Madeira Sauce, COU, Marks & Spencer*, ½ pack/180g				
162/90	30.4/16.9	2/1.1	3.6/2	1.3/0.7
Chicken, Chargrilled, Breasts, Bird's Eye*, 1 piece/93.8g				
196/208	20.9/22.2	2.4/2.5	11.4/12.1	0.1/0.1
Chicken, Chargrilled, Pasta Salsa, Healthy Eating, Tesco*, 1 pack/450g				
396/88	32.9/7.3	52.7/11.7	5.9/1.3	4.5/1

	kcal serv/100g	prot serv/100g	carb serv/100g	fat serv/100g	fibre serv/100g

Chicken, Chasseur, & Colcannon, Healthy Living, Tesco*, 1 pack/400g

348/87	38.8/9.7	26.8/6.7	9.6/2.4	2.4/0.6

Chicken, Chinese, Oriental Express*, 1 pack/350g

326/93	20/5.7	55.7/15.9	2.5/0.7	7.7/2.2

Chicken, Chinese, Wings, Sainsbury's*, 1 wing/33.9g

87/257	8.2/24.1	1.7/5	5.3/15.6	0.2/0.6

Chicken, Coronation, Marks & Spencer*, 1 serving/200g

420/210	25.2/12.6	21.2/10.6	26.4/13.2	2.6/1.3

Chicken, Escalope, Topped with Cheese, Ham & Mushrooms, Asda*,
½ pack/149.4g

259/174	37.3/25	0.9/0.6	11.9/8	0/0

Chicken, Herb, Steam Cuisine, Marks & Spencer*, 1 pack/400g

280/70	32.8/8.2	24/6	6.4/1.6	3.6/0.9

Chicken, Honey, & Mustard, Shapers, Boots*, 1 pack/241g

304/126	16.9/7	45.8/19	5.8/2.4	4.1/1.7

Chicken, Lemon, & Ginger with Apricot Rice, COU, Marks & Spencer*,
1 pack/400g

320/80	31.6/7.9	38.8/9.7	3.6/0.9	8/2

Chicken, Lemon, Breast, Fillets, BGTY, Sainsbury's*, 1 fillet/112.5g

195/173	20.8/18.4	22.5/19.9	2.4/2.1	2.1/1.9

Chicken, Lemon, Tesco*, ½ pack/175g

214/122	19.3/11	17.7/10.1	7.4/4.2	1.1/0.6

Chicken, Paprika, & Savoury Rice, BGTY, Sainsbury's*, 1 pack/401g

441/110	27.3/6.8	77/19.2	2.8/0.7	1.6/0.4

Chicken, Roast, Dinner, Bird's Eye*, 1 pack/368g

364/99	32.8/8.9	32.8/8.9	11.4/3.1	4.8/1.3

Chicken, Thai, Bird's Eye*, 1 portion/86g

189/220	15.6/18.1	2.7/3.1	12.9/15	0.1/0.1

Chicken, Tikka, Chunky, Tesco*, 1 pack/170g

221/130	46.6/27.4	0.9/0.5	3.6/2.1	0.5/0.3

Chicken &, Asparagus Pasta, Easy Steam, Healthy Living, Tesco*,
1 pack/400g

312/78	34.8/8.7	33.6/8.4	4.4/1.1	4/1

Chicken &, Black Bean, Chinese Takeaway, Tesco*, 1 serving/200g

190/95	16.6/8.3	16/8	6.6/3.3	1/0.5

Chicken &, Cashew Nuts & Veg Rice, COU, Marks & Spencer*, 1 pack/400g

320/80	27.6/6.9	34.4/8.6	8/2	4/1

	kcal serv/100g	prot serv/100g	carb serv/100g	fat serv/100g	fibre serv/100g

Chicken &, Cashew Nuts with Egg Rice, GFY, Asda*, 1 pack/396g

	384/97	23.8/6	63.4/16	4/1	23.8/6

Chicken &, Cashew Nuts, Chinese, Sainsbury's*, 1 pack/350g

	312/89	27.3/7.8	20/5.7	14/4	4.2/1.2

Chicken &, Pineapple Pasta, Shapers, Boots*, 1 pack/221g

	210/95	11.9/5.4	33.2/15	3.3/1.5	2/0.9

Chicken &, Red Wine Penne, Italiana, Weight Watchers*, 1 pack/395g

	249/63	14.6/3.7	39.9/10.1	2.8/0.7	2.4/0.6

Chicken &, White Wine with Rice, Healthy Eating, Tesco*, 1 pack/450g

	450/100	32/7.1	66.6/14.8	6.3/1.4	4.5/1

**Chicken , Honey & Mustard with Baby Potatoes, BGTY, Sainsbury's*,
1 pack/450g**

	360/80	35.6/7.9	52.2/11.6	0.9/0.2	3.6/0.8

Chicken in, Creamy Mushroom Sauce, Weight Watchers*, 1 pack/330g

	264/80	22.4/6.8	24.8/7.5	8.3/2.5	1.7/0.5

**Chicken in, Hot Ginger Sauce with Jasmine Rice, BGTY, Sainsbury's*,
1 pack/400g**

	400/100	26.4/6.6	61.6/15.4	5.6/1.4	2/0.5

Chicken in, Italian-Style Tomato & Herb Sauce, Tesco*, 1 serving/180g

	144/80	28.4/15.8	2.9/1.6	2.2/1.2	1.1/0.6

**Chicken in, Red Wine with Cabbage & Spring Onion Mash,
Marks & Spencer*, 1 pack/440g**

	265/60	44.4/10.1	10.6/2.4	6.2/1.4	15.8/3.6

Chicken in, Red Wine with Mash, Eat Smart, Safeway*, 1 pack/400g

	300/75	36.4/9.1	24.4/6.1	5.2/1.3	5.6/1.4

Chicken in, Satay Sauce, Safeway*, 1 serving/250g

	363/145	26.3/10.5	17.8/7.1	20/8	3.5/1.4

Chicken in, Sweet & Sour Sauce, GFY, Asda*, 1 pack/400g

	424/106	24/6	76/19	2.8/0.7	4.8/1.2

Chicken with, Broccoli & Pesto Pasta, BGTY, Sainsbury's*, 1 pack/299g

	296/99	30.8/10.3	36.8/12.3	2.7/0.9	7.5/2.5

**Chicken with, Mango Salsa & Potato Wedges, BGTY, Sainsbury's*,
1 pack/400g**

	336/84	28/7	41.6/10.4	6.4/1.6	6/1.5

Chicken with, Potato Wedges, BBQ, Eat Smart, Safeway*, 1 pack/350g

	368/105	33.6/9.6	49/14	3.2/0.9	6.3/1.8

Chicken with, Rice, Fiesta, Weight Watchers*, 1 pack/330g

	307/93	20.1/6.1	42.2/12.8	6.6/2	1.3/0.4

kcal serv/100g	prot serv/100g	carb serv/100g	fat serv/100g	fibre serv/100g
Chicken with, Stuffing & Roast Potatoes, Tesco*, 1 pack/440g				
480/109	44.5/10.1	50.7/11.5	11/2.5	4.3/1
Chicken with, Tagine, Cous Cous, Perfectly Balanced, Waitrose*,				
1 pack/400g				
516/129	32.8/8.2	64.8/16.2	14/3.5	4/1
Chicken with, Tomato & Basil, & Roasted Baby Potatoes, BGTY,				
Sainsbury's*, 1 pack/450g				
369/82	40.5/9	35.6/7.9	7.2/1.6	5.4/1.2
Chicken, Bacon & Leeks with Mashed Potato, BGTY, Sainsbury's*,				
1 pack/450g				
437/97	37.8/8.4	45.5/10.1	11.3/2.5	3.2/0.7
Chicken, Bang Bang, Oriental Express*, ½ pack/200g				
170/85	12.8/6.4	22/11	3.4/1.7	6.4/3.2
Chicken, BBQ Wedge, Healthy Living, Tesco*, 1 pack/196g				
321/164	19.8/10.1	53.5/27.3	3.1/1.6	2/1
Chicken, Breast, in BBQ Sauce, Weight Watchers*, 1 pack/339g				
336/99	19.7/5.8	37.3/11	11.9/3.5	3.1/0.9
Chicken, Breast, in Creamy White Wine & Mushroom Sauce,				
Marks & Spencer*, ½ pack/225g				
315/140	32/14.2	2.3/1	20.3/9	0.9/0.4
Chicken, Breast, with a Chunky Tomato Sauce, Meal for One, COU,				
Marks & Spencer*, 1 pack/400g				
360/90	31.6/7.9	37.2/9.3	9.2/2.3	3.6/0.9
Chicken, Breasts, Honey & Mustard, Bird's Eye*, 1 portion/97g				
175/180	19/19.6	4.1/4.2	9.1/9.4	0.1/0.1
Chicken, Breasts, in Sweet & Sour Sauce, Good Choice, Iceland*,				
1 pack/340g				
350/103	52/15.3	29.9/8.8	2.4/0.7	2.7/0.8
Chicken, Breasts, with Garlic Mushrooms, Simple Solution, Tesco*,				
1 serving/200g				
304/152	32.2/16.1	4/2	17.6/8.8	1/0.5
Chicken, Breasts, with Roasted Mushrooms with Wine & Pesto, Finest,				
Tesco*, 1 breast/200g				
360/180	38.2/19.1	2/1	22.2/11.1	2.8/1.4
Chicken, Breasts, with Smoked Cherry Tomatoes & Mozzarella, Gourmet,				
Healthy Living, Tesco*, 1 serving/225g				
209/93	33.3/14.8	6.1/2.7	5.9/2.6	1.1/0.5

	kcal serv/100g	prot serv/100g	carb serv/100g	fat serv/100g	fibre serv/100g

Chicken, Breasts, with Thai Green Curry, Finest, Tesco*, 1 serving/200g

292/146	33/16.5	4/2	16/8	1.4/0.7

Chicken, Breasts, with Tomato & Basil Sauce, Healthy Living, Tesco*, 1 serving/225g

221/98	32.9/14.6	9.9/4.4	5.6/2.5	2/0.9

Chicken, Cracked Pepper, Bird's Eye*, 1 portion/94.7g

196/206	20/21	3.7/3.9	11.2/11.8	0.1/0.1

Chicken, Dippers, Bird's Eye*, 5 dippers/93.3g

209/225	11.8/12.7	11.2/12	13/14	0.6/0.6

Chicken, Fillets, Sweet Chilli, Roast, Mini, Waitrose*, 1 pack/200g

216/108	46/23	7.6/3.8	0.4/0.2	1.8/0.9

Chicken, Ginger & Lemon with Apricot Rice, BGTY, Sainsbury's*, 1 pack/401.8g

438/109	39/9.7	58.3/14.5	5.6/1.4	1.2/0.3

Chicken, Japanese Teriyaki with Ramen Noodles, Sainsbury's*, 1 pack/450g

482/107	29.3/6.5	69.8/15.5	9.5/2.1	3.6/0.8

Chicken, Moroccan with Apricots & Pine Nuts, TTD, Sainsbury's*, ½ pack/200g

210/105	21.2/10.6	6.8/3.4	10.8/5.4	2.6/1.3

Chicken, Moroccan with Cous Cous & Fruity Sauce, BGTY, Sainsbury's*, 1 pack/400g

440/110	40/10	52.4/13.1	8/2	10.4/2.6

Chicken, Parmesan with Pasta, Steam Cuisine, Marks & Spencer*, 1 pack/400g

400/100	40.4/10.1	32.4/8.1	12/3	5.2/1.3

Chicken, Spatchcock Poussin, Sainsbury's*, 1 serving/122g

168/138	25.7/21.1	0.1/0.1	6.6/5.4	0.2/0.2

Chicken, Sweet Chilli, COU, Marks & Spencer*, 1 pack/400g

340/85	34.4/8.6	41.6/10.4	4/1	8.4/2.1

Chicken, Teriyaki, Asda*, 1 pack/360g

299/83	32.8/9.1	31/8.6	5/1.4	2.9/0.8

Chicken, Tomato & Basil Pasta, Asda*, 1 pack/400g

474/119	26/6.5	70/17.5	10/2.5	4.8/1.2

Chicken, Tomato & Basil, Weight Watchers*, 1 pack/330g

317/96	24.4/7.4	45.9/13.9	4/1.2	1/0.3

Chicken, with Mango Salsa & Potato Wedges, Sainsbury's*, 1 pack/400g

336/84	28/7	41.6/10.4	6.4/1.6	6/1.5

kcal serv/100g	prot serv/100g	carb serv/100g	fat serv/100g	fibre serv/100g

Chilli, & Lemongrass Prawns with Noodles, BGTY, Sainsbury's*, 1 pack/400g

328/82	20/5	55.2/13.8	2.8/0.7	5.2/1.3

Chilli, Beef & Potato Wedge Superbowl, GFY, Asda*, 1 pack/450g

477/106	27/6	63/14	13.1/2.9	6.8/1.5

Chilli, Beef, Asda*, ½ pack/200g

190/95	14/7	16/8	7.8/3.9	2.4/1.2

Chilli, Beef, Crispy, Sainsbury's*, 1 pack/400g

628/157	51.2/12.8	19.6/4.9	38.4/9.6	4.8/1.2

Chilli, Con Carne & Rice, Co-Op*, 1 pack/300g

195/65	12/4	24/8	6/2	3/1

Chilli, Con Carne & Rice, Healthy Eating, Tesco*, 1 pack/450g

446/99	41/9.1	49.1/10.9	9.5/2.1	7.2/1.6

Chilli, Con Carne with Rice, BGTY, Sainsbury's*, 1 pack/400g

432/108	24.8/6.2	67.6/16.9	6.8/1.7	4/1

Chilli, Con Carne with Rice, Eat Smart, Safeway*, 1 pack/400g

340/85	21.2/5.3	48.8/12.2	5.2/1.3	5.6/1.4

Chilli, Con Carne, Asda*, 1 can/392g

376/96	27.4/7	35.3/9	13.7/3.5	0/0

Chilli, Con Carne, Marks & Spencer*, 1 pack/285g

285/100	24.8/8.7	21.1/7.4	10.5/3.7	5.7/2

Chilli, Con Carne, Silverado Beef, Stagg*, 1 can/410g

406/99	32/7.8	44.7/10.9	11.1/2.7	6.2/1.5

Chilli, Con Carne, Tesco*, 1 can/392g

463/118	31.4/8	41.2/10.5	19.2/4.9	9.4/2.4

Chilli, Crispy Beef, Tesco*, 1 pack/250g

455/182	28.5/11.4	49.5/19.8	15.8/6.3	3/1.2

Chilli, Mexican Chilli with Potato Wedges, Weight Watchers*, 1 pack/300g

252/84	15.3/5.1	30.9/10.3	7.5/2.5	5.1/1.7

Chilli, Vegetable, & Rice, Healthy Eating, Tesco*, 1 pack/450g

392/87	12.6/2.8	72.5/16.1	5.4/1.2	6.8/1.5

Chilli, Wedge Bowl, COU, Marks & Spencer*, 1 pack/400g

380/95	28.8/7.2	45.2/11.3	9.2/2.3	7.2/1.8

Chinese House Special, Healthy Living, Tesco*, 1 pack/450g

369/82	29.3/6.5	47.3/10.5	7.2/1.6	5/1.1

Chinese Meal, For One, Safeway*, 1 serving/584g

993/170	32.1/5.5	150.7/25.8	27.4/4.7	7.6/1.3

	kcal serv/100g	prot serv/100g	carb serv/100g	fat serv/100g	fibre serv/100g

Chinese Meal, For Two, Tesco*, 1 pack/500g

| 480/96 | 22/4.4 | 80/16 | 8/1.6 | 5.5/1.1 |

Chow Mein, Beef, Sainsbury's*, 1 pack/450g

| 500/111 | 29.7/6.6 | 69.8/15.5 | 11.3/2.5 | 3.6/0.8 |

Chow Mein, Chicken, Chinese Takeaway, Sainsbury's*, 1 pack/316g

| 338/107 | 28.8/9.1 | 36.7/11.6 | 8.5/2.7 | 2.2/0.7 |

Chow Mein, Chicken, Healthy Eating, Tesco*, 1 pack/450g

| 392/87 | 36.9/8.2 | 48.6/10.8 | 5.4/1.2 | 1.8/0.4 |

Chow Mein, Chicken, Tesco*, 1 pack/350g

| 322/92 | 17.9/5.1 | 50.8/14.5 | 5.3/1.5 | 2.8/0.8 |

Chow Mein, Special, COU, Marks & Spencer*, 1 pack/400g

| 320/80 | 29.6/7.4 | 39.6/9.9 | 4/1 | 4/1 |

Chow Mein, Vegetables & Noodles in Sauce, Safeway*, 1 serving/200g

| 110/55 | 7.4/3.7 | 19/9.5 | 0.4/0.2 | 2.6/1.3 |

Colcannon, Healthy Eating, Tesco*, 1 pack/330g

| 244/74 | 6.9/2.1 | 40.3/12.2 | 6.3/1.9 | 3.3/1 |

Cous Cous, Chargrilled Red & Yellow Pepper, Tesco*, 1 pack/200g

| 212/106 | 9.2/4.6 | 35.6/17.8 | 3.6/1.8 | 1/0.5 |

Cous Cous, Chargrilled Vegetables & Olive Oil, Delphi*, ½ pot/75g

| 105/140 | 2.9/3.8 | 16.9/22.5 | 2.9/3.9 | 1.4/1.9 |

Cous Cous, Coriander & Lemon, GFY, Asda*, ½ pack/145g

| 189/130 | 6.1/4.2 | 39.2/27 | 0.9/0.6 | 2.6/1.8 |

Cous Cous, Coriander & Lemon, Sainsbury's*, ½ pack/165g

| 200/121 | 7.9/4.8 | 38.8/23.5 | 1.2/0.7 | 1.3/0.8 |

Cous Cous, Garlic & Coriander, Waitrose*, 1 serving/70g

| 235/336 | 8.2/11.7 | 44.9/64.2 | 2.5/3.6 | 4.3/6.2 |

Cous Cous, Indian-Style, Sainsbury's*, ½ pack/143g

| 204/143 | 6.4/4.5 | 35.9/25.1 | 3.9/2.7 | 1.4/1 |

Cous Cous, Lemon & Coriander, Tesco*, 1 serving/137g

| 207/151 | 5.5/4 | 38.8/28.3 | 3.3/2.4 | 2.7/2 |

Cous Cous, Mediterranean-Style, Tesco*, 1 pack/110g

| 369/335 | 13.1/11.9 | 71.6/65.1 | 3.3/3 | 6.2/5.6 |

Cous Cous, Mediterranean Tomato, GFY, Asda*, ½ pack/141g

| 192/136 | 7.1/5 | 38.1/27 | 1.3/0.9 | 2.4/1.7 |

Cous Cous, Moroccan-Style, Sainsbury's*, ½ pack/150g

| 195/130 | 7.5/5 | 32.3/21.5 | 4.1/2.7 | 1.5/1 |

Cous Cous, Mushrooms, Onion, Garlic & Herbs, Tesco*, ½ pack/50g

| 167/333 | 5.7/11.3 | 33.1/66.2 | 1.3/2.6 | 2.5/4.9 |

kcal serv/100g	prot serv/100g	carb serv/100g	fat serv/100g	fibre serv/100g

Cous Cous, Red Pepper & Chilli, Waitrose*, 1 pack/200g

| 344/172 | 9/4.5 | 46/23 | 13.8/6.9 | 2.6/1.3 |

Cous Cous, Roasted Vegetable, Finest, Tesco*, 1 serving/175g

| 263/150 | 7/4 | 30.5/17.4 | 12.4/7.1 | 2.3/1.3 |

Cous Cous, Roasted Vegetables, Waitrose*, 1 serving/200g

| 324/162 | 10.4/5.2 | 44.8/22.4 | 11.4/5.7 | 0/0 |

Cous Cous, Salad Bar, BGTY, Sainsbury's*, 1 md bowl/28g

| 29/103 | 1/3.7 | 5.2/18.5 | 0.4/1.6 | 0/0 |

Cous Cous, Spicy Moroccan Chicken & Veg, COU, Marks & Spencer*, 1 pack/400g

| 380/95 | 36.4/9.1 | 41.2/10.3 | 6.8/1.7 | 7.6/1.9 |

Cous Cous, Spicy Vegetable, GFY, Asda*, ½ pack/141g

| 183/130 | 7.1/5 | 35.3/25 | 1.6/1.1 | 2.8/2 |

Cous Cous, Spicy, Healthy Eating, Tesco*, 1 pot/250g

| 325/130 | 9/3.6 | 62.8/25.1 | 4.3/1.7 | 1.5/0.6 |

Cous Cous, Sun-Dried Tomato, Somerfield*, 1 jar/110g

| 176/160 | 3.3/3 | 27.5/25 | 5.5/5 | 0/0 |

Cous Cous, Tomato & Onion, Waitrose*, ½ pack/55g

| 188/342 | 6.9/12.6 | 35.7/64.9 | 2/3.6 | 2.8/5.1 |

Cous Cous, Wild Mushroom & Garlic, Sainsbury's*, 1 serving/166g

| 239/144 | 7/4.2 | 38/22.9 | 6.6/4 | 1/0.6 |

Cous Cous, with Lemon & Garlic, Waitrose*, ½ pack/55g

| 188/341 | 6.5/11.8 | 36/65.5 | 1.8/3.3 | 2.5/4.5 |

Curry, Bhuna Chicken, Tesco*, 1 serving/300g

| 396/132 | 34.2/11.4 | 13.5/4.5 | 22.8/7.6 | 1.5/0.5 |

Curry, Butter Chicken, Fresh, Tesco*, 1 pack/350g

| 487/139 | 41.3/11.8 | 24.9/7.1 | 24.5/7 | 6.3/1.8 |

Curry, Chicken & Rice, Asda*, 1 pack/300g

| 351/117 | 14.1/4.7 | 45/15 | 12.6/4.2 | 0.9/0.3 |

Curry, Chicken with Rice, Sainsbury's*, 1 pack/400g

| 500/125 | 21.6/5.4 | 70/17.5 | 14.8/3.7 | 3.2/0.8 |

Curry, Chicken with Rice, Tesco*, 1 pack/300g

| 300/100 | 17.1/5.7 | 43.2/14.4 | 6.6/2.2 | 1.2/0.4 |

Curry, Chicken with Rice, Weight Watchers*, 1 pack/300g

| 273/91 | 14.1/4.7 | 42.9/14.3 | 5.1/1.7 | 1.5/0.5 |

Curry, Chicken, Asda*, 1 can/200g

| 210/105 | 20/10 | 10/5 | 10/5 | 0/0 |

kcal serv/100g	prot serv/100g	carb serv/100g	fat serv/100g	fibre serv/100g
Curry, Chicken, Green Thai with Jasmine Rice, Perfectly Balanced, Waitrose*, 1 pack/400g				
512/128	26/6.5	76/19	12.8/3.2	2/0.5
Curry, Chicken, Medium Hot, Marks & Spencer*, 1 serving/200g				
310/155	15.6/7.8	28.6/14.3	14.2/7.1	1.6/0.8
Curry, Chicken, Red Thai with Jasmine Rice, Perfectly Balanced, Waitrose*, 1 pack/400g				
496/124	24.8/6.2	74/18.5	11.6/2.9	1.6/0.4
Curry, Chinese Chicken, Morrisons*, 1 pack/340g				
347/102	35/10.3	17/5	15.6/4.6	2.7/0.8
Curry, Chinese Chicken, Oriental Express*, 1 pack/340g				
286/84	16.3/4.8	55.1/16.2	2/0.6	2.7/0.8
Curry, Green Thai & Rice, GFY, Asda*, 1 pack/400g				
460/115	20/5	76/19	8.4/2.1	2/0.5
Curry, Green Thai Chicken, Sainsbury's*, 1 serving/200g				
306/153	27.2/13.6	6/3	19.2/9.6	3.2/1.6
Curry, Lamb with Rice, Bird's Eye*, 1 pack/382g				
520/136	21.4/5.6	79.5/20.8	13/3.4	3.4/0.9
Curry, Malai Prawn, Sainsbury's*, 1 serving/171g				
299/175	13.2/7.7	2.4/1.4	26.3/15.4	1.9/1.1
Curry, Prawn with Rice, Asda*, 1 pack/400g				
420/105	14/3.5	68/17	10.4/2.6	4.4/1.1
Curry, Red Thai-Style Chicken, Healthy Eating, Tesco*, 1 pack/420g				
462/110	25.2/6	74.3/17.7	7.1/1.7	0.8/0.2
Curry, Thai Green Chicken with Jasmine Rice, BGTY, Sainsbury's*, 1 pack/400g				
424/106	27.2/6.8	63.2/15.8	6.8/1.7	3.6/0.9
Curry, Thai Red Chicken with Jasmine Rice, BGTY, Sainsbury's*, 1 pack/400g				
428/107	27.6/6.9	64/16	6.8/1.7	0.8/0.2
Curry, Thai Yellow Vegetable, Sainsbury's*, ½ pack/200g				
256/128	3.4/1.7	14.2/7.1	20.6/10.3	3/1.5
Curry, Vegetable, Medium, Tesco*, 1 pack/350g				
326/93	8.1/2.3	24.9/7.1	21.7/6.2	6.7/1.9
Duck, Crispy Aromatic, Asda*, ⅓ pack/165.7g				
470/283	31.5/19	29.9/18	24.9/15	1.3/0.8
Duck, Crispy Aromatic, Ready Meals, Marks & Spencer*, 1 pack/275g				
591/215	34.7/12.6	28.3/10.3	37.4/13.6	3.3/1.2

	kcal serv/100g	prot serv/100g	carb serv/100g	fat serv/100g	fibre serv/100g
Duck, Crispy Aromatic, Tesco*, 1 serving/61g					
	131/214	8.9/14.6	7.5/12.3	7.2/11.8	0.5/0.9
Duck, Pancakes with Hoisin Sauce, Marks & Spencer*, 1 pack/80g					
	136/170	10.4/13	15.9/19.9	3.2/4	0.7/0.9
Duck, Peking, Crispy, Sainsbury's*, ½ pack/300g					
	1236/412	58.5/19.5	1.8/0.6	110.7/36.9	0/0
Dumplings, Prawn Sui Mai with Soy Sauce, Marks & Spencer*, 1 pack/130g					
	143/110	17.8/13.7	8.7/6.7	4.4/3.4	0.8/0.6
Fagottini, Mushroom, Sainsbury's*, ½ pack/155g					
	339/219	15.8/10.2	42.9/27.7	11.6/7.5	4.2/2.7
Fajita, Chicken with Salsa & Sour Cream Dips, Safeway*, 1 pack/242g					
	390/161	23.7/9.8	40.4/16.7	14.8/6.1	4.6/1.9
Fajita, Chicken, American-Style, Tesco*, 1 pack/275g					
	388/141	26.1/9.5	39.1/14.2	14/5.1	2.8/1
Fajita, Chicken, BGTY, Sainsbury's*, 1 pack/299g					
	389/130	32.9/11	54.7/18.3	4.2/1.4	4.8/1.6
Fajita, Chicken, Healthy Eating, Tesco*, ½ pack/225g					
	248/110	20.7/9.2	34.4/15.3	2.9/1.3	1.1/0.5
Fajita, Chicken, Marks & Spencer*, 1 pack/230g					
	345/150	19.8/8.6	40.7/17.7	12.2/5.3	2.3/1
Fettuccine, Cajun Chicken, COU, Marks & Spencer*, 1 pack/350g					
	368/105	27.7/7.9	48.7/13.9	7.4/2.1	3.9/1.1
Fusilli, Tomato, Weight Watchers*, 1 can/388g					
	198/51	7.4/1.9	39.2/10.1	1.6/0.4	3.1/0.8
Goulash, Beef, Bistro Range, Tesco*, 1 pack/450g					
	545/121	35.6/7.9	65.7/14.6	15.3/3.4	2.7/0.6
Haggis, Neeps & Tatties, Marks & Spencer*, 1 pack/300g					
	330/110	11.4/3.8	36.9/12.3	14.4/4.8	2.4/0.8
Hash Browns, Bird's Eye*, 1 serving/63g					
	126/200	1.3/2	13.8/21.9	7.3/11.6	1/1.6
Hash Browns, Frozen, McCain*, 1 hash brown/40g					
	70/174	1.2/3	9.6/24	2.9/7.3	0/0
Hash, Chicken Salsa, Healthy Eating, Tesco*, 1 pack/350g					
	291/83	14.4/4.1	37.1/10.6	9.5/2.7	3.9/1.1
Hash, Farmhouse, Healthy Eating, Tesco*, 1 serving/300g					
	264/88	6.6/2.2	40.8/13.6	8.1/2.7	3.3/1.1
Hot Pot, Beef, Weight Watchers*, 1 pack/320g					
	288/90	18.6/5.8	32/10	9.6/3	4.5/1.4

kcal serv/100g	prot serv/100g	carb serv/100g	fat serv/100g	fibre serv/100g
Hot Pot, Chicken, Weight Watchers*, 1 pack/340g				
306/90	18/5.3	38.4/11.3	8.8/2.6	3.1/0.9
Indian Banquet, for One, COU, Marks & Spencer*, 1 pack/500g				
400/80	33.5/6.7	51/10.2	6/1.2	15.5/3.1
Indian Meal for One, Healthy Eating, Tesco*, 1 pack/420g				
437/104	31.1/7.4	58.8/14	8.8/2.1	5.9/1.4
Jalfrezi, Chicken with Pilau Rice, BGTY, Sainsbury's*, 1 pack/450g				
432/96	31.5/7	64.4/14.3	5.4/1.2	3.6/0.8
Jalfrezi, Chicken, Sainsbury's*, 1 pack/400g				
436/109	48.4/12.1	13.6/3.4	20.8/5.2	6.8/1.7
Kebab, Chicken, Barbecue, Sainsbury's*, 1 pack/200g				
238/119	48.8/24.4	3/1.5	3.4/1.7	3.6/1.8
Kebab, Doner, Lidl*, 1 kebab/170g				
509/300	25/14.7	26/15.3	31.3/18.4	0/0
Kebab, Donner, Iceland*, 1 serving/152.3g				
268/176	14/9.2	37/24.4	7.1/4.7	3.6/2.4
Kebab, Lamb Kofta, Safeway*, 1 pack/227g				
465/205	32.5/14.3	13.2/5.8	30.4/13.4	2.3/1
Kebab, Lamb, Greek-Style, Sainsbury's*, 1 kebab/168g				
428/255	29.2/17.4	12.9/7.7	28.6/17	3.9/2.3
Kebab, Lamb, Shish, Waitrose*, 1 kebab/55.8g				
91/163	9.2/16.5	3.8/6.8	4.3/7.7	0.7/1.3
Kedgeree, COU, Marks & Spencer*, 1 pack/370g				
426/115	29.2/7.9	53.3/14.4	9.6/2.6	3/0.8
Kiev, Chicken with Garlic Butter, Tesco*, 1 Kiev/125g				
343/274	17.1/13.7	11/8.8	25.5/20.4	0.9/0.7
Kiev, Chicken, Breaded, Mini, Family, Bernard Matthews*, 1 Kiev/23g				
46/199	3.6/15.7	2.8/12.1	2.3/9.8	0/0
Kiev, Chicken, COU, Marks & Spencer*, 1 Kiev/150g				
188/125	23.7/15.8	16.2/10.8	2.7/1.8	0.8/0.5
Kiev, Chicken, Creamy Garlic, Tesco*, 1 Kiev/142g				
334/235	17.3/12.2	13.8/9.7	23.3/16.4	0.9/0.6
King Prawn, Ginger & Spring Onion, Budgens*, 1 pack/350g				
151/43	20.7/5.9	7.4/2.1	4.2/1.2	2.5/0.7
Korma, Chicken & Pilau Rice, Asda*, 1 pack/392g				
804/205	27.4/7	94.1/24	35.3/9	5.5/1.4
Korma, Chicken & Pilau Rice, New, BGTY, Sainsbury's*, 1 pack/400g				
344/86	32.4/8.1	43.2/10.8	4.8/1.2	7.6/1.9

kcal serv/100g	prot serv/100g	carb serv/100g	fat serv/100g	fibre serv/100g

Korma, Chicken & Rice, Healthy Eating, Tesco*, 1 pack/420g

| 487/116 | 30.2/7.2 | 75.2/17.9 | 7.6/1.8 | 1.3/0.3 |

Korma, Chicken, Fresh, Chilled, Tesco*, 1 pack/350g

| 819/234 | 45.9/13.1 | 22.1/6.3 | 60.9/17.4 | 8.1/2.3 |

Korma, Chicken, Sainsbury's*, 1 pack/400g

| 580/145 | 56.4/14.1 | 13.2/3.3 | 33.6/8.4 | 2.8/0.7 |

Korma, Chicken, Tesco*, 1 pack/350g

| 620/177 | 37.8/10.8 | 23.8/6.8 | 41.3/11.8 | 2.1/0.6 |

Korma, Vegetable, Sainsbury's*, 1 serving/200g

| 302/151 | 5.4/2.7 | 13.2/6.6 | 25.2/12.6 | 4.4/2.2 |

Lamb, Kofta, Kleftico, Sainsbury's*, 1 pack/401.2g

| 654/163 | 54.1/13.5 | 22.1/5.5 | 38.9/9.7 | 2/0.5 |

Lamb, Roast, Minted, in Gravy, Marks & Spencer*, 1 pack/200g

| 140/70 | 13.6/6.8 | 13.2/6.6 | 3/1.5 | 1.8/0.9 |

Lamb With, Carrot & Swede Mash, Braised, Eat Smart, Safeway*, 1 pack/388g

| 330/85 | 29.5/7.6 | 28.7/7.4 | 9.3/2.4 | 5.4/1.4 |

Lamb, Roast Dinner, Bird's Eye*, 1 pack/340g

| 357/105 | 22.4/6.6 | 38.1/11.2 | 12.9/3.8 | 4.8/1.4 |

Lasagne, Al Forno, Marks & Spencer*, 1 pack/330g

| 528/160 | 31.7/9.6 | 40.6/12.3 | 27.4/8.3 | 4.6/1.4 |

Lasagne, Asda*, 1 pack/378g

| 427/113 | 22.7/6 | 41.6/11 | 18.9/5 | 4.2/1.1 |

Lasagne, Beef, Asda*, 1 pack/400g

| 1972/493 | 116/29 | 224/56 | 68/17 | 16/4 |

Lasagne, Beef, BGTY, Sainsbury's*, 1 pack/400g

| 340/85 | 21.2/5.3 | 45.2/11.3 | 8.4/2.1 | 2.4/0.6 |

Lasagne, Beef, Frozen, Tesco*, 1 pack/400g

| 492/123 | 22.8/5.7 | 45.6/11.4 | 24.4/6.1 | 2.8/0.7 |

Lasagne, Beef, GFY, Asda*, 1 pack/350g

| 385/110 | 31.5/9 | 49/14 | 7/2 | 3.5/1 |

Lasagne, Beef, Weight Watchers*, 1 pack/300g

| 297/99 | 22.2/7.4 | 33/11 | 8.4/2.8 | 2.1/0.7 |

Lasagne, BGTY, Sainsbury's*, 1 pack/400g

| 420/105 | 23.6/5.9 | 62/15.5 | 8.8/2.2 | 2/0.5 |

Lasagne, Classic, Deep-Filled, Marks & Spencer*, 1 pack/400g

| 760/190 | 40/10 | 44.8/11.2 | 47.6/11.9 | 2.4/0.6 |

	kcal serv/100g	prot serv/100g	carb serv/100g	fat serv/100g	fibre serv/100g

Lasagne, COU, Marks & Spencer*, 1 pack/360g

| 324/90 | 24.8/6.9 | 42.1/11.7 | 6.1/1.7 | 3.6/1 |

Lasagne, Finest, Tesco*, ½ pack/300g

| 432/144 | 22.2/7.4 | 39.3/13.1 | 20.7/6.9 | 1.5/0.5 |

Lasagne, Healthy Eating, Tesco*, 1 pack/340g

| 343/101 | 17.3/5.1 | 45.6/13.4 | 10.2/3 | 3.1/0.9 |

Lasagne, Italia, Marks & Spencer*, 1 pack/400g

| 640/160 | 32.8/8.2 | 42.8/10.7 | 38/9.5 | 3.2/0.8 |

Lasagne, Italian, Sainsbury's*, 1 pack/450g

| 639/142 | 39.2/8.7 | 63.9/14.2 | 25.2/5.6 | 2.7/0.6 |

Lasagne, Mediterranean Vegetable, COU, Marks & Spencer*, 1 pack/360g

| 306/85 | 12.2/3.4 | 41.4/11.5 | 9.7/2.7 | 5/1.4 |

Lasagne, Ready Meal, Marks & Spencer*, 1 pack/360g

| 594/165 | 40.7/11.3 | 42.1/11.7 | 29.5/8.2 | 4.7/1.3 |

Lasagne, Roasted Mushroom & Spinach, COU, Marks & Spencer*, 1 pack/360g

| 288/80 | 18/5 | 43.6/12.1 | 4.3/1.2 | 4/1.1 |

Lasagne, Triangles with Chicken, COU, Marks & Spencer*, 1 pack/360g

| 324/90 | 28.1/7.8 | 42.8/11.9 | 6.5/1.8 | 3.6/1 |

Lasagne, Vegetable, BGTY, Sainsbury's*, 1 pack/400g

| 286/72 | 19.2/4.8 | 38/9.5 | 6.4/1.6 | 5.6/1.4 |

Lasagne, Vegetable, Two-Layered, BGTY, Sainsbury's*, 1 pack/400g

| 288/72 | 19.2/4.8 | 38/9.5 | 6.4/1.6 | 5.6/1.4 |

Macaroni Cheese, BGTY, Sainsbury's*, 1 pack/450g

| 504/112 | 26.1/5.8 | 77.4/17.2 | 9.9/2.2 | 5/1.1 |

Macaroni Cheese, Healthy Eating, Tesco*, 1 pack/340g

| 252/74 | 22.4/6.6 | 21.1/6.2 | 8.5/2.5 | 2/0.6 |

Macaroni Cheese, Heinz*, 1 can/400g

| 380/95 | 13.6/3.4 | 39.2/9.8 | 18.8/4.7 | 1.2/0.3 |

Macaroni Cheese, New, BGTY, Sainsbury's*, 1 pack/390g

| 441/113 | 19.9/5.1 | 72.5/18.6 | 7.8/2 | 9.4/2.4 |

Masala Dal, Waitrose*, ½ pack/150g

| 164/109 | 8.9/5.9 | 18.6/12.4 | 6/4 | 4.2/2.8 |

Meatballs, Aberdeen Angus in Sauce, Perfectly Balanced, Waitrose*, ½ pack/240g

| 228/95 | 25.2/10.5 | 15.6/6.5 | 7.2/3 | 2.6/1.1 |

	kcal serv/100g	prot serv/100g	carb serv/100g	fat serv/100g	fibre serv/100g

Meatballs, in a Spicy Tomato Sauce with Fresh Spaghetti, COU, Marks & Spencer*, 1 pack/360g

342/95	22.7/6.3	48.6/13.5	6.8/1.9	4.3/1.2

Meatballs, in Tomato Sauce, Campbell's*, 1 can/410g

340/83	22.1/5.4	39/9.5	10.7/2.6	0/0

Meatballs, Italian Pork, Al Forno, Sainsbury's*, 1 pack/450g

644/143	27.5/6.1	79.2/17.6	23.9/5.3	6.3/1.4

Melt, Mushroom & Broccoli Potato Wedge, Weight Watchers*, 1 pack/310g

285/92	10.2/3.3	39.1/12.6	9.6/3.1	3.1/1

Moussaka, COU, Marks & Spencer*, 1 pack/340g

272/80	18/5.3	28.9/8.5	9.9/2.9	4.8/1.4

Moussaka, Vegetable, Marks & Spencer*, 1 pack/300g

330/110	13.2/4.4	35.4/11.8	15.6/5.2	3.3/1.1

Noodle Bowl, Szechuan-Style Prawn, Tesco*, 1 bowl/400g

376/94	22/5.5	69.2/17.3	1.2/0.3	3.6/0.9

Noodles &, Bean Sprouts, Fresh Ideas, Tesco*, 1 pack/250g

310/124	13.5/5.4	49.5/19.8	6.5/2.6	4.8/1.9

Noodles, Char Sui, Cantonese, Sainsbury's*, 1 pack/450g

378/84	30.6/6.8	47.3/10.5	7.2/1.6	6.8/1.5

Noodles, Chicken Flavour, 3-Minute, Blue Dragon*, 1 pack/85g

403/475	7.9/9.3	52/61.2	18.2/21.4	0/0

Noodles, Chicken, Chinese-Style, GFY, Asda*, 1 pack/393g

295/75	23.6/6	35.4/9	6.7/1.7	2.4/0.6

Noodles, Chicken, Chinese, Asda*, 1 pot/302g

305/101	18.1/6	48.3/16	4.2/1.4	2.4/0.8

Noodles, Chilli Chicken, GFY, Asda*, 1 pack/415g

461/111	24.9/6	83/20	3.3/0.8	4.2/1

Noodles, Chilli Chicken, Take Away, Marks & Spencer*, 1 pack/250g

325/130	24/9.6	38/15.2	7.8/3.1	3.3/1.3

Noodles, Chow Mein, Chicken Bowl, Uncle Ben's*, 1 pack/330g

307/93	20.1/6.1	44.6/13.5	4.6/1.4	0/0

Noodles, Curry, Instant, Heinz*, 1 serving/85g

261/307	8.1/9.5	56.4/66.4	0.3/0.4	2.3/2.7

Noodles, Egg, Tossed in Sesame Oil, Asda*, ½ pack/150g

174/116	3.5/2.3	16.5/11	10.5/7	0/0

Noodles, Peking Duck, Shapers, Boots*, 1 pack/280g

395/141	20.2/7.2	70/25	3.9/1.4	5/1.8

kcal serv/100g	prot serv/100g	carb serv/100g	fat serv/100g	fibre serv/100g
Noodles, Ramen, with Chilli Beef, Marks & Spencer*, 1 pack/484g				
532/110	39.2/8.1	57.6/11.9	17.4/3.6	3.9/0.8
Noodles, Savoury Vegetable, COU, Marks & Spencer*, 1 pack/450g				
270/60	13.1/2.9	51.8/11.5	2.7/0.6	5.4/1.2
Noodles, Spicy Curry Flavour, Snack, SmartPrice, Asda*, 1 pot/76g				
358/471	8/10.5	50/65.8	14/18.4	0/0
Noodles, Super, Spicy Salsa, Dry Weight, Batchelors*, 1 pack/105g				
474/451	7.4/7	67/63.8	19.5/18.6	1.8/1.7
Noodles, Sweet Chilli, Wok, Findus*, 1 pack/300g				
300/100	9/3	60/20	1.5/0.5	0/0
Noodles, Thai-Style, GFY, Asda*, 1 pot/237.9g				
226/95	7.1/3	47.6/20	0.7/0.3	1.9/0.8
Noodles, Thai-Style, Sainsbury's*, 1 pack/340g				
381/112	11.2/3.3	66/19.4	7.8/2.3	2.4/0.7
Noodles, Thai, Waitrose*, 1 pack/300g				
357/119	20.4/6.8	55.2/18.4	6.3/2.1	5.1/1.7
Omelette, Ham & Mushroom, Farmfoods*, 1 omelette/120g				
200/167	10.4/8.7	2.2/1.8	16.7/13.9	0.1/0.1
Paella, Chicken & Chorizo, Asda*, 1 pack/390g				
432/111	35/9	55/14.1	8/2.1	9/2.3
Paella, Chicken, Healthy Eating, Tesco*, 1 pack/400g				
416/104	35.6/8.9	61.6/15.4	3.2/0.8	8.8/2.2
Pakora, Potato & Spinach, Mini, Indian Snack Selection, Waitrose*, 1 pakora/21g				
56/266	1.1/5.4	3.6/17	4.1/19.6	0.9/4.5
Pancake, Chinese-Style, Cherry Valley*, 1 pancake/8g				
25/310	0.7/9.2	4.4/54.7	0.5/6	0/0
Pancake, Vegetable Roll, 1 roll/85g				
185/218	5.6/6.6	17.9/21	10.6/12.5	0/0
Panini, Roasted Vegetables & Cheese, Starbucks*, 1 pack/215g				
542/252	18.7/8.7	44.3/20.6	32.5/15.1	0/0
Pasta Bake, Chicken, GFY, Asda*, 1 pack/400g				
424/106	24/6	56/14	11.6/2.9	2.8/0.7
Pasta Bake, Roast Vegetable, Eat Smart, Safeway*, 1 pack/330g				
380/115	12.5/3.8	64.7/19.6	6.3/1.9	4.3/1.3
Pasta Bake, Tuna, COU, Marks & Spencer*, 1 pack/360g				
378/105	28.8/8	48.2/13.4	7.2/2	4/1.1

kcal serv/100g	prot serv/100g	carb serv/100g	fat serv/100g	fibre serv/100g
Pasta Bake, Tuna, Healthy Eating, Tesco*, 1 pack/340g				
258/76	18.4/5.4	40.5/11.9	2.7/0.8	1.7/0.5
Pasta 'n' Sauce, Cheese, Leek & Ham, Batchelors*, 1 pack/126g				
478/379	17.8/14.1	86.1/68.3	6.9/5.5	2.9/2.3
Pasta 'n' Sauce, Chicken & Mushroom, Batchelors*, 1 pack/126g				
455/361	15.6/12.4	92.6/73.5	2.5/2	3.4/2.7
Pasta 'n' Sauce, Macaroni Cheese, Batchelors*, 1 pack/115g				
435/378	19.8/17.2	73.1/63.6	7/6.1	3.2/2.8
Pasta 'n' Sauce, Mild Cheese & Broccoli, Batchelors*, 1 pack/129g				
479/371	17.4/13.5	89/69	5.8/4.5	3.6/2.8
Pasta 'n' Sauce, Tomato Onion & Herb Flavour, Batchelors*, 1 pack/135g				
470/348	17.8/13.2	87.1/64.5	5.5/4.1	7.8/5.8
Pasta Salad, Chicken & Smoked Bacon, Marks & Spencer*, 1 salad/380g				
817/215	28.5/7.5	72.2/19	46.7/12.3	7.2/1.9
Pasta Salad, Feta Cheese, Sun Blush Tomatoes, Marks & Spencer*, 1 serving/190g				
361/190	10.5/5.5	32.7/17.2	21.1/11.1	4/2.1
Pasta Salad, Fusilli with Red Pesto Chicken & Santa Tomatoes, Marks & Spencer*, 1 serving/270g				
285/106	21.9/8.1	37.8/14	5.7/2.1	1.6/0.6
Pasta Salad, Torcetti with King Prawns & Vine-Ripened Tomatoes, COU, Marks & Spencer*, 1 pack/270g				
284/105	15.9/5.9	40.8/15.1	6.5/2.4	7.3/2.7
Pasta Salad, Tuna, Tesco*, 1 pot/300g				
399/133	18.6/6.2	31.5/10.5	21.9/7.3	0/0
Pasta with, Chicken, Courgette & Sun-Dried Tomato, BGTY, Sainsbury's*, 1 serving/300g				
294/98	27.3/9.1	39/13	3.3/1.1	4.5/1.5
Pasta, Tomato & Pepper, GFY, Asda*, 1 pack/400g				
344/86	12.4/3.1	56/14	7.6/1.9	4.4/1.1
Pecorino Romano, Tesco*, 1 serving/100g				
366/366	28.5/28.5	0/0	28/28	0/0
Penne, Chicken & Red Wine, Weight Watchers*, 1 pack/394g				
248/63	14.6/3.7	39.8/10.1	2.8/0.7	2.4/0.6
Penne, Tomato & Basil Sauce, Asda*, ½ pack/314g				
185/59	2.5/0.8	18.8/6	11/3.5	6.3/2
Pie, Beef Steak, Aberdeen Angus, Top Crust, Waitrose*, ½ pie/280g				
476/170	28/10	37.5/13.4	24.1/8.6	11.5/4.1

	kcal serv/100g	prot serv/100g	carb serv/100g	fat serv/100g	fibre serv/100g
Pie, Chicken & Mushroom, Asda*, 1 pie/ 150g					
	444/296	11.6/7.7	38.1/25.4	27.3/18.2	1.5/1
Pie, Chicken & Mushroom, Puff Pastry, Sainsbury's*, 1 pie/150g					
	450/300	11.7/7.8	44.4/29.6	25.1/16.7	1.4/0.9
Pie, Chicken & Mushroom, Tesco*, 1 pie/150g					
	449/299	12.9/8.6	33.6/22.4	29.1/19.4	2.6/1.7
Pie, Chicken & Vegetable, Asda*, 1 pie/130.7g					
	329/251	10.5/8	27.5/21	19.7/15	1.8/1.4
Pie, Chicken, Bird's Eye*, 1 pie/158g					
	414/262	11.4/7.2	36.5/23.1	24.6/15.6	2.1/1.3
Pie, Cottage, Aberdeen Angus, Waitrose*, 1 pie/350g					
	340/97	18.6/5.3	38.5/11	12.3/3.5	3.2/0.9
Pie, Cottage, GFY, Asda*, 1 pack/414g					
	302/73	24.8/6	37.3/9	5.8/1.4	5.4/1.3
Pie, Cottage, Healthy Eating, Tesco*, 1 pie/450g					
	347/77	21.2/4.7	44.6/9.9	9/2	3.2/0.7
Pie, Cottage, Healthy Living, Tesco*, 1 pack/400g					
	356/89	21.6/5.4	42.8/10.7	10.8/2.7	7.6/1.9
Pie, Cottage, Sainsbury's*, 1 pack/300g					
	207/69	11.4/3.8	31.2/10.4	4.2/1.4	3.6/1.2
Pie, Cottage, Tesco*, 1 pie/300g					
	300/100	9.9/3.3	37.5/12.5	12.3/4.1	1.5/0.5
Pie, Cumberland Fish, Healthy Eating, Tesco*, 1 pack/450g					
	378/84	27/6	45/10	9.9/2.2	3.6/0.8
Pie, Meat & Potato, Shortcrust, Co-Op*, ¼ pie/137g					
	403/294	10/7.3	31.9/23.3	26.2/19.1	1.9/1.4
Pie, Ocean with Cod, Weight Watchers*, 1 pack/295g					
	251/85	15.9/5.4	29.5/10	7.7/2.6	2.4/0.8
Pie, Ocean with White Fish, Weight Watchers*, 1 pack/295g					
	224/76	14.1/4.8	31.3/10.6	4.8/1.6	1.5/0.5
Pie, Pork, Crusty Bake, Mini, Sainsbury's*, 1 pie/43g					
	165/384	4.9/11.5	11.2/26	11.2/26	0.6/1.5
Pie, Pork, Crusty Bake, Sainsbury's*, 1 pie/75g					
	293/390	7.9/10.5	20.3/27	20/26.7	0.8/1
Pie, Pork, Melton Mowbray, Lattice, Sainsbury's*, 1 serving/100g					
	342/342	10.8/10.8	21.7/21.7	23.6/23.6	1.2/1.2
Pie, Potato-Topped Cottage, Marks & Spencer*, 1 pack/190g					
	238/125	11/5.8	19/10	12.9/6.8	1.3/0.7

kcal serv/100g	prot serv/100g	carb serv/100g	fat serv/100g	fibre serv/100g

Pie, Scottish Steak, Topcrust Puff Pastry, Marks & Spencer*, 1 portion/240g

| 432/180 | 31.4/13.1 | 29/12.1 | 20.4/8.5 | 1.7/0.7 |

Pie, Shepherd's with Lamb, Weight Watchers*, 1 pack/320g

| 234/73 | 12.2/3.8 | 37.1/11.6 | 3.8/1.2 | 1.6/0.5 |

Pie, Shepherd's, Marks & Spencer*, 1 pack/400g

| 380/95 | 21.2/5.3 | 38.8/9.7 | 15.6/3.9 | 5.6/1.4 |

Pie, Steak & Ale, Pub-Style, Co-Op*, 1 pie/250g

| 538/215 | 22.5/9 | 42.5/17 | 30/12 | 5/2 |

Pie, Steak & Kidney, Tinned, Fray Bentos*, ½ pie/212g

| 346/163 | 17.4/8.2 | 27.3/12.9 | 18.7/8.8 | 0/0 |

Pie, Steak, Asda*, 1 pie/150g

| 453/302 | 13.8/9.2 | 37.7/25.1 | 27.5/18.3 | 1.5/1 |

Pie, Steak, Short Crust, Sainsbury's*, ¼ pie/131g

| 392/299 | 13/9.9 | 35.5/27.1 | 22/16.8 | 1.2/0.9 |

Pie, Vegetable & Cheese, Asda*, 1 pie/131g

| 346/264 | 7.9/6 | 31.4/24 | 21/16 | 2.4/1.8 |

Pizza Pocket, Chargrilled Chicken & Veg, Healthy Eating Tesco*, 1 pack/190g

| 304/160 | 21.7/11.4 | 43.9/23.1 | 4.6/2.4 | 5.3/2.8 |

Pizza, American Hot, Pizza Express*, ½ pizza/264g

| 517/196 | 28/10.6 | 70.8/26.8 | 13.5/5.1 | 2.9/1.1 |

Pizza, American Hot, Pizza Express, Sainsbury's*, ½ pizza/147g

| 281/191 | 14.5/9.9 | 41.4/28.2 | 6.4/4.4 | 2/1.4 |

Pizza, Cajun Chicken, BGTY, Sainsbury's*, ½ pizza/165g

| 363/220 | 18.2/11 | 59.4/36 | 5.9/3.6 | 2.8/1.7 |

Pizza, Chargrilled Vegetable, COU, Marks & Spencer*, 1 pizza/294g

| 397/135 | 17.6/6 | 68.8/23.4 | 7.1/2.4 | 5.6/1.9 |

Pizza, Cheese & Tomato Slice, Ross*, 1 slice/77g

| 148/192 | 5/6.5 | 17.1/22.2 | 6.6/8.6 | 1.5/2 |

Pizza, Cheese & Tomato Thin & Crispy, Stonebaked, Tesco*, 1 pizza/155g

| 355/229 | 18/11.6 | 43.6/28.1 | 12.1/7.8 | 2/1.3 |

Pizza, Cheese & Tomato, Deep Pan, Goodfellas*, ¼ pizza/102.4g

| 258/253 | 11.7/11.5 | 30.2/29.6 | 10.7/10.5 | 3.8/3.7 |

Pizza, Cheese & Tomato, Deep Pan, Sainsbury's*, 1 pizza/182g

| 470/258 | 21.3/11.7 | 60.2/33.1 | 15.8/8.7 | 3.5/1.9 |

Pizza, Chicken Provencal, Goodfellas*, ½ pizza/142.5g

| 389/272 | 19.6/13.7 | 37/25.9 | 18/12.6 | 3/2.1 |

kcal serv/100g	prot serv/100g	carb serv/100g	fat serv/100g	fibre serv/100g
Pizza, Chicken Salsa, Healthy Eating, Tesco*, ½ pizza/169g				
313/185	22/13	51.2/30.3	2.2/1.3	2.5/1.5
Pizza, Chicken, Thin & Crispy, Somerfield*, ½ pizza/159g				
356/224	17.6/11.1	46.1/29	11.3/7.1	4.6/2.9
Pizza, Four Cheese, Thin Crust, Tesco*, ½ pizza/142g				
386/272	20.6/14.5	45.2/31.8	13.6/9.6	2.6/1.8
Pizza, Four Seasons, Pizza Express*, 1 serving/300g				
720/240	34.8/11.6	87.5/29.2	28.8/9.6	0/0
Pizza, Ham & Mushroom, BGTY, Sainsbury's*, ½ pizza/158g				
291/184	16.1/10.2	41.7/26.4	6.6/4.2	4.6/2.9
Pizza, Ham & Mushroom, COU, Marks & Spencer*, 1 pack/245g				
392/160	22.5/9.2	63/25.7	5.9/2.4	3.2/1.3
Pizza, Ham & Mushroom, Deep Pan, Waitrose*, ½ pizza/219.9g				
453/206	24/10.9	58.5/26.6	13.6/6.2	2.2/1
Pizza, Ham & Mushroom, Thin & Crispy, Asda*, 1 pizza/360g				
760/211	39.6/11	93.6/26	25.2/7	8.6/2.4
Pizza, Ham & Pineapple, American Deep Pan, Sainsbury's*, 1 pizza/412g				
1001/243	43.3/10.5	134.3/32.6	32.1/7.8	7/1.7
Pizza, Ham & Pineapple, Deep Pan, Tesco*, 1 pizza/217g				
399/184	21.3/9.8	64.7/29.8	6.3/2.9	4.1/1.9
Pizza, Ham & Pineapple, Healthy Eating, Tesco*, 1 serving/169g				
343/203	20.1/11.9	59.8/35.4	2.5/1.5	2.2/1.3
Pizza, Ham & Pineapple, Thin & Crispy, Sainsbury's*, 1 pizza/305g				
824/270	41.2/13.5	90.9/29.8	32.6/10.7	5.2/1.7
Pizza, Hawaiian, Thin Crust, Tesco*, ½ pizza/205g				
398/194	17.2/8.4	58/28.3	10.9/5.3	4.3/2.1
Pizza, Hot & Spicy Pepperoni, Stuffed Crust, Asda*, 1 pizza/245g				
666/272	34/13.9	65/26.5	30/12.2	6/2.4
Pizza, Italian Meats, Finest, Tesco*, ½ pizza/217g				
449/207	29.5/13.6	63.8/29.4	8.5/3.9	2.8/1.3
Pizza, Margherita, Pizza Express*, ½ pizza/135g				
263/195	13.8/10.2	41.2/30.5	4.9/3.6	1.9/1.4
Pizza, Margherita, Stone Baked, GFY, Asda*, ¼ pizza/73g				
158/217	8/11	28.5/39	1.4/1.9	1.3/1.8
Pizza, Mushroom, Pizza Express*, 1 pizza/400g				
627/157	30.1/7.5	87.4/21.9	20.6/5.2	0/0
Pizza, Pepperoni, Deep Pan, Goodfella's*, ¼ slice/109g				
294/270	13.8/12.7	31.5/28.9	12.6/11.6	1.7/1.6

	kcal serv/100g	prot serv/100g	carb serv/100g	fat serv/100g	fibre serv/100g

Pizza, Pepperoni, Freschetta, Schwan's*, 1 pizza/310g

| 846/273 | 33.5/10.8 | 98/31.6 | 35.7/11.5 | 0/0 |

Pizza, Pepperoni, Individual, Chicago Town*, 1 pizza/168g

| 496/295 | 16.6/9.9 | 51.9/30.9 | 24.5/14.6 | 1.3/0.8 |

Pizza, Pepperoni, Italian, Thin & Crispy, Morrisons*, 1 pizza/365g

| 843/231 | 40.5/11.1 | 91.3/25 | 35/9.6 | 0/0 |

Pizza, Pepperoni, Stonebaked, Goodfella's*, ½ pizza/181g

| 503/278 | 21.5/11.9 | 49.6/27.4 | 26.1/14.4 | 4.3/2.4 |

Pizza, Pepperoni, Thin & Crispy, Sainsbury's*, ½ pizza/132g

| 395/299 | 18.1/13.7 | 35.6/27 | 19.9/15.1 | 6.7/5.1 |

Pizza, Prosciutto, Pizzeria, Sainsbury's*, 1 pizza/325g

| 806/248 | 37.1/11.4 | 112.8/34.7 | 23.1/7.1 | 10.4/3.2 |

Pizza, Sloppy Giuseppe, Pizza Express*, ½ pizza/181g

| 310/171 | 15.2/8.4 | 50.1/27.7 | 5.4/3 | 3.4/1.9 |

Pizza, Smoked Ham & Pineapple, Weight Watchers*, 1 pizza/241g

| 429/178 | 24.8/10.3 | 66.5/27.6 | 7/2.9 | 3.6/1.5 |

Pizza, Spinach & Ricotta, BGTY, Sainsbury's*, 1 pizza/265g

| 535/202 | 27.6/10.4 | 91.2/34.4 | 6.6/2.5 | 6.9/2.6 |

Pizza, Spinach & Ricotta, Pizzeria, Sainsbury's*, 1 pizza/390g

| 1002/257 | 44.5/11.4 | 120.1/30.8 | 41.7/10.7 | 8.2/2.1 |

Pizza, Tomato, Aubergine & Spinach, Pizzeria, Waitrose*, ½ pizza/193g

| 403/209 | 15.1/7.8 | 68.3/35.4 | 7.7/4 | 7/3.6 |

Pizza, Vegetable, Asda*, 1 pizza/368.7g

| 554/150 | 25.8/7 | 88.6/24 | 10.7/2.9 | 12.5/3.4 |

Poppadums, Mildly Spiced, Sharwood's*, 1 poppadum/12.5g

| 58/444 | 2.4/18.4 | 4.6/35.5 | 3.3/25.3 | 1.4/10.5 |

Poppadums, Plain, Asda*, 1 poppadum/9g

| 44/484 | 1.6/18 | 3.6/40 | 2.5/28 | 0/0 |

Pork in, Light Mustard Sauce, COU, Marks & Spencer*, 1 serving/390g

| 312/80 | 47.6/12.2 | 12.5/3.2 | 8.2/2.1 | 1.6/0.4 |

**Pork in, Mustard Sauce with Colcannon Mash, BGTY, Sainsbury's*,
1 pack/450g**

| 369/82 | 27.9/6.2 | 45/10 | 8.6/1.9 | 2.7/0.6 |

Pork, Steaks, with Honey & Mustard Sauce, Tesco*, ½ pack/160g

| 258/161 | 26.1/16.3 | 11.7/7.3 | 11.8/7.4 | 2.2/1.4 |

Potato, Baked, with Cheese, Healthy Eating, Tesco*, 1 potato/200g

| 222/111 | 7/3.5 | 39.4/19.7 | 4/2 | 3.8/1.9 |

kcal serv/100g	prot serv/100g	carb serv/100g	fat serv/100g	fibre serv/100g
Potato, Baked, with Cheese, Tesco*, 1 pack/400g				
448/112	10.8/2.7	74.8/18.7	11.6/2.9	4/1
Potato, Baked, with Tuna & Sweetcorn, COU, Marks & Spencer*, 1 pack/300g				
270/90	15.3/5.1	38.4/12.8	5.4/1.8	4.2/1.4
Potato, Jacket, Cheese & Beans, Somerfield*, 1 pack/338.9g				
305/90	13.9/4.1	46.8/13.8	6.8/2	7.5/2.2
Potato, Jacket, Cheese & Butter, Tesco*, 1 potato/200g				
214/107	8.4/4.2	29.2/14.6	7/3.5	2/1
Potato, Jacket, Chilli Con Carne, Somerfield*, 1 pack/340g				
319/94	18.7/5.5	35/10.3	11.6/3.4	4.1/1.2
Potato, Jacket, Tuna & Sweetcorn, Deep-Filled, Marks & Spencer*, 1 pack/300g				
270/90	14.7/4.9	39.3/13.1	6.6/2.2	3.6/1.2
Potato, Jacket, Tuna & Sweetcorn, Somerfield*, 1 pack/340g				
333/98	10.9/3.2	42.5/12.5	13.3/3.9	3.4/1
Potato, Jacket, with Chilli Con Carne, COU, Marks & Spencer*, 1 potato/300g				
270/90	18/6	33/11	6.3/2.1	3.6/1.2
Potato, Jacket, with Tuna & Sweetcorn, COU, Marks & Spencer*, 1 pack/300g				
270/90	15.3/5.1	38.4/12.8	5.4/1.8	4.2/1.4
Potato, Mash, Leek & Cheese, COU, Marks & Spencer*, ½ pack/225g				
180/80	6.8/3	27/12	4.7/2.1	2.9/1.3
Potato, Roast, Home Roasts, Crispy, McCain*, 1 serving/75g				
95/126	1.7/2.2	17.7/23.6	2.7/3.6	0/0
Potato, Saute, Deep-Fried, McCain*, 1oz/28g				
47/167	0.7/2.6	6.5/23.3	2/7	0/0
Potato, Saute, Oven-Baked, McCain*, 1oz/28g				
56/199	1.2/4.4	10.3/36.9	1.1/3.8	0/0
Potato, Skins, ¼-Cut, Deep-Fried, McCain*, 1oz/28g				
52/186	0.8/3	8.4/30.1	1.7/6	0/0
Potato, Skins, Cheese & Bacon, Tesco*, 1 serving/95g				
241/254	8.7/9.2	18.5/19.5	14.7/15.5	2.9/3
Potato, Skins, Loaded, Healthy Eating, Tesco*, 1 serving/340g				
425/125	26.2/7.7	60.7/17.9	8.5/2.5	2/0.6
Potato, Smiles, Oven-Baked, McCain*, 1oz/28g				
62/220	1.1/3.9	8.9/31.9	2.4/8.6	0/0

kcal serv/100g	prot serv/100g	carb serv/100g	fat serv/100g	fibre serv/100g

Potato, Waffles, Tesco*, 1 waffle/56g

| 97/174 | 1.3/2.4 | 13.3/23.8 | 4.3/7.7 | 0.4/0.8 |

Potato, Wedges, Chunky, McCain*, 10 wedges/175g

| 242/138 | 4.2/2.4 | 40.8/23.3 | 8.2/4.7 | 0/0 |

Potato, Wedges, Hot & Spicy with Salsa Dip, Healthy Living, Tesco*, 1 serving/170g

| 112/66 | 1.9/1.1 | 21.1/12.4 | 2.2/1.3 | 2.4/1.4 |

Potato, Wedges, Southern-Fried, Asda*, 1 serving/188g

| 263/140 | 5.5/2.9 | 43.2/23 | 7.5/4 | 3.4/1.8 |

Potato, Wedges, Spicy, Oven-Baked, McCain*, 1oz/28g

| 61/219 | 1.2/4.2 | 9.7/34.8 | 2.4/8.4 | 0/0 |

Provencale, Ratatouille, Tesco*, ½ can/195g

| 72/37 | 2.1/1.1 | 8.2/4.2 | 3.5/1.8 | 1.8/0.9 |

Quiche, Baby Spinach & Gruyere, Sainsbury's*, ¼ quiche/93g

| 228/245 | 6.9/7.4 | 14/15.1 | 16/17.2 | 0.9/1 |

Quiche, Broccoli, Tesco*, 1 quiche/175g

| 340/194 | 12.3/7 | 36.6/20.9 | 16.1/9.2 | 2.5/1.4 |

Quiche, Broccoli, Tomato & Cheese, BGTY, Sainsbury's*, 1 quiche/390g

| 632/162 | 25/6.4 | 61.2/15.7 | 32/8.2 | 5.1/1.3 |

Quiche, Broccoli, Tomato & Cheese, Sainsbury's*, 1 serving/125g

| 274/219 | 7.6/6.1 | 19.4/15.5 | 18.4/14.7 | 1.6/1.3 |

Quiche, Cheese & Ham, Sainsbury's*, 1 serving/100g

| 266/266 | 9.3/9.3 | 14.4/14.4 | 19/19 | 1.2/1.2 |

Quiche, Cheese & Onion, Tesco*, 1 serving/90g

| 230/256 | 7.4/8.2 | 16.3/18.1 | 15.1/16.8 | 2.3/2.5 |

Quiche, Lorraine, Sainsbury's*, ⅓ quiche/128g

| 341/265 | 12/9.3 | 18.5/14.4 | 24.4/19 | 1.2/0.9 |

Quiche, Lorraine, Tesco*, 1 serving/81g

| 262/324 | 7.9/9.8 | 14.9/18.4 | 19/23.5 | 0.6/0.8 |

Quiche, Vegetable, Tesco*, 1 serving/100g

| 257/257 | 6.9/6.9 | 17.5/17.5 | 17.7/17.7 | 1.5/1.5 |

Ratatouille, Sainsbury's*, ½ can/190g

| 80/42 | 1.5/0.8 | 10.8/5.7 | 3.4/1.8 | 1.9/1 |

Ravioli, Five Cheese, Weight Watchers*, 1 pack/330g

| 271/82 | 10.6/3.2 | 36.6/11.1 | 9.2/2.8 | 2.6/0.8 |

Ravioli, in Tomato Sauce, Heinz*, 1 can/410g

| 299/73 | 10.7/2.6 | 53.3/13 | 4.5/1.1 | 2.5/0.6 |

kcal serv/100g	prot serv/100g	carb serv/100g	fat serv/100g	fibre serv/100g
Rice, Basmati, Pilau, Rizazz, Tilda*, 1 serving/125g				
183/146	3.1/2.5	35.9/28.7	3/2.4	0/0
Rice, Basmati, Pure, Rizazz, Tilda*, 1 bag/250g				
383/153	6.5/2.6	75.5/30.2	6/2.4	0/0
Rice, Chinese-Style, Express, Uncle Ben's*, 1 pack/250g				
338/135	7.8/3.1	68.3/27.3	3.8/1.5	0/0
Rice, Coconut & Lime, Asda*, 1 pack/360g				
695/193	16.2/4.5	117.7/32.7	17.6/4.9	3.2/0.9
Rice, Coconut, Marks & Spencer*, ½ pack/124g				
217/175	3.8/3.1	39.4/31.8	5/4	0.4/0.3
Rice, Egg Fried, Cantonese, Sainsbury's*, ½ pot/260g				
465/179	10.4/4	71.2/27.4	20.8/8	3.4/1.3
Rice, Egg Fried, Chinese-Style, Tesco*, 1 portion/250g				
418/167	11/4.4	69.8/27.9	10.5/4.2	1.8/0.7
Rice, Egg Fried, Chinese, Sainsbury's*, 1 pack/200g				
350/175	9/4.5	55.6/27.8	10.2/5.1	2.4/1.2
Rice, Egg Fried, Express, Uncle Ben's*, 1 pack/250g				
440/176	10.3/4.1	76.3/30.5	10.5/4.2	0/0
Rice, Egg Fried, Marks & Spencer*, 1 pack/200g				
420/210	8.2/4.1	64.8/32.4	14/7	0.6/0.3
Rice, Egg Fried, Rizazz, Tilda*, 1 pack/250g				
358/143	8.3/3.3	63.5/25.4	7.8/3.1	0/0
Rice, Egg Fried, Waitrose*, 1 pack/300g				
426/142	9/3	61.8/20.6	15.6/5.2	3/1
Rice, Fried, Chicken, Chinese Takeaway, Iceland*, 1 pack/340g				
510/150	22.1/6.5	70.4/20.7	15.6/4.6	2/0.6
Rice, Fried, Duck, Chicken & Pork Celebration, Sainsbury's*, 1 pack/450g				
545/121	35.6/7.9	63.9/14.2	16.2/3.6	6.8/1.5
Rice, Mexican, Ready Meals, Waitrose*, 1 pack/300g				
432/144	7.8/2.6	83.4/27.8	7.5/2.5	1.5/0.5
Rice, Mushroom & Coconut, Organic, Waitrose*, 1 pack/300g				
474/158	11.1/3.7	73.5/24.5	15/5	4.2/1.4
Rice, Pilau, Bengali, Sainsbury's*, 1 pack/200g				
330/165	8.4/4.2	53/26.5	9.4/4.7	4.4/2.2
Rice, Pilau, Express, Uncle Ben's*, ½ pack/125g				
211/169	3.9/3.1	38.8/31	4.5/3.6	0/0
Rice, Pilau, Indian Mushroom, Sainsbury's*, 1 serving/100g				
119/119	3/3	21.3/21.3	2.4/2.4	1.9/1.9

	kcal serv/100g	prot serv/100g	carb serv/100g	fat serv/100g	fibre serv/100g
Rice, Pilau, Indian Takeaway For 1, Sainsbury's*, 1 serving/201g					
	334/166	8.2/4.1	64.5/32.1	4.8/2.4	1/0.5
Rice, Pilau, Marks & Spencer*, 1 serving/250g					
	450/180	7/2.8	68.3/27.3	16/6.4	1/0.4
Rice, Pilau, Takeaway Menu For 1, BGTY, Sainsbury's*, 1 pack/151g					
	227/150	7.2/4.8	49.5/32.8	0/0	2.6/1.7
Rice, Pilau, Waitrose*, ½ pot/300g					
	534/178	12.6/4.2	105.3/35.1	6.9/2.3	5.7/1.9
Rice, Special Fried, Marks & Spencer*, 1 pack/450g					
	923/205	27.9/6.2	122.4/27.2	35.1/7.8	2.3/0.5
Rice, Special Fried, Somerfield*, 1 pack/200g					
	316/158	10/5	50/25	8/4	0/0
Rice, Special Fried, Tesco*, 1 pack/250g					
	333/133	19/7.6	44/17.6	9/3.6	4.3/1.7
Rice, Sticky Thai, Safeway*, 1 pack/200g					
	260/130	5/2.5	51.2/25.6	3.6/1.8	2.8/1.4
Rice, Sweet & Sour, Rice Bowl, Uncle Ben's*, 1 pack/350g					
	364/104	18.2/5.2	68.3/19.5	2.1/0.6	0/0
Rice, Thai, Chicken, Enjoy, Bird's Eye*, 1 pack/500g					
	535/107	34.5/6.9	66/13.2	15/3	3.5/0.7
Rice, Thai, Sticky, Sainsbury's*, 1 serving/100g					
	132/132	2.3/2.3	26.1/26.1	2/2	0.3/0.3
Rice, Tomato & Basil, Express, Uncle Ben's*, 1 pack/250g					
	450/180	9.8/3.9	78.8/31.5	10.8/4.3	0/0
Rice, Vegetable Pilau, Express, Uncle Ben's*, 1 pack/250g					
	445/178	8.5/3.4	84.5/33.8	8/3.2	0/0
Rice, Vegetable, Original, Bird's Eye*, 1oz/28g					
	29/105	1.1/4	5.8/20.8	0.2/0.6	0.3/1.1
Risotto, Cherry Tomato, COU, Marks & Spencer*, 1 pack/400g					
	320/80	7.6/1.9	66.4/16.6	3.6/0.9	7.2/1.8
Risotto, Chicken & Lemon, Weight Watchers*, 1 pack/330g					
	317/96	19.5/5.9	40.6/12.3	8.6/2.6	1.7/0.5
Risotto, Chicken, BGTY, Sainsbury's*, 1 pack/327g					
	356/109	24.5/7.5	50.7/15.5	6.2/1.9	3.3/1
Risotto, Mushroom, COU, Marks & Spencer*, 1 pack/330g					
	314/95	9.6/2.9	50.5/15.3	7.6/2.3	3.3/1
Risotto, Mushroom, Finest, Tesco*, 1 pack/350g					
	550/157	10.9/3.1	57.4/16.4	30.8/8.8	4.2/1.2

kcal serv/100g	prot serv/100g	carb serv/100g	fat serv/100g	fibre serv/100g
Risotto, Mushroom, Healthy Living, Tesco*, 1 pack/400g				
320/80	10.4/2.6	62.4/15.6	3.2/0.8	2.4/0.6
Risotto, Tomato & Cheese, GFY, Asda*, 1 pack/400g				
428/107	12.4/3.1	68/17	12/3	2.8/0.7
Rogan Josh, Prawn & Pilau Rice, BGTY, Sainsbury's*, 1 pack/401g				
353/88	19.2/4.8	61.4/15.3	3.2/0.8	7.6/1.9
Rogan Josh, Prawn, COU, Marks & Spencer*, 1 pack/400g				
360/90	19.6/4.9	64.8/16.2	2.4/0.6	3.2/0.8
Saag, Paneer, Sainsbury's*, ½ pack/200g				
380/190	17/8.5	9/4.5	30.6/15.3	2.4/1.2
Salad Bowl, Greek Style, Marks & Spencer*, 1 bowl/255g				
242/95	6.4/2.5	6.1/2.4	20.9/8.2	1.8/0.7
Salad, Bean, Three, Marks & Spencer*, 1 pack/225g				
225/100	13.1/5.8	37.6/16.7	2.9/1.3	8.8/3.9
Salad, Chargrilled Chicken Tesco*, 1 serving/300g				
384/128	18.3/6.1	45/15	14.4/4.8	7.2/2.4
Salad, Chick Pea & Cous Cous, Tesco*, 1 serving/250g				
245/98	8/3.2	38.8/15.5	6.5/2.6	0/0
Salad, Chicken & Bacon, Asda*, 1 pack/381.0g				
480/126	26.7/7	41.9/11	22.9/6	0/0
Salad, Chicken Caesar Bistro, Marks & Spencer*, ½ pack/135g				
189/140	6.8/5	8.8/6.5	14.3/10.6	0.8/0.6
Salad, Chicken Caesar, Tesco*, 1 pack/300g				
330/110	20.4/6.8	31.8/10.6	13.5/4.5	2.4/0.8
Salad, Chicken Caesar, Marks & Spencer*, ½ pack/140g				
266/190	9.4/6.7	12.2/8.7	20/14.3	1.1/0.8
Salad, Crayfish, Pret A Manger*, 1 av pack/320g				
200/63	9.7/3	2.5/0.8	16.7/5.2	0.8/0.3
Salad, Feta Cheese & Sunblushed Tomato, Marks & Spencer*, 1 serving/190g				
361/190	10.5/5.5	32.7/17.2	21.1/11.1	4/2.1
Salad, Italian Rice & Roasted Portobello Mushroom, Marks & Spencer*, ½ pack/130g				
130/100	3.6/2.8	27.6/21.2	0.7/0.5	0.8/0.6
Salad, Mixed Bean, Tesco*, 1 serving/70g				
49/70	2.2/3.2	9.2/13.1	0.4/0.5	1.3/1.9
Salad, Pasta & Pepper Side, Tesco*, 1 pack/230g				
278/121	5.5/2.4	29.9/13	15.2/6.6	3/1.3

kcal serv/100g	prot serv/100g	carb serv/100g	fat serv/100g	fibre serv/100g
Salad, Pesto Pasta, Pret A Manger*, 1 pack/320g				
442/138	12.7/4	24.5/7.7	32.9/10.3	3.4/1.1
Salad, Potato & Egg Side, Tesco*, 1 pack/300g				
192/64	7.5/2.5	12.6/4.2	12.3/4.1	3.3/1.1
Salad, Prawn Cocktail, Tesco*, 1 pack/300g				
360/120	17.1/5.7	32.7/10.9	18/6	2.4/0.8
Salad, Prawn Layered, Food To Go, Marks & Spencer*, 1 pack/220g				
176/80	10.6/4.8	21.1/9.6	5.3/2.4	2.4/1.1
Salad, Super Club, Pret A Manger*, 1 av pack/200g				
213/107	21.5/10.8	3.2/1.6	12.6/6.3	1.2/0.6
Salad, Sweet Chilli Chicken Noodle, COU, Marks & Spencer*, 1 pack/340g				
408/120	23.1/6.8	59.2/17.4	7.8/2.3	4.1/1.2
Salad, Tuna Layered, COU, Marks & Spencer*, 1 tub/450g				
360/80	30.2/6.7	37.4/8.3	9/2	3.6/0.8
Salad, Tuna Nicoise, Pret A Manger*, 1 av pack/300g				
194/65	26.7/8.9	2.9/1	8.4/2.8	2.9/1
Salad, Tuna Snack, Health Living, Tesco*, 1 serving/300g				
252/84	22.8/7.6	34.5/11.5	2.7/0.9	2.7/0.9
Samosas, Lamb, Morrisons*, 1 samosa/50g				
144/288	4.9/9.8	13.5/27	7.9/15.7	0.8/1.5
Samosas, Mini, Sainsbury's*, 1 serving/28g				
82/294	1.9/6.9	9.3/33.2	4.1/14.8	0.8/2.7
Samosas, Vegetable, Mini, Indian Snack Selection, Occasions, Sainsbury's*, 1 samosa/24.8g				
65/258	1.5/5.8	6.4/25.6	3.7/14.6	0.6/2.5
Samosas, Vegetable, Mini, Waitrose*, 2 samosas/59.8g				
146/244	2.7/4.5	17.2/28.7	7.4/12.4	1.7/2.8
Samosas, Vegetable, Northern Indian, Sainsbury's*, 1 samosa/50g				
126/252	2.9/5.8	15.3/30.6	5.9/11.8	1.3/2.6
Satay, Chicken, Sticks, Asda*, 1 stick/20g				
43/216	3.6/18	0.9/4.5	2.8/14	0/0
Sausage & Mash, Healthy Living, Tesco*, 1 pack/450g				
369/82	20.7/4.6	50.9/11.3	9.5/2.1	4.5/1
Sausage & Mash, with Onion Gravy, Healthy Eating, Tesco*, 1 pack/450g				
369/82	20.7/4.6	50.9/11.3	9.5/2.1	4.5/1
SlimFast, Pasta Carbonara with Cheese & Bacon, SlimFast*, 1 serving/70g				
240/343	15.9/22.7	34.2/48.9	4.4/6.3	4/5.7

kcal serv/100g	prot serv/100g	carb serv/100g	fat serv/100g	fibre serv/100g
Spaghetti Bolognese, BGTY, Sainsbury's*, 1 pack/450g				
392/87	21.2/4.7	66.6/14.8	4.5/1	5/1.1
Spaghetti Bolognese, GFY, Asda*, 1 serving/250g				
220/88	12.5/5	32.5/13	4.5/1.8	1.8/0.7
Spaghetti Bolognese, Heinz*, 1 can/400g				
344/86	13.6/3.4	51.2/12.8	9.2/2.3	2.8/0.7
Spaghetti Bolognese, Sainsbury's*, 1 pack/300g				
237/79	14.7/4.9	31.5/10.5	5.7/1.9	2.7/0.9
Spaghetti Bolognese, Tesco*, 1 pack/257g				
339/132	16.7/6.5	36.2/14.1	14.1/5.5	3.1/1.2
Spaghetti Bolognese, Weight Watchers*, 1 pack/320g				
301/94	18.6/5.8	46.7/14.6	4.2/1.3	3.2/1
Spaghetti Hoops, in Tomato Sauce, Heinz*, 1 can/400g				
224/56	7.6/1.9	46.8/11.7	0.8/0.2	2.4/0.6
Spaghetti Hoops, 'n' Hot Dogs, Heinz*, 1 can/400g				
304/76	11.2/2.8	44/11	9.6/2.4	1.6/0.4
Spaghetti Hoops, Tesco*, ½ can/205g				
123/60	3.3/1.6	26.4/12.9	0.4/0.2	1/0.5
Spaghetti, in Tomato Sauce with Parsley, Weight Watchers*, 1 can/400g				
196/49	7.2/1.8	40/10	0.8/0.2	2.4/0.6
Spaghetti, in Tomato Sauce, Heinz*, 1 can/400g				
244/61	6.8/1.7	52/13	0.8/0.2	2/0.5
Spaghetti, with Sausages, Heinz*, 1 can/400g				
328/82	14.8/3.7	44/11	10.4/2.6	2/0.5
Spring Rolls, Chicken, Asda*, 1 roll/58g				
115/199	2.7/4.6	14.5/25	5.2/9	2/3.4
Spring Rolls, Chinese Takeaway, Tesco*, 1 roll/50g				
101/201	2.2/4.4	13.2/26.4	4.3/8.6	0.8/1.5
Spring Rolls, Dim Sum, Sainsbury's*, 1 spring roll/12g				
26/216	0.5/4.1	3.4/28.2	1.2/9.6	0.3/2.9
Spring Rolls, Mini, Asda*, 1 roll/20g				
35/175	0.7/3.5	6.7/33.6	0.6/3	0.4/1.9
Spring Rolls, Mini, Sainsbury's, 1 roll/12g				
27/221	0.5/4.2	3.4/28.7	1.2/9.9	0.2/1.6
Spring Rolls, Mini, Tesco*, 1 roll/18g				
47/263	0.7/3.9	4.5/24.9	3/16.5	0.3/1.9
Spring Rolls, Vegetable, Asda*, 1 roll/62g				
126/203	2.2/3.5	16.7/27	5.6/9	1.7/2.7

	kcal serv/100g	prot serv/100g	carb serv/100g	fat serv/100g	fibre serv/100g

Spring Rolls, Vegetable, Chinese Takeaway, Sainsbury's*, 1 roll/59g

100/170	2.4/4	14.4/24.4	3.7/6.3	1.7/2.8

Spring Rolls, Vegetable, Chinese, Sainsbury's*, 1 roll/26g

69/193	1.5/4.1	9.7/26.9	2.8/7.7	0.5/1.4

Spring Rolls, Vegetable, Mini, Occasions, Sainsbury's*, 1 roll/24g

52/216	1/4.1	6.8/28.2	2.3/9.6	0.7/2.9

Spring Rolls, Vegetable, Mini, Party Food, Marks & Spencer*, 1 roll/17g

35/205	0.6/3.5	4.5/26.3	1.6/9.7	0.3/2

Spring Rolls, Vegetable, Tempura, Marks & Spencer*, 1 pack/140g

280/200	3.9/2.8	39.1/27.9	12/8.6	2.5/1.8

Spring Rolls, Vegetable, Tesco*, 1 roll/60g

100/166	2.4/4	12.7/21.2	4.3/7.2	1.2/2

Stew, Beef & Dumplings, Asda*, 1 pack/400g

392/98	24/6	44/11	13.2/3.3	3.2/0.8

Stew, Beef, Asda*, ½ can/196g

178/91	19.6/10	13.7/7	4.9/2.5	2.9/1.5

Stew, Beef, Meal for One, Marks & Spencer*, 1 pack/440g

350/80	30.8/7	38.3/8.7	8.4/1.9	8.8/2

Stew, Lentil & Winter Vegetable, Organic, Pure + Pronto*, 1 pack/400g

364/91	14.4/3.6	56/14	9.6/2.4	16/4

Stir-Fry, Beef & Black Bean, Sizzling, Oriental Express*, 1 pack/400g

420/105	28.8/7.2	56/14	8.4/2.1	8.4/2.1

Stir-Fry, Chinese Chicken, Sizzling, Oriental Express*, 1 pack/400g

400/100	26.4/6.6	55.2/13.8	8/2	6.8/1.7

Stir-Fry, Chinese Prawns, Sizzling, Oriental Express*, 1 pack/400g

384/96	15.6/3.9	58.8/14.7	9.6/2.4	6.4/1.6

Stir-Fry, Family, Tesco*, 1 serving/150g

51/34	3.3/2.2	8.1/5.4	0.6/0.4	2.6/1.7

Stir-Fry, Spicy Thai-Style Noodle, Tesco*, 1 pack/500g

335/67	13/2.6	42/8.4	13/2.6	6.5/1.3

Stortelli, Microwaveable, Dolmio*, 1 serving/220g

299/136	11.7/5.3	57.9/26.3	2.2/1	0/0

Stroganoff, Beef, with Rice, Tesco*, 1 pack/475g

518/109	26.6/5.6	65.1/13.7	16.6/3.5	16.2/3.4

Stroganoff, Chicken & Mushroom, COU, Marks & Spencer*, 1 pack/400g

340/85	34.4/8.6	36/9	6/1.5	4/1

Stroganoff, Mushroom with Rice, Tesco*, 1 pack/450g

500/111	13.5/3	57.6/12.8	23.9/5.3	5.9/1.3

	kcal serv/100g	prot serv/100g	carb serv/100g	fat serv/100g	fibre serv/100g
Stroganoff, Mushroom, BGTY, Sainsbury's*, 1 pack/451g					
	392/87	14.4/3.2	78.5/17.4	2.3/0.5	2.3/0.5
Stuffing Mix, Sage & Onion, Paxo*, 1 serving/60g					
	90/150	2.7/4.5	16.3/27.1	1.6/2.6	1.4/2.4
Stuffing, Sausage Meat, Balls, Aunt Bessie's*, 1 ball (baked)/26g					
	56/214	2/7.5	7.7/29.6	1.9/7.3	0.6/2.4
Sweet & Sour, Chicken Cantonese, Sainsbury's*, 1 pack/350g					
	368/105	36.4/10.4	51.1/14.6	2.1/0.6	2.1/0.6
Sweet & Sour, Chicken in Crispy Batter, Cantonese, Sainsbury's*, 1 pack/300g					
	546/182	27/9	64.2/21.4	20.1/6.7	3.3/1.1
Sweet & Sour, Chicken with Rice, Asda*, 1 pack/400g					
	440/110	18.8/4.7	88/22	1.2/0.3	2.4/0.6
Sweet & Sour, Pork, in Crispy Batter, Sainsbury's*, ½ pack/150g					
	293/195	15/10	30/20	12.5/8.3	1.7/1.1
Tagliatelle, Ham & Mushroom, BGTY, Sainsbury's*, 1 pack/450g					
	486/108	23.9/5.3	65.3/14.5	14.4/3.2	3.6/0.8
Tagliatelle, Ham & Mushroom, GFY, Asda*, 1 pack/400g					
	304/76	15.2/3.8	36/9	10.8/2.7	1.6/0.4
Tagliatelle, Ham & Mushroom, Healthy Eating, Tesco*, 1 meal/340g					
	306/90	14.6/4.3	46.2/13.6	6.8/2	3.1/0.9
Tagliatelle, Tomato & Basil Chicken, Weight Watchers*, 1 pack/330g					
	254/77	19.5/5.9	38.9/11.8	2/0.6	2.6/0.8
Tandoori Chicken Sizzler, Sainsbury's*, 1 pack/400g					
	536/134	51.2/12.8	17.2/4.3	29.2/7.3	6.8/1.7
Tandoori Chicken, Tesco*, 1 serving/175g					
	198/113	18.6/10.6	11.7/6.7	8.6/4.9	1.8/1
Tart, Goat's Cheese & Onion, Marks & Spencer*, 1 serving/161g					
	451/280	9.3/5.8	36.1/22.4	30.1/18.7	2.4/1.5
Tikka Masala, Chicken & Pilau Rice, Asda*, 1 pack/400g					
	548/137	28/7	64/16	20/5	6.4/1.6
Tikka Masala, Chicken & Rice, COU, Marks & Spencer*, 1 pack/400g					
	420/105	31.2/7.8	58.4/14.6	6.4/1.6	8.4/2.1
Tikka Masala, Chicken & Rice, Healthy Living, Tesco*, 1 pack/420g					
	483/115	31.9/7.6	68/16.2	9.7/2.3	6.7/1.6
Tikka Masala, Chicken & Rice, Takeaway, Tesco*, 1 pack/350g					
	525/150	15.4/4.4	71.1/20.3	20/5.7	4.2/1.2

kcal serv/100g	prot serv/100g	carb serv/100g	fat serv/100g	fibre serv/100g

Tikka Masala, Chicken with Pilau Rice, BGTY, Sainsbury's*, 1 pack/450g

| 428/95 | 35.1/7.8 | 57.2/12.7 | 6.3/1.4 | 4.1/0.9 |

Tikka Masala, Chicken with Pilau Rice, New, BGTY, Sainsbury's*, 1 pack/400g

| 416/104 | 32/8 | 64/16 | 3.6/0.9 | 7.2/1.8 |

Tikka Masala, Chicken, Boiled Rice & Nan, Meal For One, GFY, Asda*, 1 pack/605g

| 823/136 | 36.3/6 | 127.1/21 | 18.8/3.1 | 0/0 |

Tikka Masala, Chicken, Indian, Medium, Sainsbury's*, 1 pack/400g

| 848/212 | 52.8/13.2 | 21.2/5.3 | 61.2/15.3 | 0.4/0.1 |

Tikka Masala, Chicken, Tesco*, 1 pack/350g

| 511/146 | 38.9/11.1 | 15.1/4.3 | 32.9/9.4 | 5.3/1.5 |

Tortellini, Cheese, Weight Watchers*, 1 can/395g

| 233/59 | 8.3/2.1 | 33.6/8.5 | 7.1/1.8 | 2/0.5 |

Tortellini, Garlic & Herb, Fresh, Sainsbury's*, ½ pack/150g

| 365/243 | 16.7/11.1 | 48.3/32.2 | 11.7/7.8 | 2.7/1.8 |

Tortellini, Garlic, Basil & Ricotta, Asda*, 1 serving/150g

| 227/151 | 9/6 | 36/24 | 5.1/3.4 | 0/0 |

Tortellini, Ham & Cheese, Asda*, 1 serving/125g

| 191/153 | 8.8/7 | 25/20 | 6.3/5 | 2.3/1.8 |

Tortellini, Spinach & Ricotta, Tesco*, 1 serving/125g

| 323/258 | 14.9/11.9 | 45.3/36.2 | 9.1/7.3 | 2.4/1.9 |

Tortellini, Trio, Fresh, Tesco*, ½ pack/125g

| 323/258 | 16/12.8 | 44.8/35.8 | 8.9/7.1 | 2.5/2 |

Tortelloni, Spinach & Ricotta, Fresh, Safeway*, ½ pack/202g

| 341/169 | 14.9/7.4 | 48.5/24 | 9.7/4.8 | 4.8/2.4 |

Turkey Dinner, Roast Dinner, New, Bird's Eye*, 1 pack/340g

| 320/94 | 22.8/6.7 | 34/10 | 10.9/3.2 | 4.1/1.2 |

Wok Chinese, Findus*, 1 serving/250g

| 113/45 | 3.8/1.5 | 23.8/9.5 | 0.5/0.2 | 0/0 |

Wok Classic, Findus*, 1 serving/250g

| 113/45 | 5/2 | 18.8/7.5 | 1.3/0.5 | 0/0 |

Wonton, Prawn, Dim Sum Selection, Sainsbury's*, 1 wonton/10g

| 26/259 | 1.1/11.3 | 2.7/26.8 | 1.2/11.8 | 0.1/1.3 |

Wrap Kit, Chapati Bread, Tikka Masala, Patak's*, 1 bread/42.2g

| 121/287 | 3.2/7.5 | 22.3/53.1 | 2.7/6.4 | 1.3/3.2 |

Yorkshire Pudding 3", Baked, Aunt Bessie's*, 1 pudding/36g

| 91/252 | 3.2/9 | 13.1/36.4 | 2.8/7.9 | 0.6/1.7 |

	kcal serv/100g	prot serv/100g	carb serv/100g	fat serv/100g	fibre serv/100g

Yorkshire Pudding 7", Baked, Aunt Bessie's*, 1 pudding/110g

290/264	9.4/8.5	41.1/37.4	9.9/9	2.2/2

Yorkshire Pudding, Asda*, 1 pudding/30g

97/322	3/10	11.7/39	4.2/14	0.2/0.5

Yorkshire Pudding, Four-Minute, Aunt Bessie's*, 1 pudding/18g

59/326	1.7/9.6	6.9/38.4	2.7/14.8	0.4/2.1

Yorkshire Pudding, Giant, Aunt Bessie's*, 1 pudding/110g

290/264	9.4/8.5	41.1/37.4	9.9/9	2.2/2

Yorkshire Pudding, Individual, Asda*, 1 pudding/30.8g

50/162	1.8/5.8	7/22.7	1.6/5.2	0.2/0.6

Yorkshire Pudding, Individual, Aunt Bessie's*, 1 pudding/18g

59/326	1.7/9.6	6.9/38.4	2.7/14.8	0.4/2.1

Yorkshire Pudding, Large, Aunt Bessie's*, 1 pudding/39g

104/267	3.4/8.8	12.6/32.3	4.4/11.4	0.5/1.4

Yorkshire Pudding, Ready-To-Bake, Aunt Bessie's*, 1 pudding/17g

42/246	1.4/8.5	6/35.1	1.4/8	0.3/1.7

SANDWICHES

Bagel, Cheese & Jalapeno, Starbucks*, 1 bagel/115g

292/254	12.4/10.8	52.7/45.8	3.6/3.1	1.7/1.5

Bagel, Chicken, Lemon & Watercress, Safeway*, 1 pack/153g

329/215	19.6/12.8	43.1/28.2	6.3/4.1	0/0

Bagel, Smoked Salmon & Soft Cheese, Shapers, Boots*, 1 pack/158g

344/218	19/12	45.8/29	9.5/6	1.4/0.9

**Bagel, Soft Cheese & Smoked Salmon, American, Sainsbury's*,
1 bagel/130.9g**

356/272	10.9/8.3	41.7/31.8	16.2/12.4	2.2/1.7

Bagel, Tuna & Sweetcorn Relish, Safeway*, 1 bagel/162g

284/175	18.6/11.5	42.4/26.2	4.4/2.7	0/0

Bagel, Tuna Salad, BGTY, Sainsbury's*, 1 bagel/170g

325/191	17.7/10.4	44.2/26	7.1/4.2	1.7/1

**Bagel, Turkey, Pastrami & American Mustard, Shapers, Boots*,
1 bagel/146g**

296/203	16.1/11	46.7/32	5/3.4	2/1.4

Baguette, Cheese, Mixed, & Spring Onion, Asda*, 1 pack/190g

629/331	18.1/9.5	61/32.1	34.8/18.3	2.5/1.3

kcal serv/100g	prot serv/100g	carb serv/100g	fat serv/100g	fibre serv/100g
Baguette, Chicken & Mayonnaise, Asda*, 1 pack/190g				
407/214	18.4/9.7	58/30.5	16.5/8.7	2.5/1.3
Baguette, Chicken & Stuffing, Hot, Sainsbury's*, 1 baguette/227g				
543/239	31.1/13.7	67.2/29.6	16.3/7.2	0/0
Baguette, Chicken Tikka, Asda*, 1 pack/190g				
439/231	19.8/10.4	62.3/32.8	17.9/9.4	2.5/1.3
Baguette, Chicken Tikka, Hot, Sainsbury's*, 1 pack/190g				
386/203	16.2/8.5	54/28.4	11.6/6.1	0/0
Baguette, Egg & Tomato, Breakfast, Pret A Manger*, 1 av pack/230g				
281/122	12.4/5.4	36.5/15.9	12.1/5.3	5.7/2.5
Baguette, Egg & Tomato, Oldfields*, 1 pack/198g				
416/210	17.2/8.7	53.5/27	15/7.6	0/0
Baguette, Ham & Cheese, Snack 'n' Go, Sainsbury's*, 1 baguette/178g				
381/215	22.3/12.6	52.4/29.6	9/5.1	3.4/1.9
Baguette, Prawn Mayonnaise, Asda*, 1 pack/190g				
399/210	17.3/9.1	61.8/32.5	9.3/4.9	2.5/1.3
Baguette, Salmon & Egg, Pret A Manger*, 1 av pack/230g				
349/152	16.6/7.2	35.1/15.3	15.9/6.9	3.4/1.5
Baguette, Steak & Onion, Snack 'n' Go, Sainsbury's*, 1 baguette/177g				
396/225	25.2/14.3	53.9/30.6	8.8/5	3.9/2.2
Baguette, Tuna Mayo, Pret A Manger*, 1 av pack/230g				
535/233	24.8/10.8	57.6/25	22.9/10	3.9/1.7
Baguette, Tuna Melt, Sainsbury's*, 1 serving/204g				
373/183	23.1/11.3	52.6/25.8	8/3.9	0/0
Baton, Chicken & Bacon, Tesco*, 1 pack/201g				
511/254	18.9/9.4	49.6/24.7	26.3/13.1	3.4/1.7
Croissant, Smoked Ham & Cheese, Marks & Spencer*, 1 croissant/105g				
341/325	14.1/13.4	23.3/22.2	22.7/21.6	4.1/3.9
Flatbread, BBQ-Style Chicken, Shapers, Boots*, 1 serving/108g				
187/173	10.8/10	24.8/23	5/4.6	3/2.8
Flatbread, Cajun-Style Chicken, GFY, Asda*, 1 wrap/176.3g				
231/131	15.8/9	37/21	2.1/1.2	1.6/0.9
Flatbread, Chicken Caesar, Shapers, Boots*, 1 serving/160g				
254/159	20.8/13	35.2/22	3.4/2.1	3.2/2
Flatbread, Chicken Tikka, Shapers, Boots*, 1 flatbread/164g				
282/172	18/11	39.4/24	5.9/3.6	2.3/1.4
Flatbread, Chinese Chicken, Shapers, Boots*, 1 pack/159.3g				
273/172	17.5/11	46.1/29	2.1/1.3	2.9/1.8

kcal serv/100g	prot serv/100g	carb serv/100g	fat serv/100g	fibre serv/100g
Flatbread, Feta Cheese, Shapers, Boots*, 1 pack/165.6g				
256/154	11.1/6.7	38.2/23	6.5/3.9	2.3/1.4
Flatbread, Greek-Style Salad, Waitrose*, 1 pack/171.8g				
280/163	12.7/7.4	38.4/22.3	8.4/4.9	5.7/3.3
Flatbread, Italian Chicken, Shapers, Boots*, 1 pack/168.4g				
265/158	16.8/10	37/22	5.5/3.3	2.2/1.3
Flatbread, Mexican-Style Chicken, Safeway*, 1 pack/150g				
248/165	17.4/11.6	37.1/24.7	3.2/2.1	2.9/1.9
Flatbread, Peking Duck, Less Than 3% Fat, Shapers, Boots*, 1 pack/155.7g				
246/158	11.2/7.2	42.1/27	3.7/2.4	3/1.9
Flatbread, Prawn Korma, Shapers, Boots*, 1 pack/169.0g				
267/158	14.9/8.8	37.2/22	6.6/3.9	2.2/1.3
Flatbread, Rancher's Chicken, COU, Marks & Spencer*, 1 pack/174g				
270/155	19/10.9	40/23	3.5/2	2.6/1.5
Flatbread, Ranchers Chicken, Shapers, Boots*, 1 pack/194.2g				
303/156	23.3/12	42.7/22	4.3/2.2	2.9/1.5
Flatbread, Spicy Chicken & Salsa, Healthy Living, Tesco, 1 flatbread/183.2g				
251/137	18.5/10.1	38.6/21.1	2.6/1.4	2.2/1.2
Flatbread, Spicy Mexican, Shapers, Boots*, 1 pack/190g				
296/156	13.3/7	43.7/23	7.6/4	7/3.7
Flatbread, Sticky BBQ-Style Chicken, Shapers, Boots*, 1 pack/158.4g				
273/173	15.8/10	36.3/23	7.3/4.6	4.4/2.8
Melt, Tuna, Go Large, Asda*, 1 roll/175g				
509/291	21/12	47.3/27	26.3/15	0/0
Melt, Tuna, Marks & Spencer*, 1 pack/218g				
621/285	28.3/13	43.8/20.1	37.1/17	2.2/1
Panini, Egg & Bacon, Starbucks*, 1 panini/210g				
458/218	23.3/11.1	46.2/22	20/9.5	0/0
Panini, Ham & Swiss Cheese, Coffee Republic*, 1 panini/223g				
558/250	35/15.7	45.7/20.5	26.1/11.7	0/0
Panini, Mozzarella, Tomato & Pesto, Costa*, 1 panini/209g				
487/233	20.1/9.6	73.4/35.1	15/7.2	10.5/5
Panini, Mozzarella & Tomato, Coffee Republic*, 1 panini/255g				
566/222	28.3/11.1	60.2/23.6	25.5/10	0/0
Panini, Mozzarella & Tomato, Marks & Spencer*, 1 serving/176g				
484/275	19.9/11.3	37.5/21.3	28.5/16.2	3.7/2.1
Roll, Beef, Weight Watchers*, 1 roll/174g				
276/159	18.8/10.8	40.2/23.1	4.4/2.5	1.7/1

kcal serv/100g	prot serv/100g	carb serv/100g	fat serv/100g	fibre serv/100g
Roll, Brown, Roast Chicken & Mayonnaise, Big, Sainsbury's*, 1 pack/185g				
479/259	17.8/9.6	40.3/21.8	27.4/14.8	0/0
Roll, Cheese & Pickle, Sainsbury's*, 1 roll/136g				
359/264	14.4/10.6	47.7/35.1	13.6/10	0/0
Roll, Cheese & Tomato, Benjys*, 1 pack/263g				
742/282	32.1/12.2	78.4/29.8	33.4/12.7	0/0
Roll, Chicken & Herb, Shapers, Boots*, 1 roll/167.6g				
291/173	20.2/12	42/25	4.7/2.8	2.9/1.7
Roll, Chicken Salad, Healthy Eating, Tesco*, 1 serving/224g				
289/129	23.1/10.3	35.8/16	5.8/2.6	2.5/1.1
Roll, Egg & Tomato, Shapers, Boots*, 1 roll/166.3g				
300/181	13.3/8	49.8/30	5.3/3.2	4.3/2.6
Roll, Ham & Pineapple, Eat Smart, Safeway*, 1 serving/180g				
225/125	20.2/11.2	31/17.2	2/1.1	4.7/2.6
Roll, Ham Salad, BGTY, Sainsbury's*, 1 roll/178g				
292/164	17.8/10	41.5/23.3	6.1/3.4	0/0
Roll, Ham Salad, Good Intentions, Somerfield*, 1 pack/213.8g				
325/152	18.6/8.7	52/24.3	4.7/2.2	3.4/1.6
Roll, Leicester Ham & Cheese, Sub, Waitrose*, 1 pack/206.4ml				
581/282	26/12.6	49.4/24	31.1/15.1	26.8/13
Roll, Roast Pork, Stuffing & Apple Sauce, Boots*, 1 roll/218.1g				
602/276	21.8/10	69.8/32	26.2/12	3.9/1.8
Roll, Smoked Ham & Honey Roasted Pineapple, Marks & Spencer*, 1 roll/179g				
260/145	17.7/9.9	40.6/22.7	2.5/1.4	5.4/3
Roll, Spicy Chicken, Crusty, Marks & Spencer*, 1 roll/150g				
383/255	19.2/12.8	38.7/25.8	16.7/11.1	3/2
Roll, Tuna & Sweetcorn with Mayonnaise, Shell*, 1 pack/180g				
536/298	23.6/13.1	51.5/28.6	26.3/14.6	0/0
Sandwich, All-Day Breakfast, Finest, Tesco*, 1 pack/275g				
660/240	26.7/9.7	45.1/16.4	41.5/15.1	4.4/1.6
Sandwich, All-Day Breakfast, Ginsters*, 1 pack/241.3g				
537/223	26/10.8	48.9/20.3	26.5/11	0/0
Sandwich, All-Day Breakfast, Healthy Living, Tesco*, 1 pack/223.1g				
328/147	26.5/11.9	37.5/16.8	8/3.6	6/2.7
Sandwich, All-Day Breakfast, The Big Eat Street, Safeway*, 1 pack/213.1g				
584/274	25.8/12.1	49.2/23.1	31.5/14.8	4.5/2.1

kcal serv/100g	prot serv/100g	carb serv/100g	fat serv/100g	fibre serv/100g
Sandwich, All-Day Breakfast, Walls*, 1 pack/225.1g				
610/271	20.7/9.2	54.7/24.3	34.7/15.4	3.2/1.4
Sandwich, Apple, Cheese & Celery, Asda*, 1 pack/173.0g				
244/141	13.8/8	36.3/21	4.8/2.8	4.7/2.7
Sandwich, Avocado & Alfalfa Sprout, Pret A Manger*, 1 av pack/250g				
329/132	8.5/3.4	28.9/11.6	20/8	5.9/2.4
Sandwich, Avocado & Italian Matured Cheese, Open, Pret A Manger*,				
1 av pack/250g				
438/175	9.5/3.8	28.3/11.3	31.9/12.8	7.4/3
Sandwich, Avocado, Mozzarella & Tomato, Marks & Spencer*,				
1 pack/272.9g				
655/240	24/8.8	59.2/21.7	36/13.2	6.3/2.3
Sandwich, Bacon, Lettuce & Tomato, Daily Bread*, 1 pack/171.1g				
344/201	15.6/9.1	36.9/21.6	18.8/11	0/0
Sandwich, Bacon, Lettuce & Tomato, Ginsters*, 1 pack/192g				
516/269	30/15.6	40.7/21.2	30/15.6	0/0
Sandwich, Bacon, Lettuce & Tomato, Safeway*, 1 pack/230g				
529/230	36.6/15.9	81.4/35.4	5.3/2.3	9/3.9
Sandwich, Bacon, Chicken & Avocado, Ultimate, Marks & Spencer*,				
1 pack/241g				
552/229	25.8/10.7	43.1/17.9	30.6/12.7	6.7/2.8
Sandwich, Bacon, Chicken, Cheese Triple, BGTY, Sainsbury's*, 1 pack/263g				
534/203	30.8/11.7	51/19.4	20/7.6	11.6/4.4
Sandwich, Bacon, Chicken, Cheese, Big, Sainsbury's*, 1 pack/254g				
734/289	29.7/11.7	45.7/18	45.5/17.9	0/0
Sandwich, Bacon, Lettuce & Tomato, Asda*, 1 pack/262g				
618/236	32/12.2	53.2/20.3	31.4/12	7.9/3
Sandwich, Bacon, Lettuce & Tomato, BGTY, Sainsbury's*, 1 pack/180g				
268/149	19.4/10.8	37.4/20.8	4.5/2.5	2.9/1.6
Sandwich, Bacon, Lettuce & Tomato, COU, Marks & Spencer*, 1 pack/174g				
270/155	19.1/11	39/22.4	4/2.3	4.2/2.4
Sandwich, Bacon, Lettuce & Tomato, GFY, Asda*, 1 pack/171g				
294/172	15.4/9	44.5/26	6/3.5	2.7/1.6
Sandwich, Bacon, Lettuce & Tomato, Healthy Eating, Tesco*, 1 pack/165g				
221/134	17/10.3	32.7/19.8	2.5/1.5	3.3/2
Sandwich, Bacon, Lettuce & Tomato, Healthy Living, Tesco*, 1 pack/190g				
287/151	19.2/10.1	46.6/24.5	2.7/1.4	3/1.6

kcal serv/100g	prot serv/100g	carb serv/100g	fat serv/100g	fibre serv/100g

Sandwich, Bacon, Lettuce & Tomato, Marks & Spencer*, 1 pack/194g

| 631/325 | 22.7/11.7 | 41.1/21.2 | 40.9/21.1 | 2.5/1.3 |

Sandwich, Bacon, Lettuce & Tomato, Starbucks*, 1 pack/190g

| 437/230 | 14.6/7.7 | 53.8/28.3 | 18.2/9.6 | 0/0 |

Sandwich, Bacon, Lettuce & Tomato, Tesco*, 1 pack/203g

| 629/310 | 16.2/8 | 37.4/18.4 | 46.1/22.7 | 2.8/1.4 |

Sandwich, Bacon, Lettuce & Tomato, Waitrose*, 1 pack/210g

| 578/275 | 19.5/9.3 | 53.8/25.6 | 31.5/15 | 4.8/2.3 |

Sandwich, Bacon, Lettuce & Tomato, Weight Watchers*, 1 pack/171g

| 274/160 | 16.8/9.8 | 40.9/23.9 | 4.8/2.8 | 4.1/2.4 |

Sandwich, Bacon, Lettuce & Tomato, with Mayo, Safeway*, 1 pack/168g

| 462/275 | 17.5/10.4 | 34.8/20.7 | 28.1/16.7 | 3.9/2.3 |

Sandwich, Bap, Malted, Chargrilled Chicken, Co-Op*, 1 bap/201g

| 492/245 | 18.1/9 | 46.2/23 | 26.1/13 | 4/2 |

Sandwich, Bap, Malted, Tuna & Sweetcorn, Co-Op*, 1 bap/212g

| 530/250 | 19.1/9 | 50.9/24 | 27.6/13 | 4.2/2 |

Sandwich, Barm, White, Corned Beef & Onion, Open Choice Foods*, 1 roll/144g

| 331/230 | 18.3/12.7 | 44.2/30.7 | 8.8/6.1 | 0/0 |

Sandwich, BBQ Chicken & Flamed Veg, Calorie Conscious, Northern Bites*, 1 pack/163g

| 287/176 | 21.7/13.3 | 30/18.4 | 9/5.5 | 3.4/2.1 |

Sandwich, BBQ Chicken & Ranch Coleslaw, Big, Sainsbury's*, 1 pack/276.6g

| 474/171 | 25.5/9.2 | 62.9/22.7 | 13.3/4.8 | 0/0 |

Sandwich, BBQ Chicken on Malted Bread, Fresh Bite*, 1 pack/225.8g

| 341/151 | 20.3/9 | 52.9/23.4 | 5.4/2.4 | 0/0 |

Sandwich, BBQ Chicken Wedge, Tesco*, 1 pack/195g

| 321/165 | 19.8/10.2 | 53.5/27.4 | 3.1/1.6 | 2/1 |

Sandwich, BBQ Rib, Rustlers*, 1 pack/170g

| 444/261 | 24.8/14.6 | 40.5/23.8 | 20.2/11.9 | 0/0 |

Sandwich, Beef & Horseradish Mayonnaise, Shapers, Boots*, 1 pack/159.3g

| 266/167 | 19.1/12 | 39.8/25 | 3.3/2.1 | 4.1/2.6 |

Sandwich, Beef & Horseradish, Deep-Filled, BGTY, Sainsbury's*, 1 pack/202g

| 313/155 | 23/11.4 | 44.4/22 | 4.8/2.4 | 4.8/2.4 |

	kcal serv/100g	prot serv/100g	carb serv/100g	fat serv/100g	fibre serv/100g

Sandwich, Beef & Horseradish, Pret A Manger*, 1 av pack/250g

382/153	28/11.2	44.3/17.7	10.9/4.4	6.2/2.5

Sandwich, Beef & Roast Onion, Healthy Living, Tesco*, 1 pack/185.3g

278/150	24.6/13.3	37/20	3.5/1.9	5/2.7

Sandwich, Beef Salad, Gibsons*, 1 pack/185g

348/188	19.7/10.6	43.5/23.5	10.6/5.7	0/0

Sandwich, BLT, Eat Smart, Safeway*, 1 pack/165g

231/140	16.2/9.8	36/21.8	2.3/1.4	4/2.4

Sandwich, Breakfast, Mega Triple, Co-Op*, 1 pack/267g

750/281	31/11.6	68/25.5	40/15	9/3.4

Sandwich, Brie & Bacon, Asda*, 1 pack/181g

603/333	24.1/13.3	41.4/22.9	38.2/21.1	2.4/1.3

Sandwich, Brie & Grape, Finest, Tesco*, 1 pack/209g

527/252	17.8/8.5	43.1/20.6	31.6/15.1	3.1/1.5

Sandwich, Brie with Apple & Grapes, Sainsbury's*, 1 pack/220g

515/234	18.5/8.4	47.7/21.7	29.9/13.6	0/0

Sandwich, British Ham & Salad, COU, Marks & Spencer*, 1 pack/185g

259/140	16.3/8.8	39.6/21.4	3.5/1.9	6.5/3.5

Sandwich, Chargrilled Chicken & Watercress, BGTY, Sainsbury's*,
1 pack/172g

318/185	24.9/14.5	41.5/24.1	5.8/3.4	0/0

Sandwich, Chargrilled Chicken & Watercress, Marks & Spencer*,
1 pack/173g

285/165	22.1/12.8	41.3/23.9	2.9/1.7	3.6/2.1

Sandwich, Chargrilled Chicken Salad, Weight Watchers*, 1 pack/186g

296/159	18.4/9.9	37.9/20.4	7.8/4.2	3.5/1.9

Sandwich, Chargrilled Chicken Salsa, BGTY, Sainsbury's*, 1 pack/225g

306/136	23.9/10.6	44.8/19.9	3.6/1.6	6.5/2.9

Sandwich, Chargrilled Chicken with Honey Mustard Mayo, Spar*,
1 pack/168g

428/255	22/13.1	42/25	19.2/11.4	0/0

Sandwich, Chargrilled Chicken with Salad, Debenhams*, 1 pack/250g

325/130	19/7.6	45/18	9/3.6	0/0

Sandwich, Chargrilled Chicken, Budgens*, 1 pack/192.8g

483/250	19.9/10.3	48.1/24.9	23.4/12.1	3.5/1.8

Sandwich, Chargrilled Chicken, Ginsters*, 1 pack/209g

431/206	23.6/11.3	45.1/21.6	17.3/8.3	0/0

kcal serv/100g	prot serv/100g	carb serv/100g	fat serv/100g	fibre serv/100g

Sandwich, Cheddar Cheese Ploughman's, Deep-Fill, Asda*, 1 pack/228.6g

| 472/206 | 20.6/9 | 45.8/20 | 22.9/10 | 9.8/4.3 |

Sandwich, Cheddar Cheese Ploughman's, Marks & Spencer*, 1 pack/185g

| 435/235 | 17.8/9.6 | 43.8/23.7 | 22.9/12.4 | 4.6/2.5 |

Sandwich, Cheese & Celery, Marks & Spencer*, 1 pack/180g

| 466/259 | 19.4/10.8 | 26.5/14.7 | 31.3/17.4 | 5.2/2.9 |

Sandwich, Cheese & Coleslaw, Eat Smart, Safeway*, 1 pack/169.0g

| 245/145 | 17.1/10.1 | 35/20.7 | 3.7/2.2 | 6.8/4 |

Sandwich, Cheese & Coleslaw, Safeway*, 1 pack/187g

| 501/268 | 15.7/8.4 | 42.8/22.9 | 32/17.1 | 0.9/0.5 |

Sandwich, Cheese & Coleslaw, Shapers, Boots*, 1 pack/224g

| 338/151 | 24.6/11 | 49.3/22 | 4.7/2.1 | 7.2/3.2 |

Sandwich, Cheese & Marmite, No Mayonnaise, Boots*, 1 pack/156g

| 420/269 | 19/12.2 | 41/26.3 | 20/12.8 | 2.7/1.7 |

Sandwich, Cheese & Onion, GFY, Asda*, 1 pack/156g

| 253/162 | 20.3/13 | 35.9/23 | 3.1/2 | 0/0 |

Sandwich, Cheese & Onion, Healthy Living, Tesco, 1 pack/168g

| 314/187 | 17.3/10.3 | 39/23.2 | 9.9/5.9 | 2.9/1.7 |

Sandwich, Cheese & Onion, Heinz*, 1 pack/197g

| 563/286 | 22.1/11.2 | 47.3/24 | 31.7/16.1 | 6.3/3.2 |

Sandwich, Cheese & Onion, Tesco*, 1 pack/178g

| 621/349 | 20.5/11.5 | 30.4/17.1 | 46.5/26.1 | 3.9/2.2 |

Sandwich, Cheese & Pickle, BHS*, 1 pack/177.7g

| 504/283 | 22.3/12.5 | 52.7/29.6 | 22.6/12.7 | 3.2/1.8 |

Sandwich, Cheese & Pickle, Shapers, Boots*, 1 pack/165g

| 342/207 | 16.2/9.8 | 51.2/31 | 8.1/4.9 | 3.8/2.3 |

Sandwich, Cheese & Salad, COU, Marks & Spencer*, 1 pack/188g

| 244/130 | 22.7/12.1 | 32/17 | 3/1.6 | 4.5/2.4 |

Sandwich, Cheese & Spring Onion, Asda*, 1 pack/172g

| 635/369 | 20/11.6 | 38.9/22.6 | 44.4/25.8 | 5.3/3.1 |

Sandwich, Cheese & Tomato, Asda*, 1 pack/154g

| 388/252 | 16.9/11 | 35.7/23.2 | 19.7/12.8 | 5.7/3.7 |

Sandwich, Cheese & Tomato, Co-Op*, 1 pack/161g

| 394/245 | 16.1/10 | 37/23 | 19.3/12 | 3.2/2 |

Sandwich, Cheese & Tomato, Freshmans*, 1 pack/111g

| 248/223 | 12.2/11 | 8.9/8 | 18.6/16.8 | 0/0 |

Sandwich, Cheese & Tomato, Organic, Marks & Spencer*, 1 pack/165g

| 559/339 | 19.5/11.8 | 40.9/24.8 | 35.3/21.4 | 3.1/1.9 |

kcal serv/100g	prot serv/100g	carb serv/100g	fat serv/100g	fibre serv/100g
Sandwich, Cheese & Tomato, Tesco*, 1 pack/182g				
582/320	16.7/9.2	41.1/22.6	38.9/21.4	2/1.1
Sandwich, Cheese Coleslaw, Marks & Spencer*, 1 pack/186g				
498/268	19/10.2	32.7/17.6	32.4/17.4	6/3.2
Sandwich, Cheese Ploughman's, BGTY, Sainsbury's*, 1 pack/216.7g				
365/168	21/9.7	53.2/24.5	7.6/3.5	0/0
Sandwich, Cheese Ploughman's, Deep-Filled, Safeway*, 1 pack/231.4g				
589/255	26.3/11.4	47.8/20.7	32.6/14.1	6.5/2.8
Sandwich, Cheese Ploughman's, Healthy Living, Tesco*, 1 pack/186g				
279/150	20.8/11.2	41.5/22.3	3.3/1.8	1.7/0.9
Sandwich, Cheese Ploughman's, Marks & Spencer*, 1 pack/192.3g				
499/260	17.5/9.1	48.2/25.1	25.7/13.4	5.8/3
Sandwich, Cheese Salad, Budgens*, 1 pack/168.9g				
250/148	18.4/10.9	37/21.9	3/1.8	2.7/1.6
Sandwich, Cheese, Tomato & Spring Onion, Shapers, Boots*, 1 pack/179g				
344/192	19.7/11	39.4/22	12/6.7	5.9/3.3
Sandwich, Cheese, Apple & Grape, COU, Marks & Spencer*, 1 pack/186.2g				
270/145	15.8/8.5	46.3/24.9	2.2/1.2	3.7/2
Sandwich, Cheese, Asda*, 1 pack/262g				
618/236	32/12.2	53.2/20.3	31.4/12	7.9/3
Sandwich, Cheese, Ham, BLT, Triple pack, Asda*, 1 pack/260g				
614/236	31.7/12.2	52.8/20.3	31.2/12	7.8/3
Sandwich, Cheese, Pickle & Tomato, Somerfield*, 1 pack/166.5g				
317/191	20.8/12.5	42.5/25.6	7.1/4.3	5.8/3.5
Sandwich, Cheese, Tomato & Spring Onion, Shapers, Boots*, 1 pack/178.2g				
319/179	21.4/12	42.7/24	6.9/3.9	2.7/1.5
Sandwich, Chicken & Avocado, Pret A Manger*, 1 av pack/250g				
523/209	21/8.4	39.8/15.9	31/12.4	8.5/3.4
Sandwich, Chicken & Bacon, Club, Starbucks*, 1 pack/252g				
590/234	29/11.5	32.3/12.8	38.6/15.3	0/0
Sandwich, Chicken & Bacon, Good Intentions, Somerfield*, 1 pack/168g				
282/168	18/10.7	41.8/24.9	4.9/2.9	3.9/2.3
Sandwich, Chicken & Bacon, Healthy Eating, Tesco*, 1 pack/155g				
240/155	16.1/10.4	38.1/24.6	2.6/1.7	2.6/1.7
Sandwich, Chicken & Bacon, Marks & Spencer*, 1 pack/173g				
450/260	24.4/14.1	41.2/23.8	20.9/12.1	5.9/3.4
Sandwich, Chicken & Bacon, Shapers, Boots*, 1 pack/179g				
317/177	25.1/14	34/19	9/5	5.5/3.1

	kcal serv/100g	prot serv/100g	carb serv/100g	fat serv/100g	fibre serv/100g

Sandwich, Chicken & Bacon, Tesco*, 1 pack/195g

| 538/276 | 21.8/11.2 | 36.5/18.7 | 33.9/17.4 | 2.5/1.3 |

Sandwich, Chicken & Black Pepper Mayonnaise, Chicken Salad,
Chicken & Smoked Ham, Shapers, Boots*, 1 pack/238.3g

| 397/167 | 30.9/13 | 54.7/23 | 7.6/3.2 | 7.1/3 |

Sandwich, Chicken & Pepperonata, COU, Marks & Spencer*, 1 pack/171.4g

| 239/140 | 17.8/10.4 | 35.7/20.9 | 2.9/1.7 | 2.2/1.3 |

Sandwich, Chicken & Roast Ham, Tesco*, 1 pack/228g

| 561/246 | 30.3/13.3 | 37.8/16.6 | 31.9/14 | 2.7/1.2 |

Sandwich, Chicken & Salad, COU, Cafe, Marks & Spencer*, 1 pack/193g

| 261/135 | 18.9/9.8 | 36.7/19 | 3.7/1.9 | 3.1/1.6 |

Sandwich, Chicken & Salad, Low-Fat, Waitrose*, 1 pack/188g

| 291/155 | 19.6/10.4 | 35/18.6 | 8.1/4.3 | 3.9/2.1 |

Sandwich, Chicken & Salad, Marks & Spencer*, 1 pack/200g

| 408/204 | 18.4/9.2 | 35.2/17.6 | 21.6/10.8 | 3/1.5 |

Sandwich, Chicken & Stuffing, Marks & Spencer*, 1 pack/166g

| 412/248 | 20.3/12.2 | 33.4/20.1 | 21.9/13.2 | 4.8/2.9 |

Sandwich, Chicken & Stuffing, Tesco*, 1 pack/323g

| 1043/323 | 33.6/10.4 | 95/29.4 | 58.8/18.2 | 3.2/1 |

Sandwich, Chicken & Stuffing, Waitrose*, 1 pack/183g

| 450/246 | 23.4/12.8 | 46.8/25.6 | 18.8/10.3 | 2.7/1.5 |

Sandwich, Chicken & Sweetcorn, Marks & Spencer*, 1 pack/186g

| 394/212 | 20.3/10.9 | 36.8/19.8 | 18.6/10 | 3.7/2 |

Sandwich, Chicken & Sweetcorn, Shapers, Boots*, 1 pack/180g

| 324/180 | 21.6/12 | 45/25 | 6.3/3.5 | 3.6/2 |

Sandwich, Chicken & Sweetcorn, Tesco*, 1 pack/194g

| 433/223 | 18.2/9.4 | 42.9/22.1 | 21/10.8 | 3.3/1.7 |

Sandwich, Chicken Caesar, Boots*, 1 pack/226.0g

| 531/235 | 22.1/9.8 | 49.7/22 | 27.1/12 | 3.8/1.7 |

Sandwich, Chicken Caesar, Finest, Tesco*, 1 pack/199g

| 454/228 | 30.6/15.4 | 38.2/19.2 | 19.9/10 | 2.8/1.4 |

Sandwich, Chicken Mayonnaise with Tomato, Lettuce & Cucumber,
Oldfields*, 1 pack/171.8g

| 372/216 | 18.2/10.6 | 35.3/20.5 | 17.7/10.3 | 0/0 |

Sandwich, Chicken No Mayo, Marks & Spencer*, 1 pack/142g

| 220/155 | 21.3/15 | 24.9/17.5 | 4.3/3 | 4.4/3.1 |

Sandwich, Chicken Pesto with Rocket, Woolworths*, 1 pack/195g

| 326/167 | 9.8/5 | 33/16.9 | 17.2/8.8 | 0/0 |

kcal serv/100g	prot serv/100g	carb serv/100g	fat serv/100g	fibre serv/100g

Sandwich, Chicken Salad on Malted Bread with Mayo, Safeway*, 1 pack/195g

| 392/201 | 21.3/10.9 | 36.5/18.7 | 17.9/9.2 | 4.1/2.1 |

Sandwich, Chicken Salad with Mayo, BGTY, Sainsbury's*, 1 serving/200g

| 314/157 | 24/12 | 43.8/21.9 | 4.8/2.4 | 0/0 |

Sandwich, Chicken Salad, BGTY, Sainsbury's*, 1 pack/197g

| 278/141 | 20.3/10.3 | 36.6/18.6 | 5.9/3 | 0/0 |

Sandwich, Chicken Salad, Big Fill, Somerfield*, 1 pack/247.8g

| 513/207 | 28.5/11.5 | 50.6/20.4 | 21.8/8.8 | 5/2 |

Sandwich, Chicken Salad, COU, Marks & Spencer*, 1 pack/194g

| 256/132 | 19/9.8 | 36.9/19 | 3.7/1.9 | 3.1/1.6 |

Sandwich, Chicken Salad, Deep-Filled, Safeway*, 1 pack/211.9g

| 445/210 | 23.3/11 | 44.7/21.1 | 18.7/8.8 | 7.8/3.7 |

Sandwich, Chicken Salad, Eat Smart, Safeway*, 1 pack/183g

| 265/145 | 25.1/13.7 | 31.3/17.1 | 4.2/2.3 | 1.5/0.8 |

Sandwich, Chicken Salad, GFY, Asda*, 1 pack/194g

| 239/123 | 21.3/11 | 36.9/19 | 1.7/0.9 | 5.4/2.8 |

Sandwich, Chicken Salad, Healthy Eating, Tesco*, 1 pack/195g

| 255/131 | 20.7/10.6 | 32.4/16.6 | 4.8/2.5 | 7.7/3.9 |

Sandwich, Chicken Salad, Healthy Living, Co-Op*, 1 pack/180g

| 297/165 | 18/10 | 41.4/23 | 7.2/4 | 5.4/3 |

Sandwich, Chicken Salad, Heinz*, 1 pack/165.5g

| 246/148 | 19.6/11.8 | 37/22.3 | 2.2/1.3 | 8.8/5.3 |

Sandwich, Chicken Salad, Low-Fat, Healthy, Spar*, 1 pack/191g

| 300/157 | 15.1/7.9 | 40.5/21.2 | 8.6/4.5 | 0/0 |

Sandwich, Chicken Salad, Prawn Mayo, Egg & Bacon, Waitrose*, 1 pack/246g

| 608/247 | 24.1/9.8 | 43.8/17.8 | 37.4/15.2 | 5.9/2.4 |

Sandwich, Chicken Salad, Scottish Slimmers*, 1 pack/168.7g

| 275/163 | 16.1/9.5 | 38.5/22.8 | 6.4/3.8 | 3/1.8 |

Sandwich, Chicken Salad, Waitrose*, 1 pack/208g

| 406/195 | 21.4/10.3 | 35.6/17.1 | 19.8/9.5 | 5.2/2.5 |

Sandwich, Chicken Tandoori, Waitrose*, 1 pack/181g

| 302/167 | 21/11.6 | 41.6/23 | 5.6/3.1 | 7.4/4.1 |

Sandwich, Chicken Tikka & Cucumber on Brown Bread, Royal London Hospital*, 1 pack/200g

| 330/165 | 18.8/9.4 | 35/17.5 | 12.8/6.4 | 0/0 |

kcal serv/100g	prot serv/100g	carb serv/100g	fat serv/100g	fibre serv/100g

Sandwich, Chicken Tikka Masala, GO Foods Wonderfill*, 1 pack/136g

| 343/252 | 15.5/11.4 | 32/23.5 | 17.4/12.8 | 0/0 |

Sandwich, Chicken Tikka, Asda*, 1 pack/186g

| 316/170 | 20.5/11 | 39.1/21 | 8.7/4.7 | 2.8/1.5 |

Sandwich, Chicken Tikka, COU, Marks & Spencer*, 1 pack/185g

| 268/145 | 22.4/12.1 | 37.9/20.5 | 3.3/1.8 | 5.9/3.2 |

Sandwich, Chicken Tikka, Eat Smart, Safeway*, 1 pack/159g

| 240/151 | 18.8/11.8 | 34.3/21.6 | 3/1.9 | 4/2.5 |

Sandwich, Chicken Tikka, Improved Recipe, COU, Marks & Spencer*, 1 pack/186g

| 270/145 | 22.5/12.1 | 38.1/20.5 | 3.3/1.8 | 6/3.2 |

Sandwich, Chicken Tikka, Marks & Spencer*, 1 pack/180g

| 391/217 | 18.7/10.4 | 35.1/19.5 | 19.6/10.9 | 3.6/2 |

Sandwich, Chicken Tikka, Taste!*, 1 pack/195.7g

| 368/188 | 22.9/11.7 | 42.5/21.7 | 11.8/6 | 0/0 |

Sandwich, Chicken Tikka, Thai-Style, Korma, Big, Sainsbury's*, 1 pack/268g

| 581/217 | 31.9/11.9 | 54.9/20.5 | 26/9.7 | 0/0 |

Sandwich, Chicken Tikka, Weight Watchers*, 1 pack/158g

| 289/183 | 20.2/12.8 | 37/23.4 | 6.8/4.3 | 2.5/1.6 |

Sandwich, Chicken with Sour Cream on Malted Brown Bread, Weight Watchers*, 1 pack/143g

| 265/185 | 21/14.7 | 36.9/25.8 | 3.7/2.6 | 2.8/2 |

Sandwich, Chicken, Bacon & Tomato, BGTY, Sainsbury's*, 1 pack/190g

| 270/142 | 21.7/11.4 | 36.1/19 | 4.4/2.3 | 0/0 |

Sandwich, Chicken, Healthier Choice, Ginsters*, 1 pack/183g

| 247/135 | 18.7/10.2 | 37.5/20.5 | 2.6/1.4 | 0/0 |

Sandwich, Chicken, Lightly Spiced, Starbucks*, 1 pack/200g

| 286/143 | 22.4/11.2 | 36.4/18.2 | 4.8/2.4 | 0/0 |

Sandwich, Chicken, Lime & Coriander, BP*, 1 pack/154.5g

| 291/189 | 19.3/12.5 | 38.8/25.2 | 6.5/4.2 | 0/0 |

Sandwich, Chicken, No Mayo, Daily Bread*, 1 pack/160.3g

| 278/174 | 13.8/8.6 | 38.1/23.8 | 7/4.4 | 0/0 |

Sandwich, Chicken, Prawn, Ham Salad Triple, Healthy Eating, Tesco*, 1 pack/248g

| 350/141 | 25.8/10.4 | 51.6/20.8 | 4.5/1.8 | 5.2/2.1 |

kcal serv/100g	prot serv/100g	carb serv/100g	fat serv/100g	fibre serv/100g

Sandwich, Chicken, Tikka, Coronation, Thai-Style, Classic, Somerfield*, 1 pack/230g

| 614/267 | 29/12.6 | 63/27.4 | 27.4/11.9 | 7.8/3.4 |

Sandwich, Chilli Chicken, Taste!*, 1 pack/77.2g

| 112/145 | 4.3/5.6 | 18/23.4 | 2.5/3.2 | 0/0 |

Sandwich, Chinese Chicken, Esso*, 1 pack/177.8g

| 409/230 | 23.1/13 | 40.6/22.8 | 16/9 | 7.1/4 |

Sandwich, Chinese Chicken, Jalfrezi Chicken, Red Thai Chicken, Shapers, Boots*, 1 pack/230g

| 439/191 | 25.3/11 | 57.5/25 | 12/5.2 | 3.9/1.7 |

Sandwich, Chinese Chicken, Malted Brown Bread, Waitrose*, 1 pack/164g

| 333/203 | 22.1/13.5 | 35.9/21.9 | 11.2/6.8 | 5.4/3.3 |

Sandwich, Christmas, Shell*, 1 pack/182.7g

| 414/226 | 20.3/11.1 | 46.7/25.5 | 15/8.2 | 3.8/2.1 |

Sandwich, Ciabatta, Chicken & Herb, Shapers, Boots*, 1 pack/168g

| 290/173 | 20/11.9 | 42/25 | 4.7/2.8 | 2.9/1.7 |

Sandwich, Club, Pret A Manger*, 1 av pack/250g

| 542/217 | 31.9/12.8 | 46.8/18.7 | 25.2/10.1 | 5.7/2.3 |

Sandwich, Corned Beef with Onion & Tomato, The Salad Garden*, 1 pack/137g

| 338/247 | 19.5/14.2 | 31.5/23 | 14.8/10.8 | 0/0 |

Sandwich, Coronation Chicken, Marks & Spencer*, 1 pack/210g

| 420/200 | 23.5/11.2 | 42.4/20.2 | 20.4/9.7 | 6.5/3.1 |

Sandwich, Coronation Chicken, Pret A Manger*, 1 av pack/250g

| 415/166 | 19.8/7.9 | 53.1/21.2 | 13.6/5.4 | 0.5/0.2 |

Sandwich, Cottage Cheese & Tomato, Shapers, Boots*, 1 pack/150g

| 219/146 | 11.7/7.8 | 27/18 | 7.2/4.8 | 3.6/2.4 |

Sandwich, Crab Marie Rose, Brown Bread, Royal London Hospital*, 1 pack/158g

| 293/185 | 15.3/9.7 | 34.8/22 | 11.2/7.1 | 0/0 |

Sandwich, Crayfish & Lemon Mayonnaise, Daily Bread*, 1 pack/173.0g

| 391/226 | 16.4/9.5 | 53.6/31 | 11.4/6.6 | 0/0 |

Sandwich, Crayfish & Rocket, Pret A Manger, 1 av pack/250g

| 435/174 | 23.5/9.4 | 41.8/16.7 | 19.4/7.8 | 3.7/1.5 |

Sandwich, Cream Cheese & Peppers, Taste!*, 1 pack/154.2g

| 296/192 | 11.2/7.3 | 39.3/25.5 | 10.5/6.8 | 0/0 |

Sandwich, Cream Cheese, Red Pepper & Spinach, Daily Bread*, 1 pack/156g

| 273/175 | 11.5/7.4 | 37.4/24 | 8.1/5.2 | 0/0 |

kcal serv/100g	prot serv/100g	carb serv/100g	fat serv/100g	fibre serv/100g

Sandwich, Danish Ham Salad, Lean, COU, Marks & Spencer*, 1 pack/192g

| 250/130 | 20.4/10.6 | 37.4/19.5 | 1.7/0.9 | 2.7/1.4 |

Sandwich, Edam Cheese, Oldfields*, 1 pack/175g

| 326/186 | 17.2/9.8 | 41.9/23.9 | 9.9/5.7 | 0/0 |

Sandwich, Egg & Bacon, Boots*, 1 pack/179g

| 480/268 | 21.5/12 | 34/19 | 28.6/16 | 2.5/1.4 |

Sandwich, Egg & Bacon, Ginsters*, 1 pack/210g

| 523/249 | 27.7/13.2 | 46.2/22 | 24.4/11.6 | 0/0 |

Sandwich, Egg & Bacon, Tesco*, 1 pack/179g

| 530/298 | 18.9/10.6 | 36/20.2 | 34.5/19.4 | 2.3/1.3 |

Sandwich, Egg & Cress, BGTY, Sainsbury's*, 1 pack/166g

| 317/191 | 15.9/9.6 | 43.2/26 | 9/5.4 | 0/0 |

Sandwich, Egg & Cress, Co-Op*, 1 pack/159g

| 398/250 | 14.3/9 | 33.4/21 | 23.9/15 | 3.2/2 |

Sandwich, Egg & Cress, COU, Marks & Spencer*, 1 pack/192g

| 240/125 | 18.8/9.8 | 29.8/15.5 | 5.2/2.7 | 5.4/2.8 |

Sandwich, Egg & Cress, Free-Range, Marks & Spencer*, 1 pack/192g

| 374/195 | 18.6/9.7 | 32.1/16.7 | 19.4/10.1 | 2.9/1.5 |

Sandwich, Egg & Cress, Free-Range, Safeway*, 1 pack/190.4g

| 473/249 | 17.9/9.4 | 37.1/19.5 | 28.3/14.9 | 4/2.1 |

Sandwich, Egg & Cress, Free-Range, Tesco*, 1 pack/195g

| 402/206 | 20.3/10.4 | 25.2/12.9 | 24.4/12.5 | 5.9/3 |

Sandwich, Egg & Cress, Heinz*, 1 pack/162g

| 241/149 | 15.6/9.6 | 36.8/22.7 | 3.6/2.2 | 8.7/5.4 |

Sandwich, Egg & Cress, Marks & Spencer*, 1 pack/182g

| 331/182 | 18.4/10.1 | 24.8/13.6 | 17.7/9.7 | 5.8/3.2 |

Sandwich, Egg & Cress, Reduced-Fat, Waitrose*, 1 pack/162g

| 262/162 | 15.7/9.7 | 26.7/16.5 | 10.4/6.4 | 10.4/6.4 |

Sandwich, Egg & Cress, Sainsbury's*, 1 pack/170g

| 357/210 | 15.6/9.2 | 37.6/22.1 | 16.2/9.5 | 0/0 |

Sandwich, Egg & Tomato, on Softgrain Bread, Daily Bread*, 1 pack/160.3g

| 278/174 | 13.8/8.6 | 38.1/23.8 | 7/4.4 | 0/0 |

Sandwich, Egg & Tomato, Tesco*, 1 pack/172g

| 341/198 | 15.1/8.8 | 37.8/22 | 14.3/8.3 | 3.3/1.9 |

Sandwich, Egg & Watercress, Free-Range, Marks & Spencer*, 1 pack/191.9g

| 355/185 | 17.7/9.2 | 34.8/18.1 | 15.7/8.2 | 5.6/2.9 |

Sandwich, Egg Mayo & Cress, Starbucks*, 1 pack/202g

| 450/223 | 19.2/9.5 | 37.4/18.5 | 24.8/12.3 | 0/0 |

kcal serv/100g	prot serv/100g	carb serv/100g	fat serv/100g	fibre serv/100g
Sandwich, Egg Mayonnaise & Cress, Co-Op*, 1 pack/159g				
405/255	14/8.8	33/20.8	24/15.1	3/1.9
Sandwich, Egg Mayonnaise & Cress, Go Simple, Asda*, 1 pack/169g				
370/219	16.9/10	33.8/20	18.6/11	2.9/1.7
Sandwich, Egg Mayonnaise & Cress, Millers*, 1 pack/166g				
369/222	15.6/9.4	31.2/18.8	20.3/12.2	0/0
Sandwich, Egg Mayonnaise & Cress, Shapers, Boots*, 1 pack/161g				
304/189	15.1/9.4	38.6/24	9.8/6.1	0/0
Sandwich, Egg Mayonnaise & Cress, Wheatgerm, Tesco*, 1 pack/146g				
368/252	14.3/9.8	26.9/18.4	22.6/15.5	1.9/1.3
Sandwich, Egg Mayonnaise & Cress, Wholemeal Bread, Oldfields*, 1 pack/128g				
301/235	12.4/9.7	30.7/24	14.3/11.2	4.6/3.6
Sandwich, Egg Mayonnaise & Salad, Superdrug*, 1 pack/169g				
286/169	12.8/7.6	30.9/18.3	12.3/7.3	4.1/2.4
Sandwich, Egg Mayonnaise with Cress, Reduced-Fat, Waitrose*, 1 pack/162g				
300/185	16.8/10.4	29.3/18.1	12.8/7.9	5.5/3.4
Sandwich, Egg Mayonnaise, Boots*, 1 pack/183.6g				
449/244	17.8/9.7	40.5/22	23.9/13	4.2/2.3
Sandwich, Egg Mayonnaise, Healthy Living, Tesco*, 1 pack/162.2g				
253/156	15.1/9.3	34.7/21.4	6/3.7	4.5/2.8
Sandwich, Egg Mayonnaise, Pret A Manger*, 1 av pack/250g				
394/158	16.2/6.5	37.8/15.1	19.8/7.9	3.8/1.5
Sandwich, Egg Mayonnaise, Shell*, 1 pack/189g				
522/276	18.5/9.8	46.7/24.7	29.1/15.4	0/0
Sandwich, Egg Mayonnaise, Snack & Shop, Esso*, 1 pack/240g				
624/260	22.6/9.4	61.2/25.5	32.2/13.4	0/0
Sandwich, Egg Mayonnaise, Waitrose*, 1 pack/180g				
396/220	18.2/10.1	34.4/19.1	20.5/11.4	6.1/3.4
Sandwich, Egg Salad, Co-Op*, 1 pack/190g				
285/150	13.3/7	41.8/22	7.6/4	7.6/4
Sandwich, Egg Salad, Free-Range, Good Intentions, Somerfield*, 1 pack/173g				
260/150	12.5/7.2	37.4/21.6	6.7/3.9	5/2.9
Sandwich, Egg Salad, Free-Range, Sainsbury's*, 1 pack/224.5g				
450/200	19.1/8.5	55.1/24.5	16.9/7.5	0/0

kcal serv/100g	prot serv/100g	carb serv/100g	fat serv/100g	fibre serv/100g

Sandwich, Egg Salad, Free-Range, Waitrose*, 1 pack/180g

| 257/143 | 14.9/8.3 | 29.7/16.5 | 8.8/4.9 | 6.5/3.6 |

Sandwich, Egg Salad, GFY, Asda*, 1 pack/156.8g

| 229/146 | 12.6/8 | 34.5/22 | 4.6/2.9 | 4.6/2.9 |

Sandwich, Egg Salad, Healthy Living, Tesco*, 1 pack/182g

| 264/145 | 13.1/7.2 | 33.9/18.6 | 7.6/4.2 | 3.3/1.8 |

Sandwich, Egg Salad, Shapers, Boots*, 1 pack/184g

| 304/165 | 12.7/6.9 | 44.2/24 | 8.5/4.6 | 2/1.1 |

Sandwich, Egg Salad, Weight Watchers*, 1 pack/171.6g

| 255/148 | 12.9/7.5 | 39.2/22.8 | 5.2/3 | 2.4/1.4 |

Sandwich, Egg Tomato & Salad Cream, Cafe Revive, Marks & Spencer*, 1 pack/206.5g

| 476/230 | 17.2/8.3 | 46.8/22.6 | 25.9/12.5 | 3.9/1.9 |

Sandwich, Egg, Co-Op*, 1 pack/190g

| 285/150 | 13/6.8 | 42/22.1 | 7/3.7 | 7/3.7 |

Sandwich, Feta Cheese with Tomatoes & Rocket on Mediterranean Loaf, Daily Bread*, 1 pack/217.9g

| 366/168 | 13.3/6.1 | 40.3/18.5 | 16.6/7.6 | 0/0 |

Sandwich, Fire-Roasted Red Pepper & Herbed Soft Cheese, Marks & Spencer*, 1 pack/148.9g

| 335/225 | 10.4/7 | 36.7/24.6 | 15.9/10.7 | 4/2.7 |

Sandwich, Flame-Grilled Chicken, Rustlers*, 1 pack/150g

| 347/231 | 24.5/16.3 | 30.2/20.1 | 14.3/9.5 | 0/0 |

Sandwich, Fresh Salad & Salad Cream, Fulfilled*, 1 pack/172g

| 244/142 | 8.4/4.9 | 37/21.5 | 7.1/4.1 | 0/0 |

Sandwich, Gammon & Egg, Safeway*, 1 pack/233.3g

| 489/210 | 30.1/12.9 | 47.5/20.4 | 18.6/8 | 0/0 |

Sandwich, Gourmet Prawn, Pret A Manger*, 1 av pack/250g

| 454/182 | 19.4/7.8 | 38.1/15.2 | 25.4/10.2 | 4.4/1.8 |

Sandwich, Ham & Cheddar, Marks & Spencer*, 1 pack/165g

| 396/240 | 24.9/15.1 | 33/20 | 18.6/11.3 | 2.8/1.7 |

Sandwich, Ham & Cheese Toasted, Coffee Republic*, 1 pack/160g

| 429/268 | 25.1/15.7 | 39/24.4 | 20.3/12.7 | 0/0 |

Sandwich, Ham & Cheese, Baxter & Platts*, 1 pack/168g

| 408/243 | 19/11.3 | 34.4/20.5 | 21.8/13 | 2.9/1.7 |

Sandwich, Ham & Cheese, Eat Smart, Safeway*, 1 pack/230g

| 311/135 | 26/11.3 | 44.4/19.3 | 3/1.3 | 7.4/3.2 |

	kcal serv/100g	prot serv/100g	carb serv/100g	fat serv/100g	fibre serv/100g

Sandwich, Ham & Chicken, Healthy Living, Co-Op*, 1 pack/150g

285/190	18/12	42/28	6/4	4.5/3

Sandwich, Ham & Dijon Mustard, Healthy Selection, Budgens*, 1 pack/120g

190/158	11.6/9.7	26.3/21.9	3/2.5	2.4/2

Sandwich, Ham & Mustard, Eat Smart, Safeway*, 1 pack/139g

250/180	19/13.7	36.6/26.3	3.1/2.2	2.8/2

Sandwich, Ham & Mustard, Tesco*, 1 pack/147g

437/297	15.6/10.6	30.6/20.8	27.9/19	1.8/1.2

Sandwich, Ham & Swiss Cheese, Marks & Spencer*, 1 pack/159g

393/247	23.4/14.7	30.1/18.9	20/12.6	5.2/3.3

Sandwich, Ham & Swiss Cheese, Safeway*, 1 pack/201.1g

533/265	29.1/14.5	39.6/19.7	28.7/14.3	3/1.5

Sandwich, Ham & Tomato, GFY, Asda*, 1 pack/173g

254/147	17.3/10	39.8/23	2.9/1.7	2.4/1.4

Sandwich, Ham & Turkey Salad, Co-Op*, 1 pack/188g

263/140	16.9/9	39.5/21	5.6/3	3.8/2

Sandwich, Ham Cheese & Pickle, Sutherland*, 1 pack/230g

727/316	26/11.3	47.4/20.6	48.1/20.9	0/0

Sandwich, Ham Salad Wedge, Healthy Eating, Tesco*, 1 pack/198g

269/136	14.1/7.1	45.5/23	3.4/1.7	2/1

Sandwich, Ham Salad, Big Fill, Somerfield*, 1 pack/222g

515/232	20.9/9.4	50.8/22.9	25.3/11.4	5.1/2.3

Sandwich, Ham Salad, Coffee Republic*, 1 pack/224g

309/138	19.3/8.6	44.6/19.9	6/2.7	0/0

Sandwich, Ham Salad, Co-Op*, 1 pack/193g

299/155	17.4/9	36.7/19	9.7/5	1.9/1

Sandwich, Ham Salad, Ginsters*, 1 pack/179g

220/123	15.8/8.8	29.4/16.4	4.5/2.5	0/0

Sandwich, Ham Salad, Healthy Eating, Tesco*, 1 pack/163g

215/132	17.3/10.6	28.5/17.5	3.6/2.2	3.3/2

Sandwich, Ham Salad, Prawn Mayo & Chicken, Healthy Eating, Tesco*, 1 pack/248g

350/141	25.8/10.4	51.6/20.8	4.5/1.8	5.2/2.1

Sandwich, Ham Salad, Safeway*, 1 pack/272g

403/148	22.6/8.3	66.6/24.5	4.9/1.8	5.2/1.9

Sandwich, Ham Salad, Snack & Shop*, 1 pack/191.2g

304/159	17.6/9.2	43.7/22.9	6.5/3.4	9.6/5

kcal serv/100g	prot serv/100g	carb serv/100g	fat serv/100g	fibre serv/100g

Sandwich, Ham Salad, Woolworths*, 1 pack/181g

| 286/158 | 15.2/8.4 | 41.1/22.7 | 6.7/3.7 | 0/0 |

Sandwich, Ham, Asda*, 1 pack/262g

| 618/236 | 32/12.2 | 53.2/20.3 | 31.4/12 | 7.9/3 |

Sandwich, Ham, Cheese & Pickle, Healthy Living, Co-Op*, 1 pack/185g

| 370/200 | 24.1/13 | 50/27 | 7.4/4 | 5.6/3 |

Sandwich, Ham, Cheese & Pickle, Marks & Spencer*, 1 pack/197g

| 459/233 | 25.6/13 | 31.3/15.9 | 25.8/13.1 | 4.7/2.4 |

Sandwich, Ham, Cheese & Pickle, Pret A Manger*, 1 av pack/250g

| 592/237 | 29.7/11.9 | 62.6/25 | 27.6/11 | 6/2.4 |

Sandwich, Ham, Marks & Spencer*, 1 pack/200g

| 220/110 | 34.4/17.2 | 6.4/3.2 | 5.2/2.6 | 0/0 |

Sandwich, Ham, Subway*, 1 x 6" pack/223g

| 288/129 | 18/8.1 | 45.9/20.6 | 5/2.3 | 4/1.8 |

Sandwich, Houmous & Crunchy Salad, Oldfields*, 1 pack/180g

| 256/142 | 11.3/6.3 | 36/20 | 7.6/4.2 | 0/0 |

Sandwich, Houmous with Crunchy Vegetables, Starbucks*, 1 pack/218.9g

| 359/164 | 10.3/4.7 | 57.8/26.4 | 9.6/4.4 | 6.4/2.9 |

**Sandwich, Houmous with Mixed Leaves & Carrot, BGTY, Sainsbury's*,
1 pack/175g**

| 275/157 | 10.7/6.1 | 46.7/26.7 | 5.1/2.9 | 0/0 |

Sandwich, Italian-Style Mozzarella, Taste*, 1 pack/183.1g

| 390/213 | 16.8/9.2 | 36.8/20.1 | 19.4/10.6 | 3.7/2 |

Sandwich, Lean Danish Ham & Salad, COU, Marks & Spencer*, 1 pack/182g

| 255/140 | 19.3/10.6 | 34/18.7 | 4.4/2.4 | 3.5/1.9 |

Sandwich, Lemon & Mint Chicken, Delilite*, 1 pack/178.6g

| 326/182 | 22/12.3 | 41.3/23.1 | 6.4/3.6 | 3/1.7 |

**Sandwich, Lemon Chicken & Relish, Perfectly Balanced, Waitrose*,
1 pack/151g**

| 243/161 | 18.6/12.3 | 32.3/21.4 | 4.4/2.9 | 5.3/3.5 |

Sandwich, Lime & Coriander Chicken, BGTY, Sainsbury's*, 1 pack/168g

| 282/168 | 17.8/10.6 | 39.5/23.5 | 5.9/3.5 | 0/0 |

**Sandwich, Mature Cheddar Cheese & Tomato, Big, Sainsbury's*,
1 pack/233g**

| 596/256 | 30.1/12.9 | 61.3/26.3 | 25.6/11 | 0/0 |

Sandwich, Mature Cheddar Cheese Salad, Upper Crust*, 1 pack/225.1g

| 466/207 | 21.4/9.5 | 45.7/20.3 | 22.1/9.8 | 0/0 |

kcal serv/100g	prot serv/100g	carb serv/100g	fat serv/100g	fibre serv/100g

**Sandwich, Mature Cheddar, Soft Cheese & Celery, Sainsbury's*,
1 pack/183g**

| 576/315 | 18.7/10.2 | 39.9/21.8 | 35.3/19.3 | 0/0 |

Sandwich, Mediterranean Tuna Salad, Waitrose*, 1 pack/207g

| 253/122 | 14.9/7.2 | 35.4/17.1 | 5.8/2.8 | 5.4/2.6 |

Sandwich, Mediterranean Tuna, COU, Marks & Spencer*, 1 pack/260g

| 364/140 | 26.8/10.3 | 51/19.6 | 5.7/2.2 | 4.2/1.6 |

**Sandwich, Mozzarella, Tomato & Basil, Healthy Options, Oldfields*,
1 pack/175g**

| 285/163 | 14.2/8.1 | 38.6/22.1 | 8.4/4.8 | 5.7/3.3 |

Sandwich, Mozzarella & Tomato Calzone, Waitrose*, 1 pack/175g

| 410/234 | 18.9/10.8 | 39.7/22.7 | 19.4/11.1 | 3.9/2.2 |

Sandwich, New York Deli, Boots*, 1 pack/245g

| 603/246 | 27/11 | 46.6/19 | 34.3/14 | 5.4/2.2 |

Sandwich, Pastrami & Gherkin, BGTY, Sainsbury's*, 1 pack/230g

| 357/155 | 22.5/9.8 | 53.1/23.1 | 6/2.6 | 6.9/3 |

Sandwich, Peking Duck, No Mayo, Boots*, 1 pack/221.7g

| 400/180 | 17.1/7.7 | 59.9/27 | 10.2/4.6 | 3.8/1.7 |

**Sandwich, Pitta Pocket, Chargrilled Chicken, Marks & Spencer*,
1 pack/208g**

| 279/134 | 23.3/11.2 | 30.2/14.5 | 7.3/3.5 | 3.3/1.6 |

Sandwich, Plain Salad, Northern Bites*, 1 pack/210g

| 193/92 | 8.6/4.1 | 32.1/15.3 | 4.2/2 | 6.3/3 |

Sandwich, Ploughman's, Deep-Fill, Ginsters*, 1 pack/232g

| 636/274 | 22.3/9.6 | 48.3/20.8 | 40.8/17.6 | 0/0 |

Sandwich, Ploughman's, Shell*, 1 pack/225.9g

| 540/239 | 20.3/9 | 43.8/19.4 | 31.4/13.9 | 2.3/1 |

Sandwich, Poached Salmon & Rocket, Marks & Spencer*, 1 pack/180g

| 495/275 | 24.3/13.5 | 38.2/21.2 | 26.8/14.9 | 3.8/2.1 |

Sandwich, Poached Salmon & Rocket, Pret A Manger*, 1 Av pack/260g

| 516/198 | 26.7/10.3 | 38.8/14.9 | 27.7/10.7 | 4.9/1.9 |

Sandwich, Poached Salmon, Marks & Spencer*, 1 pack/171g

| 397/232 | 22.1/12.9 | 27.7/16.2 | 21.9/12.8 | 4.4/2.6 |

Sandwich, Poached Salmon, Prawn & Rocket, Waitrose*, 1 pack/165.6g

| 309/186 | 18.6/11.2 | 39/23.5 | 8.6/5.2 | 3.5/2.1 |

Sandwich, Prawn & Egg, Safeway*, 1 pack/216g

| 400/185 | 20.3/9.4 | 40.6/18.8 | 17.3/8 | 2.2/1 |

kcal serv/100g	prot serv/100g	carb serv/100g	fat serv/100g	fibre serv/100g
Sandwich, Prawn & Mayonnaise, BGTY, Sainsbury's*, 1 pack/165g				
312/189	17.2/10.4	33.5/20.3	12/7.3	5.1/3.1
Sandwich, Prawn & Mayonnaise, COU, Marks & Spencer*, 1 pack/141g				
254/180	16.8/11.9	28.6/20.3	3.8/2.7	2.4/1.7
Sandwich, Prawn & Mayonnaise, Healthy Selection, Budgens*, 1 pack/143g				
296/207	15.7/11	31.5/22	11.9/8.3	2.6/1.8
Sandwich, Prawn & Mayonnaise, on Oatmeal Bread, Big, Sainsbury's*, 1 pack/259g				
686/265	26.2/10.1	54.6/21.1	40.4/15.6	0/0
Sandwich, Prawn & Mayonnaise, Reduced-Fat, Waitrose*, 1 pack/146g				
276/189	13.4/9.2	35.2/24.1	9.1/6.2	3.7/2.5
Sandwich, Prawn & Mayonnaise, Safeway*, 1 pack/168g				
402/239	15.1/9	35.4/21.1	22.2/13.2	5.2/3.1
Sandwich, Prawn & Rocket, Pret A Manger*, 1 pack/280g				
435/155	23.5/8.4	41.8/14.9	19.4/6.9	3.7/1.3
Sandwich, Prawn Cocktail Salad, Shapers, Boots*, 1 pack/167g				
296/177	16.7/10	30.1/18	12/7.2	4.8/2.9
Sandwich, Prawn Cocktail, Classic, Heinz*, 1 pack/193g				
409/212	16.2/8.4	48.3/25	16.8/8.7	4.8/2.5
Sandwich, Prawn Cocktail, Healthy Eating, Tesco*, 1 pack/154g				
245/159	16.9/11	33.9/22	4.2/2.7	2.8/1.8
Sandwich, Prawn Cocktail, Weight Watchers*, 1 pack/168g				
252/150	15/8.9	30.4/18.1	7.7/4.6	4.7/2.8
Sandwich, Prawn Marie Rose, Waitrose*, 1 pack/164g				
303/185	15.4/9.4	28.4/17.3	14.3/8.7	4.4/2.7
Sandwich, Prawn Mayo, Chicken Salad, Ham Salad, Healthy Living, Tesco*, 1 pack/250.7g				
341/136	32.4/12.9	43.9/17.5	4/1.6	3.5/1.4
Sandwich, Prawn Mayonnaise, Healthy Living, Tesco*, 1 pack/157g				
245/156	16/10.2	34.2/21.8	4.9/3.1	0.8/0.5
Sandwich, Prawn Mayonnaise on Oatmeal Bread, Co-Op*, 1 pack/159g				
445/280	17.5/11	44.5/28	22.3/14	3.2/2
Sandwich, Prawn Mayonnaise on Oatmeal Bread, Weight Watchers*, 1 pack/158g				
254/161	16.4/10.4	37.4/23.7	4.3/2.7	3.6/2.3
Sandwich, Prawn Mayonnaise, BGTY, Sainsbury's*, 1 pack/175g				
275/157	21.5/12.3	36.9/21.1	4.6/2.6	0/0

	kcal serv/100g	prot serv/100g	carb serv/100g	fat serv/100g	fibre serv/100g

Sandwich, Prawn Mayonnaise, Co-Op*, 1 pack/154g

285/185   15/9.7   42/27.3   6/3.9   5/3.2

Sandwich, Prawn Mayonnaise, Daily Bread*, 1 pack/156.5g

373/239   18.6/11.9   35.9/23   17.2/11   0/0

Sandwich, Prawn Mayonnaise, Eat Smart, Safeway*, 1 pack/165g

256/155   17.2/10.4   38/23   3.8/2.3   3.3/2

Sandwich, Prawn Mayonnaise, Ginsters*, 1 pack/152g

415/273   18.8/12.4   27.1/17.8   27.1/17.8   0/0

Sandwich, Prawn Mayonnaise, GFY, Asda*, 1 pack/160g

270/169   16/10   35.2/22   7.4/4.6   3.4/2.1

Sandwich, Prawn Mayonnaise, Healthy Eating, Tesco*, 1 pack/154g

270/175   18.3/11.9   35/22.7   6.3/4.1   2.9/1.9

Sandwich, Prawn Mayonnaise, Heinz*, 1 pack/180g

493/274   16/8.9   43.2/24   28.4/15.8   4.5/2.5

Sandwich, Prawn Mayonnaise, Reduced-Fat, Waitrose*, 1 pack/155g

284/183   13.8/8.9   31/20   11.6/7.5   4.3/2.8

Sandwich, Prawn Mayonnaise, Shapers, Boots*, 1 pack/161g

291/181   16.1/10   40.3/25   7.4/4.6   3.1/1.9

Sandwich, Prawn Mayonnaise, Woolworths*, 1 pack/144g

321/223   18.1/12.6   35/24.3   12/8.3   0/0

Sandwich, Rare Roast Beef & Horseradish, Marks & Spencer*, 1 pack/168g

311/185   24.9/14.8   35.4/21.1   7.2/4.3   4/2.4

Sandwich, Red Salmon & Cucumber, BGTY, Sainsbury's*, 1 pack/178.1g

276/155   19.4/10.9   40.4/22.7   4.1/2.3   0/0

Sandwich, Red Salmon & Cucumber, Marks & Spencer*, 1 pack/183g

375/205   20.3/11.1   33.9/18.5   17/9.3   2.6/1.4

Sandwich, Red Thai Chicken, Iceberg Lettuce & Mayonnaise, Woolworths*, 1 pack/160g

328/205   18.4/11.5   41.8/26.1   9.6/6   0/0

Sandwich, Reformed Smoked Ham & Salad on Oatmeal Bread, Woolworths*, 1 pack/187g

286/153   17/9.1   34.4/18.4   9/4.8   0/0

Sandwich, Roast Beef on White, No Cheese or Sauce, Subway*, 1 pack/222g

289/130   18.9/8.5   44.4/20   5/2.3   4/1.8

Sandwich, Roast Beef with Cheese, Subway*, 6" Sandwich/222g

291/131   19/8.6   45.1/20.3   5/2.3   4/1.8

kcal serv/100g	prot serv/100g	carb serv/100g	fat serv/100g	fibre serv/100g

Sandwich, Roast Beef with Horseradish Mayonnaise, Finest, Tesco*, 1 pack/222.8g

439/197	27.9/12.5	46.2/20.7	15.8/7.1	3.6/1.6

Sandwich, Roast Beef, Daily Bread*, 1 pack/199.3g

281/141	17.3/8.7	39.8/20	5.4/2.7	0/0

Sandwich, Roast Beef, English Mustard Mayonnaise, Oldfields*, 1 pack/150g

405/270	24/16	43.5/29	17.9/11.9	0/0

Sandwich, Roast Beef, Healthy, Woolworths*, 1 pack/191g

283/148	20.1/10.5	34.2/17.9	7.4/3.9	0/0

Sandwich, Roast Chicken & Bacon, Boots*, 1 pack/250g

599/240	29/11.6	42/16.8	35/14	3.5/1.4

Sandwich, Roast Chicken & Salad With Mayo, Big, Sainsbury's*, 1 pack/268.8g

560/208	29.6/11	56.2/20.9	23.9/8.9	24.2/9

Sandwich, Roast Chicken & Salad, COU, Marks & Spencer*, 1 pack/196g

265/135	20/10.2	34.9/17.8	4.1/2.1	6.9/3.5

Sandwich, Roast Chicken & Stuffing, Marks & Spencer*, 1 pack/182g

519/285	24/13.2	42.6/23.4	27.8/15.3	5.5/3

Sandwich, Roast Chicken & Stuffing, Tesco*, 1 pack/164g

313/191	23.9/14.6	33.3/20.3	9.3/5.7	2.8/1.7

Sandwich, Roast Chicken Breast, BGTY, Sainsbury's*, 1 pack/161.0g

277/172	24/14.9	35.7/22.2	4.2/2.6	0/0

Sandwich, Roast Chicken Salad, Marks & Spencer*, 1 pack/221g

420/190	23/10.4	51.7/23.4	13.9/6.3	2.4/1.1

Sandwich, Roast Chicken Salad, Shapers, Boots*, 1 pack/193g

284/147	21.2/11	36.7/19	5.8/3	4.4/2.3

Sandwich, Roast Chicken with Black Pepper Mayo, Boots*, 1 pack/160g

296/185	24/15	32/20	8/5	2.9/1.8

Sandwich, Roast Chicken, Bacon & Salad, Big, Sainsbury's*, 1 pack/249g

610/245	27.6/11.1	54/21.7	31.6/12.7	0/0

Sandwich, Roast Chicken, No Mayo, COU, Marks & Spencer*, 1 serving/147g

250/170	21.3/14.5	31/21.1	3.8/2.6	2.1/1.4

Sandwich, Roast Chicken, Shapers, Boots*, 1 pack/163g

289/177	24.5/15	31/19	7.5/4.6	2.4/1.5

Sandwich, Roast Peppers & Goat's Cheese Focaccia, Finest, Tesco*, 1 focaccia/150g

419/279	10.5/7	32.3/21.5	27.5/18.3	2.6/1.7

	kcal serv/100g	prot serv/100g	carb serv/100g	fat serv/100g	fibre serv/100g

Sandwich, Roast Turkey Salad, Roast Chicken, Tuna & Tomato, Shapers, Boots*, 1 pack/261.5g

375/143	26.2/10	55/21	5.5/2.1	5.2/2

Sandwich, Roasted Vegetable & Chilli Bean, Marks & Spencer*, 1 pack/200g

340/170	10.4/5.2	49/24.5	11.4/5.7	4.2/2.1

Sandwich, Roasted Vegetable, Open, COU Marks & Spencer*, 1 pack/150g

260/173	12.6/8.4	46.9/31.3	2.2/1.5	6.6/4.4

Sandwich, Salad & Pepper Salsa, Hackens*, 1 pack/157.0g

197/126	8/5.1	34.2/21.8	3.1/2	0/0

Sandwich, Salmon & Cucumber, Healthy Choice, Sutherland*, 1 pack/164g

321/196	16.1/9.8	43.6/26.6	9.2/5.6	0/0

Sandwich, Salmon & Cucumber, Shapers, Boots*, 1 pack/164.9g

310/188	19.8/12	38/23	8.7/5.3	5.6/3.4

Sandwich, Salmon & Cucumber, White Bread, Waitrose*, 1 pack/161.4g

304/189	15.8/9.8	41.1/25.5	8.5/5.3	2.7/1.7

Sandwich, Salt Beef, Gherkins & Mustard Mayo, Sainsbury's*, 1 pack/242g

486/201	22.5/9.3	58.3/24.1	18.2/7.5	7.5/3.1

Sandwich, Sausage, Onion Chutney & Tomato, Softgrain Bread, Daily Bread*, 1 pack/166.5g

359/215	11.7/7	44.4/26.6	16.2/9.7	0/0

Sandwich, Sausage, Triple pack, GFY, Asda*, 1 pack/215g

424/197	19.4/9	64.5/30	9.7/4.5	4.9/2.3

Sandwich, Seafood Cocktail, Waitrose*, 1 pack/210.2g

267/127	15.3/7.3	37/17.6	6.3/3	17/8.1

Sandwich, Simply Chicken, Eat Smart, Safeway*, 1 pack/147g

250/170	21.3/14.5	33.8/23	3.2/2.2	2.1/1.4

Sandwich, Simply Egg Mayonnaise, Ginsters*, 1 pack/161g

309/192	13.7/8.5	38.8/24.1	10.9/6.8	0/0

Sandwich, Simply Prawn Mayonnaise, Boots*, 1 pack/261g

736/282	28.7/11	49.6/19	47/18	5.7/2.2

Sandwich, Simply Salad, Shapers, Boots*, 1 pack/216g

300/139	11.2/5.2	49.7/23	6.3/2.9	3.9/1.8

Sandwich, Simply Tuna Mayonnaise & Cucumber, Boots*, 1 pack/200g

498/249	24/12	42/21	26/13	4.8/2.4

Sandwich, Smoked Ham & Cheese, Co-Op*, 1 pack/167g

334/200	25.1/15	40.1/24	8.4/5	3.3/2

	kcal serv/100g	prot serv/100g	carb serv/100g	fat serv/100g	fibre serv/100g

Sandwich, Smoked Ham & Cheese, Tesco*, 1 pack/204g

620/304	28.8/14.1	40.2/19.7	38.1/18.7	3.3/1.6

Sandwich, Smoked Ham & Edam, Shapers, Boots*, 1 pack/183g

315/172	17/9.3	34.8/19	11.9/6.5	4.9/2.7

Sandwich, Smoked Ham & Mustard, Marks & Spencer*, 1 pack/149g

347/233	15/10.1	28/18.8	19.4/13	3/2

Sandwich, Smoked Ham & Mustard, Sainsbury's*, 1 pack/175g

406/232	18.6/10.6	38.3/21.9	19.8/11.3	0/0

Sandwich, Smoked Ham Salad, Weight Watchers*, 1 pack/181g

244/135	19.7/10.9	29.9/16.5	5.1/2.8	5.1/2.8

Sandwich, Smoked Ham With Pineapple & Soft Cheese, BGTY, Sainsbury's*, 1 pack/188g

301/160	16.4/8.7	50.6/26.9	3.8/2	0/0

Sandwich, Smoked Ham, Cheese & Pickle, COU, Marks & Spencer*, 1 pack/174g

270/155	25.1/14.4	34.8/20	3.1/1.8	6.4/3.7

Sandwich, Smoked Ham, Cheese & Pickle, Shapers, Boots*, 1 pack/172g

296/172	22.4/13	32.7/19	8.4/4.9	5/2.9

Sandwich, Smoked Salmon & Black Pepper, Fulfilled*, 1 pack/120g

293/244	16.6/13.8	34.8/29	10.3/8.6	0/0

Sandwich, Smoked Salmon & Cream Cheese, Marks & Spencer*, 1 pack/162g

437/270	19/11.7	31.3/19.3	26.2/16.2	4.1/2.5

Sandwich, Smoked Salmon Crème Fraîche, Safeway*, 1 pack/171.4g

359/210	18.8/11	40.4/23.6	13.3/7.8	4.3/2.5

Sandwich, Smoked Salmon with Soft Cheese, Waitrose*, 1 pack/154g

300/195	22.8/14.8	29.6/19.2	10/6.5	6.5/4.2

Sandwich, Smoked Salmon, Crème Fraîche & Watercress on Seed Loaf, Fresh, Gourmet Organics*, 1 pack/152.3g

302/199	20.4/13.4	37.2/24.5	7.8/5.1	0/0

Sandwich, Smoked Salmon, Luxury, Marks & Spencer*, 1 pack/137g

333/243	20.6/15	26/19	16.3/11.9	2.5/1.8

Sandwich, Smoked Salmon, Pret A Manger*, 1 Av pack/250g

370/148	9.5/3.8	50.7/20.3	14.4/5.8	4.4/1.8

Sandwich, Smoked Turkey Summer Salad, Starbucks*, 1 pack/198g

303/153	21.4/10.8	44.2/22.3	4.8/2.4	3/1.5

Sandwich, Spicy Aubergine & Soft Cheese, Pret A Manger*, 1 av pack/250g

319/128	11.6/4.6	52.9/21.2	6.8/2.7	7/2.8

kcal serv/100g	prot serv/100g	carb serv/100g	fat serv/100g	fibre serv/100g

Sandwich, Spicy Chicken, Deep-Filled, Co-Op*, 1 pack/216g

| 421/195 | 21.6/10 | 51.8/24 | 15.1/7 | 6.5/3 |

Sandwich, Sub, Beef & Onion, Marks & Spencer*, 1 pack/207g

| 611/295 | 27.5/13.3 | 53/25.6 | 31.7/15.3 | 3.1/1.5 |

Sandwich, Sub, Chargrilled Chicken Caesar, Sainsbury's*, 1 pack/216g

| 611/283 | 28.9/13.4 | 55.3/25.6 | 30.5/14.1 | 0/0 |

Sandwich, Sub, Egg Mayonnaise, Daily Bread*, 1 pack/165.2g

| 441/267 | 15.8/9.6 | 48.8/29.6 | 22.3/13.5 | 0/0 |

Sandwich, Sub, Meatball with Cheese & Salad, Subway*, 1 pack/286g

| 526/184 | 24/8.4 | 52.9/18.5 | 26/9.1 | 6/2.1 |

Sandwich, Sub, Nacho-Style Chicken Sub, Global, Somerfield*, 1 Roll/226g

| 513/227 | 16.7/7.4 | 69.6/30.8 | 18.8/8.3 | 9.5/4.2 |

Sandwich, Sub, The Big Chicken & Bacon, Marks & Spencer*, 1 pack/218g

| 545/250 | 34/15.6 | 54.3/24.9 | 21.8/10 | 3.1/1.4 |

Sandwich, Sweet Chilli Prawn Salad, Healthy Eating, Wild Bean Cafe*, 1 pack/198g

| 297/150 | 16.2/8.2 | 50.7/25.6 | 3.2/1.6 | 6.9/3.5 |

Sandwich, Three Cheese & Onion, New Style, Weight Watchers*, 1 pack/148g

| 275/186 | 21.9/14.8 | 38.8/26.2 | 3.6/2.4 | 2.1/1.4 |

Sandwich, Tiger Prawn & Thai Dressing, Waitrose*, 1 pack/200g

| 342/171 | 19.2/9.6 | 47.2/23.6 | 8.6/4.3 | 4.4/2.2 |

Sandwich, Tuna & Celery, Perfectly Balanced, Waitrose*, 1 pack/172g

| 272/158 | 20.1/11.7 | 35.3/20.5 | 5.5/3.2 | 6.7/3.9 |

Sandwich, Tuna & Cucumber, BGTY, Sainsbury's*, 1 pack/164g

| 275/169 | 19.6/12 | 35.2/21.6 | 6.4/3.9 | 4.9/3 |

Sandwich, Tuna & Cucumber, Ginsters*, 1 pack/171g

| 238/139 | 16.9/9.9 | 33.2/19.4 | 5.5/3.2 | 0/0 |

Sandwich, Tuna & Cucumber, Healthy Choice, Asda*, 1 pack/164g

| 315/192 | 17.9/10.9 | 36.6/22.3 | 10.8/6.6 | 1.8/1.1 |

Sandwich, Tuna & Cucumber, Heinz*, 1 pack/183.4g

| 276/151 | 22.5/12.3 | 39.5/21.6 | 2.9/1.6 | 12.4/6.8 |

Sandwich, Tuna & Cucumber, Marks & Spencer*, 1 pack/170g

| 430/253 | 20.4/12 | 30.6/18 | 25.2/14.8 | 4.1/2.4 |

Sandwich, Tuna & Cucumber, Red Cal Mayonnaise, BGTY, Sainsbury's*, 1 pack/182g

| 288/158 | 22.2/12.2 | 41/22.5 | 4.2/2.3 | 0/0 |

	kcal serv/100g	prot serv/100g	carb serv/100g	fat serv/100g	fibre serv/100g

Sandwich, Tuna & Cucumber, Shapers, Boots*, 1 pack/179g

322/180	19.7/11	43/24	7.9/4.4	3/1.7

Sandwich, Tuna & Cucumber, Shell*, 1 pack/188g

431/229	23.1/12.3	41.2/21.9	19.2/10.2	0/0

Sandwich, Tuna & Green Pesto, BGTY, Sainsbury's*, 1 pack/211.4g

279/132	23.2/11	35.9/17	4.6/2.2	0/0

Sandwich, Tuna & Lemon Mayo, Shapers, Boots*, 1 pack/206g

318/154	20.6/10	37.2/18	9.7/4.7	3.5/1.7

Sandwich, Tuna & Sweetcorn, Asda*, 1 pack/205g

592/289	23.6/11.5	44.7/21.8	35.3/17.2	5.5/2.7

Sandwich, Tuna & Sweetcorn, COU, Marks & Spencer*, 1 pack/180g

270/150	22.7/12.6	34.2/19	4.3/2.4	6.8/3.8

Sandwich, Tuna & Sweetcorn, Eat Smart, Safeway*, 1 pack/152g

251/165	20.4/13.4	33.3/21.9	3.8/2.5	4.3/2.8

Sandwich, Tuna & Sweetcorn, Ginsters*, 1 pack/163.3g

306/188	17.1/10.5	41.1/25.2	8.2/5	0/0

Sandwich, Tuna & Sweetcorn, Healthy Eating, Tesco*, 1 pack/154g

263/171	17.6/11.4	39.4/25.6	3.9/2.5	3.2/2.1

Sandwich, Tuna & Sweetcorn, Heinz*, 1 pack/208g

528/254	21.6/10.4	48.9/23.5	27.5/13.2	3.3/1.6

Sandwich, Tuna & Sweetcorn, Marks & Spencer*, 1 pack/185g

453/245	20.4/11	38.7/20.9	24.1/13	3.9/2.1

Sandwich, Tuna & Sweetcorn, New Recipe, Healthy Living, Tesco*, 1 pack/209.6g

330/157	27.3/13	47.3/22.5	3.6/1.7	4.8/2.3

Sandwich, Tuna & Sweetcorn, Safeway*, 1 pack/154.5g

256/165	19.8/12.8	36/23.2	2.8/1.8	2.6/1.7

Sandwich, Tuna & Sweetcorn, Sainsbury's*, 1 pack/183g

441/241	19.4/10.6	42.5/23.2	21.4/11.7	0/0

Sandwich, Tuna & Sweetcorn, Shapers, Boots*, 1 pack/170g

306/180	20.4/12	45.9/27	4.6/2.7	3.6/2.1

Sandwich, Tuna & Sweetcorn, Tesco*, 1 pack/174g

432/248	19.7/11.3	42.5/24.4	20.4/11.7	3.1/1.8

Sandwich, Tuna Crème Fraîche & Spring Onion, Healthy Options, Oldfields*, 1 pack/185.2g

287/155	16.7/9	37.7/20.4	7.8/4.2	5.6/3

Sandwich, Tuna Crunch, Healthy Living, Tesco*, 1 pack/180g

261/145	19.8/11	35.8/19.9	4.3/2.4	0.9/0.5

kcal serv/100g	prot serv/100g	carb serv/100g	fat serv/100g	fibre serv/100g
Sandwich, Tuna Mayo, Pret A Manger*, 1 av pack/250g				
622/249	29.2/11.7	60.9/24.4	29/11.6	4/1.6
Sandwich, Tuna Mayonnaise with Spring Onions, Starbucks*, 1 pack/209g				
318/152	18.8/9	41.6/19.9	8.4/4	3.1/1.5
Sandwich, Tuna Melt, Swedish Bread, Shapers, Boots*, 1 pack/163g				
254/156	22.8/14	32.6/20	3.6/2.2	3.4/2.1
Sandwich, Tuna Salad Wedge, Tesco*, 1 pack/204.9g				
291/142	16.6/8.1	49/23.9	3.1/1.5	1.6/0.8
Sandwich, Tuna Salad with Sour Cream Dressing, Weight Watchers*, 1 pack/201g				
260/129	19.7/9.8	35.5/17.7	4.2/2.1	5.7/2.8
Sandwich, Tuna Salad, Marks & Spencer*, 1 pack/250g				
575/230	31.3/12.5	42/16.8	31.5/12.6	5.3/2.1
Sandwich, Tuna Salad, on White, Tesco*, 1 pack/190g				
352/185	18.6/9.8	39.5/20.8	13.3/7	2.1/1.1
Sandwich, Tuna Salad, Tesco*, 1 pack/197g				
427/217	18.7/9.5	41.2/20.9	20.9/10.6	2.2/1.1
Sandwich, Tuna Salad, Weight Watchers*, 1 pack/191g				
248/130	20.2/10.6	30.2/15.8	5.2/2.7	5/2.6
Sandwich, Tuna With Salad, Debenhams*, 1 pack/249g				
309/124	19.2/7.7	42.1/16.9	8.5/3.4	0/0
Sandwich, Tuna, Healthy Options, Spar*, 1 pack/150g				
269/179	21.5/14.3	37.4/24.9	3.6/2.4	0/0
Sandwich, Tuna, Tomato & Onion, COU, Marks & Spencer*, 1 pack/177g				
250/141	19.6/11.1	33.3/18.8	4.2/2.4	3.9/2.2
Sandwich, Turkey & Bacon, COU, Marks & Spencer*, 1 pack/165g				
256/155	19.8/12	34.7/21	4/2.4	2.8/1.7
Sandwich, Turkey & Coleslaw, Cafe, Asda*, 1 pack/193g				
457/237	19.3/10	38.6/20	25.1/13	0/0
Sandwich, Turkey & Cranberry, COU, Marks & Spencer*, 1 pack/180g				
279/155	21.8/12.1	41/22.8	3.1/1.7	5.2/2.9
Sandwich, Turkey & Ham Salad, Sutherland*, 1 pack/185g				
303/164	18.1/9.8	46.6/25.2	4.8/2.6	0/0
Sandwich, Turkey & Stuffing, Marks & Spencer*, 1 pack/190g				
352/185	23.4/12.3	43.9/23.1	9.3/4.9	3.6/1.9
Sandwich, Turkey Breast & Ham Sandwich, Subway*, 1 pack/235g				
294/125	20/8.5	46.1/19.6	4.9/2.1	4/1.7

	kcal serv/100g	prot serv/100g	carb serv/100g	fat serv/100g	fibre serv/100g

Sandwich, Turkey, Lettuce & Tomato, Shapers, Boots*, 1 pack/217g

310/143	21.3/9.8	45.6/21	4.8/2.2	6.3/2.9

Sandwich, Turkey, Pork & Herb, Starbucks*, 1 pack/198g

465/235	23.2/11.7	44.7/22.6	21.4/10.8	4.2/2.1

Sandwich, Turkey, Stuffing & Cranberry Sauce, Shapers, Boots*,
1 pack/167g

316/189	16.7/10	43.4/26	8.4/5	2.5/1.5

Sandwich, Veggie Delite, Subway*, 1 pack/166g

226/136	9/5.4	44/26.5	3/1.8	4/2.4

Sandwich, Wensleydale & Carrot, Marks & Spencer*, 1 pack/183g

430/235	18.1/9.9	39.2/21.4	22.5/12.3	5.1/2.8

Sandwich, York Ham, Starbucks*, 1 pack/208g

341/164	21.6/10.4	44.1/21.2	8.7/4.2	6/2.9

Wrap, American Deli, Shapers, Boots*, 1 pack/171.7g

249/145	16.3/9.5	36.1/21	4.5/2.6	3.4/2

Wrap, Avocado & Salad, Pret a Manger*, 1 serving/200g

605/303	10.5/5.3	36.1/18.1	46.5/23.3	5.8/2.9

Wrap, BBQ Steak, Marks & Spencer*, 1 pack/253g

506/200	26.8/10.6	62.7/24.8	17.2/6.8	4.6/1.8

Wrap, Beef in Black Bean, Marks & Spencer*, 1 pack/150g

338/225	15.3/10.2	30.8/20.5	17.1/11.4	2.4/1.6

Wrap, Brie & Cranberry, Marks & Spencer*, 1 pack/224.5g

549/245	13.7/6.1	61.2/27.3	27.8/12.4	3.8/1.7

Wrap, Cajun Chicken Louisiana-Style, Sainsbury's*, 1 pack/190g

395/209	21/11.1	45.2/23.9	14.4/7.6	0/0

Wrap, Cajun, GFY, Asda*, 1 pack/176.3g

231/131	15.8/9	37/21	2.1/1.2	1.6/0.9

Wrap, Chargrilled Chicken, Perfectly Balanced, Waitrose*, 1 pack/230g

361/157	23.7/10.3	52.2/22.7	6.7/2.9	6.7/2.9

Wrap, Chicken Caesar, Boots*, 1 pack/160.4g

254/159	20.8/13	35.2/22	3.4/2.1	3.2/2

Wrap, Chicken Caesar, Healthy Eating, Tesco*, 1 pack/170g

296/174	20.4/12	44.6/26.2	4/2.4	4.4/2.6

Wrap, Chicken Caesar, Marks & Spencer*, 1 pack/225g

675/300	26.8/11.9	46.1/20.5	43/19.1	3.2/1.4

Wrap, Chicken Caesar, Tesco*, 1 pack/110g

252/229	10.8/9.8	27.5/25	11/10	0.1/0.1

kcal serv/100g	prot serv/100g	carb serv/100g	fat serv/100g	fibre serv/100g

Wrap, Chicken Fajita Red, Yellow Peppers, Weight Watchers*, 1 pack/177g

| 297/168 | 15.9/9 | 43.7/24.7 | 6.5/3.7 | 3/1.7 |

Wrap, Chicken Fajita, Asda*, 1 pack/180g

| 369/205 | 16.9/9.4 | 37.1/20.6 | 16.9/9.4 | 0.7/0.4 |

Wrap, Chicken Fajita, Tesco*, 1 pack/220g

| 381/173 | 21.3/9.7 | 49.7/22.6 | 10.6/4.8 | 0.7/0.3 |

Wrap, Chicken Fajita, Waitrose*, 1 pack/174g

| 279/160 | 14.5/8.3 | 36.9/21.2 | 8.2/4.7 | 3.5/2 |

Wrap, Chicken Fillet with Cheese & Bacon, Asda*, 1 pack/164.1g

| 366/223 | 41/25 | 2.3/1.4 | 21.3/13 | 0/0 |

Wrap, Chicken Salad, Pret A Manger*, 1 av pack/230g

| 323/140 | 16.9/7.4 | 31.2/13.6 | 14.6/6.4 | 1.6/0.7 |

Wrap, Chicken Salsa, Healthy Eating, Tesco*, 1 pack/240g

| 348/145 | 19.9/8.3 | 52.8/22 | 6.2/2.6 | 1.2/0.5 |

Wrap, Chicken Thai-Style, Boots*, 1 pack/156g

| 290/186 | 17.2/11 | 32.8/21 | 10/6.4 | 3.4/2.2 |

Wrap, Chicken Tikka Masala, Patak's*, 1 pack/150g

| 252/168 | 11.7/7.8 | 29/19.3 | 9.9/6.6 | 0/0 |

Wrap, Chicken Tikka, Ginsters*, 1 pack/150g

| 278/185 | 13.4/8.9 | 38.3/25.5 | 8/5.3 | 2.4/1.6 |

Wrap, Chicken Tikka, Mattessons*, 1 pack/150g

| 284/189 | 14.7/9.8 | 32.3/21.5 | 10.5/7 | 4.8/3.2 |

Wrap, Chilli Beef, COU, Marks & Spencer*, 1 pack/179g

| 260/145 | 17.4/9.7 | 40.6/22.7 | 2.5/1.4 | 3.4/1.9 |

Wrap, Chilli Chicken, BGTY, Sainsbury's*, 1 pack/180g

| 313/174 | 18.4/10.2 | 50.4/28 | 4.3/2.4 | 0/0 |

Wrap, Chinese Chicken, Marks & Spencer*, 1 pack/155g

| 239/154 | 21.7/14 | 34.6/22.3 | 1.6/1 | 3.1/2 |

Wrap, Coronation Chicken, Waitrose*, 1 pack/163.6g

| 284/173 | 16.6/10.1 | 34.9/21.3 | 8.4/5.1 | 3.6/2.2 |

Wrap, Dhansak Prawn, Marks & Spencer*, 1 pack/208.1g

| 385/185 | 14.8/7.1 | 48.5/23.3 | 15/7.2 | 5/2.4 |

Wrap, Duck, Food To Go, Marks & Spencer*, 1 pack/257g

| 474/185 | 21.8/8.5 | 65.3/25.5 | 13.8/5.4 | 2.6/1 |

Wrap, Egg Mayonnaise, Tomato & Cress, Sainsbury's*, 1 pack/255g

| 592/232 | 18.6/7.3 | 45.1/17.7 | 38.3/15 | 0/0 |

Wrap, Feta Cheese Flat Bread, COU, Marks & Spencer*, 1 pack/180g

| 225/125 | 11.3/6.3 | 37.1/20.6 | 4/2.2 | 3.4/1.9 |

kcal serv/100g	prot serv/100g	carb serv/100g	fat serv/100g	fibre serv/100g

Wrap, Feta Cheese, GFY, Asda*, 1 pack/165g

| 256/155 | 11.6/7 | 36.3/22 | 7.1/4.3 | 3.5/2.1 |

Wrap, Fiery Mexican Cheese, Ginsters*, 1 pack/150g

| 437/291 | 16.7/11.1 | 56.3/37.5 | 16.4/10.9 | 4.1/2.7 |

Wrap, Goat's Cheese & Tomato, TTD, Sainsbury's*, 1 pack/204g

| 420/206 | 14.3/7 | 52.2/25.6 | 17.1/8.4 | 0/0 |

Wrap, Greek Salad, COU, Marks & Spencer*, 1 pack/180g

| 225/125 | 11.3/6.3 | 37.1/20.6 | 4/2.2 | 3.4/1.9 |

Wrap, Green Thai Chicken, Sainsbury's*, 1 pack/212g

| 422/199 | 20.1/9.5 | 54.1/25.5 | 13.8/6.5 | 0/0 |

Wrap, Gressingham Duck & Hoi Sin Sauce, TTD, Sainsbury's*, 1 pack/199g

| 354/178 | 18.5/9.3 | 49.4/24.8 | 9.2/4.6 | 0/0 |

Wrap, Ham, Cheese & Pickle Tortilla, Weight Watchers*, 1 pack/170.1g

| 296/174 | 18.5/10.9 | 44.9/26.4 | 4.8/2.8 | 2/1.2 |

Wrap, Hoisin Duck, Marks & Spencer*, 1 pack/232g

| 510/220 | 23/9.9 | 56.6/24.4 | 21.6/9.3 | 3/1.3 |

Wrap, Houmous Salad, Pret A Manger*, 1 av pack/230g

| 351/153 | 11.5/5 | 41.1/17.9 | 15.6/6.8 | 7.9/3.4 |

Wrap, Italian Chicken, Sainsbury's*, ½ pack/211g

| 395/187 | 33.1/15.7 | 13.1/6.2 | 23.2/11 | 1.9/0.9 |

Wrap, Mediterranean Tuna with Chargrilled Veg & Mixed Leaves, Boots*, 1 pack/208g

| 412/198 | 18.9/9.1 | 49.9/24 | 15.2/7.3 | 3.1/1.5 |

Wrap, Mediterranean-Style Chicken, Waitrose*, 1 pack/182.7g

| 296/162 | 15.2/8.3 | 34/18.6 | 11/6 | 4.2/2.3 |

Wrap, Mexican Bean & Potato in Spinach Tortilla, Daily Bread*, 1 pack/195.8g

| 329/168 | 9.6/4.9 | 49/25 | 10.6/5.4 | 0/0 |

Wrap, Mexican Chicken, Marks & Spencer*, 1 serving/218g

| 447/205 | 18.7/8.6 | 42.9/19.7 | 22.5/10.3 | 2.8/1.3 |

Wrap, Mexican-Style Chicken, Co-Op*, 1 pack/163g

| 367/225 | 17.9/11 | 42.4/26 | 14.7/9 | 4.9/3 |

Wrap, Mexican Sweet Potato & Three Bean, Marks & Spencer*, 1 pack/222g

| 522/235 | 16.9/7.6 | 58.6/26.4 | 24.4/11 | 3.1/1.4 |

Wrap, Mexican Three Bean, Marks & Spencer*, 1 pack/246.8g

| 580/235 | 18.8/7.6 | 65.2/26.4 | 27.2/11 | 3.5/1.4 |

Wrap, Mild Chicken Curry, Patak's*, 1 pack/150g

| 239/159 | 12.2/8.1 | 32/21.3 | 9/6 | 4.2/2.8 |

	kcal serv/100g	prot serv/100g	carb serv/100g	fat serv/100g	fibre serv/100g

Wrap, Moroccan-Style Cous Cous, Tesco*, 1 serving/240g

	370/154	12.7/5.3	65.4/27.3	6.5/2.7	3/1.3

Wrap, Moroccan Chicken, Shapers, Boots*, 1 serving/154g

	271/176	14.8/9.6	40/26	5.7/3.7	2.6/1.7

Wrap, Nacho Chicken, COU, Marks & Spencer*, 1 pack/181.5g

	244/135	17.4/9.6	35.7/19.7	3.8/2.1	2.5/1.4

Wrap, Parma Ham Chicken, Perfectly Balanced, Waitrose*, ½ pack/198g

	212/107	39.8/20.1	5/2.5	3.6/1.8	1.8/0.9

Wrap, Peking Duck, Asda*, 1 pack/172g

	427/248	16.2/9.4	49/28.5	18.4/10.7	1.9/1.1

Wrap, Peking Duck, Boots*, 1 pack/229g

	440/192	19/8.3	68.7/30	9.8/4.3	6/2.6

Wrap, Peking Duck, Waitrose*, 1 pack/182g

	319/175	18.2/10	47.2/25.9	6.4/3.5	2.9/1.6

Wrap, Roasted Vegetable & Feta, BGTY, Sainsbury's*, 1 serving/200g

	318/159	11.6/5.8	50/25	8/4	0/0

Wrap, Sausage & Bacon, Asda*, 1 pack/21g

	52/249	3.8/18	3.2/15	2.7/13	0.1/0.5

Wrap, Smoked Salmon & Prawn, Finest, Tesco*, 1 serving/58.5g

	84/143	8.4/14.3	0.6/1	5.4/9.1	0/0

Wrap, Spanish Chorizo Sausage, Black Olive & Bean, TTD, Sainsbury's*, 1 pack/237g

	517/218	18.2/7.7	63.3/26.7	21.1/8.9	0/0

Wrap, Sushi Salmon & Cucumber, Waitrose*, 1 pack/180g

	299/166	11.3/6.3	49/27.2	6.5/3.6	2.9/1.6

Wrap, Sweet & Sour Prawn, Eat Smart, Safeway*, 1 pack/204g

	275/135	13.1/6.4	49/24	2.4/1.2	2.9/1.4

Wrap, Tandoori Chicken, GFU, Asda*, 1 pack/167g

	281/168	16.7/10	43.4/26	4.5/2.7	2.8/1.7

Wrap, Thai Prawn, COU, Marks & Spencer*, 1 pack/181g

	235/130	11/6.1	40.5/22.4	2.4/1.3	3.3/1.8

Wrap, Tortilla, Chicken Fajita, Sutherland*, 1 pack/158g

	379/240	20.5/13	42.7/27	14.2/9	0/0

Wrap, Tortilla, Vegetable, Asda*, 1 pack/125g

	245/196	8.5/6.8	46.5/37.2	2.8/2.2	1/0.8

Wrap, Tuna Nicoise, Healthy Eating, Tesco*, 1 pack/117g

	160/137	9.7/8.3	24.1/20.6	2.7/2.3	0.6/0.5

kcal serv/100g	prot serv/100g	carb serv/100g	fat serv/100g	fibre serv/100g

Wrap, Tuna Salsa, Healthy Eating, Wild Bean Cafe*, 1 pack/159g

| 245/154 | 18/11.3 | 37.4/23.5 | 2.7/1.7 | 2.4/1.5 |

Wrap, Tuna, Sweetcorn & Red Pepper, BGTY, Sainsbury's*, 1 pack/178g

| 306/172 | 20.5/11.5 | 37.7/21.2 | 8.2/4.6 | 3.7/2.1 |

Wrap, Turkey, Bacon & Cranberry, COU, Marks & Spencer*, 1 pack/143.8g

| 230/160 | 13.8/9.6 | 39/27.1 | 2.2/1.5 | 3.3/2.3 |

SAUCES, DIPS AND DRESSINGS

Chutney, Albert's Victorian, Baxters*, 1 serving/25g

| 38/150 | 8.8/35 | 1.5/6 | 0/0.1 | 0/0 |

Chutney, Cranberry & Caramelised Red Onion, Baxters*, 1 serving/20g

| 31/154 | 0.1/0.3 | 7.6/38 | 0/0.1 | 0.1/0.3 |

Chutney, Fruit, Spiced, Baxters*, 1 tsp/16g

| 23/143 | 1/6 | 5.6/34.8 | 0/0.1 | 0/0 |

Chutney, Major Grey Mango, Patak's*, 1oz/28g

| 71/255 | 0.1/0.4 | 18.5/66 | 0.1/0.2 | 0.2/0.7 |

Chutney, Mango & Apple, Sharwood's*, 1oz/28g

| 65/233 | 0.1/0.4 | 16.1/57.6 | 0/0.1 | 0.3/1.1 |

Chutney, Mango & Lime, Sharwood's*, 1oz/28g

| 58/206 | 0.1/0.4 | 14.1/50.5 | 0.1/0.3 | 0.2/0.8 |

Chutney, Mango, Green Label, Sharwood's*, 1 serving/10g

| 23/234 | 0/0.3 | 5.8/57.8 | 0/0.2 | 0.1/0.9 |

Chutney, Mango, Hot, Patak's*, 1oz/28g

| 72/258 | 0.1/0.4 | 18.8/67.1 | 0.1/0.2 | 0.2/0.7 |

Chutney, Tomato, TTD, Sainsbury's*, 1 tbsp/15g

| 29/193 | 0.3/2 | 6.7/44.7 | 0.2/1.3 | 0.4/2.7 |

Dip, Applewood Cheddar & Onion, Fresh, BGTY, Sainsbury's*, ½ pot/85g

| 85/100 | 6.2/7.3 | 6.2/7.3 | 3.9/4.6 | 0.4/0.5 |

Dip, Aubergine, Fresh, Waitrose*, 1 serving/85g

| 159/187 | 2.1/2.5 | 8.9/10.5 | 12.8/15 | 1.4/1.7 |

Dip, Cajun Red Pepper, Sainsbury's*, 1 serving/50g

| 25/50 | 0.7/1.4 | 3.5/7 | 0.9/1.8 | 0.7/1.4 |

Dip, Celery, Marks & Spencer*, 1 pot/130g

| 163/125 | 2.3/1.8 | 5.7/4.4 | 14.3/11 | 1.6/1.2 |

Dip, Cheddar & Onion, Marks & Spencer*, 1oz/28g

| 88/315 | 1.4/5.1 | 2.1/7.5 | 8.3/29.5 | 0.1/0.5 |

	kcal serv/100g	prot serv/100g	carb serv/100g	fat serv/100g	fibre serv/100g
Dip, Cheese & Bacon with Breadsticks, Weight Watchers*, 1 pack/50g					
	98/196	8/16	12/24	2.1/4.2	0.7/1.4
Dip, Cheese & Chive, 50% Less Fat, Asda*, 1 pot/125g					
	261/209	5.6/4.5	11.3/9	21.5/17.2	0/0
Dip, Cheese & Chive, Classic, Tesco*, 1 serving/32g					
	164/511	1.1/3.3	1/3.1	17.3/54	0/0.1
Dip, Cheese & Chive, Healthy Eating, Tesco*, 1 tsp/10g					
	23/228	0.6/5.7	0.6/6.4	2/19.9	0/0
Dip, Cheese & Chive, Healthy Selection, Somerfield*, 1oz/28g					
	67/239	1.7/6	1.4/5	6.2/22	0/0
Dip, Chilli, Marks & Spencer*, 1 pot/35g					
	103/295	0.1/0.4	25.6/73.2	0.1/0.2	0.1/0.4
Dip, Chunky Tomato Salsa, Tesco*, 1 pot/170g					
	68/40	1.9/1.1	10/5.9	2.2/1.3	1.9/1.1
Dip, Cranberry, Asda*, ½ pot/40g					
	53/132	0.2/0.4	11.6/29	0.6/1.6	0.3/0.8
Dip, Creamy Roasted Tomato & Herb, COU, Marks & Spencer*, 1 serving/40g					
	30/75	3.1/7.7	2.9/7.2	0.7/1.7	0.4/0.9
Dip, Cucumber & Mint, Eat Smart, Safeway*, ½ pot/85g					
	55/65	6.2/7.3	4.2/4.9	1.1/1.3	0.7/0.8
Dip, Cucumber & Mint, Fresh, Sainsbury's*, 1oz/28g					
	34/123	1.3/4.5	1/3.7	2.8/10	0/0
Dip, Doritos Mild Salsa, Walkers*, 1oz/28g					
	11/40	0.3/0.9	2.4/8.5	0.1/0.2	0.6/2.2
Dip, Feta Cheese, Fresh, Tesco*, 1oz/28g					
	81/288	1.9/6.8	2.2/7.9	7.1/25.5	0.2/0.7
Dip, Garlic & Herb, Marks & Spencer*, 1oz/28g					
	88/315	0.7/2.4	2/7.1	8.6/30.6	0.1/0.5
Dip, Garlic & Herb, Reduced-Fat, Marks & Spencer*, 1 serving/10g					
	10/95	0.6/6	0.8/8.1	0.4/4	0.1/0.5
Dip, Garlic & Herb, Tesco*, ¼ pack/42.5g					
	260/604	0.4/0.9	1.4/3.2	28.1/65.4	0.1/0.3
Dip, Mature Cheddar Cheese & Chive, Fresh, Waitrose*, ½ pot/85g					
	393/462	4.9/5.8	2/2.4	40.5/47.7	1.4/1.7
Dip, Mexican Bean, Doritos*, 1 tbsp/20g					
	18/89	0.5/2.7	2.4/12.1	0.7/3.3	0.5/2.4
Dip, Mustard & Honey, Fresh, Sainsbury's*, 1oz/28g					
	100/356	0.6/2.2	1.4/5.1	10.2/36.3	0/0

	kcal serv/100g	prot serv/100g	carb serv/100g	fat serv/100g	fibre serv/100g

Dip, Onion & Garlic, 50% Less Fat, Asda*, 1oz/28g

59/209	1.3/4.5	2.5/9	4.8/17.2	0/0

Dip, Onion & Garlic, Fresh, BGTY, Sainsbury's*, 1oz/28g

56/201	1.2/4.4	1.3/4.8	5.1/18.2	0.2/0.8

Dip, Onion & Garlic, Healthy Eating, Tesco*, 1 pot/170g

345/203	5.6/3.3	13.4/7.9	29.9/17.6	0.2/0.1

Dip, Onion & Garlic, Healthy Selection, Somerfield*, 1oz/28g

62/222	0.8/3	1.4/5	5.9/21	0/0

Dip, Peanut, Satay Selection, Occasions, Sainsbury's*, 1 serving/2g

4/186	0.1/7.1	0.3/13.8	0.2/11.4	0/1.1

Dip, Pecorino, Basil & Pine Nut, Fresh, Waitrose*, ½ pot/85g

338/398	4.3/5.1	4.3/5.1	33.7/39.7	0/0

Dip, Philadelphia & Breadsticks, Light, Kraft*, 1 portion/50g

119/238	4.3/8.5	12.3/24.5	6/12	0.6/1.1

Dip, Philadelphia Light with Italian Breadsticks, Kraft*, 1 pack/50g

123/245	4.2/8.4	11.5/23	6.5/13	0.8/1.5

Dip, Roast Onion, Garlic & Rocket, Reduced-Fat, Waitrose*, 1 serving/25g

51/202	0.7/2.7	1.4/5.4	4.7/18.8	0.4/1.5

Dip, Salsa, Kettle*, 1 serving/25g

10/39	0.4/1.7	2/8	0/0	0/0

Dip, Smoked Salmon & Dill, Fresh, Waitrose*, ½ pot/85g

373/439	4.3/5.1	3.5/4.1	38/44.7	0.1/0.1

Dip, Smoked Salmon & Dill, Reduced-Fat, Waitrose*, ½ pot/85g

184/217	3.3/3.9	5.2/6.1	16.7/19.7	0.9/1.1

Dip, Sour Cream & Chive, Asda*, ⅕ pot/33g

116/350	0.8/2.4	1.3/4	11.9/36	0/0.1

Dip, Sour Cream & Chive, BGTY, Sainsbury's, 1oz/28g

46/165	1.4/4.9	1/3.4	4.1/14.6	0.2/0.7

Dip, Sour Cream & Chive, Doritos*, 1 tbsp/20g

64/322	0.5/2.5	0.6/3.1	6.7/33.3	0/0.1

Dip, Sour Cream & Chive, Fresh, Tesco*, ½ pot/75g

305/407	1.6/2.1	3.1/4.1	31.8/42.4	0/0

Dip, Sour Cream & Chive, Primula*, 1oz/28g

97/346	1.4/5	0.5/1.8	9.9/35.3	0/0

Dip, Spicy Moroccan, BGTY, Sainsbury's*, ½ pot/84.8g

56/66	1.8/2.1	8.5/10	1.7/2	1.4/1.7

Dip, Thousand Island, Marks & Spencer*, 1oz/28g

69/245	0.6/2.1	2.6/9.4	6.2/22.2	0.2/0.7

kcal serv/100g	prot serv/100g	carb serv/100g	fat serv/100g	fibre serv/100g
Dip, Tikka, Classic, Fresh, Healthy Choice, Safeway*, 1oz/28g				
38/137	2.9/10.2	1.7/6	2.2/8	0.4/1.3
Dip, Tomato Salsa, Fresh, Waitrose*, 1 serving/50g				
24/47	0.8/1.5	2.5/5	1.2/2.3	0.9/1.7
Dip, Tzatziki, Somerfield*, 1oz/28g				
37/131	1.7/6	0.8/3	3.1/11	0/0
Dip, Yoghurt & Cucumber Mint, Tesco*, 1oz/28g				
34/121	2/7	2/7.2	2/7.1	0.2/0.6
Dressing, Balsamic Vinegar & Oregano, Waitrose*, 1 serving/25g				
101/404	0.2/0.6	2.1/8.2	10.3/41	0.1/0.4
Dressing, Balsamic Vinegar & Smoked Garlic, Safeway*, 1 tbsp/15ml				
19/125	0/0.1	4.2/28.3	0.1/0.9	0.1/0.5
Dressing, Balsamic Vinegar, Asda*, 1 pack/44ml				
121/275	0.4/0.9	3.1/7	11.9/27	0/0
Dressing, Balsamic with Garlic & Herbs, Finest, Tesco*, 1 serving/10ml				
13/133	0/0.3	0.3/3.4	1.3/13.1	0/0.1
Dressing, Balsamic, Extra Virgin Olive Oil, TTD, Sainsbury's*, 1 tsp/5ml				
19/376	0/0.5	0.6/12.8	1.8/36	0/0.4
Dressing, Blue Cheese, BGTY, Sainsbury's*, 1 tbsp/15ml				
16/108	0.4/2.9	0.5/3.6	0.9/6	0.1/0.7
Dressing, Blue Cheese, Fresh, Sainsbury's*, 1 dtsp/10ml				
42/423	0.2/2.3	0.1/0.5	4.6/45.7	0/0.1
Dressing, Blue Cheese, Healthy Eating, Tesco*, 1 tsp/5g				
4/82	0.2/4.4	0.5/9	0.2/3.1	0/0.1
Dressing, Blue Cheese, Hellmann's*, 1 tbsp/15g				
69/459	0.1/0.7	0.9/6.3	7.1/47.2	0.2/1.1
Dressing, Blue Cheese, Low-Fat, Weight Watchers*, 1oz/28g				
17/59	0.4/1.5	1.6/5.8	1/3.4	0/0
Dressing, Caesar-Style, GFY, Asda*, 1 sachet/44ml				
34/77	2.2/5	4/9	1/2.3	0/0
Dressing, Caesar-Style, Kraft*, 1 tbsp/15ml				
15/102	0.3/2.1	2.3/15	0.5/3.5	0/0.1
Dressing, Caesar-Style, Low-Fat, Weight Watchers*, 1 tsp/6g				
4/60	0.1/1.6	0.3/5.8	0.2/3.4	0/0
Dressing, Caesar, 95% Fat-Free, Tesco*, 1 tsp/6g				
5/88	0.2/4.1	0.5/8.9	0.2/3.7	0/0.3
Dressing, Caesar, BGTY, Sainsbury's*, 1 serving/25ml				
27/108	0.3/1.3	2.1/8.3	2/7.8	0.2/0.9

	kcal serv/100g	prot serv/100g	carb serv/100g	fat serv/100g	fibre serv/100g
Dressing, Caesar, Chilled, Reduced-Fat, Tesco*, 1 tsp/5ml					
	13/252	0.3/6.5	0.2/3.1	1.2/23.7	0/0.1
Dressing, Caesar, Finest, Tesco*, 1 tbsp/15ml					
	72/477	0.3/1.9	0.4/2.8	7.6/50.9	0/0.2
Dressing, Caesar, Fresh, Asda*, 1 dtsp/10ml					
	45/445	0.3/2.5	0.1/0.7	4.8/48	0/0
Dressing, Caesar, Fresh, Marks & Spencer*, 1 tsp/6g					
	32/525	0.1/2	0.1/1.8	3.4/56.4	0/0.2
Dressing, Caesar, Fresh, Sainsbury's*, 1 tsp/6g					
	29/479	0.2/3	0.1/1.1	3.1/51.4	0/0.2
Dressing, Caesar, Gourmet, Fresh, Waitrose*, 1 tbsp/15ml					
	72/479	0.7/4.5	0.1/0.9	7.6/50.8	0.1/0.5
Dressing, Caesar, Healthy Eating, Tesco*, 1 tbsp/15ml					
	11/74	0.5/3	1.3/8.4	0.4/2.8	0/0.2
Dressing, Caesar, Hellmann's*, 1 tsp/6g					
	30/499	0.2/2.5	0.3/4.5	3.1/51.7	0/0.3
Dressing, French Classic, Marks & Spencer*, 1 tbsp/15ml					
	77/516	0.1/0.6	1.2/8.2	8/53.1	0/0.2
Dressing, French Dressing, Fresh, Co-Op*, 1 tbsp/15ml					
	70/467	0/0	0/0	7/46.7	0/0
Dressing, French-Style Calorie-Wise Salad, Kraft*, 1 tbsp/15ml					
	24/160	0/0	2.8/18.7	1.6/10.7	0/0
Dressing, French-Style, Eat Smart, Safeway*, 1 serving/15ml					
	22/145	0.1/0.7	4.3/28.9	0.4/2.5	0.1/0.7
Dressing, French-Style, Oil-Free, Healthy Eating, Tesco*, 1 tbsp/15g					
	5/30	0/0.3	0.9/6	0/0.2	0.2/1.4
Dressing, French, BGTY, Sainsbury's*, 1 tbsp/15ml					
	12/79	0.2/1.1	1.3/8.8	0.7/4.4	0.1/0.5
Dressing, French, Chilled, Tesco*, 1 tbsp/15ml					
	63/421	0.2/1.1	2.3/15.1	5.9/39.6	0/0
Dressing, French, COU, Marks & Spencer*, ⅓ bottle/105g					
	74/70	0.7/0.7	12.1/11.5	2.7/2.6	0.7/0.7
Dressing, French, Fresh, Healthy Eating, Tesco*, 1 tbsp/15ml					
	8/56	0.2/1.1	1/6.7	0.4/2.8	0/0
Dressing, French, Fresh, Morrisons*, 1 tbsp/15ml					
	75/499	0.2/1.5	2/13.6	7.3/48.7	0/0
Dressing, French, Fresh, Safeway*, 1 tbsp/15ml					
	77/510	0.2/1.5	2.1/13.8	7.5/49.9	0/0

	kcal serv/100g	prot serv/100g	carb serv/100g	fat serv/100g	fibre serv/100g
Dressing, French, Fresh, Sainsbury's*, 1 tbsp/15ml					
	64/429	0.1/0.6	1/6.6	6.7/44.6	0.1/0.6
Dressing, French, Fresh, Somerfield*, 1 tbsp/15ml					
	74/490	0.2/1	1.1/7	7.7/51	0/0
Dressing, French, GFY, Asda*, 1 tbsp/15g					
	8/50	0.1/0.7	1.1/7	0.3/2.1	0/0.1
Dressing, French, Healthy Eating, Tesco*, 1 tbsp/15ml					
	3/23	0.1/0.8	0.5/3.1	0.1/0.8	0/0
Dressing, French, Less Than 3% Fat, Marks & Spencer*, 1 tbsp/15ml					
	10/68	0.1/0.7	1.7/11.5	0.4/2.6	0.1/0.7
Dressing, French, Low-Fat, Hellmann's*, 1 tbsp/15g					
	9/62	0/0.1	1.6/10.8	0.2/1.6	0.1/0.5
Dressing, French, Luxury, Hellmann's*, 1 tbsp/15g					
	45/297	0.1/0.4	2.2/14.9	3.9/25.9	0/0.3
Dressing, French, Oil-Free, Perfectly Balanced, Waitrose*, 1 serving/15ml					
	11/72	0.3/2.2	1.8/12.2	0.2/1.6	0.2/1.1
Dressing, Garlic & Herb, Perfectly Balanced, Waitrose*, 1 serving/50ml					
	68/135	0.3/0.6	15/29.9	0.7/1.4	0.4/0.8
Dressing, Garlic & Herb, Reduced-Calorie, Hellmann's*, 1 tbsp/15ml					
	35/232	0.1/0.6	1.9/12.8	2.9/19.3	0.1/0.4
Dressing, Green Olive, Marks & Spencer*, 1oz/28g					
	40/144	0.4/1.5	0.6/2.2	4/14.4	0.4/1.3
Dressing, Green Thai, Coconut & Lemon Grass, Loyd Grossman*, 1oz/28g					
	49/174	0.1/0.2	5.4/19.3	3/10.6	0.1/0.5
Dressing, Honey & Mustard, Finest, Tesco*, 1 serving/25ml					
	72/288	0.4/1.7	4.9/19.6	5.6/22.5	0.2/0.7
Dressing, Honey & Mustard, Fresh, Marks & Spencer*, 1 serving/10ml					
	43/430	0.2/1.7	1/9.7	4.2/42.4	0.1/0.5
Dressing, Honey & Mustard, Fresh, Safeway*, 1 serving/80ml					
	309/386	1/1.3	10.7/13.4	29/36.3	0/0
Dressing, Honey & Mustard, GFY, Asda*, 1 tbsp/15g					
	13/89	0.2/1.5	2/13	0.5/3.4	0.1/0.8
Dressing, Honey & Mustard, Healthy Eating, Tesco*, 1 tbsp/15g					
	12/79	0.2/1.5	1.8/12.1	0.4/2.7	0.1/0.9
Dressing, Honey & Mustard, Sainsbury's*, 1 serving/10ml					
	37/366	0.1/1	1.5/15.4	3.3/33	0/0.1
Dressing, Honey, Orange & Mustard, BGTY, Sainsbury's*, 1 tbsp/15ml					
	16/105	0.3/1.8	2.8/18.6	0.4/2.5	0.3/1.8

	kcal serv/100g	prot serv/100g	carb serv/100g	fat serv/100g	fibre serv/100g

Dressing, Hot Lime & Coconut, BGTY, Sainsbury's*, 1 tbsp/15ml

| 8/51 | 0.1/0.7 | 0.9/5.7 | 0.4/2.9 | 0.2/1.2 |

Dressing, Italian Balsamic, Loyd Grossman*, 1 serving/10g

| 36/357 | 0.1/0.9 | 1.3/13.1 | 3.4/33.5 | 0/0.1 |

Dressing, Italian Salad, Hellmann's*, 1 serving/50g

| 103/206 | 0.4/0.7 | 6.4/12.8 | 8.4/16.7 | 0/0 |

Dressing, Italian, Waistline, 99% Fat-Free, Crosse & Blackwell*, 1 tsp/6g

| 2/39 | 0/0.7 | 0.4/7 | 0.1/0.9 | 0/0.3 |

**Dressing, Lemon & Black Pepper, Good Intentions, Somerfield*,
1 tbsp/15ml**

| 36/241 | 0.4/2.6 | 1.6/10.5 | 3.2/21 | 0.1/0.4 |

Dressing, Lemon & Cracked Black Pepper, GFY, Asda*, 1 tbsp/15g

| 9/57 | 0/0.2 | 2.1/14 | 0/0 | 0/0.3 |

Dressing, Lemon & Tarragon, Healthy Eating, Tesco*, 1 serving/10ml

| 11/113 | 0.1/1.1 | 2.2/21.6 | 0.2/2.4 | 0/0 |

Dressing, Lime & Coriander, EPC*, 1 serving/50g

| 29/57 | 0.2/0.3 | 6.7/13.3 | 0.2/0.3 | 0/0 |

Dressing, Lime & Coriander, Sainsbury's*, 1 tbsp/15ml

| 61/409 | 0.1/0.4 | 1.5/10 | 6.1/40.8 | 0.1/0.5 |

Dressing, Lime Sublime Creamy, Ainsley Harriott*, 1 serving/28g

| 95/338 | 0/0 | 2.8/10 | 9.1/32.5 | 0/0 |

Dressing, Mayonnaise-Style, 90% Fat-Free, Weight Watchers*, 1 tsp/11g

| 14/125 | 0.2/1.7 | 1/8.9 | 1/9.2 | 0/0 |

Dressing, Mild Mustard, Low-Fat, Weight Watchers*, 1 tbsp/10g

| 6/63 | 0.2/2 | 0.6/5.7 | 0.4/3.6 | 0/0 |

Dressing, Miracle Whip, Kraft*, 1 tbsp/15ml

| 60/400 | 0/0.3 | 1.7/11 | 5.9/39 | 0/0.1 |

Dressing, Mustard & Dill, Perfectly Balanced, Waitrose*, 1 tbsp/15ml

| 24/159 | 0.2/1.1 | 4.7/31.5 | 0.5/3.2 | 0.2/1.1 |

Dressing, Orange & Honey, Luxury, Hellmann's*, 1 serving/15ml

| 17/110 | 0.1/0.8 | 2.6/17.5 | 0.5/3.5 | 0.1/0.8 |

Dressing, Parmesan & Peppercorn, Loyd Grossman*, 1oz/28g

| 98/349 | 0.6/2.1 | 1.7/5.9 | 9.9/35.2 | 0.1/0.5 |

Dressing, Passion Fruit & Mango, Healthy Eating, Tesco*, 1 tbsp/15ml

| 25/169 | 0.1/0.6 | 5.5/36.7 | 0.3/2.2 | 0.1/0.4 |

Dressing, Porcini Mushroom, TTD, Sainsbury's*, 1 tbsp/15g

| 46/308 | 0.2/1.3 | 0.5/3.3 | 4.8/32.1 | 0.8/5.4 |

	kcal serv/100g	prot serv/100g	carb serv/100g	fat serv/100g	fibre serv/100g

Dressing, Provencal Roasted Vegetable, Healthy Eating, Tesco*, 1 serving/10ml

| | 8/75 | 0.1/1 | 1.2/12.1 | 0.3/2.5 | 0/0.4 |

Dressing, Ranch-Style, Asda*, 1 serving/44ml

| | 37/85 | 1.5/3.5 | 4/9 | 1.7/3.9 | 0/0 |

Dressing, Raspberry Balsamic Vinegar, EPC*, 1 serving/50g

| | 34/67 | 0.2/0.4 | 7.9/15.7 | 0.1/0.1 | 0.3/0.6 |

Dressing, Red Pepper, Marks & Spencer*, 1 tbsp/15ml

| | 58/385 | 0.1/0.6 | 1.1/7.6 | 5.9/39.2 | 0.1/0.5 |

Dressing, Roasted Garlic, More Than A Dressing, EPC*, 1 serving/100ml

| | 55/55 | 0.6/0.6 | 12.4/12.4 | 0.3/0.3 | 0/0 |

Dressing, Roasted Red Pepper, TTD, Sainsbury's*, 1 tbsp/15ml

| | 52/347 | 0.2/1.3 | 1.5/10 | 5.1/34 | 0.2/1.3 |

Dressing, Salad Cream-Style, Weight Watchers*, 1 tbsp/10g

| | 12/115 | 0.2/1.5 | 1.6/16.2 | 0.4/4.4 | 0/0 |

Dressing, Salad, BGTY, Sainsbury's*, 1 tbsp/15g

| | 21/140 | 0.1/0.8 | 1.6/10.8 | 1.5/9.9 | 0/0.3 |

Dressing, Salad, Italian, Newman's Own*, 1 tbsp/10g

| | 55/545 | 0/0.2 | 0.1/1 | 6/59.8 | 0/0 |

Dressing, Salad, Light, Heinz*, 1 serving/9.8g

| | 24/244 | 0.2/1.8 | 1.4/13.5 | 2/19.9 | 0/0 |

Dressing, Salad, Low-Fat, Weight Watchers*, 1 tbsp/10g

| | 11/106 | 0.2/1.5 | 1.5/15.4 | 0.4/4.3 | 0/0 |

Dressing, Seafood, Marks & Spencer*, 1 tsp/7g

| | 39/555 | 0.1/0.9 | 0.3/4.9 | 4.2/59.3 | 0.1/0.9 |

Dressing, Smoked Garlic & Parmesan, Sainsbury's*, 1 serving/20ml

| | 83/415 | 0.6/3 | 0.8/4 | 8.2/41.1 | 0.1/0.3 |

Dressing, Sun-Dried Tomato, Safeway*, 1 serving/40ml

| | 126/314 | 0.4/1.1 | 5.5/13.8 | 11.3/28.3 | 0/0 |

Dressing, Sun-Dried Tomato, Sainsbury's, 1 serving/15ml

| | 27/179 | 0.2/1.5 | 1.6/10.9 | 2.2/14.4 | 0.1/0.6 |

Dressing, Sweet Chilli, COU, Marks & Spencer*, 1 tbsp/15ml

| | 9/60 | 0.1/0.5 | 2.2/14.5 | 0.1/0.5 | 0.1/0.4 |

Dressing, Sweetfire Pepper, Healthy Eating, Tesco*, 1 serving/10ml

| | 7/67 | 0.1/0.6 | 1.6/15.7 | 0/0.3 | 0/0.1 |

Dressing, Texas Ranch, Frank Cooper*, 1 pot/28g

| | 128/457 | 0.5/1.9 | 2.6/9.4 | 12.8/45.8 | 0.1/0.2 |

	kcal serv/100g	prot serv/100g	carb serv/100g	fat serv/100g	fibre serv/100g
Dressing, Thai Lime & Coriander, EPC*, 1 serving/25g					
	26/104	0.4/1.6	5.6/22.3	0.2/0.9	0.3/1.1
Dressing, Thousand Island, 1 tsp/6g					
	19/323	0.1/1.1	0.8/12.5	1.8/30.2	0/0.4
Dressing, Thousand Island, BGTY, Sainsbury's*, 1 serving/50g					
	53/105	0.6/1.2	10.8/21.6	0.6/1.1	1.5/2.9
Dressing, Thousand Island, COU, Marks & Spencer*, 1 serving/30g					
	26/85	0.4/1.4	4.3/14.2	0.8/2.6	0.3/1.1
Dressing, Thousand Island, Fat-Free, Kraft*, 1fl oz/30ml					
	27/90	0.2/0.5	6.2/20.5	0/0.2	0.8/2.8
Dressing, Thousand Island, Frank Cooper*, 1 pot/28g					
	122/437	0.3/1.2	2/7.2	12.5/44.8	0.1/0.3
Dressing, Thousand Island, Healthy Eating, Tesco*, 1 serving/25ml					
	47/189	0.7/2.9	2.5/10	3.8/15.1	0/0
Dressing, Thousand Island, Original, Kraft*, 1oz/28g					
	102/365	0.3/0.9	5.3/19	8.8/31.5	0.1/0.4
Dressing, Thousand Island, Reduced-Calorie, 1 tsp/6g					
	12/195	0/0.7	0.9/14.7	0.9/15.2	0/0
Dressing, Thousand Island, Tesco*, 1 serving/30ml					
	130/433	0.3/1	3.7/12.3	12.7/42.2	0/0
Dressing, Tomato & Basil, Fresh, Somerfield*, 1 tbsp/15ml					
	52/348	0.3/2	1.1/7	5.3/35	0/0
Dressing, Tomato & Basil, Healthy Eating, Tesco*, 1 serving/10ml					
	7/73	0.1/0.5	1.3/12.9	0.2/2	0.1/0.5
Dressing, Tomato & Herb, Less Than 1% Fat, Asda*, 1 tbsp/15g					
	6/43	0.1/0.7	1.2/8	0.1/0.9	0.1/0.4
Dressing, Tomato & Olive, Eat Smart, Safeway*, 1 tbsp/15ml					
	15/100	0.1/0.7	3.4/22.8	0.1/0.7	0.3/1.8
Dressing, Tomato & Red Pepper, BGTY, Sainsbury's*, 1 serving/50ml					
	42/83	0.6/1.1	5/10	2.2/4.3	0.3/0.6
Dressing, Waistline, Reduced-Fat, Crosse & Blackwell*, 1oz/28g					
	29/105	0.2/0.8	3.2/11.6	1.7/6	0.1/0.3
Dressing, Yoghurt & Mint, GFY, Asda*, 1 tbsp/15ml					
	9/60	0.6/3.9	1.2/8	0.2/1.4	0/0
Dressing, Yoghurt & Mint, Healthy Eating, Tesco*, 1 tbsp/15g					
	20/135	0.2/1.5	3.9/26.2	0.4/2.7	0/0
Dressing, Yoghurt & Mint, Perfectly Balanced, Waitrose*, 1 serving/100ml					
	130/130	4.6/4.6	22.1/22.1	2.6/2.6	0.7/0.7

	kcal serv/100g	prot serv/100g	carb serv/100g	fat serv/100g	fibre serv/100g
Gravy, Beef, Fresh, Sainsbury's*, 1 serving/83ml					
	45/54	2.6/3.1	2.7/3.2	2.7/3.3	0.4/0.5
Gravy, Chicken, Fresh, Marks & Spencer*, 1oz/28g					
	10/35	0.7/2.5	1.4/5	0/0.1	0.1/0.3
Gravy, For Poultry, Marks & Spencer*, 1 jar/400g					
	136/34	10/2.5	20/5	1.6/0.4	1.2/0.3
Gravy, Fresh, Somerfield*, 1 pack/300g					
	69/23	0/0	12/4	3/1	0/0
Gravy, Onion, Fresh, Asda*, ⅙ pot/77g					
	30/39	1.3/1.7	2.5/3.3	1.6/2.1	0.3/0.4
Gravy, Onion, Rich, Marks & Spencer*, ½ pack/150g					
	60/40	3/2	8.9/5.9	1.8/1.2	0.5/0.3
Guacamole, Asda*, ½ pot/56.5g					
	105/184	0.9/1.6	2.3/4	10.3/18	0/0
Guacamole, Chunky, Marks & Spencer*, 1 serving/50g					
	65/130	0.8/1.5	2.6/5.1	5.7/11.3	1.9/3.7
Guacamole, Doritos*, 1 tbsp/20g					
	32/159	0.2/1.2	0.5/2.6	3.2/16	0/0.1
Guacamole, Fresh, Sainsbury's*, 1oz/28g					
	59/210	0.5/1.8	1.5/5.3	5.7/20.2	0.7/2.5
Guacamole, Fresh, Waitrose*, ½ pot/85.1g					
	172/202	1.4/1.7	2.8/3.3	17.2/20.2	2.9/3.4
Guacamole, GFY, Asda*, 1 pack/113g					
	144/127	3.2/2.8	4.9/4.3	12.4/11	2.5/2.2
Guacamole, Reduced-Fat, Sainsbury's*, ½ pot/65g					
	86/133	1/1.5	2.3/3.5	8.2/12.6	2.6/4
Guacamole, Reduced-Fat, Waitrose*, 1 serving/25g					
	32/129	0.8/3	0.7/2.7	3/11.8	1.2/4.7
Guacamole, Tesco*, 1 serving/35g					
	67/190	0.7/1.9	1.4/4.1	6.4/18.4	0.9/2.5
Ketchup, BBQ, Heinz*, 1 serving/10g					
	14/137	0.1/1.3	3.1/31.3	0/0.3	0/0.3
Ketchup, Tomato, 25% Less Sugar, Asda*, 1 tbsp/10g					
	7/71	0.2/1.6	1.6/16	0/0.1	0/0
Ketchup, Tomato, Frank Cooper*, 1 sachet/12g					
	14/119	0.1/1	3.3/27.9	0/0.3	0.1/0.6
Ketchup, Tomato, Heinz*, 1 tbsp/15g					
	16/107	0.2/1	3.7/24.7	0/0.1	0.1/0.6

kcal serv/100g	prot serv/100g	carb serv/100g	fat serv/100g	fibre serv/100g
Ketchup, Tomato, Sainsbury's*, 1 tbsp/15g				
19/128	0.1/0.9	4.3/28.7	0.1/0.5	0.2/1
Ketchup, Tomato, Value, Tesco*, 1 tbsp/15ml				
21/139	0.3/2.3	4.8/32.2	0/0.1	0.2/1.4
Ketchup, Wicked Orange, Heinz*, 1 serving/11g				
12/108	0.1/1	2.7/24.7	0/0.1	0.1/0.6
Mayonnaise, Finest, Tesco*, 1 dtsp/22g				
155/703	0.2/1.1	0.3/1.5	16.9/77	0/0
Mayonnaise, French-Style, BGTY, Sainsbury's*, 1 tbsp/15ml				
55/366	0.1/0.6	1.1/7.5	5.5/36.9	0/0
Mayonnaise, French with Course Ground Mustard, Sainsbury's*, 1 serving/15ml				
93/618	0.1/0.8	0.3/1.7	10.1/67.3	0/0.3
Mayonnaise, French, Sainsbury's*, 1 tsp/6ml				
41/678	0.1/1.2	0.1/2.4	4.4/73.6	0.1/1.4
Mayonnaise, Garlic & Herb, Marks & Spencer*, 1 tsp/6g				
43/712	0.2/3.4	0.1/2.4	4.6/76.9	0.1/0.9
Mayonnaise, Garlic & Herb, Reduced-Calorie, Hellmann's*, 1 serving/25ml				
58/233	0.2/0.7	3.3/13.1	4.8/19.3	0.1/0.4
Mayonnaise, Garlic-Flavoured, Frank Cooper*, 1 tsp/6g				
28/460	0.1/2.2	0.5/8.8	2.8/46.2	0/0.1
Mayonnaise, Garlic, Asda*, 1 serving/20g				
136/678	0.3/1.3	1.2/6	14.4/72	0/0
Mayonnaise, Garlic, Morrisons*, 1 tbsp/15ml				
55/365	0.1/0.7	1.3/8.8	5.4/36	0/0
Mayonnaise, Garlic, Waitrose*, 1 tsp/6g				
21/346	0/0.6	0.5/8.6	2.1/34.3	0/0
Mayonnaise, Good Intentions, Somerfield*, 1 serving/30g				
93/309	0.2/0.5	2.2/7.4	9.2/30.8	0/0
Mayonnaise, Half-Fat, Healthy Choice, Safeway*, 1 tsp/11g				
35/319	0.1/0.8	1.2/10.8	3.3/30.3	0/0
Mayonnaise, Hellmann's*, 1 tsp/11g				
79/722	0.1/1.1	0.1/1.3	8.7/79.1	0/0
Mayonnaise, Lemon, Waitrose*, 1 tsp/8ml				
56/694	0.1/1.2	0.1/1.3	6.1/76	0.4/5.4
Mayonnaise, Light, Morrisons*, 1 tsp/11g				
32/287	0.2/1.4	0.9/8.5	3/27.5	0/0

kcal serv/100g	prot serv/100g	carb serv/100g	fat serv/100g	fibre serv/100g
Mayonnaise, Light, BGTY, Sainsbury's*, 1 tsp/11g				
33/296	0.1/0.5	0.8/7.2	3.2/29.3	0/0
Mayonnaise, Light, Hellmann's*, 1 serving/10g				
30/299	0.1/0.7	0.7/6.7	3/29.8	0/0
Mayonnaise, Light, Kraft*, 1 serving/25g				
61/245	0.2/0.6	3.8/15	5/20	0/0
Mayonnaise, Mediterranean, Hellmann's*, 1 tsp/11g				
79/722	0.1/1.1	0.1/1.3	8.7/79.1	0/0
Mayonnaise, Mild Dijon Mustard, Frank Cooper*, 1 pot/28g				
114/406	0.9/3.3	2.6/9.3	11.1/39.5	0/0.1
Mayonnaise, Onion & Chive, BGTY, Sainsbury's*, 1 tbsp/15ml				
19/127	0.3/2	1.8/11.8	1.2/8	0.1/0.7
Mayonnaise, Real, Hellmann's*, 1 tbsp/15ml				
101/676	0.2/1	0.2/1.2	11.1/74	0/0
Mayonnaise, Reduced-Calorie, Hellmann's*, 1 serving/30g				
90/299	0.2/0.7	2/6.7	8.9/29.8	0/0
Mayonnaise, Reduced-Calorie, Tesco*, 1 tbsp/15g				
49/326	0.1/0.8	1.5/9.8	4.7/31.5	0/0
Mayonnaise, Reduced-Calorie, Waitrose*, 1 tsp/11g				
32/287	0.2/1.4	0.9/8.5	3/27.5	0/0
Mayonnaise, Weight Watchers*, 1 tbsp/15g				
42/280	0.2/1	1.1/7.3	4.2/27.7	0.1/0.7
Mint, Jelly, Baxters*, 1oz/28g				
74/264	0/0	18.5/66	0/0	0/0
Mustard, American, French's*, 1 tbsp/15g				
27/180	0.9/6	2.4/16	1.8/12	0/0
Mustard, Cajun, Colman's*, 1 tsp/6g				
11/187	0.4/7	1.4/23	0.4/6.5	0.2/2.7
Mustard, Coarse Grain, Frank Cooper*, 1 tsp/6g				
12/206	0.5/8.9	1/17	0.7/11.4	0/0
Mustard, Dijon, Frank Cooper*, 1 tsp/6g				
11/179	0.4/7.2	0.6/10	0.7/12.3	0/0
Mustard, Dijon, Marks & Spencer*, 1 tsp/6g				
9/153	0.6/10	0.4/7.2	0.6/9.5	0.1/1
Mustard, English, Frank Cooper*, 1 tsp/6g				
11/188	0.3/5.7	1.3/22	0.5/8.6	0/0.2
Mustard, English, Marks & Spencer*, 1 tsp/6g				
14/226	0.8/12.6	0.5/8.7	1/15.9	0.1/1

	kcal serv/100g	prot serv/100g	carb serv/100g	fat serv/100g	fibre serv/100g
Mustard, English, Powder, Colman's*, 1 tsp/5g					
	26/518	1.5/29	1.2/24	1.7/34	0.3/6.2
Mustard, English, Safeway*, 1 tsp/6g					
	10/163	0.4/6.1	1.1/18.3	0.4/6.7	0/0
Mustard, English, with Chillies, Sainsbury's*, 1 tsp/5g					
	10/204	0.4/8.3	0.9/18.1	0.5/10.9	0.3/6.4
Mustard, French Classic Yellow, Colman's*, 1 tsp/6g					
	4/73	0.3/4.3	0.2/2.6	0.3/4.2	0/0
Mustard, French Mild, Colman's*, 1 tsp/6g					
	6/104	0.4/6.3	0.2/4	0.4/7	0.2/3.8
Mustard, French, Frank Cooper*, 1 tsp/6g					
	7/113	0.3/4.6	0.4/7	0.4/7.4	0/0
Mustard, Honey, Colman's*, 1 tsp/6g					
	12/208	0.4/7.4	1.4/24	0.5/8.2	0/0
Mustard, Wholegrain, Colman's*, 1 tsp/6g					
	10/173	0.5/8.5	0.5/8.5	0.7/11	0.4/5.9
Pasta Sauce, Arrabbiata, Fresh, Tesco*, 1 serving/110ml					
	29/26	0.8/0.7	4.1/3.7	1/0.9	1/0.9
Pasta Sauce, Arrabbiata, Italiano, Tesco*, ½ pot/175g					
	65/37	3/1.7	10.7/6.1	1.1/0.6	1.8/1
Pasta Sauce, Arrabbiata, Sainsbury's*, 1oz/28g					
	13/45	0.4/1.4	0.9/3.3	0.8/2.9	0.4/1.6
Pasta Sauce, Basil & Oregano for Bolognese, Ragu*, 1 serving/200g					
	76/38	4/2	15.2/7.6	0/0	1.6/0.8
Pasta Sauce, Beef Bolognese, Fresh, Asda*, ¼ pot/82g					
	78/95	3.5/4.3	2.8/3.4	6/7.3	0.3/0.4
Pasta Sauce, Bolognese, Dolmio*, ¼ jar/175g					
	91/52	3.2/1.8	18/10.3	0/0	0/0
Pasta Sauce, Bolognese, Finest, Tesco*, 1 serving/175g					
	170/97	12.3/7	6.7/3.8	10.7/6.1	0.9/0.5
Pasta Sauce, Bolognese, Fresh, Sainsbury's*, ½ pot/150g					
	120/80	9/6	7.1/4.7	6.2/4.1	1.8/1.2
Pasta Sauce, Bolognese, Original, Asda*, 1 serving/157.5g					
	73/46	2.2/1.4	11/7	2.2/1.4	1.3/0.8
Pasta Sauce, Bolognese, Original, Light, Dolmio*, 1 serving/125g					
	44/35	2/1.6	8.6/6.9	0.1/0.1	0/0
Pasta Sauce, Bolognese, Traditional, Ragu, 1 jar/515g					
	345/67	10.3/2	51/9.9	10.8/2.1	6.2/1.2

	kcal serv/100g	prot serv/100g	carb serv/100g	fat serv/100g	fibre serv/100g

Pasta Sauce, Chargrilled Vegetable with Extra Virgin Olive Oil, Bertolli*, ½ jar/250g

150/60	5.3/2.1	21.8/8.7	4.8/1.9	6/2.4

Pasta Sauce, Cheese & Bacon Bake, Homepride*, 1oz/28g

27/95	0.6/2	0.7/2.5	2.4/8.6	0/0

Pasta Sauce, Cherry Tomato & Basil, Sacla*, 1 serving/96g

90/94	1.2/1.2	5.1/5.3	7.1/7.4	0/0

Pasta Sauce, Cream & Mushroom, Marks & Spencer*, 1oz/28g

45/160	0.4/1.5	1.8/6.6	4/14.3	0.2/0.6

Pasta Sauce, Creamy Mushroom, Dolmio*, 1 pack/150g

167/111	2/1.3	5.6/3.7	15/10	0/0

Pasta Sauce, Creamy Tomato & Bacon Bake, Homepride*, 1 serving/110g

99/90	2.1/1.9	7.2/6.5	6.9/6.3	0/0

Pasta Sauce, Creamy Tomato & Herb Bake, Homepride*, 1 jar/455g

464/102	9.1/2	34.1/7.5	32.3/7.1	0/0

Pasta Sauce, Dolmio*, 1 serving/100g

133/133	4.3/4.3	22.5/22.5	2.5/2.5	0/0

Pasta Sauce, Extra Mushrooms Bolognese, Dolmio*, 1 jar/500g

235/47	8/1.6	46.5/9.3	0.5/0.1	0/0

Pasta Sauce, Extra Spicy Bolognese, Dolmio*, 1 serving/250g

133/53	4.3/1.7	23/9.2	2.8/1.1	0/0

Pasta Sauce, Four Cheese, GFY, Asda*, ½ pot/175g

144/82	7/4	11/6.3	8/4.6	0.9/0.5

Pasta Sauce, Four Cheese, Sainsbury's*, 1 serving/150g

296/197	9.9/6.6	6.8/4.5	25.5/17	1.2/0.8

Pasta Sauce, Ham & Mushroom, Creamy, Stir & Serve, Homepride*, 1 serving/92g

124/135	1.7/1.8	5.1/5.5	10.8/11.7	0/0

Pasta Sauce, Italian Tomato & Herb, for Pasta, Sainsbury's*, ½ jar/146g

102/70	2.9/2	16.2/11.1	2.9/2	2/1.4

Pasta Sauce, Napoletana, Fresh, Sainsbury's*, 1oz/28g

25/91	0.5/1.9	2.2/7.9	1.6/5.8	0.3/1.1

Pasta Sauce, Olive & Tomato, Sacla*, 1 serving/95g

87/92	1.2/1.3	3.4/3.6	7.6/8	0/0

Pasta Sauce, Onion & Garlic, Tesco*, 1 serving/225g

83/37	2.7/1.2	17.1/7.6	0.7/0.3	1.8/0.8

Pasta Sauce, Original, for Bolognese, Ragu*, 1 jar/525g

268/51	8.9/1.7	56.2/10.7	0.5/0.1	5.3/1

kcal serv/100g	prot serv/100g	carb serv/100g	fat serv/100g	fibre serv/100g
Pasta Sauce, Original, Healthy Eating, Tesco*, 1 jar/455g				
155/34	5.5/1.2	29.6/6.5	0.5/0.1	3.6/0.8
Pasta Sauce, Porcini Mushroom Stir-In, BGTY, Sainsbury's*, ½ jar/75g				
57/76	2.9/3.8	4.3/5.7	3.2/4.2	1.4/1.9
Pasta Sauce, Roasted Vegetable, Sainsbury's*, ½ pot/151g				
103/68	2.4/1.6	10.1/6.7	5.9/3.9	0.6/0.4
Pasta Sauce, Spicy Italian Chilli, Microwaveable, Dolmio*, 1 sachet/170g				
92/54	2.4/1.4	12.9/7.6	3.4/2	0/0
Pasta Sauce, Spicy Pepper & Tomato, Sacla*, ½ jar/95g				
132/139	1.3/1.4	6.5/6.8	11.2/11.8	0/0
Pasta Sauce, Spicy with Peppers, Tesco*, 1 jar/455g				
177/39	5.5/1.2	35.9/7.9	1.4/0.3	5/1.1
Pasta Sauce, Spinach & Ricotta, BGTY, Sainsbury's*, 1 serving/150g				
74/49	4.1/2.7	5.1/3.4	4.1/2.7	3.3/2.2
Pasta Sauce, Sun-Dried Tomato, Stir-In, Light, Dolmio*, ½ tub/75g				
62/83	1.3/1.7	7.4/9.8	3.5/4.7	0/0
Pasta Sauce, Sun-Ripened Tomato & Basil, Microwaveable, Dolmio*,				
½ pack/190g				
106/56	2.7/1.4	15/7.9	4/2.1	0/0
Pasta Sauce, Sweet Red Pepper, Loyd Grossman*, 1oz/28g				
24/87	0.5/1.7	2/7.3	1.6/5.6	0.3/1.2
Pasta Sauce, Tomato & Basil, Bertolli*, 1 serving/250g				
118/47	3.8/1.5	19.8/7.9	2.8/1.1	4/1.6
Pasta Sauce, Tomato & Basil, Dolmio*, 1 serving/170g				
95/56	2.4/1.4	13.4/7.9	3.6/2.1	0/0
Pasta Sauce, Tomato & Basil, Loyd Grossman*, ½ jar/175g				
152/87	3/1.7	12.8/7.3	9.8/5.6	2.1/1.2
Pasta Sauce, Tomato & Basil, Organic, Seeds Of Change*, 1 jar/390g				
234/60	5.5/1.4	33.2/8.5	8.6/2.2	4.3/1.1
Pasta Sauce, Tomato & Chargrilled Vegetable, Loyd Grossman*,				
1 serving/150g				
134/89	2.7/1.8	11.9/7.9	8.4/5.6	1.4/0.9
Pasta Sauce, Tomato & Chilli, Loyd Grossman*, ½ jar/175g				
154/88	3/1.7	12.8/7.3	10/5.7	1.6/0.9
Pasta Sauce, Tomato & Herb, Organic, Sainsbury's*, 1 serving/75g				
38/51	0.9/1.2	5/6.6	1.5/2	0.4/0.5
Pasta Sauce, Tomato & Mascarpone, Asda*, 1 serving/175g				
210/120	2.8/1.6	10.5/6	17.5/10	0/0

kcal serv/100g	prot serv/100g	carb serv/100g	fat serv/100g	fibre serv/100g
Pasta Sauce, Tomato & Mascarpone, BGTY, Sainsbury's*, ½ pot/150g				
75/50	3/2	5.4/3.6	4.5/3	5.4/3.6
Pasta Sauce, Tomato & Mascarpone, Fresh, Sainsbury's*, 1 serving/150g				
177/118	3.3/2.2	6.3/4.2	15.5/10.3	1.7/1.1
Pasta Sauce, Tomato & Mascarpone, Tesco*, 1 serving/175g				
194/111	4.9/2.8	9.5/5.4	15.2/8.7	1.1/0.6
Pasta Sauce, Tomato Red Wine Shallots, Bertolli*, ½ jar/250g				
113/45	4.3/1.7	18/7.2	4.3/1.7	3.8/1.5
Pasta Sauce, Tomato, Basil & Parmesan Stir-In, BGTY, Sainsbury's*, 1 serving/75g				
69/92	2.2/2.9	5.9/7.8	4.1/5.5	0.8/1
Piccalilli, Haywards*, 1 serving/28g				
18/66	0.4/1.4	3.9/13.9	0.1/0.5	0/0
Piccalilli, Marks & Spencer*, 1 tbsp/15g				
11/70	0.3/1.9	2/13.5	0.2/1.2	0.2/1.1
Pickle, Branston, Crosse & Blackwell*, 1 tsp/10g				
14/140	0.1/0.7	3.4/34.2	0/0.3	0.1/1.3
Pickle, Lime, Hot, Patak's*, 1 tsp/16g				
30/186	0.4/2.6	0.7/4.2	3/18.7	0/0.3
Pickle, Lime, Sharwood's*, 1 tsp/16g				
24/152	0.4/2.2	2.4/15	1.5/9.3	0.5/2.9
Pickle, Sandwich, Branston*, 1 tsp/10g				
14/140	0.1/0.7	3.4/34.2	0/0.3	0.1/1.3
Redcurrant Jelly, Baxters*, 1oz/28g				
73/260	0/0	18.2/65	0/0	0/0
Relish, Caramelised Onion & Chilli, Marks & Spencer*, 1 serving/20g				
47/235	0.3/1.4	11/55.1	0.2/1.1	0.2/1
Relish, Caramelised Red Onion, Tesco*, 1 serving/10g				
28/280	0.1/0.6	6.9/69.1	0/0.1	0.1/0.7
Relish, Hamburger, Bick's*, 1oz/28g				
27/96	0.4/1.3	6.2/22.3	0.1/0.2	0/0
Relish, Onion, Marks & Spencer*, 1oz/28g				
46/165	0.3/1	9/32.1	0.8/3	0.3/1.1
Relish, Sweetcorn, Bicks*, 1 tbsp/22g				
23/103	0.3/1.3	5.3/24.3	0/0.2	0/0
Salad Cream, 60% Less Fat, Asda*, 1 serving/10g				
14/138	0.1/0.8	1.1/11	1/10	0/0

	kcal serv/100g	prot serv/100g	carb serv/100g	fat serv/100g	fibre serv/100g
Salad Cream, Heinz*, 1 tbsp/10g					
	33/331	0.1/1.4	2/20.3	2.7/26.7	0/0
Salad Cream, Light, Heinz*, 1 tbsp/10g					
	24/244	0.2/1.8	1.4/13.5	2/19.9	0/0
Salad Cream, Waistline, Crosse & Blackwell*, 1 tbsp/10g					
	12/120	0.1/1	1.4/14.4	0.6/6.4	0/0.2
Salad Cream, Weight Watchers*, 1 serving/14g					
	16/115	0.2/1.5	2.3/16.2	0.6/4.4	0/0
Salsa, Fresh, Sainsbury's*, 1oz/28g					
	15/54	0.5/1.7	2/7	0.6/2.1	0.3/0.9
Salsa, Fresh, Somerfield*, 1oz/28g					
	12/44	0.3/1	2/7	0.3/1	0/0
Salsa, Fresh, Waitrose*, 1oz/28g					
	16/57	0.3/1.2	1.9/6.9	0.8/2.7	0.3/1
Salsa, GFY, Asda*, ½ pot/236g					
	85/36	2.4/1	16.5/7	0.9/0.4	4.7/2
Salsa, Hot, Fresh, Tesco*, 1oz/28g					
	17/62	0.5/1.8	2.2/7.9	0.7/2.6	0.3/0.9
Salsa, Marks & Spencer*, ½ jar/136g					
	95/70	1.6/1.2	16.3/12	3.3/2.4	2/1.5
Salsa, Smokey BBQ, Weight Watchers*, 1 serving/56g					
	20/36	0.6/1.1	4.3/7.6	0.1/0.1	1.3/2.3
Salsa, Spiced Mango, Ginger & Chilli, Weight Watchers*, ½ pot/50g					
	43/85	0.5/1	10/19.9	0.1/0.2	1.3/2.6
Salsa, Spicy, Less Than 3% Fat, Marks & Spencer*, ½ pot/85g					
	30/35	1.1/1.3	4.8/5.6	0.7/0.8	0.7/0.8
Salsa, Spicy, Marks & Spencer*, 1oz/28g					
	17/60	0.4/1.3	2/7.2	0.8/2.7	0.3/1.2
Salsa, Tomato, Waitrose*, 1 serving/50g					
	24/47	0.8/1.5	2.5/5	1.2/2.3	0.9/1.7
Sauce Mix, Beef Stroganoff, Colman's*, 1 pack/40g					
	160/399	5/12.4	19.4/48.4	6.9/17.3	2.6/6.4
Sauce Mix, Cheddar Cheese, Colman's*, 1 serving/40g					
	158/394	7.9/19.7	18.1/45.2	6/14.9	0.6/1.5
Sauce Mix, Chicken Chasseur, Colman's*, 1 pack/45g					
	123/273	5.4/12	23.9/53	0.5/1	0/0
Sauce Mix, Chicken Supreme, Colman's*, ½ pack/20g					
	72/362	2.4/12.1	10.6/53.2	2.2/11.2	1.3/6.5

	kcal serv/100g	prot serv/100g	carb serv/100g	fat serv/100g	fibre serv/100g
Sauce Mix, Chilli Con Carne, Colman's*, 1 serving/13g					
	40/305	1/7.5	7.6/58.4	0.6/4.6	1/7.7
Sauce Mix, Coq Au Vin, Colman's*, 1 pack/50g					
	141/281	3.8/7.5	29.5/59	0.5/1	0/0
Sauce Mix, Parsley, Knorr*, 1 sachet/48g					
	210/437	2/4.2	24.3/50.6	11.6/24.2	0.4/0.8
Sauce Mix, Pepper, Instant, Safeway*, 1 serving/22g					
	77/348	0.7/3.2	14.6/66.3	1.7/7.5	0.9/4.1
Sauce, Apple, Baxters*, 1 tsp/15g					
	7/49	0/0.1	1.7/11.1	0.1/0.4	0.1/0.7
Sauce, Apple, Bramley, Colman's*, 1 tsp/15ml					
	16/108	0/0.2	3.9/26	0/0	0/0
Sauce, Apple, Heinz*, 1 tsp/15g					
	8/56	0/0.3	2/13.4	0/0.2	0.2/1.5
Sauce, Balti, Cooking, Sharwood's*, 1 jar/420g					
	370/88	4.6/1.1	38.2/9.1	21.8/5.2	2.1/0.5
Sauce, Barbeque, Cook-In, Homepride*, 1 serving/130g					
	96/74	1/0.8	18.2/14	2.1/1.6	0/0
Sauce, BBQ Original, Heinz*, 1 serving/9.5g					
	12/137	0.1/1.3	2.8/31	0/0.3	0/0.3
Sauce, BBQ, HP*, 1 serving/20ml					
	29/143	0.2/0.8	6.6/33.1	0/0.2	0/0
Sauce, BBQ, Tesco*, 1 serving/50g					
	63/125	0.7/1.3	14.9/29.7	0.1/0.1	0.4/0.7
Sauce, Black Bean, Canton, Stir-Fry, Blue Dragon*, 1 pack/100g					
	88/88	2.8/2.8	14.8/14.8	2/2	1.5/1.5
Sauce, Black Bean, Stir-Fry, Fresh Ideas, Tesco*, ½ sachet/25g					
	33/132	1.1/4.2	5.7/22.6	0.7/2.8	0.2/0.8
Sauce, Black Bean, Stir-Fry, Safeway*, ⅓ pack/33g					
	43/129	1.2/3.7	6.7/20.2	1.2/3.7	0.3/0.9
Sauce, Bolognese, Loyd Grossman*, ¼ jar/106g					
	80/75	2.1/2	10.8/10.2	3.1/2.9	1.5/1.4
Sauce, Bolognese, Original, Dolmio*, 1 serving/250g					
	130/52	4.3/1.7	22/8.8	2.8/1.1	0/0
Sauce, Brazilian Chicken, Chicken Tonight*, 1 serving/125g					
	49/39	1.5/1.2	8.8/7	0.9/0.7	1.6/1.3
Sauce, Brown, Daddies Favourite, HP*, 1 tsp/6g					
	6/102	0.1/0.9	1.5/24.3	0/0.1	0/0

	kcal serv/100g	prot serv/100g	carb serv/100g	fat serv/100g	fibre serv/100g
Sauce, Carbonara, GFY, Asda,*, 1 serving/170g					
	167/98	8.5/5	10.2/6	10.2/6	0/0
Sauce, Carbonara, Pasta, Tesco*, 1 serving/150g					
	182/121	4.2/2.8	4.8/3.2	16.2/10.8	0/0
Sauce, Chasseur, Cook-In, Homepride*, 1 can/390g					
	156/40	2.7/0.7	35.9/9.2	0.4/0.1	0/0
Sauce, Chasseur, Classic, Chicken Tonight*, 1 serving/100g					
	45/45	0.7/0.7	3.9/3.9	2.9/2.9	1.3/1.3
Sauce, Cheese, Fresh, Waitrose*, 1 pot/350g					
	459/131	17.9/5.1	20/5.7	34.3/9.8	0/0
Sauce, Chicken, Spanish, Chicken Tonight*, 1 serving/250g					
	123/49	4.3/1.7	20/8	3.3/1.3	2.5/1
Sauce, Chilli & Garlic, Amoy*, 1oz/28g					
	31/112	3.4/12	7.6/27	0/0	0/0
Sauce, Chilli & Garlic, Lea & Perrins*, 1 tsp/6g					
	4/60	0.1/1	0.9/14.9	0/0	0/0
Sauce, Chilli Con Carne, Cook-In, Homepride*, 1 can/390g					
	234/60	9.8/2.5	43.7/11.2	2.3/0.6	0/0
Sauce, Chilli, Amoy*, 1 tsp/6g					
	2/25	0.1/1	0.3/5.2	0/0	0.1/1
Sauce, Chilli, HP*, 1 tsp/6g					
	8/134	0.1/1.2	1.9/32.3	0/0.1	0/0
Sauce, Chinese Sweet & Sour, Cooking, Sainsbury's*, ¼ jar/125g					
	109/87	0.9/0.7	25.1/20.1	0.1/0.1	0.9/0.7
Sauce, Chinese, Curry, Farmfoods*, 1 sachet/200g					
	220/110	1.2/0.6	14.2/7.1	17.6/8.8	1.4/0.7
Sauce, Chinese, Stir-Fry, Sachet, Fresh, Sainsbury's*, ½ sachet/51ml					
	83/163	0.9/1.7	7.2/14.1	5.7/11.1	0.9/1.8
Sauce, Chocolate, Sainsbury's*, 1 serving/30g					
	108/360	0.4/1.3	18.8/62.8	3.5/11.6	0.3/0.9
Sauce, Chow Mein, Stir-Fry, Blue Dragon*, 1 sachet/120g					
	110/92	1.3/1.1	18.5/15.4	3.5/2.9	0.5/0.4
Sauce, Country French, Chicken Tonight*, ¼ jar/125g					
	123/98	0.9/0.7	4.1/3.3	11.4/9.1	0.9/0.7
Sauce, Country French, Low-Fat, Chicken Tonight*, 1 serving/125g					
	58/46	1.1/0.9	5.3/4.2	3.5/2.8	0.9/0.7
Sauce, Cracked Black Pepper, Marks & Spencer*, 1 jar/300g					
	345/115	8.1/2.7	20.1/6.7	26.7/8.9	1.2/0.4

kcal serv/100g	prot serv/100g	carb serv/100g	fat serv/100g	fibre serv/100g
Sauce, Cranberry Jelly, Baxters*, 1 tsp/15g				
40/268	0/0	10.1/67	0/0	0/0
Sauce, Creamy Lemon & Dill, Fresh, Sainsbury's*, ½ pot/150g				
242/161	2.4/1.6	6.3/4.2	23/15.3	2.3/1.5
Sauce, Creamy Mushroom, Low-Fat, Chicken Tonight*, 1 serving/250g				
108/43	3.3/1.3	7.3/2.9	7.3/2.9	2.5/1
Sauce, Creamy Peppercorn & Whisky, Baxters*, 1 pack/320g				
422/132	6.1/1.9	21.4/6.7	34.6/10.8	0.6/0.2
Sauce, Creamy White Wine & Herb, 95% Fat-Free, Homepride*, 1 serving/220g				
150/68	1.3/0.6	13.9/6.3	9.9/4.5	1.5/0.7
Sauce, Curry, 98% Fat-Free, Homepride*, 1oz/28g				
15/54	0.4/1.4	2.6/9.2	0.4/1.5	0.2/0.6
Sauce, Curry, Cook-In, Homepride*, ½ can/250g				
270/108	1.8/0.7	22.8/9.1	19/7.6	1.5/0.6
Sauce, Curry, Medium, Uncle Ben's*, 1 serving/100g				
66/66	0.9/0.9	11.1/11.1	2/2	0/0
Sauce, Curry, Mild, Tesco*, 1 jar/500g				
420/84	5.5/1.1	67/13.4	14/2.8	4/0.8
Sauce, Curry, Sweet, 1oz/28g				
25/91	0.3/1.2	2.7/9.6	1.6/5.6	0.4/1.4
Sauce, Dark Soya, Amoy*, 1 serving/10g				
9/85	0.1/1.2	2/20	0/0	0/0
Sauce, Diane, Safeway*, ½ pot/85g				
40/47	0.7/0.8	2.8/3.3	3/3.5	0.3/0.3
Sauce, Dipping for Dim Sum, Amoy*, 1 tbsp/15ml				
29/190	0/0	7.2/48	0/0	0/0
Sauce, Dopiaza, Patak's*, 1 serving/212g				
235/111	3.6/1.7	19.3/9.1	16.1/7.6	2.8/1.3
Sauce, Enchilada, Medium, Old El Paso*, 1 can/270g				
92/34	0/0	13.5/5	4.6/1.7	0/0
Sauce, Fajita, Asda*, ¼ jar/125g				
79/63	1.3/1	6.3/5	5.4/4.3	1.3/1
Sauce, for Bolognese, Light, Original, Ragu*, 1 jar/515g				
196/38	7.2/1.4	42.2/8.2	0.5/0.1	6.2/1.2
Sauce, for Bolognese, Original, Ragu*, 1 jar/515g				
242/47	7.2/1.4	42.2/8.2	4.6/0.9	6.2/1.2

kcal serv/100g	prot serv/100g	carb serv/100g	fat serv/100g	fibre serv/100g
Sauce, Fruity, HP*, 1 tsp/6g				
8/141	0.1/1.2	2.1/35.1	0/0.1	0/0
Sauce, Garlic, Lea & Perrins*, 1 tsp/6g				
20/337	0.1/1.8	1.1/17.8	1.7/29	0/0
Sauce, Golden Honey Mustard, Lite, Continental, Chicken Tonight*, 1 serving/122g				
104/85	1/0.8	11.3/9.3	6.1/5	0/0
Sauce, Green Thai, Curry, Asda*, 1 jar/340g				
309/91	1.7/0.5	14.6/4.3	27.2/8	0.7/0.2
Sauce, Green Thai, Loyd Grossman*, ½ jar/175g				
228/130	4/2.3	17.7/10.1	15.8/9	2.1/1.2
Sauce, Hoi Sin & Spring Onion, Stir-Fry, Sharwood's*, 1 jar/165g				
223/135	4.3/2.6	45.9/27.8	2.5/1.5	1.5/0.9
Sauce, Hoi Sin, Sharwood's*, 1 tbsp/20g				
42/211	0.5/2.7	9.9/49.5	0.1/0.3	0.1/0.6
Sauce, Hollandaise, Marks & Spencer*, 1oz/28g				
56/200	0.4/1.6	0.7/2.4	5.7/20.5	0/0.1
Sauce, Hollandaise, Sainsbury's*, 1 tbsp/15ml				
77/515	0.1/0.5	0.6/4.2	8.3/55	0/0
Sauce, Hollandaise, Schwartz*, 1 pack/25g				
98/392	2.8/11.3	15.4/61.5	2.8/11.2	0/0
Sauce, Honey & Coriander, Stir-Fry, Blue Dragon*, 1 pack/120g				
115/96	0.6/0.5	26.5/22.1	0.7/0.6	0.4/0.3
Sauce, Honey & Mustard, Chicken Tonight*, ¼ jar/130g				
139/107	2.1/1.6	17.6/13.5	6.8/5.2	1.7/1.3
Sauce, Honey & Mustard, COU, Marks & Spencer*, ½ jar/160g				
112/70	3.7/2.3	14.7/9.2	4.6/2.9	1.1/0.7
Sauce, Horseradish, Asda*, 1oz/28g				
38/135	0.6/2.2	3.9/14	2/7	0.6/2
Sauce, Horseradish, Creamed, Colman's*, 1 tsp/16g				
37/229	0.7/4.3	3.4/21.4	2.1/13.3	0/0
Sauce, Horseradish, Hot, Colman's*, 1 tbsp/15ml				
16/105	0.3/1.8	1.5/9.7	0.9/5.7	0/0
Sauce, Hot Chilli, Sharwood's*, 1fl oz/30ml				
36/120	0.2/0.5	8.8/29.4	0.2/0.6	0.4/1.3
Sauce, Hot Pepper, Encona*, 1 tsp/5ml				
3/52	0/0.5	0.5/10.5	0.1/1.2	0/0

	kcal serv/100g	prot serv/100g	carb serv/100g	fat serv/100g	fibre serv/100g

Sauce, Jalfrezi, Mild, Sharwood's*, 1 jar/445g

347/78	6.2/1.4	47.2/10.6	14.7/3.3	5.8/1.3

Sauce, Korma, Cooking, BGTY, Sainsbury's*, ¼ jar/129g

119/92	1.4/1.1	13.9/10.8	6.3/4.9	1.8/1.4

Sauce, Korma, Cooking, Healthy Eating, Tesco*, ¼ jar/125g

120/96	2.4/1.9	9.3/7.4	8/6.4	0.8/0.6

Sauce, Korma, Sharwood's*, 1 serving/105g

150/143	1.5/1.4	12.8/12.2	10.3/9.8	1.9/1.8

Sauce, Korma, Uncle Ben's*, 1 jar/500g

625/125	6/1.2	57/11.4	39/7.8	0/0

Sauce, Lemon Butter, Schwartz*, 1 serving/9g

35/388	0.9/10.2	5.5/61.4	1/11.3	0/0

Sauce, Lemon, Amoy*, 1 tsp/5ml

5/104	0/0	1.3/26	0/0	0/0

Sauce, Madras, Curry, Sharwood's*, 1 jar/420g

521/124	7.1/1.7	37.4/8.9	38.2/9.1	5.9/1.4

Sauce, Mediterranean Vegetable, Waitrose*, ⅓ pot/120g

60/50	1.6/1.3	5.4/4.5	3.6/3	1.9/1.6

Sauce, Mint Jelly, Sweet, Colman's*, 1 serving/14ml

35/249	0/0.2	8.5/61	0/0	0/0

Sauce, Mint, Baxters*, 1oz/28g

17/62	0.5/1.7	3.7/13.2	0.1/0.3	0/0

Sauce, Mint, Sainsbury's*, 1 dtsp/10g

13/126	0.3/2.5	2.9/28.7	0/0.1	0.4/4

Sauce, Moroccan Seven Vegetable Cous Cous, Sainsbury's*, 1 serving/50g

89/178	1.3/2.6	3/5.9	8/16	0/0

Sauce, Mushroom & Garlic, 95% Fat-Free, Homepride*, 1 serving/220g

154/70	2/0.9	15.4/7	9.2/4.2	0.7/0.3

Sauce, Napoletana, Italiano, New Improved Recipe, Tesco*, ½ pot/175g

126/72	2.8/1.6	15.2/8.7	6/3.4	1.9/1.1

Sauce, Oyster & Spring Onion, Stir-Fry, Blue Dragon*, 1 serving/80g

74/92	1.3/1.6	15.9/19.9	0.6/0.7	0.9/1.1

Sauce, Oyster-Flavoured, Amoy*, 1 tsp/5ml

5/108	0.1/2	1.3/25	0/0	0/0

Sauce, Oyster, Stir-Fry, Sainsbury's, 1 tbsp/15g

9/61	0.2/1.6	2/13.3	0/0.1	0/0.2

Sauce, Parsley, Colman's*, 1 sachet/20g

64/320	2.1/10.4	13.2/66	0.3/1.7	0/0

	kcal serv/100g	prot serv/100g	carb serv/100g	fat serv/100g	fibre serv/100g
Sauce, Parsley, Fresh, Sainsbury's*, ½ pot/150g					
	183/122	3.8/2.5	10.5/7	14/9.3	2/1.3
Sauce, Parsley, Made Up, Semi-Skim Milk, Sainsbury's*, ¼ sachet/51ml					
	34/67	1.8/3.5	4.4/8.6	1.1/2.1	0.1/0.1
Sauce, Passata, Italian, Sainsbury's*, ¼ jar/175g					
	51/29	1.9/1.1	10.5/6	0.2/0.1	1.4/0.8
Sauce, Passata, Italian, Tesco*, 1 pack/500g					
	170/34	5.5/1.1	32/6.4	1/0.2	5/1
Sauce, Peking Lemon, Stir-Fry, Blue Dragon*, 1 serving/35g					
	58/166	0.1/0.3	12.9/36.8	0.7/1.9	0/0.1
Sauce, Pepper & Brandy, Pour Over, Knorr*, 1oz/28g					
	29/104	0.3/1	1.1/4	2.5/9	0/0
Sauce, Pepper, Creamy, Colman's*, 1 pack/25g					
	88/352	3.3/13	12.5/50	2.8/11	0/0
Sauce, Pepper, Creamy, Schwartz*, 1 serving/25g					
	92/368	4.4/17.6	15.3/61	1.5/5.9	0/0
Sauce, Peppercorn, Creamy, Chicken Tonight*, ¼ jar/125g					
	100/80	1.3/1	4.8/3.8	8.4/6.7	0.6/0.5
Sauce, Pesto, Chargrilled Aubergine, Sacla*, 1 serving/47.6g					
	79/164	0.9/1.9	1.7/3.5	7.7/16	0/0
Sauce, Pesto, Classic Green, Sacla*, 1oz/28g					
	142/507	1.1/4.1	2.4/8.5	14.2/50.7	0/0
Sauce, Pesto, Classic, Sacla*, 1 serving/45g					
	209/465	2.5/5.5	2.5/5.6	21/46.7	0/0
Sauce, Pesto, Fresh, Waitrose*, 1 tbsp/26g					
	120/463	3.3/12.8	2.1/8.2	10.9/42.1	0.4/1.4
Sauce, Pesto, Green, Bertolli*, 1 serving/47g					
	202/429	2.5/5.4	2/4.2	20.2/43	0.6/1.3
Sauce, Pesto, Green, Sainsbury's*, 1oz/28g					
	120/430	1.5/5.4	2.3/8.3	11.7/41.7	0/0
Sauce, Pesto, Red, Sacla*, 1 serving/25g					
	82/327	1.1/4.3	2.2/8.9	7.6/30.4	0/0
Sauce, Pesto, Red, Sainsbury's*, 1 serving/60g					
	242/404	2.9/4.8	10.2/17	21.3/35.5	0.5/0.8
Sauce, Plum, Sharwood's*, 1 serving/50g					
	121/241	0.3/0.5	29.7/59.4	0.1/0.2	0.3/0.6
Sauce, Prawn Cocktail, Frank Cooper*, 1 tbsp/15g					
	47/316	0.1/0.8	2.7/18.3	4/26.7	0/0.1

kcal serv/100g	prot serv/100g	carb serv/100g	fat serv/100g	fibre serv/100g
Sauce, Real Oyster, Sharwood's*, 1 jar/150ml				
113/75	2/1.3	25.5/17	0.3/0.2	0.5/0.3
Sauce, Red Wine & Herbs, Ragu*, ¼ jar/130g				
81/62	2.7/2.1	11.4/8.8	2.6/2	1.4/1.1
Sauce, Red Wine & Onion, Rich, Simply Sausages, Colman's*, ¼ jar/125g				
49/39	1.1/0.9	10.6/8.5	0.3/0.2	1.6/1.3
Sauce, Red Wine, Cook-In, Homepride*, ¼ can/98g				
47/48	0.5/0.5	9.9/10.1	0.6/0.6	0/0
Sauce, Redcurrant, Colman's*, 1 tsp/12g				
44/368	0.1/0.7	10.8/90	0/0	0/0
Sauce, Roasted Vegetable, Stir-In, Dolmio*, 1oz/28g				
38/135	0.4/1.5	2.5/9.1	2.9/10.3	0/0
Sauce, Rogan Josh, 99% Fat-Free, Homepride*, ⅓ jar/153g				
92/60	2.8/1.8	17.7/11.6	1.1/0.7	3.1/2
Sauce, Rogan Josh, Patak's*, 1 serving/270g				
192/71	4.9/1.8	25.4/9.4	7.8/2.9	0/0
Sauce, Satay, Amoy*, 1 tsp/5ml				
10/198	0.5/10.2	0.6/11.6	0.6/12.3	0/0
Sauce, Satay, Indonesian, Sharwood's*, 1oz/28g				
31/112	0.8/2.8	3.3/11.8	1.7/6	0.2/0.6
Sauce, Seafood, Asda*, 1 serving/10g				
47/474	0.1/1.2	1.6/16	4.5/45	0/0
Sauce, Seafood, Baxters*, 1oz/28g				
149/533	0.4/1.5	2.8/9.9	15.2/54.2	0.2/0.7
Sauce, Seafood, BGTY, Sainsbury's*, 1 serving/15ml				
23/150	0.1/0.8	2.3/15.1	1.4/9.3	0/0.1
Sauce, Seafood, Colman's*, 1 serving/14ml				
47/335	0.1/0.9	2.8/20	3.9/28	0/0
Sauce, Seafood, Sainsbury's*, 1 tbsp/15g				
50/330	0.1/0.7	2.6/17.6	4.2/28.2	0/0.1
Sauce, Smokey Bacon & Tomato, Stir-In, Dolmio*, 1 pot/150g				
248/165	8.3/5.5	10.4/6.9	19.2/12.8	0/0
Sauce, Soy, Dark, Amoy*, 1 tsp/5ml				
4/73	0.1/1.9	0.8/16.3	0/0	0/0
Sauce, Soy, Light, Amoy*, 1 tsp/5ml				
3/55	0.2/3.2	0.6/11.5	0/0	0/0
Sauce, Soy, Light, Sharwood's*, 1 tsp/5ml				
1/18	0.2/4.4	0/0.2	0/0	0/0.3

kcal serv/100g	prot serv/100g	carb serv/100g	fat serv/100g	fibre serv/100g

Sauce, Soy, Reduced Salt, Amoy*, 1 tsp/5ml

| 3/56 | 0.2/4 | 0.5/10 | 0/0 | 0/0 |

Sauce, Soy, Rich, Sharwood's*, 1 tsp/5ml

| 2/48 | 0.2/4.6 | 0.4/7.5 | 0/0 | 0/0.3 |

Sauce, Soy, Superior Dark, Amoy*, 1 tsp/5ml

| 3/63 | 0.1/1.9 | 0.8/16.3 | 0/0 | 0/0 |

Sauce, Spaghetti Bolognese, Colman's*, 1 pack/45g

| 149/330 | 4/8.9 | 29.9/66.5 | 1.4/3.1 | 2.8/6.2 |

Sauce, Spaghetti Bolognese, Dolmio*, 1 serving/100g

| 39/39 | 1.6/1.6 | 8/8 | 0/0 | 0/0 |

Sauce, Spicy Tikka, Cooking, Sharwood's*, 1oz/28g

| 27/95 | 0.4/1.3 | 2.6/9.4 | 1.7/5.9 | 0.2/0.8 |

Sauce, Sun-Dried Tomato For Pasta, Stir & Serve, Homepride*, 1 serving/100g

| 62/62 | 1/1 | 7.6/7.6 | 3/3 | 0/0 |

Sauce, Sun-Dried Tomato, Stir-In, Light, Dolmio*, 1 serving/75g

| 62/83 | 1.3/1.7 | 7.4/9.8 | 3.5/4.7 | 0/0 |

Sauce, Sun-Dried Tomato, Stir-In, Dolmio*, 1 serving/75g

| 124/165 | 1.1/1.5 | 7/9.3 | 10.5/14 | 0/0 |

Sauce, Sweet & Sour, Chinese, Sainsbury's*, ½ jar/150g

| 222/148 | 0.3/0.2 | 54.9/36.6 | 0.2/0.1 | 0.2/0.1 |

Sauce, Sweet & Sour, Colman's*, 1 pack/40g

| 134/334 | 1.4/3.4 | 31.2/78 | 0/0.1 | 0/0 |

Sauce, Sweet & Sour, Cook-In, New, Homepride*, 1 serving/125g

| 115/92 | 0.4/0.3 | 28.1/22.5 | 0.1/0.1 | 1.3/1 |

Sauce, Sweet & Sour, Cooking, GFY, Asda*, 1 jar/500g

| 310/62 | 4.5/0.9 | 70/14 | 1.5/0.3 | 3/0.6 |

Sauce, Sweet & Sour, Cooking, Healthy Choice, Asda*, 1 jar/500g

| 175/35 | 3/0.6 | 40/8 | 0.5/0.1 | 2.5/0.5 |

Sauce, Sweet & Sour, Homepride*, 1 serving/195g

| 193/99 | 0.8/0.4 | 47.6/24.4 | 0.2/0.1 | 0/0 |

Sauce, Sweet & Sour, Oriental, Chicken Tonight*, ¼ jar/125g

| 115/92 | 0.8/0.6 | 26.1/20.9 | 0.9/0.7 | 1.1/0.9 |

Sauce, Sweet & Sour, Original, Uncle Ben's*, 1 pack/300g

| 264/88 | 1.5/0.5 | 65.1/21.7 | 0/0 | 0/0 |

Sauce, Sweet & Sour, Stir-Fry, Blue Dragon*, 1 serving/120g

| 150/125 | 0.8/0.7 | 28/23.3 | 3.8/3.2 | 1.1/0.9 |

	kcal serv/100g	prot serv/100g	carb serv/100g	fat serv/100g	fibre serv/100g
Sauce, Sweet & Sour, Stir-Fry, GFY, Asda*, ½ pack/51ml					
	43/85	0.5/0.9	5.6/11	2.1/4.1	1.7/3.4
Sauce, Sweet & Sour, Stir-Fry, Healthy Eating, Tesco*, 1 jar/440g					
	167/38	2.6/0.6	35.2/8	0.4/0.1	3.5/0.8
Sauce, Sweet & Sour, Stir-Fry, Sharwood's*, 1 jar 160g					
	160/100	1.3/0.8	38.6/24.1	0.2/0.1	1.6/1
Sauce, Sweet & Sour, Uncle Ben's*, 1 serving/200g					
	168/84	0.8/0.4	43.4/21.7	0/0	0/0
Sauce, Sweet Chilli & Coriander, Sharwood's*, 1 pack/370g					
	407/110	1.1/0.3	90.3/24.4	4.4/1.2	0.4/0.1
Sauce, Sweet Chilli Dipping, Blue Dragon*, 1 tsp/5ml					
	12/230	0/0	2.8/56	0/0	0/0
Sauce, Sweet Chilli, Asda*, 1 tbsp/15ml					
	18/123	0.1/0.4	4.5/30	0/0.1	0.1/0.8
Sauce, Szechuan Spicy Tomato, Stir-Fry, Blue Dragon*, 1 sachet/120g					
	151/126	1.6/1.3	21.1/17.6	6.7/5.6	2.4/2
Sauce, Szechuan-Style, Stir-Fry, Fresh Ideas, Tesco*, 1 sachet/50g					
	114/228	1/1.9	16.7/33.4	4.9/9.7	0.1/0.1
Sauce, Szechuan, Stir-Fry, Tesco*, ½ jar/220g					
	205/93	2.2/1	32.3/14.7	7/3.2	2/0.9
Sauce, Tartar, Kraft*, 2 tbsp/30ml					
	162/539	0.4/1.3	0/0	17.5/58.3	0/0
Sauce, Tartare, Baxters*, 1oz/28g					
	144/515	0.3/1	2.2/8	14.9/53.3	0.1/0.3
Sauce, Tartare, Colman's*, 1 serving/14ml					
	37/263	0.2/1.1	2/14	3/21.7	0/0
Sauce, Teriyaki, Blue Dragon*, ½ pack/60g					
	104/173	1.2/2	17.2/28.6	0/0	0/0
Sauce, Texan Barbeque, Stir It Up, Chicken Tonight*, ½ pot/40g					
	241/602	1.8/4.4	13.5/33.8	21/52.5	2.3/5.8
Sauce, Thai Fish, Amoy*, 1 tbsp/15ml					
	12/80	2/13.4	1/6.7	0/0	0/0
Sauce, Thai Green, Curry, Express, Uncle Ben's*, 1 pack/170g					
	131/77	1.9/1.1	9.2/5.4	9.9/5.8	0/0
Sauce, Thai Red, Curry, Sharwood's*, 1 serving/138g					
	150/109	1.7/1.2	10.9/7.9	11/8	0.3/0.2
Sauce, Tikka Masala, Cooking, Sharwood's*, 1 tsp/2g					
	2/122	0/1.2	0.2/11.9	0.2/7.8	0/0.9

kcal serv/100g	prot serv/100g	carb serv/100g	fat serv/100g	fibre serv/100g

Sauce, Tikka Masala, Deliciously Good, Homepride*, ¼ jar/149g

| 121/81 | 3.1/2.1 | 14.9/10 | 5.4/3.6 | 2.2/1.5 |

Sauce, Tikka Masala, GFY, Asda*, ½ jar/250g

| 190/76 | 7.3/2.9 | 22.5/9 | 8/3.2 | 1.3/0.5 |

Sauce, Tikka Masala, Jar, Sharwood's*, 1 jar/435g

| 492/113 | 6.1/1.4 | 41.8/9.6 | 33.1/7.6 | 6.1/1.4 |

Sauce, Toffee, GFY, Asda*, 1 serving/5g

| 15/306 | 0.1/2.2 | 3.4/68 | 0.1/2.8 | 0/0 |

Sauce, Tomato & Basil for Pasta, Stir & Serve, Homepride*, 1 jar/480g

| 278/58 | 5.8/1.2 | 32.2/6.7 | 13.9/2.9 | 0/0 |

Sauce, Tomato & Basil, Fresh, Organic, Waitrose*, ¼ pot/175g

| 77/44 | 1.8/1 | 10.9/6.2 | 3/1.7 | 1.4/0.8 |

Sauce, Tomato & Roasted Garlic, Stir-In, Dolmio*, ½ pack/75g

| 94/125 | 0.9/1.2 | 5.8/7.7 | 7.7/10.2 | 0/0 |

Sauce, Tomato, Organic, Heinz*, 1 tsp/5g

| 5/105 | 0.1/1.3 | 1.2/24 | 0/0.1 | 0/0.9 |

Sauce, Tomato, Value, Tesco*, 1 serving/10g

| 14/139 | 0.2/2.3 | 3.2/32.2 | 0/0.1 | 0.1/1.4 |

Sauce, White Wine & Cream, Homepride*, 1 jar/500g

| 405/81 | 5.5/1.1 | 45/9 | 22.5/4.5 | 0/0 |

Sauce, White, Savoury, Made with Semi-Skimmed Milk, 1oz/28g

| 36/128 | 1.2/4.2 | 3.1/11.1 | 2.2/7.8 | 0.1/0.2 |

Sauce, White, Savoury, Made with Whole Milk, 1oz/28g

| 42/150 | 1.1/4.1 | 3.1/10.9 | 2.9/10.3 | 0.1/0.2 |

Sauce, Worcestershire, Lea & Perrins*, 1 tsp/5ml

| 4/88 | 0.1/1.1 | 1.1/22 | 0/0 | 0/0 |

Tapenade, Green Olive, Best, Safeway*, 1 tsp/15g

| 71/470 | 0.2/1.6 | 1.5/10.2 | 7.1/47 | 0.3/1.7 |

Taramasalata, Fresh, BGTY, Sainsbury's*, 1oz/28g

| 71/253 | 1.2/4.3 | 3.8/13.5 | 5.7/20.2 | 0.2/0.7 |

Taramasalata, Fresh, Healthy Eating, Tesco*, 1 pot/170g

| 430/253 | 7.3/4.3 | 23/13.5 | 34.3/20.2 | 1.2/0.7 |

Taramasalata, Marks & Spencer*, 1oz/28g

| 140/500 | 1.1/3.9 | 1.5/5.5 | 14.3/51.2 | 0.5/1.7 |

Taramasalata, Tesco*, 1 serving/50g

| 220/440 | 3.7/7.4 | 4.4/8.8 | 20.9/41.7 | 0.2/0.3 |

Taramasalata, Reduced-Fat, Waitrose*, 1 pot/170g

| 598/352 | 7.1/4.2 | 16.3/9.6 | 56.1/33 | 1/0.6 |

	kcal serv/100g	prot serv/100g	carb serv/100g	fat serv/100g	fibre serv/100g
Tomato Frito, Heinz*, 1oz/28g					
	20/73	0.4/1.3	2.2/7.7	1.1/4.1	0.2/0.8
Tzatziki, Fresh, Sainsbury's*, 1oz/28g					
	35/126	1.1/4	1/3.7	3/10.6	0.1/0.3
Tzatziki, Marks & Spencer*, 1oz/28g					
	41/145	1.6/5.6	1.7/5.9	3.1/10.9	0.1/0.4
Tzatziki, Tesco*, 1 serving/85g					
	121/142	4.3/5.1	3.5/4.1	9.9/11.7	0.9/1
Tzatziki, Total*, 1oz/28g					
	27/98	1.4/4.9	1.1/4.1	2/7	0/0
Tzatziki, Waitrose*, 1 serving/50g					
	57/113	3.4/6.8	2.5/5	3.7/7.3	0.4/0.7
Vinaigrette, Balsamic Vinegar & Pistachio, Finest, Tesco*, 1 tbsp/15ml					
	56/370	0/0.2	0.4/2.8	5.9/39.2	0/0
Vinaigrette, BGTY, Sainsbury's*, 1fl oz/30ml					
	23/78	0.2/0.6	2.5/8.4	1.4/4.7	0.2/0.7
Vinaigrette, Finest, Tesco*, 1 serving/50ml					
	248/495	0.5/0.9	6.6/13.2	24.4/48.7	0.3/0.5
Vinaigrette, Frank Cooper*, 1 pot/28g					
	46/163	0.3/1	3.9/14.1	3.2/11.4	0.1/0.3
Vinaigrette, French-Style, Finest, Tesco*, 1 tbsp/15ml					
	69/461	0.1/0.8	0.9/5.9	7.1/47.4	0/0.2
Vinaigrette, French, Full-Flavoured, Fat-Free, Kraft*, 1 tbsp/15ml					
	7/47	0/0.1	1.6/10.5	0/0	0/0.3
Vinaigrette, Luxury French, Hellmann's*, 1 tsp/5ml					
	15/305	0/0.8	0.8/16	1.3/26.1	0/0.4
Vinaigrette, Newman's Own*, ½ tbsp/5g					
	17/333	0/0.5	0.2/3.9	1.8/35	0/0
Vinaigrette, Oil-Free, Tesco*, 1 tbsp/15ml					
	5/30	0/0.3	0.9/6	0/0.1	0.2/1.4
Vinaigrette, Perfectly Balanced, Waitrose*, 1 tsp/5ml					
	4/89	0/0.4	1/20.9	0/0.4	0/0.5

SOUPS

	kcal serv/100g	prot serv/100g	carb serv/100g	fat serv/100g	fibre serv/100g
Asparagus with Croutons, in a Cup, Sainsbury's*, 1 serving/200ml					
	103/52	1.9/1	12.7/6.4	5/2.5	3.3/1.7

	kcal serv/100g	prot serv/100g	carb serv/100g	fat serv/100g	fibre serv/100g
Asparagus, Fresh, New Covent Garden Soup Co*, 1 carton/600g					
	324/54	12.6/2.1	10.8/1.8	25.8/4.3	5.4/0.9
Asparagus, Healthy Eating, Tesco*, 1 serving/19g					
	67/351	0.7/3.6	11.5/60.3	2/10.6	0.6/3.2
Aubergine & Red Pepper, New Covent Garden Soup Co*, ½ pint/296ml					
	71/24	2.7/0.9	14.2/4.8	0.3/0.1	1.2/0.4
Autumn Vegetable, Baxters*, 1 can/425g					
	170/40	7.7/1.8	34/8	0.9/0.2	6.4/1.5
Bean, Italian-Style, Tesco*, 1 can/300g					
	153/51	8.4/2.8	21.9/7.3	3.6/1.2	3.3/1.1
Beef & Tomato Cup a Soup, Batchelors*, 1 serving/215g					
	71/33	1.3/0.6	15.7/7.3	0.4/0.2	1.1/0.5
Beef & Vegetable Big, Heinz*, ½ can/200g					
	90/45	4.8/2.4	14.6/7.3	1.4/0.7	1.8/0.9
Beef & Vegetable Mighty, Asda*, ½ can/81g					
	32/40	1.9/2.3	4.9/6	0.6/0.8	0.5/0.6
Beef Broth Big, Heinz*, ½ can/200g					
	82/41	4/2	13.6/6.8	1.2/0.6	1.4/0.7
Beef Consommé, Sainsbury's*, 1 can/415g					
	46/11	8.3/2	2.9/0.7	0/0	0/0
Blended Autumn Vegetable, Heinz*, ½ can/200g					
	114/57	2.4/1.2	12.8/6.4	6/3	1.4/0.7
Blended Carrot & Coriander, Heinz*, ½ can/200g					
	104/52	1.4/0.7	12.4/6.2	5.4/2.7	1.2/0.6
Blended Red Pepper with Tomato, Heinz*, ½ can/200g					
	102/51	1.6/0.8	10.4/5.2	5.8/2.9	1.4/0.7
Broccoli & Blue Stilton, New Covent Garden Soup Co*, 1 carton/600g					
	378/63	21/3.5	17.4/2.9	25.2/4.2	0/0
Broccoli & Cauliflower, Slim A Soup, Made Up, Batchelors*, 1 serving/203g					
	59/29	1/0.5	9.9/4.9	1.6/0.8	0.8/0.4
Broccoli & Cauliflower, Thick & Creamy, Cup a Soup, Batchelors*, 1 sachet/279g					
	120/43	2/0.7	17.3/6.2	4.7/1.7	0.6/0.2
Broccoli & Stilton, Asda*, 1 pack/302g					
	172/57	6.6/2.2	18.1/6	8.2/2.7	0/0
Broccoli & Stilton, Canned, Tesco*, 1 can/400g					
	224/56	7.2/1.8	16.8/4.2	14/3.5	1.2/0.3

	kcal serv/100g	prot serv/100g	carb serv/100g	fat serv/100g	fibre serv/100g
Broccoli & Stilton, Fresh, Safeway*, 1 serving/250g					
	133/53	6/2.4	8.8/3.5	8.3/3.3	1.3/0.5
Broccoli & Stilton, Fresh, Sainsbury's*, ½ bottle/300ml					
	156/52	6.3/2.1	11.7/3.9	9.3/3.1	2.7/0.9
Broccoli & Stilton, Fresh, Tesco*, ½ pot/300g					
	219/73	9.9/3.3	15/5	13.2/4.4	2.1/0.7
Broccoli, Baxters*, 1 can/425g					
	191/45	5.5/1.3	25.1/5.9	7.7/1.8	1.7/0.4
Butternut Squash & Red Pepper, Baxters*, 1 can/425g					
	153/36	3/0.7	25.9/6.1	4.3/1	2.6/0.6
Cajun Spicy Vegetable, Slim A Soup, Batchelors*, 1 sachet/211g					
	57/27	1.7/0.8	10.6/5	1.1/0.5	1.3/0.6
Cantonese Chicken & Sweetcorn, Fresh, Sainsbury's*, ½ bottle/300ml					
	135/45	6.3/2.1	23.7/7.9	1.5/0.5	1.5/0.5
Cantonese Hot & Sour Noodle, Baxters*, 1 serving/215g					
	133/62	3/1.4	23.9/11.1	2.8/1.3	1.1/0.5
Carrot & Butterbean, Baxters*, 1 can/425g					
	234/55	6.8/1.6	33.6/7.9	8.1/1.9	7.2/1.7
Carrot & Coriander, Baxters*, 1 can/425g					
	162/38	3.4/0.8	23.4/5.5	6/1.4	3.4/0.8
Carrot & Coriander, BGTY, Sainsbury's*, ½ can/200g					
	48/24	0.6/0.3	9.6/4.8	0.8/0.4	0.2/0.1
Carrot & Coriander, Classic Homestyle, Marks & Spencer*, 1 can/425g					
	170/40	2.6/0.6	23.8/5.6	8.5/2	3/0.7
Carrot & Coriander, Fresh, Improved, Sainsbury's*, ½ bottle/300ml					
	84/28	1.5/0.5	9/3	4.8/1.6	7.8/2.6
Carrot & Coriander, Fresh, Marks & Spencer*, ½ pot/300g					
	90/30	1.2/0.4	12.6/4.2	4.5/1.5	1.5/0.5
Carrot & Coriander, Fresh, Sainsbury's*, ½ bottle/300ml					
	150/50	4.2/1.4	12.3/4.1	9.3/3.1	1.8/0.6
Carrot & Coriander, Fresh, Tesco*, 1 pack/600g					
	270/45	3.6/0.6	35.4/5.9	12.6/2.1	5.4/0.9
Carrot & Coriander, GFY, Asda*, ½ pot/251g					
	88/35	3/1.2	10/4	4/1.6	1/0.4
Carrot & Coriander, Heinz*, 1 can/400g					
	208/52	2.8/0.7	24.8/6.2	10.8/2.7	2.4/0.6
Carrot & Coriander, New Covent Garden Soup Co*, 1fl oz/30ml					
	13/42	0.2/0.8	1.2/3.9	0.8/2.6	0.2/0.6

kcal serv/100g	prot serv/100g	carb serv/100g	fat serv/100g	fibre serv/100g
Carrot & Coriander, Sainsbury's*, ½ bottle/300ml				
84/28	1.5/0.5	9/3	4.8/1.6	7.8/2.6
Carrot & Coriander, Tesco*, ½ can/210g				
92/44	1.5/0.7	11.3/5.4	4.6/2.2	1.7/0.8
Carrot & Coriander, Vie Country, Knorr*, 1 pack/500ml				
190/38	3/0.6	19.5/3.9	11/2.2	5/1
Carrot & Ginger, Perfectly Balanced, Waitrose*, ½ pot/300g				
66/22	1.2/0.4	9.3/3.1	2.7/0.9	3/1
Carrot & Lentil, Weight Watchers*, 1 can/295g				
91/31	4.1/1.4	17.7/6	0.3/0.1	2.1/0.7
Carrot & Parsnip, Marks & Spencer*, 1oz/28g				
9/32	0.1/0.5	1.4/4.9	0.3/1.2	0.3/0.9
Carrot, Onion & Chick Pea, Healthy Choice, Baxters*, 1 can/425g				
145/34	7.2/1.7	30.2/7.1	0.4/0.1	6.4/1.5
Celeriac & Bacon, New Covent Garden Soup Co*, 1 serving/300g				
228/76	3.3/1.1	9/3	21.3/7.1	4.8/1.6
Chicken & Broccoli, Soup a Cups, GFY, Asda*, 1 cup/226ml				
52/23	1.1/0.5	9/4	1.4/0.6	0.9/0.4
Chicken & Golden Sweetcorn, Microwaveable Cup, Heinz*, 1 cup/275ml				
149/54	3.9/1.4	15.4/5.6	8.3/3	0.6/0.2
Chicken & Ham, Big, Heinz*, ½ can/200g				
92/46	4.6/2.3	13.8/6.9	2/1	1.4/0.7
Chicken & Leek, Big, Heinz*, ½ can/200g				
118/59	4.6/2.3	15.6/7.8	4/2	1/0.5
Chicken & Leek, Cup a Soup, Batchelors*, 1 serving/213g				
77/36	1.3/0.6	14.3/6.7	1.9/0.9	0.6/0.3
Chicken & Mushroom with Pasta Cup a Soup, Batchelors*, 1 serving/250g				
115/46	3.3/1.3	17.8/7.1	3.5/1.4	1.3/0.5
Chicken & Mushroom, Slim A Soup, Batchelors*, 1 sachet/203g				
59/29	1.4/0.7	8.3/4.1	2.2/1.1	0.6/0.3
Chicken & Mushroom, Tesco*, 1 serving/100g				
53/53	0.8/0.8	5.7/5.7	3/3	0.4/0.4
Chicken & Sweetcorn, Baxters*, 1 can/425g				
166/39	6.8/1.6	26.4/6.2	3.8/0.9	2.6/0.6
Chicken & Sweetcorn, BGTY, Sainsbury's*, 1 serving/200g				
42/21	2.4/1.2	7/3.5	0.4/0.2	0.2/0.1
Chicken & Sweetcorn, Fresh, Asda*, 1 pack/500g				
260/52	13/2.6	30/6	9.5/1.9	0/0

	kcal serv/100g	prot serv/100g	carb serv/100g	fat serv/100g	fibre serv/100g

Chicken & Sweetcorn, Fresh, Sainsbury's*, ½ bottle/300ml

135/45	6.3/2.1	23.7/7.9	1.5/0.5	1.5/0.5

Chicken & Sweetcorn, GFY, Asda*, 1 can/400g

108/27	6/1.5	16.8/4.2	2/0.5	0.8/0.2

Chicken & Sweetcorn, Healthy Eating, Tesco*, 1 serving/200ml

64/32	3/1.5	10.6/5.3	1/0.5	0.4/0.2

Chicken & Sweetcorn, in a Cup, BGTY, Sainsbury's*, 1 sachet/200ml

50/25	1.4/0.7	7.6/3.8	1.6/0.8	1.2/0.6

Chicken & Sweetcorn, Slim A Soup, Batchelors*, 1 sachet/203g

59/29	1.2/0.6	9.1/4.5	1.8/0.9	0.2/0.1

Chicken & Vegetable, Big, Heinz*, 1 can/400g

188/47	9.6/2.4	29.2/7.3	4/1	3.6/0.9

Chicken & Vegetable, Cup a Soup with Croutons, Batchelors*, 1 serving/222g

133/60	1.6/0.7	17.3/7.8	6.7/3	3.3/1.5

Chicken & Vegetable, Cup a Soup, Batchelors*, 1 sachet/30g

131/437	1.4/4.8	18.8/62.7	5.6/18.6	0.3/1.1

Chicken & Vegetable, Cup, Tesco*, 1 sachet/29ml

122/422	1.6/5.6	17.8/61.3	5/17.1	0.1/0.5

Chicken & Vegetable, Fresh, Somerfield*, ½ pot/300g

177/59	8.7/2.9	16.8/5.6	8.4/2.8	9/3

Chicken & Vegetable, Healthy Choice, Baxters*, 1 can/426g

132/31	5.5/1.3	23.9/5.6	2.1/0.5	6.8/1.6

Chicken & Vegetable, Marks & Spencer*, 1oz/28g

17/59	1.5/5.3	1.6/5.7	0.5/1.7	0.3/1.1

Chicken & Vegetable, Perfectly Balanced, Waitrose*, 1 can/68g

23/34	1.2/1.8	3.7/5.4	0.4/0.6	0.7/1

Chicken & Vegetable, Thick, Heinz*, 1 can/400g

152/38	4.8/1.2	24.8/6.2	3.6/0.9	2.4/0.6

Chicken Broth, Baxters*, 1 can/425g

145/34	5.1/1.2	22.5/5.3	3.8/0.9	2.6/0.6

Chicken Broth, Fresh, Baxters*, 1 serving/300g

117/39	14.7/4.9	6.3/2.1	3.6/1.2	2.1/0.7

Chicken Broth, Traditional, Baxters*, ½ can/207g

62/30	2.5/1.2	11/5.3	0.8/0.4	1.2/0.6

Chicken Fusion, Fresh, New Covent Garden Co*, ½ carton/300g

162/54	7.8/2.6	14.4/4.8	8.1/2.7	1.2/0.4

	kcal serv/100g	prot serv/100g	carb serv/100g	fat serv/100g	fibre serv/100g

Chicken Mulligatawny, Perfectly Balanced, Waitrose*, 1 serving/300g

138/46	5.1/1.7	15.9/5.3	6/2	1.2/0.4

Chicken Mulligatawny, Tesco*, 1 pack/600g

570/95	21.6/3.6	32.4/5.4	39.6/6.6	2.4/0.4

Chicken Noodle & Vegetable, Slim A Soup, Batchelors*, 1 serving/203g

59/29	1.6/0.8	9.9/4.9	1.4/0.7	0.6/0.3

Chicken Noodle, Asda*, 1 can/410g

107/26	6.6/1.6	16.4/4	1.6/0.4	0.4/0.1

Chicken Noodle, Cup a Soup, Batchelors*, 1 serving/217g

89/41	3.7/1.7	16.1/7.4	1.3/0.6	0.4/0.2

Chicken Noodle, Cup, Asda*, 1 sachet/13g

40/305	1.2/9	8.2/63	0.2/1.9	0.5/3.6

Chicken Noodle, Heinz*, 1oz/28g

8/27	0.3/1.1	1.4/4.9	0.1/0.3	0.1/0.2

Chicken Noodle, Old Fashioned, EAT*, 1 can/400ml

240/60	24/6	22/5.5	6.4/1.6	2.4/0.6

Chicken Noodle, Weight Watchers*, 1 can/295g

50/17	2.1/0.7	9.1/3.1	0.3/0.1	0.6/0.2

Chicken, Campbell's*, 1 can/295g

142/48	3.2/1.1	10.3/3.5	10.6/3.6	0/0

Chicken, Coconut & Lemon Grass, Fresh, Waitrose*, ½ pot/300g

303/101	7.8/2.6	12.3/4.1	24.9/8.3	2.4/0.8

Chicken, Condensed, 99% Fat-Free, Campbell's*, 1 can/295g

100/34	4.7/1.6	14.8/5	2.7/0.9	0/0

Chicken, Cup a Soup, Batchelors*, 1 serving/213g

98/46	1.5/0.7	12.4/5.8	4.7/2.2	0.6/0.3

Chicken, Mushroom & Potato, Big, Heinz*, ½ can/200g

122/61	5.8/2.9	14.6/7.3	4.4/2.2	0.8/0.4

Chicken, Mushroom & Rice, Chilled, Marks & Spencer*, ½ pot/300g

240/80	10.2/3.4	25.8/8.6	11.4/3.8	1.8/0.6

Chicken, Our Best, New Covent Garden Food Co*, 1 carton/600ml

804/134	28.2/4.7	73.2/12.2	44.4/7.4	5.4/0.9

Chicken, Sweetcorn & Potato, Heinz*, 1 can/400g

204/51	4.8/1.2	22/5.5	11.2/2.8	1.2/0.3

Chicken, Weight Watchers*, 1 can/295g

89/30	3.5/1.2	12.1/4.1	3/1	0.3/0.1

Chilli Bean, Marks & Spencer*, ½ carton/300g

150/50	7.5/2.5	14.1/4.7	7.5/2.5	8.1/2.7

	kcal serv/100g	prot serv/100g	carb serv/100g	fat serv/100g	fibre serv/100g

Chilli Pumpkin, Sainsbury's*, 1 serving/300g

120/40	1.8/0.6	12/4	7.2/2.4	3.9/1.3

Chunky Chicken & Vegetable, Marks & Spencer*, 1 can/425g

276/65	22.1/5.2	28.1/6.6	7.7/1.8	2.6/0.6

Chunky Chicken, Leek & Potato, Heinz*, 1 can/400g

236/59	9.2/2.3	31.2/7.8	8/2	2/0.5

Chunky Minestrone Meal, Tesco*, ½ can/205g

78/38	2.7/1.3	13.9/6.8	1.2/0.6	1.8/0.9

Chunky Tomato, New Covent Garden Soup Co*, ½ pack/300g

135/45	5.4/1.8	15.9/5.3	5.4/1.8	3.3/1.1

Chunky Tuscan-Style Bean & Sausage, Marks & Spencer*, 1 can/415g

249/60	10/2.4	32/7.7	9.1/2.2	4.2/1

Chunky Vegetable, Big, Heinz*, 1 serving/400g

208/52	6/1.5	34.8/8.7	5.2/1.3	4.8/1.2

Chunky Vegetable, Eat Smart, Safeway*, 1 can/415g

95/23	2.9/0.7	19.1/4.6	0.8/0.2	5/1.2

Chunky Vegetable, Fresh, Baxters*, 1 serving/300ml

117/39	4.8/1.6	23.4/7.8	0.6/0.2	3.3/1.1

Chunky Vegetable, Fresh, Sainsbury's*, ½ bottle/296ml

77/26	1.5/0.5	14.2/4.8	1.5/0.5	3.6/1.2

Chunky Vegetable, Fresh, Tesco*, 1 serving/300g

123/41	1.8/0.6	16.5/5.5	5.7/1.9	3/1

Chunky Winter Vegetable, Marks & Spencer*, 1 can/415ml

166/40	6.2/1.5	31.1/7.5	1.2/0.3	1.7/0.4

Classic Tomato, Pret A Manger*, 1 serving/336g

179/53	3.1/0.9	25.3/7.5	7.1/2.1	2.5/0.7

Cock-a-Leekie Traditional, Baxters*, 1 can/425g

98/23	4.3/1	17.4/4.1	1.3/0.3	1.3/0.3

Country Garden, Baxters*, 1 can/425g

149/35	3.8/0.9	27.6/6.5	2.6/0.6	3/0.7

Country Mushroom, Selection, Campbell's*, 1 serving/250ml

80/32	1.5/0.6	8.5/3.4	4.5/1.8	1.3/0.5

Country Vegetable, Chilled, Marks & Spencer*, ½ pot/300g

105/35	1.5/0.5	9.6/3.2	6.3/2.1	3/1

Country Vegetable, Fresh, Chilled, Marks & Spencer*, 1 pot/600g

210/35	3/0.5	19.2/3.2	12.6/2.1	6/1

Country Vegetable, Fresh, Waitrose*, 1 serving/300g

165/55	6.3/2.1	21.3/7.1	6/2	4.8/1.6

kcal serv/100g	prot serv/100g	carb serv/100g	fat serv/100g	fibre serv/100g
Country Vegetable, Heinz*, 1oz/28g				
14/51	0.6/2.3	2.6/9.3	0.1/0.5	0.3/1.1
Country Vegetable, Vie Knorr*, 1 pack/500ml				
160/32	4.5/0.9	27.5/5.5	3.5/0.7	6/1.2
Country Vegetable, Weight Watchers*, 1 can/295g				
89/30	3.2/1.1	17.4/5.9	0.6/0.2	3/1
Cream of Chicken & Mushroom, Heinz*, 1oz/28g				
14/49	0.4/1.3	1.3/4.6	0.8/2.9	0/0.1
Cream of Chicken, Asda*, 1 can/410g				
209/51	4.9/1.2	16.4/4	13.9/3.4	0.4/0.1
Cream of Chicken, Fresh, Tesco*, 1 serving/300g				
294/98	9.9/3.3	18.9/6.3	19.8/6.6	0.6/0.2
Cream of Chicken, Heinz*, 1oz/28g				
14/51	0.4/1.3	1.2/4.4	0.9/3.2	0/0.1
Cream of Leek, Traditional, Baxters*, 1 can/425g				
196/46	3/0.7	22.1/5.2	10.6/2.5	1.7/0.4
Cream of Mushroom Cup a Soup, Batchelors*, 1 serving/219g				
125/57	1.3/0.6	16.4/7.5	6.1/2.8	0.9/0.4
Cream of Mushroom, Condensed, 99% Fat-Free, Campbell's*, 1 can/295g				
71/24	1.8/0.6	10.3/3.5	2.7/0.9	0/0
Cream of Mushroom, Condensed, Campbell's*, 1 can/295ml				
204/69	5/1.7	15.6/5.3	13.3/4.5	0/0
Cream of Mushroom, Fresh, Tesco*, ½ pot/250g				
108/43	2.5/1	10/4	6.5/2.6	0.5/0.2
Cream of Mushroom, Fresh, Waitrose*, ½ pot/300g				
210/70	3.9/1.3	11.1/3.7	16.5/5.5	1.5/0.5
Cream of Mushroom, Heinz*, 1oz/28g				
14/51	0.4/1.4	1.4/5.1	0.8/2.7	0/0.1
Cream of Mushroom, Sainsbury's*, 1 can/400g				
220/55	2.4/0.6	5.6/1.4	20.8/5.2	0.4/0.1
Cream of Mushroom, Tesco*, 1 serving/200g				
108/54	1.8/0.9	9.2/4.6	7/3.5	0.2/0.1
Cream of Potato & Leek, Sainsbury's*, ½ can/200g				
116/58	1.8/0.9	13.6/6.8	6/3	0.8/0.4
Cream of Tomato & Basil, Somerfield*, 1 pack/450g				
279/62	4.5/1	22.5/5	18/4	0/0
Cream of Tomato, Asda*, ½ can/205g				
150/73	1.6/0.8	18.5/9	7.6/3.7	1/0.5

kcal serv/100g	prot serv/100g	carb serv/100g	fat serv/100g	fibre serv/100g
Cream of Tomato, Campbell's*, 1 can/295g				
195/66	2.1/0.7	22.4/7.6	10.6/3.6	0/0
Cream of Tomato, For One, Heinz*, 1 can/300g				
192/64	2.7/0.9	21.3/7.1	10.8/3.6	1.2/0.4
Cream of Tomato, Fresh, Sainsbury's*, ½ bottle/300ml				
126/42	2.7/0.9	21/7	3.6/1.2	1.8/0.6
Cream of Tomato, Fresh, Waitrose*, ½ pot/300g				
210/70	3/1	14.7/4.9	15.3/5.1	1.5/0.5
Cream of Tomato, Heinz*, 1oz/28g				
18/64	0.3/0.9	2/7.1	1/3.6	0.1/0.4
Cream of Tomato, Improved, Tesco*, ½ can/200g				
142/71	1.8/0.9	17.4/8.7	7.2/3.6	1/0.5
Cream of Tomato, Microwave, Heinz*, 1oz/28g				
19/68	0.3/0.9	2.1/7.5	1.1/3.8	0.1/0.4
Cream of Tomato, Organic, Heinz*, 1 can/400g				
220/55	3.6/0.9	28.8/7.2	10/2.5	1.6/0.4
Cream of Vegetable Cup a Soup, Batchelors*, 1 sachet/33g				
134/406	1.9/5.8	19.7/59.8	5.3/16	2/6.2
English Asparagus, New Covent Garden Soup Co*, ½ pack/300g				
114/38	2.1/0.7	16.5/5.5	4.5/1.5	0.3/0.1
French Onion, 1oz/28g				
11/40	0.1/0.2	1.6/5.7	0.6/2.1	0.3/1
French Onion & Gruyere Cheese, Finest, Tesco*, ½ pot/300g				
210/70	4.2/1.4	14.1/4.7	15.3/5.1	1.5/0.5
French Onion, Baxters*, 1 can/425g				
94/22	3/0.7	17.9/4.2	0.9/0.2	1.7/0.4
French Onion, Chilled, Marks & Spencer*, ½ pot/300g				
150/50	6/2	21.6/7.2	4.5/1.5	3/1
French Onion, GFY, Asda*, ½ pot/253g				
91/36	4.8/1.9	15.2/6	1.3/0.5	1/0.4
French Onion, Heinz*, 1 pack/400g				
100/25	2/0.5	22.8/5.7	0.4/0.1	1.6/0.4
Goats Cheese & Rocket, Sainsbury's*, 1 serving/300g				
180/60	6/2	9.6/3.2	13.2/4.4	0.9/0.3
Golden Vegetable, Cup a Soup, Batchelors*, 1 serving/212g				
70/33	1.1/0.5	15.5/7.3	0.4/0.2	0.8/0.4
Golden Vegetable, Knorr*, 1 pack/76g				
299/394	7.9/10.4	34.5/45.4	14.4/19	2.5/3.3

kcal serv/100g	prot serv/100g	carb serv/100g	fat serv/100g	fibre serv/100g

Golden Vegetable, Slim A Soup, Batchelors*, 1 sachet/207g

| 58/28 | 1/0.5 | 9.7/4.7 | 1.7/0.8 | 1.4/0.7 |

Golden Vegetable, Soup-A-Slim, Asda*, 1 sachet/15g

| 50/336 | 0.9/6 | 9/60 | 1.2/8 | 0.3/1.9 |

Green Thai Chicken, Waitrose*, 1 pack/400g

| 324/81 | 15.2/3.8 | 22.8/5.7 | 19.2/4.8 | 1.1/0.3 |

Haddock, Chowder, Smoked, Asda*, 1 serving/300g

| 135/45 | 7.1/2.4 | 18/6 | 3.9/1.3 | 2.1/0.7 |

Hearty Vegetable, 99% Fat-Free, Campbells*, 1 can/295g

| 91/31 | 2.4/0.8 | 18/6.1 | 1.2/0.4 | 0/0 |

Italian Plum Tomato & Basil, Perfectly Balanced, Waitrose*, ½ pot/300g

| 69/23 | 2.7/0.9 | 11.4/3.8 | 1.5/0.5 | 2.7/0.9 |

Italian-Style Tomato & Chicken, BGTY, Sainsbury's*, 1 can/400g

| 148/37 | 12.4/3.1 | 22/5.5 | 1.2/0.3 | 1.6/0.4 |

Jamaican Jerk Chicken & Pumpkin, Sainsbury's*, 1 pack/600g

| 282/47 | 16.2/2.7 | 30.6/5.1 | 10.2/1.7 | 1.2/0.2 |

Lamb & Vegetable, Big, Heinz*, 1oz/28g

| 16/56 | 0.7/2.4 | 2.6/9.3 | 0.3/1 | 0.3/1.1 |

Leek & Potato, Chilled, Marks & Spencer*, 1 serving/300g

| 240/80 | 2.7/0.9 | 15.6/5.2 | 18.6/6.2 | 1.8/0.6 |

Leek & Potato, Fresh, Sainsbury's*, 1 bowl/300ml

| 189/63 | 3.3/1.1 | 11.7/3.9 | 14.4/4.8 | 1.5/0.5 |

Leek & Potato, Fresh, Tesco*, ½ pack/300g

| 201/67 | 4.2/1.4 | 18.9/6.3 | 12/4 | 2.4/0.8 |

Leek & Potato, GFY, Asda*, 1 sachet/220g

| 55/25 | 0.7/0.3 | 11/5 | 0.9/0.4 | 0.7/0.3 |

Leek & Potato, in a Cup, BGTY, Sainsbury's*, 1 sachet/196ml

| 55/28 | 0.6/0.3 | 9.6/4.9 | 1.6/0.8 | 1.6/0.8 |

Leek & Potato, New Covent Garden Soup Co*, ½ carton/284g

| 105/37 | 3.4/1.2 | 20.2/7.1 | 4.3/1.5 | 2.3/0.8 |

Leek & Potato, Organic, Sainsbury's*, ½ can/200g

| 84/42 | 3.2/1.6 | 11.4/5.7 | 2.8/1.4 | 1.8/0.9 |

Leek & Potato, Slim A Soup, Batchelors*, 1 serving/204g

| 57/28 | 0.8/0.4 | 10.2/5 | 1.4/0.7 | 0.4/0.2 |

Leek & Potato, Weight Watchers*, 1 sachet/214.8ml

| 58/27 | 1.1/0.5 | 11/5.1 | 1.1/0.5 | 0.2/0.1 |

Lentil & Bacon, Baxters*, 1 can/425g

| 255/60 | 11.5/2.7 | 33.6/7.9 | 8.1/1.9 | 3.4/0.8 |

kcal serv/100g	prot serv/100g	carb serv/100g	fat serv/100g	fibre serv/100g
Lentil & Bacon, Marks & Spencer*, 1oz/28g				
18/63	1.1/4.1	2.4/8.6	0.4/1.6	0.2/0.7
Lentil & Chick Pea, Organic, Tesco*, 1 serving/300ml				
117/39	5.7/1.9	18.3/6.1	2.4/0.8	1.5/0.5
Lentil & Tomato, New Covent Garden Soup Co*, ½ pack/284g				
162/57	10.2/3.6	23/8.1	3.1/1.1	2/0.7
Lentil & Vegetable, Baxters*, 1 can/423g				
144/34	8/1.9	28.8/6.8	0.4/0.1	6.3/1.5
Lentil, Heinz*, 1 can/300g				
117/39	6.9/2.3	21.3/7.1	0.6/0.2	3/1
Lobster Bisque, Baxters*, 1 can/415g				
220/53	14.1/3.4	21.6/5.2	8.7/2.1	0.4/0.1
Mexican Black Bean, Extra Special, Asda*, ½ pot/262.5g				
195/74	6/2.3	18.4/7	10.8/4.1	4.5/1.7
Minestrone with Wholemeal Pasta, Baxters*, 1 can/415g				
133/32	3.7/0.9	27.8/6.7	0.8/0.2	4.2/1
Minestrone, Asda*, ½ can/200g				
54/27	1.8/0.9	8.8/4.4	1.2/0.6	1.2/0.6
Minestrone, Baxters*, 1 can/425g				
145/34	5.5/1.3	25.5/6	2.6/0.6	3.4/0.8
Minestrone, Chilled, Marks & Spencer*, ½ pot/300g				
66/22	4.2/1.4	7.5/2.5	2.1/0.7	3.6/1.2
Minestrone, Cup a Soup, Batchelors*, 1 serving/217g				
100/46	2/0.9	18/8.3	2.4/1.1	1.1/0.5
Minestrone, Cup a Soup, BGTY, Sainsbury's*, 1 serving/200ml				
54/27	1.6/0.8	12/6	0.2/0.1	1.2/0.6
Minestrone, For One, Heinz*, 1 can/303g				
97/32	4.2/1.4	15.8/5.2	2.1/0.7	2.1/0.7
Minestrone, Fresh, Baxters*, 1 box/568ml				
233/41	10.2/1.8	35.2/6.2	5.7/1	3.4/0.6
Minestrone, Fresh, Sainsbury's*, ½ bottle/300ml				
93/31	3.6/1.2	13.2/4.4	2.7/0.9	2.7/0.9
Minestrone, Fresh, Tesco*, 1 serving/300g				
126/42	4.2/1.4	20.7/6.9	3/1	1.8/0.6
Minestrone, Fresh, Waitrose*, 1 pack/600g				
240/40	6.6/1.1	34.8/5.8	8.4/1.4	4.8/0.8
Minestrone, Healthy Choice, Baxters*, ½ can/207.5g				
67/32	1.9/0.9	13.9/6.7	0.4/0.2	2.5/1.2

kcal serv/100g	prot serv/100g	carb serv/100g	fat serv/100g	fibre serv/100g
Minestrone, Heinz*, 1 can/300g				
96/32	4.2/1.4	15.6/5.2	2.1/0.7	2.1/0.7
Minestrone, in a Cup, BGTY, Sainsbury's*, 1 serving/200ml				
54/27	1.6/0.8	12/6	0.2/0.1	1.2/0.6
Minestrone, in a Cup, Sainsbury's*, 1 serving/227ml				
84/37	3.2/1.4	14.3/6.3	1.6/0.7	0.5/0.2
Minestrone, In a Mug, Healthy Eating, Tesco*, 1 sachet/21g				
72/342	0.8/3.6	14.2/67.7	1.3/6.3	0.7/3.2
Minestrone, Packet, Knorr*, 1 pack/61g				
178/292	5.6/9.2	32.9/53.9	2.7/4.4	4/6.5
Minestrone, Slim A Soup, Batchelors*, 1 serving/203g				
53/26	1.4/0.7	9.1/4.5	1.2/0.6	1.2/0.6
Minestrone, Weight Watchers*, 1 can/295g				
59/20	2.4/0.8	9.7/3.3	1.2/0.4	1.5/0.5
Minted Lamb Hot Pot, Big, Heinz*, 1oz/28g				
14/51	0.6/2.2	2.4/8.5	0.3/1	0.3/0.9
Mulligatawny Beef Curry, Heinz*, 1oz/28g				
17/60	0.5/1.8	2/7.2	0.8/2.7	0.1/0.5
Mushroom & Garlic, Slimming Cup a Soup, Tesco*, 1 serving/16g				
58/360	0.9/5.8	9.8/61.1	1.6/10.3	0.5/3.2
Mushroom Crème Fraîche, Waistline, Crosse & Blackwell*, 1 carton/300g				
69/23	3.6/1.2	8.4/2.8	2.4/0.8	0.9/0.3
Mushroom, Cream of, Canned, 1 serving/220g				
101/46	2.4/1.1	8.6/3.9	6.6/3	0.2/0.1
Mushroom, Fresh, Sainsbury's*, 1 serving/300g				
204/68	4.8/1.6	14.1/4.7	14.4/4.8	2.4/0.8
Mushroom, Weight Watchers*, 1 can/295g				
86/29	3.5/1.2	16.5/5.6	0.6/0.2	0.3/0.1
New England Clam Chowder, Select, Campbell's*, 1 cup/240ml				
221/92	6/2.5	14.4/6	14.4/6	1.9/0.8
Oxtail, Heinz*, 1oz/28g				
11/41	0.5/1.9	1.9/6.7	0.2/0.8	0.1/0.3
Oxtail, Sainsbury's*, ½ can/200g				
66/33	4.6/2.3	10.2/5.1	0.8/0.4	0.4/0.2
Parsnip, Leek & Ginger, New Covent Garden Food Co*, 1 carton/600g				
162/27	7.2/1.2	29.4/4.9	1.8/0.3	7.8/1.3
Pea & Ham, 1oz/28g				
20/70	1.1/4	2.6/9.2	0.6/2.1	0.4/1.4

	kcal serv/100g	prot serv/100g	carb serv/100g	fat serv/100g	fibre serv/100g
Pea & Ham, Asda*, ½ can/205g					
	107/52	5.3/2.6	18.5/9	1.2/0.6	1.2/0.6
Pea & Ham, Baxters*, 1 can/425g					
	247/58	12.3/2.9	34.4/8.1	6.8/1.6	5.1/1.2
Pea & Ham, Fresh, Sainsbury's*, ½ bottle/302ml					
	136/45	7.9/2.6	14.8/4.9	5.1/1.7	3.3/1.1
Pea & Ham, Marks & Spencer*, 1oz/28g					
	17/62	1.1/4	2.6/9.2	0.3/1	0.3/1.2
Pea & Ham, Thick, Heinz*, 1 can/400g					
	204/51	12.8/3.2	34.8/8.7	1.6/0.4	4/1
Pea, in a Cup, Symingtons*, 1 sachet/30.5g					
	97/311	2.2/7.2	16.8/54.1	2.2/7.2	2.1/6.9
Plum Tomato & Crème Fraîche, New Covent Garden Soup Co*, ½ carton/300g					
	141/47	3/1	10.8/3.6	9.6/3.2	2.7/0.9
Potato & Leek, 1oz/28g					
	15/52	0.4/1.5	1.7/6.2	0.7/2.6	0.2/0.8
Potato & Leek, Baxters*, 1 can/425g					
	170/40	4.3/1	26.8/6.3	5.1/1.2	2.1/0.5
Potato & Leek, Thick, Heinz*, 1 can/400g					
	136/34	2.8/0.7	26/6.5	2.4/0.6	2/0.5
Potato, Leek & Chicken, BGTY, Sainsbury's*, 1 can/400g					
	152/38	8.4/2.1	21.6/5.4	3.6/0.9	2/0.5
Pumpkin, New Covent Garden Soup Co*, ½ pint/296ml					
	95/32	3.3/1.1	14.2/4.8	2.7/0.9	3/1
Pumpkin, Pepper & Paprika, New Covent Garden Soup Co*, 1 pack/600g					
	108/18	3.6/0.6	15/2.5	4.2/0.7	2.4/0.4
Red Pepper & Tomato, Perfectly Balanced, Waitrose*, 1 can/415g					
	154/37	3.3/0.8	18.7/4.5	7.5/1.8	3.7/0.9
Red Pepper & Tomato, Vie Country, Knorr*, 1 pack/500ml					
	195/39	4/0.8	32/6.4	6/1.2	5/1
Red Pepper, Tomato & Basil, Marks & Spencer*, 1 can/415g					
	83/20	5.4/1.3	11.2/2.7	1.2/0.3	3.3/0.8
Roast Pumpkin, EAT*, 1 can/400ml					
	260/65	4.4/1.1	23.6/5.9	16.8/4.2	3.2/0.8
Roasted Parsnip, Chunky Carrot & Sweet Potato, Baxters*, ½ pot/300g					
	186/62	2.7/0.9	25.5/8.5	8.1/2.7	4.2/1.4

	kcal serv/100g	prot serv/100g	carb serv/100g	fat serv/100g	fibre serv/100g
Roasted Red Pepper, Fresh, Waitrose*, 1 pack/600g					
	172/29	4.6/0.8	18/3	9/1.5	5.8/1
Roasted Vegetable, Fresh, Sainsbury's*, ½ pot/273ml					
	71/26	1.4/0.5	13.1/4.8	1.4/0.5	3.3/1.2
Scotch Broth, Baxters*, 1 can/425g					
	200/47	8.1/1.9	30.2/7.1	5.1/1.2	3.8/0.9
Scotch Broth, Tesco*, 1 can/400g					
	152/38	6/1.5	26.8/6.7	2.4/0.6	3.2/0.8
Scotch Broth, Thick, Heinz*, ½ can/200g					
	94/47	4.2/2.1	16.2/8.1	1.4/0.7	1.8/0.9
Smoked Haddock Chowder, New Covent Garden Soup Co*, ½ pint/284ml					
	142/50	6.2/2.2	23/8.1	2.8/1	1.4/0.5
Smoked Haddock Chowder, Sainsbury's*, 1 serving/100ml					
	203/203	3.6/3.6	15.3/15.3	14.1/14.1	0.3/0.3
Spiced Cauliflower, Pea & Imperial Rice, New Covent Garden Soup Co*, 1 serving/100ml					
	55/55	1.3/1.3	3.3/3.3	4.1/4.1	0.6/0.6
Spicy Corn Chowder, New Covent Garden Soup Co*, ½ pint/284ml					
	133/47	4/1.4	16.8/5.9	5.7/2	2.6/0.9
Spicy Lentil & Tomato, Soup-a-Slim, Asda*, 1 serving/17g					
	56/327	2/12	10.7/63	0.5/3	0.8/4.6
Spicy Lentil & Vegetable, Chilled, Marks & Spencer*, ½ serving/600g					
	300/50	16.2/2.7	48/8	4.8/0.8	6.6/1.1
Spicy Lentil, Seeds Of Change*, 1 pack/500g					
	345/69	14/2.8	47/9.4	11/2.2	4/0.8
Spicy Parsnip, Baxters*, 1 can/425g					
	217/51	4.7/1.1	25.9/6.1	10.6/2.5	6.4/1.5
Spicy Parsnip, BGTY, Sainsbury's*, 1 pack/400g					
	180/45	8.8/2.2	28.4/7.1	3.6/0.9	4/1
Spicy Parsnip, Fresh, Tesco*, 1 serving/300g					
	102/34	1.8/0.6	13.5/4.5	4.8/1.6	4.8/1.6
Spicy Parsnip, Perfectly Balanced, Waitrose*, 1 can/415g					
	125/30	4.2/1	19.9/4.8	2.9/0.7	4.6/1.1
Spicy Pumpkin, Sainsbury's*, ½ bottle/300ml					
	96/32	1.2/0.4	11.4/3.8	5.1/1.7	1.8/0.6
Spicy Red Lentil & Tomato, Marks & Spencer*, ½ pack/300g					
	150/50	8.1/2.7	24/8	2.4/0.8	3.3/1.1

	kcal serv/100g	prot serv/100g	carb serv/100g	fat serv/100g	fibre serv/100g
Spicy Thai Chicken, Baxters*, 1 can/415g					
	278/67	7.5/1.8	29.5/7.1	14.5/3.5	1.2/0.3
Spicy Tomato & Lentil, Asda*, 1 can/410g					
	156/38	4.1/1	24.6/6	4.5/1.1	1.6/0.4
Spicy Tomato & Lentil, BGTY, Sainsbury's*, 1 can/400g					
	240/60	12.8/3.2	41.6/10.4	2.8/0.7	0.4/0.1
Spicy Tomato & Lentil, Tesco*, 1 can/400g					
	180/45	8.4/2.1	34.8/8.7	0.8/0.2	3.2/0.8
Spicy Tomato & Rice with Sweetcorn, Baxters*, ½ can/207g					
	93/45	2.7/1.3	19/9.2	0.6/0.3	1.2/0.6
Spinach & Watercress, New Covent Garden Soup Co*, ½ carton/298g					
	60/20	3.9/1.3	8.3/2.8	1.2/0.4	2.4/0.8
Spring Vegetable, Heinz*, 1 can/400g					
	124/31	3.2/0.8	24.8/6.2	1.6/0.4	2.8/0.7
Sun-Dried Tomato & Basil, Heinz*, 1 serving/275ml					
	124/45	1.7/0.6	17.9/6.5	5.2/1.9	0.3/0.1
Super Chicken Noodle, Knorr*, 1 pack/56g					
	182/325	8/14.3	31.4/56	2.7/4.9	1/1.8
Sweet Cherry Tomato, TTD, Sainsbury's*, 1 pack/300g					
	120/40	2.1/0.7	18/6	4.5/1.5	3/1
Sweetcorn Chowder, New Covent Garden Soup Co*, ½ carton/250ml					
	118/47	3.5/1.4	14.8/5.9	5/2	2.3/0.9
Tangy Tomato, Slim A Soup, Batchelors*, 1 serving/230ml					
	81/35	2.5/1.1	15.4/6.7	1/0.4	1.1/0.5
Thai Chicken Fusion, New Covent Garden Soup Co.*, 111g					
	59/54	2.9/2.6	5.3/4.8	3/2.7	0.4/0.4
Thai Chicken, GFY, Asda*, 1 serving/200g					
	85/43	3.4/1.7	11/5.5	3/1.5	1/0.5
Three Bean, Organic, Seeds of Change*, 1 pack/500g					
	285/57	8.5/1.7	49.5/9.9	6/1.2	5.5/1.1
Tomato & Basil, Chilled, Marks & Spencer*, 1 serving/300g					
	105/35	2.7/0.9	18.6/6.2	2.1/0.7	2.1/0.7
Tomato & Basil, Delicious, Tesco*, 1 serving/300ml					
	150/50	3/1	22.2/7.4	5.7/1.9	2.1/0.7
Tomato & Basil, Finest, Tesco*, ½ pot/300g					
	204/68	3/1	12.3/4.1	15.6/5.2	1.8/0.6
Tomato & Basil, Fresh, Improved, Sainsbury's*, ½ bottle/300ml					
	105/35	4.2/1.4	12.3/4.1	4.2/1.4	1.8/0.6

	kcal serv/100g	prot serv/100g	carb serv/100g	fat serv/100g	fibre serv/100g

Tomato & Basil, Fresh, Sainsbury's*, 1 pack/300ml

| | 78/26 | 2.4/0.8 | 12/4 | 2.1/0.7 | 2.1/0.7 |

Tomato & Basil, Fresh, Tesco*, 1 pack/300g

| | 129/43 | 3/1 | 17.1/5.7 | 5.4/1.8 | 2.1/0.7 |

Tomato & Basil, GFY, Asda*, 1 serving/250ml

| | 103/41 | 3.5/1.4 | 9.8/3.9 | 5.5/2.2 | 1/0.4 |

Tomato & Basil, New Covent Garden Soup Co*, 1 pack/568g

| | 187/33 | 10.2/1.8 | 32.4/5.7 | 2.3/0.4 | 2.8/0.5 |

Tomato & Basil, Soup-a-Slim, Asda*, 1 sachet/16g

| | 52/326 | 1.1/7 | 11.2/70 | 0.3/2 | 0.6/3.9 |

Tomato & Basil, Vie Country, Knorr*, 1 pack/500ml

| | 145/29 | 4/0.8 | 27.5/5.5 | 2/0.4 | 4.5/0.9 |

Tomato & Basil, Waitrose*, 1 serving/300ml

| | 123/41 | 1.8/0.6 | 13.5/4.5 | 6.9/2.3 | 1.8/0.6 |

Tomato & Brown Lentil, Baxters*, 1 can/425g

| | 166/39 | 10.2/2.4 | 37/8.7 | 0.4/0.1 | 6.4/1.5 |

Tomato & Butterbean, Baxters*, 1 can/425g

| | 234/55 | 8.5/2 | 37.4/8.8 | 5.5/1.3 | 7.7/1.8 |

Tomato & Lentil, Heinz*, 1 can/400g

| | 216/54 | 10.8/2.7 | 41.6/10.4 | 0.8/0.2 | 4/1 |

Tomato & Lentil, Marks & Spencer*, ½ can/211.1g

| | 95/45 | 4.9/2.3 | 17.7/8.4 | 0.4/0.2 | 3.2/1.5 |

Tomato & Orange, Baxters*, 1 can/425g

| | 183/43 | 4.7/1.1 | 35.7/8.4 | 2.1/0.5 | 2.1/0.5 |

Tomato & Red Pepper, Weight Watchers*, 1 serving/205g

| | 25/12 | 0.8/0.4 | 5.1/2.5 | 0.2/0.1 | 0.8/0.4 |

Tomato & Three Bean, BGTY, Sainsbury's*, 1 can/400g

| | 216/54 | 11.6/2.9 | 34/8.5 | 3.6/0.9 | 3.2/0.8 |

Tomato, 99% Fat-Free, Campbell's*, 1 can/200g

| | 88/44 | 1.4/0.7 | 16/8 | 2/1 | 0/0 |

Tomato, Aubergine & Grilled Pepper, New Covent Garden Soup Co*, ½ carton/300g

| | 48/16 | 1.8/0.6 | 5.7/1.9 | 2.1/0.7 | 2.1/0.7 |

Tomato, Cup a Soup, Batchelors*, 1 serving/212g

| | 85/40 | 0.8/0.4 | 17.2/8.1 | 1.5/0.7 | 1.3/0.6 |

Tomato, Fresh Country, New Covent Garden Soup Co*, ½ pint/284ml

| | 114/40 | 5.4/1.9 | 18.2/6.4 | 2.3/0.8 | 2.3/0.8 |

kcal serv/100g	prot serv/100g	carb serv/100g	fat serv/100g	fibre serv/100g
Tomato, in a Cup, Tesco*, 1 serving/23g				
75/328	1.5/6.4	15.8/68.5	0.7/3.2	0/0.1
Tomato, Mixed Bean & Vegetable, Chunky, Sainsbury's*, 1 can/400g				
232/58	8.8/2.2	46/11.5	1.2/0.3	6.4/1.6
Tomato, Mixed Bean & Vegetable, Tesco, 1oz/28g				
18/64	0.7/2.4	2.7/9.8	0.1/0.3	0.4/1.6
Tomato, Onion & Basil, GFY, Asda*, 1 can/400g				
116/29	3.2/0.8	20/5	2.4/0.6	1.2/0.3
Tomato, Weight Watchers*, 1 can/295g				
74/25	2.1/0.7	13.6/4.6	1.5/0.5	0.9/0.3
Tuscan Bean, GFY, Asda*, 1 carton/400ml				
224/56	11.6/2.9	36/9	3.6/0.9	3.2/0.8
Tuscan Bean, New Covent Garden Soup Co*, ½ carton/300g				
171/57	11.7/3.9	26.4/8.8	2.1/0.7	7.2/2.4
Tuscan Bean, Organic, Sainsbury's*, 1 pack/400g				
148/37	8.8/2.2	20.8/5.2	3.2/0.8	5.2/1.3
Tuscan Bean, Perfectly Balanced, Waitrose*, ½ pot/300g				
147/49	6/2	18.3/6.1	5.4/1.8	5.4/1.8
Vegetable & Beef, Sainsbury's*, 1 can/400g				
260/65	8.4/2.1	34/8.5	10/2.5	5.2/1.3
Vegetable & Lentil, Fresh, Somerfield*, ½ pack/300g				
183/61	8.1/2.7	25.2/8.4	5.7/1.9	4.5/1.5
Vegetable Broth, Healthy Eating, Tesco*, 1 can/400g				
148/37	4.8/1.2	29.6/7.4	0.8/0.2	4/1
Vegetable Broth, Marks & Spencer*, 1 pack/213g				
85/40	2.1/1	13.4/6.3	3/1.4	1.7/0.8
Vegetable Chowder, New Covent Garden Soup Co*, ½ carton/300g				
159/53	8.7/2.9	19.8/6.6	5.1/1.7	3.3/1.1
Vegetable, Chunky, Simply Organic*, 1 pot/500g				
200/40	8/1.6	26.5/5.3	7/1.4	7/1.4
Vegetable, Extra Thick, Sainsbury's*, 1 can/400g				
176/44	6.4/1.6	32/8	2.4/0.6	5.2/1.3
Vegetable, Fresh, Co-Op*, 1 pack/600g				
150/25	3.6/0.6	24/4	6/1	6/1
Vegetable, Heinz*, 1 can/400g				
188/47	5.6/1.4	33.6/8.4	3.6/0.9	4.4/1.1
Vegetable, in a Cup, BGTY, Sainsbury's*, 1 sachet/200g				
52/26	1/0.5	8.8/4.4	1.6/0.8	1.8/0.9

kcal serv/100g	prot serv/100g	carb serv/100g	fat serv/100g	fibre serv/100g

Vegetable, In a Mug, Healthy Eating, Tesco*, 1 mug/18g

| 66/365 | 1.3/7 | 11.9/66.3 | 1.4/8 | 0.5/2.6 |

Vegetable, New Covent Garden Soup Co*, ½ pint/284ml

| 88/31 | 3.1/1.1 | 16.8/5.9 | 1.1/0.4 | 3.1/1.1 |

Vegetable, Tesco*, ½ can/200g

| 88/44 | 2.6/1.3 | 18.6/9.3 | 0.4/0.2 | 2/1 |

Vegetable, Weight Watchers*, 1 serving/295ml

| 83/28 | 2.7/0.9 | 16.5/5.6 | 0.6/0.2 | 2.4/0.8 |

Winter Vegetable & Lentil, New Covent Garden Soup Co*, 1 serving/300g

| 243/81 | 15.3/5.1 | 36/12 | 4.2/1.4 | 7.8/2.6 |

Winter Warmer, New Covent Garden Soup Co*, 1 serving/300g

| 180/60 | 7.5/2.5 | 31.5/10.5 | 2.7/0.9 | 6.9/2.3 |

Won Ton, Blue Dragon*, 1 can/410g

| 62/15 | 5.7/1.4 | 8.6/2.1 | 0.4/0.1 | 0/0 |

SPREADS

Butter, Half-Fat, Anchor*, thin spread/7g

| 25/363 | 0/0.1 | 0.1/0.8 | 2.8/40 | 0.1/0.8 |

Butter, Half-Fat, Marks & Spencer*, thin spread/7g

| 26/370 | 0.1/1.8 | 0.1/2 | 2.8/39.5 | 0/0.5 |

Butter, Half-Fat, Tesco*, thin spread/7g

| 25/361 | 0.1/2.1 | 0/0.4 | 2.7/39 | 0/0.6 |

Butter, I Can't Believe It's Not Butter*, thin spread/7g

| 44/625 | 0/0.4 | 0/0.7 | 4.8/69 | 0/0 |

Cheese Spread, Cheese & Garlic, Primula*, 1 serving/20g

| 49/247 | 3.1/15.7 | 0.9/4.3 | 3.7/18.6 | 0/0 |

Cheese Spread, Cheese & Salmon with Dill, Primula*, ⅓oz/10g

| 26/261 | 1.8/17.6 | 0.4/3.8 | 2/19.5 | 0/0 |

Cheese Spread, Cheez Whiz, Original, Light, 41% Less Fat, Kraft*, 2 tbsp/30g

| 63/210 | 4.7/15.7 | 3.5/11.7 | 3.4/11.3 | 0/0 |

Cheese Spread, Chunky Triangles, BGTY, Sainsbury's*, 1 triangle/25g

| 43/171 | 3.7/14.8 | 2.5/10 | 2/8 | 0/0 |

Cheese Spread, Chunky, Triangles, Kerrygold*, 2 triangles/47g

| 119/254 | 4.3/9.1 | 4.5/9.5 | 9.4/20 | 0/0 |

	kcal serv/100g	prot serv/100g	carb serv/100g	fat serv/100g	fibre serv/100g
Cheese Spread, Dairylea Light, Half-Fat, Kraft*, 1 serving/25g					
	40/161	3/12	2.1/8.2	2.2/8.7	0/0
Cheese Spread, Dairylea, Kraft*, 1oz/28g					
	71/255	2.1/7.6	2.2/8	6/21.5	0/0
Cheese Spread, Garlic & Herbs, Light, Benecol*, 1 serving/20g					
	35/174	1.6/7.8	0.8/4.2	2.8/14	0.1/0.7
Cheese Spread, Garlic & Herbs, Light, Philadelphia, Kraft*, 1oz/28g					
	50/180	2/7.2	1/3.4	4.3/15.5	0.1/0.2
Cheese Spread, Healthy Eating, Tesco*, ¼ pot/25g					
	47/187	5/20	1.6/6.5	2.3/9	0/0
Cheese Spread, Kerrygold*, 1oz/28g					
	60/213	3.1/11	2.4/8.5	4.2/15	0/0
Cheese Spread, Light, Laughing Cow*, 1 triangle/18g					
	25/141	2.4/13.5	1.2/6.5	1.3/7	0/0
Cheese Spread, Light, Philadelphia, Kraft*, 1oz/28g					
	53/190	2.1/7.6	1/3.4	4.5/16	0.1/0.3
Cheese Spread, Light, Primula*, 1oz/28g					
	48/171	4.5/16	1.8/6.6	2.5/9	0/0
Cheese Spread, Low-Fat, Weight Watchers*, 1 serving/50g					
	56/112	9.1/18.1	1.7/3.4	1.5/2.9	0.6/1.2
Cheese Spread, Mediterranean Soft & Creamy, Extra Light, Asda*, 1 serving/32g					
	42/130	4.2/13	1.9/6	1.9/6	0/0
Cheese Spread, Philadelphia, Extra Light, Kraft*, 1oz/28g					
	28/101	3.1/11	0.8/3	1.4/5	0.2/0.6
Cheese Spread, Portions, GFY, Asda*, 1 triangle/22.4g					
	35/161	3.1/14	1.3/6	2/9	0/0
Cheese Spread, Triangles, Chunky, Dairylea, Kraft*, 1 triangle/14g					
	32/225	1.4/9.9	1/7.3	2.5/17.5	0/0
Cheese Spread, with Chives, Primula*, 1oz/28g					
	71/253	4.2/15	0.3/1	5.9/21	0/0
Cheese Spread, with Shrimp, Primula*, 1 tbsp/15g					
	38/253	2.3/15	0.2/1	3.2/21	0/0
Chocolate Spread, Cadbury's*, 1 tsp/12g					
	69/575	0.5/4.5	6.6/55	4.6/38	0/0
Chocolate Spread, Milk, Belgian, Sainsbury's*, 1 serving/10g					
	56/559	1.2/11.9	4.7/47.2	3.6/35.8	0.1/1.4

kcal serv/100g	prot serv/100g	carb serv/100g	fat serv/100g	fibre serv/100g

Chocolate Spread, Milk, SmartPrice, Asda*, 1 tbsp/16g

| 92/573 | 0.6/4 | 9/56 | 5.9/37 | 0.3/2 |

Chocolate Spread, Nutella, Ferrero*, 1 tsp/12g

| 64/533 | 0.8/6.5 | 6.8/57 | 3.7/31 | 0/0 |

Chocolate Spread, Value, Tesco*, 1 serving/20g

| 116/581 | 0.6/3 | 10.9/54.5 | 7.8/39 | 0.3/1.5 |

Paste, BBQ Bean, Princes*, 1 serving/33g

| 35/106 | 1.9/5.7 | 6.5/19.8 | 0.1/0.4 | 0/0 |

Paste, Beef, Asda*, 1 serving/37g

| 72/194 | 6.3/17 | 0/0.1 | 5.2/14 | 0/0 |

Paste, Beef, Princes*, 1 serving/18g

| 40/220 | 2.6/14.4 | 0.9/5.2 | 2.8/15.8 | 0/0 |

Paste, Beef, Sainsbury's*, 1 jar/75g

| 142/189 | 12/16 | 1.1/1.5 | 9.9/13.2 | 1.1/1.4 |

Paste, Chicken & Ham, Asda*, ½ jar/38g

| 82/217 | 5.3/14 | 0.8/2.1 | 6.5/17 | 0/0 |

Paste, Chicken & Stuffing, Asda*, ½ jar/35g

| 71/203 | 5.6/16 | 1.2/3.3 | 4.9/14 | 0/0 |

Paste, Chicken, Tesco*, 1 serving/12g

| 30/248 | 1.8/14.8 | 0.3/2.3 | 2.4/20 | 0/0.1 |

Paste, Crab, Classic, Shippam*, 1 jar/35g

| 48/138 | 4.9/14.1 | 2.1/6 | 2.2/6.4 | 0/0 |

Paste, Crab, Princes*, 1 pot/35g

| 36/104 | 4.7/13.4 | 1.7/4.8 | 1.2/3.5 | 0/0 |

Paste, Crab, Tesco*, 1 jar/75g

| 89/119 | 10.5/14 | 3.5/4.6 | 3.8/5 | 0.1/0.1 |

Paste, Salmon & Shrimp, Tesco*, 1 jar/75g

| 83/111 | 11.3/15.1 | 3.8/5 | 2.6/3.4 | 0.1/0.1 |

Paste, Salmon, Princes*, 1 serving/30g

| 59/195 | 4.1/13.5 | 2/6.5 | 3.8/12.8 | 0/0 |

Paste, Sardine & Tomato, Co-Op*, 1 serving/25g

| 34/135 | 4/16 | 0.8/3 | 1.5/6 | 0.5/2 |

Paste, Sardine & Tomato, Princes*, 1 jar/75g

| 110/146 | 11.6/15.4 | 3.8/5 | 5.4/7.2 | 0/0 |

Paste, Sardine & Tomato, Sainsbury's*, 1 mini pot/35g

| 60/170 | 5.9/16.9 | 0.4/1.2 | 3.8/10.8 | 0.5/1.3 |

Paste, Tuna & Mayonnaise, Princes*, 1 pot/75g

| 158/210 | 12.5/16.6 | 1/1.3 | 11.6/15.4 | 0/0 |

	kcal serv/100g	prot serv/100g	carb serv/100g	fat serv/100g	fibre serv/100g

Paste, Tuna & Mayonnaise, Sainsbury's*, 1 tbsp/17g

| 41/242 | 3.3/19.2 | 0.1/0.6 | 3.1/18.1 | 0.3/1.6 |

Paste, Tuna & Mayonnaise, Tesco*, 1 serving/15g

| 31/209 | 2.2/14.9 | 0.3/2.1 | 2.4/15.7 | 0/0.1 |

Paste, Vegetable, Sainsbury's*, 1 serving/17g

| 26/154 | 1.3/7.4 | 1/5.9 | 1.9/11.2 | 0.6/3.4 |

Pâté, Apricot, Asda*, 1 serving/50g

| 156/312 | 6/12 | 1.5/3 | 14/28 | 0/0 |

Pâté, Ardennes, BGTY, Sainsbury's*, 1 serving/50g

| 95/189 | 9.1/18.1 | 1.2/2.4 | 6/11.9 | 0.1/0.1 |

Pâté, Ardennes, Healthy Eating, Tesco*, 1 serving/50g

| 119/238 | 8.3/16.5 | 1.3/2.6 | 9/17.9 | 0.8/1.6 |

Pâté, Ardennes, Healthy Living, Tesco*, 1 serving/50g

| 116/231 | 7.3/14.6 | 3.9/7.7 | 7.9/15.8 | 0.8/1.5 |

Pâté, Ardennes, Reduced-Fat, Safeway*, 1 serving/50g

| 97/194 | 9.3/18.5 | 1.6/3.1 | 6/11.9 | 0.1/0.1 |

Pâté, Ardennes, Reduced-Fat, Waitrose*, ¼ pack/42g

| 94/224 | 6.5/15.4 | 1.1/2.6 | 7.1/16.9 | 0.2/0.5 |

Pâté, Ardennes, Safeway*, 1 serving/50g

| 166/331 | 6.4/12.8 | 3/6 | 14.2/28.4 | 0.4/0.8 |

Pâté, Ardennes, Sainsbury's*, 1 serving/20g

| 60/299 | 3.3/16.5 | 0.4/2.1 | 5/24.9 | 0/0.1 |

Pâté, Ardennes, Tesco*, 1 tbsp/15g

| 53/354 | 2/13.3 | 0.1/0.5 | 5/33.2 | 0.2/1.2 |

Pâté, Asparagus, Sainsbury's*, ½ pot/57g

| 88/153 | 2/3.4 | 3.1/5.4 | 7.5/13.1 | 0.6/1 |

Pâté, Breton Course Country With Apricots, Sainsbury's*, 1 serving/21g

| 60/285 | 2.8/13.5 | 1.5/7 | 4.7/22.5 | 0.1/0.5 |

Pâté, Brie & Cranberry, Marks & Spencer*, 1 serving/55g

| 160/290 | 4.1/7.5 | 10.4/18.9 | 11.3/20.5 | 0.3/0.5 |

Pâté, Brussels & Mushroom, 25% Less Fat, Asda*, 1 serving/40g

| 88/220 | 5.6/14 | 1.1/2.7 | 6.8/17 | 0/0 |

Pâté, Brussels, 25% Less Fat, Morrisons*, ¼ pack/42.5g

| 107/249 | 6.1/14.2 | 0.3/0.7 | 8.9/20.6 | 0/0 |

Pâté, Brussels, BGTY, Sainsbury's*, 1 serving/50g

| 137/273 | 6.3/12.6 | 3.1/6.2 | 11/22 | 0.1/0.1 |

Pâté, Brussels, Co-Op*, 1 serving/15g

| 51/340 | 1.7/11 | 0.6/4 | 4.7/31 | 0.3/2 |

kcal serv/100g	prot serv/100g	carb serv/100g	fat serv/100g	fibre serv/100g
Pâté, Brussels, Healthy Eating, Tesco*, 1 serving/28g				
66/235	4.6/16.4	0.6/2.3	5/17.8	0.5/1.9
Pâté, Brussels, Marks & Spencer*, 1 pot/170g				
519/305	22.6/13.3	4.8/2.8	45.2/26.6	1.7/1
Pâté, Brussels, Reduced Fat, Asda*, 1 serving/44g				
88/199	6.6/15	0.9/2.1	6.6/15	0.8/1.9
Pâté, Brussels, Sainsbury's*, 1 pack/170g				
663/390	18/10.6	1.9/1.1	64.9/38.2	0.2/0.1
Pâté, Brussels, Tesco*, 1 serving/28g				
92/330	3.1/11	0.8/3	8.5/30.5	0.3/1.1
Pâté, Carrot, Ginger & Spring Onion, Marks & Spencer*, 1 serving/50g				
73/145	0.8/1.5	4.8/9.6	5.5/11	0.5/0.9
Pâté, Celery, Stilton & Walnut, Waitrose*, 1 pot/115g				
294/256	10.4/9	3.7/3.2	26.5/23	2.5/2.2
Pâté, Chargrilled Vegetable, BGTY Sainsbury's*, ½ pot/57.3g				
43/75	2.8/4.9	6.2/10.8	0.7/1.3	1.5/2.7
Pâté, Chicken Liver & Brandy, Asda*, 1 serving/50g				
177/353	4.5/9	2.8/5.5	16.4/32.8	1.6/3.2
Pâté, Chicken Liver, Marks & Spencer*, 1oz/28g				
79/281	3.9/14	0.5/1.9	6.7/24.1	0/0.1
Pâté, Chicken Liver, Organic, Waitrose*, ½ tub/87.5g				
205/233	11.1/12.6	1.6/1.8	16.2/18.4	1.2/1.4
Pâté, Coarse Farmhouse, Organic, Sainsbury's*, 1 serving/56g				
138/246	7.4/13.3	2.1/3.7	11/19.7	0.4/0.8
Pâté, Coarse Pork Liver With Garlic, Asda*, 1 pack/40g				
130/326	5.2/13	0.4/1	12/30	0/0
Pâté, Country Style Coarse, Quorn*, ½ pot/65g				
68/104	6/9.2	4.7/7.3	2.7/4.2	1.8/2.7
Pâté, Crab, Marks & Spencer*, 1oz/28g				
63/225	3.4/12.1	1.7/5.9	4.8/17.3	0/0
Pâté, Crab, Waitrose*, 1oz/28g				
59/209	4.1/14.5	0.1/0.5	4.6/16.6	0/0
Pâté, Duck & Champagne, Luxury, Marks & Spencer*, 1oz/28g				
106/380	2.3/8.3	2.3/8.3	9.9/35.2	2.2/7.8
Pâté, Duck & Orange, Asda*, 1 serving/40g				
94/235	6.4/16	0.9/2.2	7.2/18	0/0
Pâté, Duck & Orange, Marks & Spencer*, 1oz/28g				
88/315	3/10.6	0.8/2.8	8.1/29	0.1/0.5

kcal serv/100g	prot serv/100g	carb serv/100g	fat serv/100g	fibre serv/100g
Pâté, Duck Liver With Champagne & Truffles, TTD, Sainsbury's*, **1 serving/50g**				
212/423	4.1/8.2	1.3/2.5	21.1/42.2	0/0
Pâté, Farmhouse Mushroom, Asda*, 1 serving/50g				
126/252	6.5/13	2.5/5	10/20	0.4/0.7
Pâté, Farmhouse-Style, Finest, Tesco*, 1 serving/28g				
83/295	3.3/11.9	1/3.6	7.3/25.9	0.3/1
Pâté, Farmhouse-Style, Marks & Spencer*, ¼ pack/42g				
90/215	6/14.4	0.8/1.9	7.1/16.9	0.5/1.2
Pâté, Farmhouse with Mushrooms & Garlic, Tesco*, 1 serving/90g				
257/285	12.4/13.8	0.5/0.6	22.8/25.3	1.2/1.3
Pâté, Herb, Organic, Suma*, 1 serving/25g				
59/234	3/12	1.5/6	4.5/18	0/0
Pâté, Isle of Skye Smoked Salmon, TTD, Sainsbury's*, ½ pot/58g				
161/277	9.6/16.5	0.5/0.8	13.4/23.1	0.1/0.1
Pâté, Liver & Pork, Healthy Eating, Tesco*, 1 serving/28g				
64/229	4/14.4	2.4/8.4	4.3/15.3	0.4/1.3
Pâté, Liver Spreading, Somerfield*, 1oz/28g				
77/275	3.9/14	0.8/3	6.4/23	0/0
Pâté, Liver, Value, Tesco*, 1 serving/50g				
151/302	6.5/13	2.1/4.1	13/26	0.3/0.5
Pâté, Mackerel, Smoked, 1oz/28g				
103/368	3.8/13.4	0.4/1.3	9.6/34.4	0/0
Pâté, Mackerel, Tesco*, 1 serving/29g				
102/353	4.1/14.3	0.1/0.5	9.5/32.6	0/0
Pâté, Mediterranean Roast Vegetable, Tesco*, 1 serving/28g				
31/112	0.7/2.4	1.2/4.3	2.6/9.4	0.3/1.2
Pâté, Mexican Red Pepper & Wild Chilli Organic Yeast, Tartex*, 1 pot/50g				
99/198	3.2/6.4	3.5/7	8/16	0/0
Pâté, Mushroom, BGTY, Sainsbury's*, ½ pot/58g				
29/50	2.7/4.6	3.9/6.7	0.3/0.5	1.7/3
Pâté, Mushroom, COU, Marks & Spencer*, 1oz/28g				
17/60	0.8/2.9	2.1/7.4	0.5/1.9	0.3/0.9
Pâté, Mushroom, Marks & Spencer*, 1 pot/115g				
224/195	4.8/4.2	5.5/4.8	20.1/17.5	1.5/1.3
Pâté, Mushroom, Sainsbury's*, 1oz/28g				
47/168	0.9/3.1	1.7/5.9	4.3/15.2	0.4/1.3

kcal serv/100g	prot serv/100g	carb serv/100g	fat serv/100g	fibre serv/100g
Pâté, Mushroom, Tesco*, 1oz/28g				
42/151	0.9/3.2	2.5/9.1	3.2/11.3	0.3/0.9
Pâté, Poached Salmon & Watercress, Tesco*, 1 serving/25g				
60/238	4.8/19.2	0.1/0.4	4.4/17.7	0.1/0.2
Pâté, Pork & Garlic, Somerfield*, 1oz/28g				
83/295	3.9/14	0.8/3	7/25	0/0
Pâté, Pork & Mushroom, Somerfield*, 1oz/28g				
95/339	3.1/11	0.8/3	8.7/31	0/0
Pâté, Pork with Port & Cranberry, Tesco*, 1 serving/28g				
83/296	3.4/12.1	1.2/4.3	7.2/25.6	0.2/0.6
Pâté, Pork, with Peppercorns, Tesco*, 1 serving/28g				
84/300	3.6/12.9	0.4/1.4	7.5/26.8	0.2/0.7
Pâté, Ricotta, Sun-dried Tomato & Basil, Princes*, 1 jar/110g				
343/312	5.7/5.2	9.1/8.3	31.6/28.7	0/0
Pâté, Salmon, Organic, Marks & Spencer*, 1oz/28g				
76/270	4.7/16.9	0/0	6.3/22.5	0/0
Pâté, Salmon, Smoked, Marks & Spencer*, 1oz/28g				
74/265	4.7/16.9	0/0	6.2/22	0/0
Pâté, Smoked Mackerel, Marks & Spencer*, 1oz/28g				
104/370	3.8/13.4	0.2/0.7	9.7/34.7	0.1/0.3
Pâté, Smoked Mackerel, Sainsbury's*, ½ pot/57g				
201/352	8.7/15.2	1.1/1.9	18/31.5	0.2/0.3
Pâté, Smoked Salmon, Healthy Eating, Tesco*, 1 serving/50g				
65/130	8.8/17.5	1.3/2.6	2.8/5.5	0/0
Pâté, Smoked Salmon, Organic, Waitrose*, 1oz/28g				
83/296	3.9/13.9	0.7/2.4	7.2/25.6	0/0
Pâté, Smoked Salmon, Waitrose*, ½ pot/56g				
122/217	9.9/17.7	0.8/1.5	8.7/15.6	0.3/0.6
Pâté, Spiced Parsnip & Carrot, Organic, Asda*, ½ pot/58g				
63/109	2.1/3.7	5.8/10	3.5/6	1.5/2.6
Pâté, Spicy Bean, Princes*, ½ pot/55g				
46/84	2/3.6	9.2/16.7	0.2/0.3	0/0
Pâté, Tuna With Butter & Lemon Juice, Sainsbury's*, ½ pot/58g				
209/360	11/19	0.1/0.1	18.3/31.6	0.2/0.3
Pâté, Tuna, Marks & Spencer*, 1oz/28g				
99/355	5/18	0/0	8.8/31.3	0/0
Pâté, Tuna, Tesco*, 1 pack/115g				
332/289	22.8/19.8	0.3/0.3	26.7/23.2	0.2/0.2

	kcal serv/100g	prot serv/100g	carb serv/100g	fat serv/100g	fibre serv/100g

Sandwich Filler, Chicken & Bacon With Sweetcorn, Sainsbury's*,
1 serving/60g

187/312	7.9/13.2	1.6/2.6	16.6/27.6	0.7/1.1

Sandwich Filler, Chicken Tikka & Citrus Raita, COU, Marks & Spencer*,
½ pot/85g

77/90	10.7/12.6	4.2/4.9	1.7/2	0.8/0.9

Sandwich Filler, Chicken Tikka, BGTY, Sainsbury's*, ½ pot/85g

99/117	14/16.5	5.1/6	2.6/3	0.9/1

Sandwich Filler, Chicken Tikka, Mild, Heinz*, 1 serving/52g

102/196	2.7/5.2	6.4/12.3	7.3/14	0.4/0.7

Sandwich Filler, Chicken with Salad Vegetables, Heinz*, 1 filling/56g

114/203	2.9/5.1	6.6/11.7	8.5/15.1	0.3/0.5

Sandwich Filler, Chicken, Stuffing & Bacon, COU, Marks & Spencer*,
1 pack/170g

170/100	22.3/13.1	10.5/6.2	3.7/2.2	2.2/1.3

Sandwich Filler, Chicken, Sweetcorn & Sage, Healthy Eating, Tesco*,
1 serving/125g

105/84	11.8/9.4	11/8.8	1.6/1.3	1.6/1.3

Sandwich Filler, Chicken, Tomato & Sweetcure Bacon, Marks & Spencer*,
1 pot/170g

502/295	19.4/11.4	4.8/2.8	44.9/26.4	1.2/0.7

Sandwich Filler, Coronation Chicken, Somerfield*, 1 serving/85g

326/383	7.1/8.4	8.2/9.7	29.3/34.5	0.7/0.8

Sandwich Filler, Coronation Chicken, Tesco*, 1 tbsp/30g

84/279	4.4/14.7	1.8/6.1	6.5/21.8	0.2/0.7

Sandwich Filler, Egg Mayonnaise, BGTY, Sainsbury's*, 1 serving/85g

102/120	9.3/10.9	0.8/0.9	6/7.1	1/1.2

Sandwich Filler, Egg Mayonnaise, Chunky Free Range, Tesco*,
1 serving/50g

104/208	6.2/12.3	0.1/0.2	8.8/17.6	0.2/0.3

Sandwich Filler, Egg Mayonnaise, Deli, Somerfield*, 1 serving/40g

120/301	3.9/9.7	0.1/0.2	11.7/29.2	0/0

Sandwich Filler, Egg Mayonnaise, Sainsbury's*, 1 serving/50g

138/275	5.1/10.1	0.6/1.1	12.8/25.6	0.3/0.5

Sandwich Filler, Egg Mayonnaise, Tesco*, 1 serving/50g

122/243	5.3/10.5	1.3/2.5	10.6/21.2	0.4/0.8

Sandwich Filler, Ham & Salad Vegetables, Heinz*, 1oz/28g

57/204	1.5/5.3	2.8/10	4.5/15.9	0.1/0.4

kcal serv/100g	prot serv/100g	carb serv/100g	fat serv/100g	fibre serv/100g

Sandwich Filler, Prawn Mayonnaise, GFY, Asda*, 1 serving/57g

| 101/177 | 6.8/12 | 1.7/3 | 7.4/13 | 0.1/0.1 |

Sandwich Filler, Prawn Mayonnaise, Marks & Spencer*, 1oz/28g

| 91/325 | 2.4/8.7 | 0.2/0.7 | 8.9/31.7 | 0.2/0.8 |

Sandwich Filler, Prawn Mayonnaise, Waitrose*, 1 pot/170g

| 537/316 | 15.1/8.9 | 0.3/0.2 | 52.9/31.1 | 0/0 |

Sandwich Filler, Seafood Cocktail, Marks & Spencer*, 1oz/28g

| 76/272 | 1.8/6.4 | 2.3/8.2 | 6.7/23.8 | 0.1/0.2 |

Sandwich Filler, Tuna & Sweetcorn with Salad Vegetables, Heinz*, 1oz/28g

| 53/191 | 1.6/5.8 | 3.4/12.1 | 3.7/13.2 | 0.2/0.7 |

Sandwich Filler, Tuna & Sweetcorn, COU, Marks & Spencer*, ½ pot/85g

| 77/90 | 9.9/11.6 | 4.8/5.7 | 1.7/2 | 1.1/1.3 |

Sandwich Filler, Tuna & Sweetcorn, Marks & Spencer*, 1oz/28g

| 70/250 | 4/14.2 | 0.6/2.3 | 5.8/20.7 | 0.4/1.3 |

Sandwich Spread, Chicken & Bacon, Asda*, 1 jar/170g

| 610/359 | 30.6/18 | 3.4/2 | 52.7/31 | 1.7/1 |

Sandwich Spread, Chicken Tikka, Asda*, 1 serving/50g

| 77/154 | 3.5/7 | 4.5/9 | 5/10 | 0.1/0.2 |

Sandwich Spread, Cucumber, Heinz*, 1oz/28g

| 46/164 | 0.5/1.7 | 3.6/12.7 | 3.2/11.6 | 0.2/0.6 |

Sandwich Spread, Original, Heinz*, 1oz/28g

| 66/237 | 0.5/1.7 | 4.3/15.2 | 5.2/18.6 | 0.2/0.7 |

Sandwich Spread, Somerfield*, 1oz/28g

| 59/212 | 0.3/1 | 7.3/26 | 3.1/11 | 0/0 |

Spread, 63% Fat, Benecol*, 1 serving/12g

| 69/573 | 0.1/0.6 | 0.1/1 | 7.6/63 | 0/0 |

Spread, Butter & Olive, Olivio*, thin spread/7g

| 38/536 | 0/0.5 | 0/0.7 | 4.1/59 | 0/0 |

Spread, Butterlicious, Sainsbury's*, thin spread/7g

| 44/628 | 0/0.6 | 0.1/1.1 | 4.8/69 | 0/0.1 |

Spread, Buttery Gold, Somerfield*, 1 tbsp/15g

| 94/627 | 0.1/0.5 | 0.2/1 | 10.4/69 | 0/0 |

Spread, Buttery Taste, Benecol*, 1 tsp/7g

| 40/573 | 0/0.6 | 0.1/1 | 4.4/63 | 0/0 |

Spread, Chocolate Hazelnut, Tesco*, 1 tsp/10g

| 54/542 | 0.7/7 | 5.1/50.8 | 3.5/34.5 | 0.4/3.7 |

Spread, Diet, Delight*, 1oz/28g

| 64/228 | 1/3.6 | 0.4/1.6 | 6.4/23 | 0/0 |

	kcal serv/100g	prot serv/100g	carb serv/100g	fat serv/100g	fibre serv/100g
Spread, Fat, Carapelli, St Ivel*, thin spread/7g					
	38/537	0/0.6	0.1/0.8	4.1/59	0/0
Spread, Flora Buttery, Flora*, thin spread/7g					
	45/637	0.1/1.1	0/0.5	4.9/70	0/0
Spread, Flora Diet Light, Flora*, 1 tbsp/10g					
	23/227	0.4/3.5	0.2/1.6	2.3/23	0/0
Spread, Flora Light, Flora*, 1oz/28g					
	100/357	0/0.1	1/3.7	10.6/38	0.2/0.6
Spread, Flora Original, Flora*, 1 serving/10g					
	63/630	0/0.1	0/0.1	7/70	0/0
Spread, Flora Pro-Activ, Flora*, 1 serving/10g					
	33/328	0/0.1	0.3/3.2	3.5/35	0/0.3
Spread, Flora, Low Salt, Flora*, 1oz/28g					
	176/630	0/0.1	0/0.1	19.6/70	0/0
Spread, Gold, Low-Fat, St Ivel*, thin spread/7g					
	26/365	0.1/2.1	0.2/2.9	2.7/38	0/0
Spread, Gold, Lowest, Low-Fat, St Ivel*, thin spread/7g					
	18/259	0/0.7	0.2/3.3	1.9/27	0/0
Spread, Golden, Light, Healthy Eating, Tesco*, 1 serving/10g					
	35/354	0.2/1.5	0.2/1.5	3.8/38	0/0
Spread, Light, Benecol*, 2 tsp/12g					
	38/318	0.3/2.8	0/0.2	4.1/34	0/0
Spread, Light, Olivio*, thin spread/7g					
	34/486	0/0	0/0	3.9/55	0/0
Spread, Low-Fat 32%, Benecol*, 1 serving/12g					
	36/300	0.3/2.8	0/0.2	3.8/32	0/0
Spread, Olive Gold, With Olive Oil, Low-Fat, Asda*, 1 serving/10g					
	54/537	0/0.2	0.1/1.2	5.9/59	0/0
Spread, Olive Light, Low-Fat, BGTY, Sainsbury's*, thin spread/ 7g					
	25/356	0.1/2	0.1/1.5	2.7/38	0/0
Spread, Olive Light, Low-Fat, Tesco*, 1 serving/15g					
	52/348	0.2/1.5	0/0	5.7/38	0/0
Spread, Olive Light, Safeway*, 1 tsp/10g					
	35/346	0.1/1	0/0	3.8/38	0/0
Spread, Olive Oil, 55% Reduced-Fat, Benecol*, thin spread/7g					
	35/498	0/0.3	0/0.5	3.9/55	0/0
Spread, Olive Oil, 59% Reduced Fat, Safeway*, thin spread/7g					
	37/532	0/0.1	0/0.1	4.1/59	0/0

	kcal serv/100g	prot serv/100g	carb serv/100g	fat serv/100g	fibre serv/100g

Spread, Olive Oil, 59% Vegetable Fat, Olivio*, thin spread/7g

38/536	0/0.2	0.1/1	4.1/59	0/0

Spread, Olive, BGTY, Sainsbury's*, 1 tsp/14g

50/356	0.3/2	0.2/1.5	5.3/38	0/0

Spread, Olive, Reduced-Fat, Asda*, thin spread/7g

38/537	0/0.2	0.1/1.2	4.1/59	0/0

Spread, Olive, Reduced-Fat, Sainsbury's*, 1 serving/10g

54/536	0/0.1	0.1/1.2	5.9/59	0/0

Spread, Olive, Tesco*, 1 serving/28g

150/537	0.1/0.2	0.3/1.2	16.5/59	0/0

Spread, Olivite, Low-Fat, Weight Watchers*, thin spread/7g

25/351	0/0	0/0.2	2.7/38.9	0/0

Spread, Pure Gold, GFY, Asda*, 1 serving/10g

35/353	0.2/1.7	0.1/1	3.8/38	0/0

Spread, Pure Gold, Light, 65% Less Fat, Asda*, 1 serving/10g

24/239	0.3/2.5	0.1/1	2.5/25	0/0

Spread, Sunflower, Asda*, 1 serving/10g

64/635	0/0.2	0.1/1	7/70	0/0

Spread, Sunflower, Co-Op*, thin spread/7g

44/635	0/0.2	0.1/1	4.9/70	0/0

Spread, Sunflower, Light, 38% Less Fat, Asda*, thin spread/7g

24/342	0/0	0/0	2.7/38	0/0

Spread, Sunflower, Light, Better For You, Morrisons*, 1 tsp/5g

17/342	0/0	0/0	1.9/38	0/0

Spread, Sunflower, Light, BGTY, Sainsbury's*, 1 serving/10g

35/352	0.1/1	0.2/1.5	3.8/38	0/0

Spread, Sunflower, Light, GFY, Asda*, 1 serving/10g

35/351	0/0	0/0	3.9/39	0/0

Spread, Sunflower, Light, Healthy Eating, Tesco*, 1 serving/6g

21/347	0/0.3	0.1/1	2.3/38	0/0

Spread, Sunflower, Light, Summerlite, Aldi*, 1 serving/10g

34/344	0/0.2	0/0.3	3.8/38	0/0

Spread, Sunflower, Low-Fat, Good Intentions, Somerfield*, 1 serving/10g

35/347	0/0	0/0	3.9/38.6	0/0

Spread, Sunflower, Low-Fat, Marks & Spencer*, 1 serving/14g

48/342	0/0	0/0	5.3/38	0.1/1

Spread, Sunflower, Low-Fat, Somerfield*, 1 serving/10g

34/342	0/0	0/0	3.8/38	0/0

	kcal serv/100g	prot serv/100g	carb serv/100g	fat serv/100g	fibre serv/100g

Spread, Sunflower, Marks & Spencer*, thin spread/7g

	44/635	0/0.2	0.1/1	4.9/70	0/0

Spread, Sunflower, Reduced-Fat, Asda*, thin spread/7g

	37/531	0/0.2	0.1/1	4.1/58.5	0/0

Spread, Sunflower, Sainsbury's*, thin spread/7g

	44/631	0/0.2	0/0.1	4.9/70	0/0.1

Spread, Sunflower, Tesco*, 1 serving/15g

	95/631	0/0	0/0.2	10.5/70	0/0

Spread, Vitalite, Lite, St Ivel*, thin spread/7g

	24/348	0.1/1.5	0/0	2.7/38	0/0

Spread, Vitalite, St Ivel*, thin spread/7g

	40/578	0/0.4	0.1/1.2	4.4/63	0/0

Toast Toppers, Chicken & Mushroom, Heinz*, 1 serving/56g

	31/56	2.9/5.1	3.2/5.7	0.8/1.4	0.1/0.2

Toast Toppers, Mushroom & Bacon, Heinz*, 1 serving/56g

	53/94	3.9/6.9	3.7/6.6	2.5/4.4	0.2/0.3

Vegemite, Australian, Kraft*, 1 tsp/5g

	9/173	1.2/23.5	1/19.7	0/0	0/0

SWEETS AND CHOCOLATE

Aero, Creamy White Centre, Nestle, 1 bar/46g

	244/530	3.5/7.6	26.4/57.4	13.8/30	0/0

Aero, Honeycomb, Nestle*, 1 serving/40g

	199/497	2.4/5.9	24.9/62.2	10/25	0/0

Aero, Minis, Nestle*, 1 bar/11g

	57/518	0.8/7.6	6.3/57.2	3.2/28.8	0/0

Aero, Mint, Nestle*, 1 bar/48g

	252/526	3.1/6.5	28.9/60.2	13.8/28.8	0/0

Aero, Nestle*, 1 bar/46g

	238/518	3.5/7.6	26.3/57.2	13.2/28.8	0/0

Boost, Cadbury's*, 1 bar/55g

	297/540	3.2/5.9	34.3/62.3	16.1/29.3	0/0

Boost, Treat-Size, Cadbury's*, 1 bar/24.3g

	128/535	1.3/5.3	14.3/59.6	7.3/30.5	0/0

Boost, with Glucose & Guarana, Cadbury's*, 1 bar/61g

	323/530	3.5/5.8	36.8/60.3	18.1/29.6	0/0

kcal serv/100g	prot serv/100g	carb serv/100g	fat serv/100g	fibre serv/100g
Boost, with Glucose, Cadbury's*, 1 bar/61g				
326/535	3.2/5.3	36.4/59.6	18.6/30.5	0/0
Bounty, Calapuno, Mars*, 1 pack/175g				
919/525	11/6.3	95/54.3	55/31.4	0/0
Bounty, Dark, Mars*, 1 funsize/29g				
137/471	0.9/3.2	15.7/54.1	7.8/26.8	0/0
Bounty, Milk, Mars*, 1 funsize/29g				
137/471	1.1/3.7	16.4/56.4	7.4/25.6	0/0
Buttons, Cadbury's*, 1 treat pack/14g				
74/525	1.1/7.8	8/56.8	4.1/29.4	0/0
Buttons, White, Cadbury's*, 1 bag/32g				
171/535	2.8/8.8	18.1/56.5	9.7/30.3	0/0
Campino, Oranges & Cream, Bendicks*, 1oz/28g				
116/416	0/0.1	24/85.8	2.3/8.1	0/0
Campino, Strawberries & Cream, Bendicks*, 1oz/28g				
117/418	0/0.1	24.1/86.2	2.3/8.1	0/0
Caramac, Nestle*, 1 bar/30g				
163/563	1.7/5.8	15.8/54.4	10.4/35.8	0/0
Caramel, Cadbury's*, 1 bar/50g				
240/480	2.2/4.3	30.7/61.3	12.2/24.3	0/0
Caramel, Egg, Cadbury's*, 1 egg/39g				
191/490	1.7/4.3	23/58.9	10.2/26.1	0/0
Chewing Gum, Airwaves, Wrigleys*, 1 piece/1g				
2/150	0/0	0.6/62	0/0	0/0
Chewing Gum, Orbit, Spearmint, Wrigleys*, 1 piece/3g				
6/190	0/0	1.9/62	0/0	0/0
Chocolate Cream, Fry's*, 1 serving/50g				
215/430	1.3/2.6	34.3/68.6	7.7/15.4	0/0
Chocolate Eclairs, Cadbury's*, 1 sweet/8g				
39/485	0.4/4.6	6/75	1.5/18.8	0/0
Chocolate Orange, Milk, Mini Segments, Terry's*, 1 segment/8g				
42/527	0.6/7.7	4.6/57.9	2.4/29.4	0.2/2.1
Chocolate Orange, Milk, Terry's*, 1 orange/175g				
928/530	13.1/7.5	100.3/57.3	52.5/30	3.7/2.1
Chocolate Orange, Plain, Terry's*, 1 orange/175g				
889/508	6.7/3.8	99.4/56.8	51.5/29.4	10.9/6.2
Chocolate Orange, White, Terry's*, 1 segment/11.4g				
59/535	0.7/6.3	6.7/60.9	3.2/29.4	0/0

kcal serv/100g	prot serv/100g	carb serv/100g	fat serv/100g	fibre serv/100g
Chocolate, A Darker Shade of Milk, Green & Black's*, 1 serving/20g				
108/542	1.9/9.5	10.8/54	6.4/32	0/0
Chocolate, Animal Bar, Nestle*, 1 bar/19g				
97/513	1.1/5.8	12.1/63.6	5/26.1	0/0
Chocolate, Assortment, Diabetic, Thorntons*, 1oz/28g				
108/385	1.2/4.3	16/57	6.7/24	0.7/2.5
Chocolate, Belgian Dark, Extra Special, Asda*, 2 squares/20g				
102/508	2.2/11	5.2/26	8/40	3.2/16
Chocolate, Belgian Milk, TTD, Sainsbury's*, 2 squares/20g				
108/540	2/9.8	10.2/50.9	6.6/33	0.5/2.3
Chocolate, Belgian Plain with Ginger, TTD, Sainsbury's*, 2 squares/20g				
114/571	1.4/7.2	6.2/31.2	9.3/46.4	2.2/10.9
Chocolate, Belgian Seashells, Woolworths*, 1 box/63g				
347/550	3.5/5.5	33.3/52.9	19.6/31.1	0/0
Chocolate, Belgian White with Coffee, TTD, Sainsbury's*, 2 squares/20g				
110/548	1.3/6.5	11.4/56.9	6.5/32.7	0/0
Chocolate, Belgian White with Lemon, TTD, Sainsbury's*, 2 squares/20g				
109/546	1.1/5.7	12.2/61.2	6.2/30.9	0/0.1
Chocolate, Belgian, Finest, Tesco*, 1 chocolate/12g				
62/520	0.7/5.9	6.7/55.6	3.4/28.4	0.6/5.2
Chocolate, Big Purple One, Nestle*, 1 chocolate/38.7g				
191/489	2/5	23.5/60.2	9.9/25.4	0.2/0.6
Chocolate, Black Magic, Nestle*, 1oz/28g				
128/456	1.2/4.4	17.5/62.6	5.8/20.8	0.4/1.6
Chocolate, Bournville, Cadbury's*, 1 bar/50g				
248/495	2.3/4.6	29.8/59.6	13.4/26.7	0/0
Chocolate, Brandy Liqueurs, Asda*, 1 chocolate/8.3g				
33/409	0.3/4	4.8/60	1.4/17	0.1/0.8
Chocolate, Bubble bar, Marks & Spencer*, 1 bar/25g				
136/542	2.4/9.5	13/51.8	8.3/33.1	0.6/2.2
Chocolate, Cafe au Lait, Thorntons*, 1 chocolate/16g				
77/481	0.8/5.3	9.3/58.1	4/25	0.1/0.6
Chocolate, Cappuccino bar, Thorntons*, 1 bar/38g				
201/529	2/5.2	18.9/49.7	13.2/34.7	0.2/0.5
Chocolate, Chomp, Cadbury's*, 1 treat-size bar/12g				
56/465	0.4/3.5	8.1/67.9	2.4/19.8	0/0
Chocolate, Coconut, White, Excellence, Lindt*, 1 square/10g				
61/610	0.6/6	4.8/48	4.4/44	0/0

	kcal serv/100g	prot serv/100g	carb serv/100g	fat serv/100g	fibre serv/100g
Chocolate, Continental, Cappuccino, Thorntons*, 1 bar/38.0g					
	201/529	2/5.2	18.9/49.7	13.2/34.7	0/0.1
Chocolate, Creamy Vanilla White, Green & Black's*, 1 serving/20g					
	115/577	1.5/7.5	10.5/52.5	7.5/37.5	0/0
Chocolate, Dairy Milk, Bubbly, Cadbury's*, 1 bar/35.2g					
	184/525	2.7/7.6	19.7/56.4	10.4/29.7	0/0
Chocolate, Dairy Milk, Cadbury's*, 1 treat-size bar/15g					
	80/530	1.2/7.8	8.6/57.1	4.5/29.9	0/0
Chocolate, Dairy Milk, Caramel Centre, Cadbury's*, 1 square/10g					
	50/495	0.6/5.7	6.1/61.1	2.5/25.3	0/0
Chocolate, Dairy Milk, Mint Chips, Cadbury's*, 1 serving/50g					
	253/505	3.3/6.5	30.6/61.2	13.1/26.1	0/0
Chocolate, Dairy Milk, Snack-Size, Cadbury's*, 1 bar/30g					
	159/530	2.3/7.8	17.1/57.1	9/29.9	0/0
Chocolate, Dark, Bar, Thorntons*, 1 sm bar/48g					
	245/511	4.5/9.3	15.2/31.6	18.6/38.8	7.6/15.9
Chocolate, Dark, Orange with Slivered Almonds, Excellence, Lindt*, 1 square/10g					
	50/500	0.6/6	4.6/46	3/30	0/0
Chocolate, Dark, with 70% Cocoa Solids, Organic, Green & Black's*, 1 serving/20g					
	115/576	1.5/7.5	9.1/45.5	8.1/40.5	0/0
Chocolate, Dark, with a Soft Mint Centre, Green & Black's*, 4 squares/30g					
	136/452	1.4/4.8	16.8/56	7/23.2	0/0
Chocolate, Dark, with Cherries, Green & Black's*, 1 serving/75g					
	390/520	5.3/7	43/57.3	24.6/32.8	0/0
Chocolate, Dark, with Hazelnuts & Currants, Green & Black's*, 1 serving/60g					
	323/539	5/8.4	31/51.6	21.8/36.4	0/0
Chocolate, Excellence, 85% Cocoa Solids, Lindt*, 1 square/8.3g					
	44/530	0.9/11	2.7/32	3.8/46	0/0
Chocolate, Ferrero Rocher, Ferrero*, 1 chocolate/12.5g					
	74/593	0.9/7	6.1/49	5.1/41	0/0
Chocolate, Freddo, Dairy Milk, Cadbury's*, 1 frog/20g					
	106/530	1.6/7.8	11.4/57.1	6/29.9	0/0
Chocolate, Fruit & Nut, Cadbury's*, 1 bar/49g					
	240/490	3.9/8	27.3/55.7	12.9/26.3	0/0

kcal serv/100g	prot serv/100g	carb serv/100g	fat serv/100g	fibre serv/100g
Chocolate, Fruit & Nut, Dark, Tesco*, 4 squares/25g				
124/494	1.5/5.8	13.7/54.8	7/27.9	1.6/6.5
Chocolate, Fudge, Keto bar*, 1 serving/65g				
250/385	24/36.9	24/36.9	7/10.8	21/32.3
Chocolate, Jazz Orange Bar, Thorntons*, 1 bar/56g				
304/543	3.8/6.8	31.2/55.7	18.1/32.3	0.7/1.2
Chocolate, Kinder Bueno, Ferrero*, 1 twin bar/43g				
245/570	3.7/8.5	20.5/47.6	16.6/38.5	0/0
Chocolate, Kinder Maxi, Ferrero*, 1 bar/21g				
116/550	2.1/10	10.7/51	7.1/34	0/0
Chocolate, Kinder Surprise, Ferrero*, 1 egg/20g				
110/550	2/10	10.2/51	6.8/34	0.1/0.4
Chocolate, Kinder, Ferrero*, 1 bar/12.5g				
69/550	1.3/10	6.4/51	4.3/34	0/0
Chocolate, Kinder, Riegel, Ferrero*, 1 bar/21g				
117/558	2.1/10	11.1/53	7.1/34	0/0
Chocolate, Limes, Pascall*, 1 sweet/8g				
27/333	0/0.3	6.2/77.2	0.2/2.5	0/0
Chocolate, Milk Caramel, Green & Black's*, 1 serving/20g				
92/461	1.2/5.9	11.5/57.5	4.6/22.9	0/0
Chocolate, Milk, Thorntons*, 1 sm bar/50g				
269/538	3.8/7.5	27.4/54.8	16/32	0.5/1
Chocolate, Milk, with Whole Almonds, Green & Black's*, 1 serving/20g				
114/572	2.3/11.5	8.3/41.5	8/40	0/0
Chocolate, Mini Bites, Chunky, Moments, Fox's*, 1 roll/20g				
90/450	1.1/5.7	10.5/52.4	4.9/24.6	0.4/2.2
Chocolate, Mini Eggs, Milk, Cadbury's*, 1 egg/3g				
15/495	0.2/5.6	2/67.7	0.7/22.2	0/0
Chocolate, Mint Crisp, Sainsbury's*, 4 squares/19g				
95/501	1/5	12.1/63.7	4.8/25	0.7/3.6
Chocolate, Mint Crisps, Marks & Spencer*, 1 mint/8g				
40/494	0.4/5.4	4.4/54.8	2.4/29.6	0.2/3.1
Chocolate, Mint Thins, Plain, Safeway*, 1 thin/10g				
48/480	0.2/2.3	6.8/67.5	2.2/22.3	0.1/0.7
Chocolate, Nuts About Caramel, Cadbury's*, 1 bar/55g				
272/495	3.2/5.8	31.1/56.6	15.1/27.4	0/0
Chocolate, Peppermint Patty, Hershey*, 3 patties/41g				
160/390	1/2.4	33/80.5	3/7.3	0/0

kcal serv/100g	prot serv/100g	carb serv/100g	fat serv/100g	fibre serv/100g
Chocolate, Taz Chocolate Bar, Cadbury's*, 1 bar/25g				
121/485	1.2/4.8	15.5/62	6/24	0/0
Chocolate, Teddy, Milk, Thorntons*, 1 teddy/250g				
1358/543	19/7.6	131.5/52.6	83.8/33.5	2.5/1
Chocolate, White, Thorntons*, 1 bar/50g				
273/546	3.4/6.7	29.7/59.4	15.7/31.4	0/0
Chocolate, Whole Nut, Cadbury's*, 1 bar/49g				
270/550	4.6/9.3	23.9/48.8	17.2/35.2	0/0
Chocolate, with Orange & Spices, Green & Black's*, 1 serving/20g				
110/552	1.2/6	11.3/56.5	6.7/33.5	0/0
Chocolates, Alpini, Thorntons*, 1 chocolate/13g				
70/538	0.9/7	7.1/54.6	4.2/32.3	0.3/2.3
Chocolates, Cappuccino, Thorntons*, 1 chocolate/13g				
70/538	0.8/5.9	6.3/48.5	4.7/36.2	0.1/0.8
Chocolates, Champagne, Thorntons*, 1 chocolate/16g				
76/475	1.1/6.9	6.9/43.1	4.7/29.4	0.4/2.5
Chocolates, Chocolate Mousse, Thorntons*, 1 chocolate/13g				
67/515	1/7.5	5.2/40	4.7/36.2	0.4/3.1
Chocolates, Coffee Creme, Dark, Thorntons*, 1 chocolate/13g				
52/400	0.4/3	9.3/71.5	1.4/10.8	0.1/0.8
Chocolates, Coffee Creme, Milk, Thorntons*, 1 chocolate/13g				
52/400	0.4/2.8	9.7/74.6	1.3/10	0.1/0.8
Chocolates, Country Caramel, Milk, Thorntons*, 1 chocolate/9g				
45/500	0.4/4.6	5.6/62.2	2.4/26.7	0/0
Chocolates, Dairy Box, Milk, Nestle*, 1 sm box/227g				
1085/478	12.9/5.7	138/60.8	53.3/23.5	1.8/0.8
Chocolates, Dark, Elegant, Elizabeth Shaw*, 1 chocolate/8g				
38/469	0.2/2.9	5/62.5	1.8/23.1	0/0
Chocolates, Liqueurs, Cognac Truffle, Thorntons*, 1 chocolate/14g				
65/464	1/7.3	5.6/40	3.8/27.1	0.4/2.9
Chocolates, Mingles, Bendicks*, 1 chocolate/5g				
26/528	0.3/6.5	2.8/55	1.6/32.9	0/0
Chocolates, Mint Crisp, Bendicks*, 1 mint/7.7g				
40/494	0.4/5.2	4.4/55	2.4/29.9	0/0
Chocolates, Mint Crisp, Dark, Elizabeth Shaw*, 1 chocolate/6g				
27/458	0.1/1.9	4.1/68	1.2/20.7	0/0
Chocolates, Mint Crisp, Milk, Elizabeth Shaw*, 1 chocolate/6g				
30/493	0.2/4	4.3/70.9	1.3/21.4	0/0

	kcal serv/100g	prot serv/100g	carb serv/100g	fat serv/100g	fibre serv/100g
Chocolates, Mint Crisp, Thorntons*, 1 chocolate/7g					
	34/486	0.5/7.7	2.8/40	2.2/31.4	0.3/4.3
Chocolates, Praline, Roast Hazelnut, Thorntons*, 1 chocolate/13g					
	70/538	0.8/6	6.7/51.5	4.4/33.8	0.4/3.1
Chocolates, Truffle, Amaretto, Thorntons*, 1 chocolate/14g					
	66/471	0.8/5.5	7.7/55	3.6/25.7	0.4/2.9
Chocolates, Truffle, Brandy, Thorntons*, 1 chocolate/14g					
	68/486	0.9/6.1	7.3/52.1	3.8/27.1	0.1/0.7
Chocolates, Truffle, Caramel, Thorntons*, 1 chocolate/14g					
	67/479	0.6/4.2	8.1/57.9	3.6/25.7	0.3/2.1
Chocolates, Truffle, Cherry, Thorntons*, 1 chocolate/14g					
	58/414	0.6/4.2	7.1/50.7	3/21.4	0.2/1.4
Chocolates, Truffle, Rum, Thorntons*, 1 chocolate/13g					
	63/485	0.6/4.8	7.6/58.5	3.2/24.6	0.6/4.8
Creme Egg, Cadbury's, 1 egg/39g					
	174/445	1.6/4	27.6/70.8	6.2/15.9	0/0
Crispies, Dairy Milk, Cadbury's*, 1 bar/49g					
	250/510	3.7/7.6	28.7/58.6	13.4/27.4	0/0
Crunchie, Cadbury's, 1 standard bar/41g					
	193/470	1.8/4.4	29.6/72.1	7.4/18.1	0/0
Crunchie, Nuggets, Cadbury's*, 1 bag/125g					
	569/455	4.8/3.8	91.4/73.1	20.5/16.4	0/0
Curly Wurly, Cadbury's*, 1 bar/28g					
	126/450	1.3/4.8	19.6/69.9	4.7/16.7	0/0
Curly Wurly, Squirlies, Cadbury's*, 1 squirl/3g					
	14/450	0.1/3.9	2.1/69	0.5/17.8	0/0
Double Decker, Cadbury's*, 1 bar/51g					
	237/465	2.7/5.2	33.1/64.9	10.6/20.7	0/0
Dream, Cadbury's*, 1 bar/45g					
	250/555	2/4.5	26.9/59.7	15/33.3	0/0
Drifter, Nestle*, 1 finger/31g					
	144/479	1.2/4.1	20/66.7	6.5/21.7	0.3/0.9
Flake, Cadbury's*, 1 standard bar/34g					
	180/530	2.8/8.1	18.9/55.7	10.4/30.7	0/0
Flyte, Mars*, 1 bar/45g					
	196/435	1.6/3.6	32.5/72.3	6.6/14.7	0/0
Flyte, Snacksize, Mars*, 1 bar/22.5g					
	98/436	0.9/3.8	16.3/72.5	3.3/14.5	0/0

	kcal serv/100g	prot serv/100g	carb serv/100g	fat serv/100g	fibre serv/100g
Fruit Gums, No-Added-Sugar, Boots*, 1 sweet/1.6g					
	2/88	0/0	0.4/22	0/0	0/0
Fruit Gums, Rowntree's*, 1 pack/48g					
	164/342	2.3/4.7	38.8/80.8	0.1/0.2	0/0
Fruit Pastilles, Rowntree's*, 1 tube/53g					
	184/348	2.3/4.3	43.9/82.9	0/0	0/0
Fruities, Weight Watchers*, 1 serving/2g					
	3/135	0/0	1.1/54	0/0	0.7/34
Fudge, Cadbury's*, 1 standard bar/26g					
	116/445	0.7/2.8	18.8/72.3	4.2/16.3	0/0
Fudge, Dairy, Co-Op*, 1 sweet/9g					
	39/430	0.2/2	6.8/76	1.2/13	0/0
Fudge, Pure Indulgence, Thorntons*, 1 bar/45g					
	210/466	0.8/1.8	29.7/65.9	9.9/21.9	0/0
Fuse, Cadbury's*, 1 standard bar/49g					
	238/485	3.7/7.6	28.5/58.2	12.2/24.8	0/0
Galaxy, Amicelli, Mars*, 1 serving/13g					
	66/507	0.8/6.2	7.8/59.7	3.5/27.1	0/0
Galaxy, Caramel, Mars*, 1 bar/49g					
	239/488	2.6/5.3	29.4/60.1	12.3/25.1	0/0
Galaxy, Chocolate, Mars*, 1 bar/47g					
	250/532	4.2/9	26.6/56.6	14.1/30	0/0
Galaxy, Fruit & Hazelnut, Milk, Mars*, 1 bar/47g					
	235/501	3.3/7.1	25.9/55.2	13.2/28	0/0
Galaxy, Liaison, Mars*, 1 bar/48g					
	233/485	2.6/5.4	28.9/60.3	11.9/24.7	0/0
Galaxy, Ripple, Mars*, 1 bar/33g					
	169/528	2.2/6.9	19/59.3	9.4/29.3	0/0
Galaxy, Swirls, Mars*, 1 bag/150g					
	747/498	7.4/4.9	90.3/60.2	39.8/26.5	0/0
Haribo* Mix, Fantasy, 1 sm pack/100g					
	360/360	6.6/6.6	79/79	2/2	0.3/0.3
Haribo* Mix, Horror, 1 sm pack/100g					
	360/360	6.6/6.6	79/79	2/2	0.3/0.3
Haribo* Mix, Kiddies Super, 1 pack/100g					
	401/401	1.1/1.1	95.3/95.3	1.7/1.7	0.8/0.8
Haribo* Mix, Milky, 1 pack/175g					
	644/368	12.4/7.1	139.3/79.6	4/2.3	0.7/0.4

kcal serv/100g	prot serv/100g	carb serv/100g	fat serv/100g	fibre serv/100g
Haribo*, American Hard Gums, 1 pack/175g				
630/360	0.5/0.3	149.6/85.5	3.3/1.9	0.4/0.2
Haribo*, Cola Bottles, 1 sm pack/16g				
57/358	1.2/7.7	12.6/78.9	0.2/1.3	0/0.3
Haribo*, Cola Bottles, Fizzy, 1 med pack/175g				
628/359	11/6.3	137/78.3	4/2.3	0.9/0.5
Haribo*, Dolly Mixtures, 1 pack/175g				
719/411	3.2/1.8	157.9/90.2	8.4/4.8	0.4/0.2
Haribo*, Gold Bears, 1 pack/100g				
358/358	7.7/7.7	78.9/78.9	1.3/1.3	0.3/0.3
Haribo*, Jelly Beans, 1 pack/100g				
360/360	3.8/3.8	89.2/89.2	1.2/1.2	0/0
Haribo*, Mint Imperials, 1 pack/175g				
695/397	0.7/0.4	172.9/98.8	0.9/0.5	0.2/0.1
Haribo*, Starmix, 1 pack/100g				
360/360	6.6/6.6	79/79	2/2	0.3/0.3
Haribo*, Tangfastics, 1 pack/100g				
359/359	6.3/6.3	78.3/78.3	2.3/2.3	0.5/0.5
Haribo*, Wine Gums, 1 pack/175g				
655/374	10.9/6.2	150.3/85.9	1.1/0.6	0.2/0.1
Heroes, Miniature, Cadbury's*, 3 sweets/30g				
147/490	1.7/5.6	17.8/59.2	7.7/25.6	0/0
Jelly Babies, Bassett's*, 1 baby/6g				
20/335	0.2/4	4.8/79.5	0/0	0/0
Jelly Beans, Rowntree's*, 1 pack/35g				
128/367	0/0	32.1/91.8	0/0	0/0
Jelly Tots, Rowntree's*, 1 pack/42g				
145/346	0/0.1	36.3/86.5	0/0	0/0
Kit Kat, 2 Finger, Nestle*, 2 finger bar/21g				
106/506	1.4/6.7	12.7/60.6	5.5/26.3	0/0
Kit Kat, 4 Finger, Nestle*, 4 finger bar/48g				
243/507	3.3/6.8	28.9/60.2	12.7/26.5	0.6/1.2
Kit Kat, Chunky, Nestle*, 1 bar/55g				
283/514	3.6/6.5	32.9/59.8	15.2/27.6	0/0
Kit Kat, Chunky, Snack Size, Nestle*, 1 bar/26g				
133/513	1.7/6.6	15.7/60.4	7.1/27.2	0.3/1.1
Kit Kat, Kubes, Nestle*, 1 pack/50g				
258/515	3/5.9	30.5/60.9	13.8/27.5	0.5/1

kcal serv/100g	prot serv/100g	carb serv/100g	fat serv/100g	fibre serv/100g
Kit Kat, Mint, Nestle*, 4 finger bar/48g				
243/506	2.9/6	29.5/61.4	12.6/26.3	0.5/1.1
Kit Kat, Orange, 2 Finger, Nestle*, 2 finger bar/20g				
101/506	1.3/6.7	12.1/60.6	5.3/26.3	0/0
Kit Kat, White, Nestle*, 1 chunky bar/53g				
278/525	4.2/8	30.9/58.3	15.3/28.9	0/0
Lion bar, Mini, Nestle*, 1 bar/16g				
80/486	0.8/4.6	11.1/67.7	3.6/21.7	0/0
Lion bar, Nestle*, 1 bar/55g				
260/472	2.6/4.7	35.5/64.5	11.9/21.7	0/0
Lion bar, Peanut, Nestle*, 1 bar/49g				
256/522	3.5/7.1	27.9/56.9	14.5/29.6	0/0
Liquorice, Allsorts, Bassett's*, 1 pack/225g				
792/352	5.2/2.3	169.9/75.5	10.1/4.5	3.6/1.6
Lollipops, Assorted Flavours, Asda*, 1 lolly/7g				
27/380	0/0	6.7/95	0/0	0/0
Lollipops, Assorted, Co-Op*, 1 lolly/10g				
40/400	0/0	9.7/97	0/0	0/0
Lollipops, Chupa Chups*, 1 lolly/18g				
72/400	0.1/0.6	17.5/97.2	0.1/0.6	0/0
Lollipops, Marks & Spencer*, 1oz/28g				
107/383	0/0	26.7/95.4	0/0	0/0
M&M's, Mars*, 1 funsize/20g				
97/487	0.9/4.7	13.9/69.6	4.2/21.1	0/0
M&M's, Mini, Mars*, 1 sm pack/36g				
176/489	2.3/6.3	22.9/63.6	8.4/23.2	0/0
M&M's, Peanut, Mars*, 1 pack/45g				
231/514	4.6/10.2	25.8/57.3	12.2/27.1	0/0
M&M's, Plain, Mars*, 1 pack/48g				
240/499	2/4.1	33.9/70.7	10/20.8	1/2.1
Magic Stars, Milky Way, Mars*, 1 pack/33.0g				
172/522	2.3/6.9	19.3/58.5	9.5/28.9	0/0
Maltesers, Mars*, 1 sm pack/37g				
183/494	3.7/10	22.7/61.4	8.5/23.1	0/0
Maltesers, White Chocolate, Mars*, 1 pack/37g				
186/504	2.9/7.9	22.6/61	9.4/25.4	0/0
Mars Bar, 5 Little Ones, Mars*, 1 piece/8g				
38/477	0.4/4.5	5.9/73.6	1.5/18.3	0/0

	kcal serv/100g	prot serv/100g	carb serv/100g	fat serv/100g	fibre serv/100g
Mars Bar, Mars*, 1 standard bar/42g					
	190/452	1.7/4	29.2/69.6	7.4/17.5	0/0
Milky Bar, Buttons, Nestle*, 1 mini bag/16g					
	87/542	1.2/7.6	9.2/57.5	5/31.3	0/0
Milky Bar, Crunchies, Nestle*, 1 pack/30g					
	168/560	2.1/7	16.5/54.9	10.4/34.7	0/0
Milky Bar, Nestle*, 1 bar/12g					
	65/542	0.9/7.6	6.9/57.5	3.8/31.3	0/0
Milky Way, Celebrations Chocolate, Mars*, 1 sweet/8g					
	35/438	0/0	6/75	1.5/18.8	0/0
Milky Way, Magic Stars, Mars*, 1 bag/33g					
	184/557	2.9/8.8	17.1/51.8	11.6/35	0/0
Milky Way, Mars*, 1 single bar/26g					
	118/454	1.1/4.2	18.7/72	4.3/16.6	0/0
Minstrels, Galaxy, Mars*, 1 pack/42g					
	206/491	2.5/6	29.2/69.5	8.8/21	0/0
Mintoes, Morrisons*, 1 sweet/8.1g					
	33/411	0/0.1	6.8/84.4	0.6/8.1	0/0
Mints, Soft, Trebor*, 1 pack/48g					
	182/380	0/0	45.6/94.9	0/0	0/0
Munchies, Mint, Rowntree, Nestle*, 1 pack/61g					
	268/433	2.4/3.8	41.7/67.4	10.2/16.5	0/0
Munchies, Nestle*, 1 pack/52g					
	255/490	2.4/4.7	33.2/63.9	12.5/24	0/0
Peppermint Cream, Fry's*, 1 bar/51g					
	217/425	1.3/2.6	35.1/68.8	7.9/15.4	0/0
Picnic, Cadbury's*, 1 bar/48g					
	228/475	3.6/7.5	28/58.3	11.3/23.6	0/0
Polo Fruits, Nestle*, 1 tube/37g					
	142/383	0/0	35.5/96	0/0	0/0
Polo, Citrus Sharp, Nestle*, 1 tube/34g					
	134/393	0/0	32.8/96.6	0.3/1	0/0
Polo, Mints, Original, Nestle*, 1 mint/2g					
	8/404	0/0	2/98.9	0/1.1	0/0
Polo, Smoothies, Nestle*, 1 polo/4g					
	16/408	0/0.1	3.5/86.9	0.3/6.8	0/0
Polo, Spearmint, Nestle*, 1 tube/35g					
	139/397	0/0	33.8/96.6	0.4/1.1	0/0

	kcal serv/100g	prot serv/100g	carb serv/100g	fat serv/100g	fibre serv/100g
Revels, Mars*, 1 sm bag/35g					
	173/495	2.2/6.2	23/65.6	8.1/23.1	0/0
Rolo, Giant, Nestle*, 1 rolo/9g					
	42/468	0.3/3.2	6.3/70	1.8/19.5	0/0
Rolo, Minis, Nestle*, 1 pack/26g					
	124/473	0.9/3.5	18.1/69.1	5.3/20.3	0/0
Rolo, Nestle*, 1 rolo/5g					
	24/473	0.2/3.5	3.5/69.1	1/20.3	0/0
Skittles, Mars*, 1 pack/55g					
	220/400	0/0	49.8/90.5	2.3/4.2	0/0
Smarties, Mini Cones, Nestle*, 1 serving/44g					
	145/330	2/4.5	19.8/45	5.8/13.1	0/0
Smarties, Mini Eggs, Nestle*, 1 lge pack/112g					
	533/476	5.3/4.7	77.7/69.4	22.3/19.9	0.8/0.7
Smarties, Minis, Nestle*, 1 serving/14.8g					
	69/458	0.6/4.1	11/73.5	2.5/16.4	0.1/0.6
Snickers, Cruncher, Mars*, 1 bar/40g					
	209/523	3.6/9	22.8/57	12/30	0.9/2.3
Snickers, Mars*, 1 standard/61g					
	311/510	6.2/10.2	33.7/55.3	16.8/27.6	0/0
Snow Flake, Cadbury's*, 1 bar/36g					
	198/550	2.6/7.2	21.6/60.1	11.1/30.9	0/0
Softmints, Trebor*, 1 tube/40g					
	156/391	0/0	37.3/93.3	0.8/2	0/0
Spira, Cadbury's*, 2 twists/40g					
	210/525	3.1/7.8	22.7/56.8	11.8/29.4	0/0
Starbar, Cadbury's*, 1 bar/53g					
	286/540	4.8/9.1	29.2/55	16.7/31.6	0/0
Starburst Joosters, Mars*, 1 pack/45g					
	160/356	0/0	40/88.8	0/0.1	0/0
Starburst Tropical Fruit Chews, Mars*, 1 tube/45g					
	168/373	0/0	34.6/76.9	3.3/7.3	0/0
Starburst, Mars*, 1 pack/45g					
	185/411	0.1/0.3	38.4/85.3	3.4/7.6	0/0
Tic Tac, Fresh Mint, Ferrero*, 2 Tic Tacs/1g					
	4/390	0/0	1/97.5	0/0	0/0
Tic Tac, Lime & Orange, Ferrero*, 2 Tic Tacs/1g					
	4/386	0/0	1/95.5	0/0	0/0

kcal serv/100g	prot serv/100g	carb serv/100g	fat serv/100g	fibre serv/100g
Tic Tac, Spearmint, Ferrero*, 1 box/16g				
62/390	0/0	15.6/97.5	0/0	0/0
Time Out, Cadbury's*, 2 fingers/35g				
189/540	1.9/5.4	21.6/61.8	10.5/29.9	0/0
Time Out, Orange, Snack Size, Cadbury's*, 1 finger/11g				
61/555	0.6/5	6.5/59.4	3.6/32.9	0/0
Toffee Crisp, Mini, Nestle*, 1 bar/18g				
92/507	0.7/4.1	11/60.8	5/27.5	0/0
Toffee Crisp, Nestle*, 1 bar/48g				
237/494	2/4.1	29.8/62.1	12.2/25.5	0/0
Toffee, Devon Butter, Thorntons*, 1 sweet/9g				
40/444	0.2/1.7	6.5/72.2	1.5/16.7	0/0
Topic, Mars*, 1 bar/47g				
232/493	2.8/6	27.3/58.1	12.4/26.3	0/0
Tropical Tunes, Mars*, 1 pack/37g				
143/387	0/0	35.7/96.6	0/0	0/0
Turkish Delight, Fry's*, 1 bar/51g				
186/365	1/2	37.4/73.3	3.7/7.2	0/0
Twirl, Cadbury's*, 1 finger/22g				
116/525	1.8/8.1	12.3/55.9	6.6/30.1	0/0
Twix, Mars*, 1 single bar/29g				
144/495	1.7/5.8	18.4/63.5	7/24.2	0/0
Twixels, Mars*, 1 finger/6g				
31/513	0.3/5	3.8/64	1.6/26.1	0/0
Wagon Wheel, Burton's*, 1 wheel/36g				
159/441	1.8/4.9	24.2/67.3	6.1/16.9	0.5/1.3
Walnut Whip, Vanilla, Nestle*, 1 whip/34g				
160/486	1.9/5.7	20/60.5	8.1/24.6	0/0
Wine Gums, Maynards*, 1 sweet/5g				
17/331	0.3/6	3.8/76.6	0/0	0/0
Wispa, Bite, with Biscuit in Caramel, Cadbury's*, 1 bar/47g				
240/510	3/6.4	26.7/56.9	13.4/28.6	0/0
Wispa, Cadbury's*, 1 treat-size bar/15g				
83/550	1.1/7.1	8.1/53.9	5.1/34.2	0/0
Wispa, Gold, Cadbury's*, 1 bar/52g				
263/505	3/5.7	29.6/57	14.6/28	0/0
Wispa, Mint, Cadbury's*, 1 bar/50g				
275/550	3.5/7	27.4/54.7	16.8/33.6	0/0

kcal serv/100g	prot serv/100g	carb serv/100g	fat serv/100g	fibre serv/100g
York Fruits, Terry's*, 1 sweet/9g				
30/328	0/0	7.3/81.4	0/0	0.1/1
Yorkie, Honeycomb, Nestle*, 1 bar/65g				
331/509	3.7/5.7	41.3/63.6	16.8/25.8	0/0
Yorkie, Original, Nestle*, 1 bar/70g				
368/525	4.6/6.5	41/58.6	20.6/29.4	0/0
Yorkie, Raisin & Biscuit, Nestle, 1 bar/63g				
307/487	3.7/5.9	38.1/60.5	15.5/24.6	0/0

VEGETABLE PRODUCTS

kcal serv/100g	prot serv/100g	carb serv/100g	fat serv/100g	fibre serv/100g
Artichoke, Hearts, Chargrilled in Olive Oil, TTD, Sainsbury's*, ¼ jar/73g				
150/205	0.7/1	2.5/3.4	15.2/20.8	0/0
Aubergine, Baked Topped, Marks & Spencer*, 1 serving/150g				
165/110	3.6/2.4	11.1/7.4	11.6/7.7	1.4/0.9
Aubergine, Marinated & Grilled, Waitrose*, ½ pack/100g				
106/106	1/1	3/3	10/10	2/2
Carrot & Swede Mash, Fresh, Tesco*, 1oz/28g				
22/80	0.3/1.2	3.1/11.1	1/3.4	0.4/1.4
Cauliflower Cheese, Asda*, 1 pack/454g				
431/95	21.8/4.8	14.1/3.1	31.8/7	3.2/0.7
Cauliflower Cheese, COU, Marks & Spencer*, 1 pack/300g				
195/65	15.9/5.3	17.1/5.7	6.6/2.2	3.9/1.3
Cauliflower Cheese, Healthy Eating, Tesco*, 1 pack/500g				
345/69	29.5/5.9	24/4.8	14.5/2.9	9.5/1.9
Cauliflower, Florets, in a Cheese Sauce, Healthy Living, Tesco*, ½ pack/250g				
160/64	16.3/6.5	9.5/3.8	6.5/2.6	2.5/1
Cauliflower, Florets, in Cheese Sauce, Tesco*, 1 pack/500g				
345/69	29.5/5.9	24/4.8	14.5/2.9	9.5/1.9
Chips, 11mm Fresh, Deep-Fried, McCain*, 1oz/28g				
66/235	0.9/3.2	8.9/31.8	3/10.6	0/0
Chips, 14mm Fresh, Deep-Fried, McCain*, 1oz/28g				
59/209	0.8/2.7	9.6/34.2	1.9/6.8	0/0
Chips, 14mm Fryer's Choice, Deep-Fried, McCain*, 1oz/28g				
56/199	1/3.5	8.2/29.3	2.2/8	0/0

kcal serv/100g	prot serv/100g	carb serv/100g	fat serv/100g	fibre serv/100g
Chips, American-Style Oven, Safeway*, 1 serving/125g				
288/230	5.1/4.1	47.8/38.2	8.5/6.8	3.8/3
Chips, American-Style Oven, Sainsbury's*, 1 serving/165g				
314/190	8.9/5.4	38.9/23.6	13.7/8.3	2.1/1.3
Chips, American-Style Southern-Fried, Iceland*, 1 serving/100g				
251/251	4/4	34/34	11/11	3/3
Chips, American-Style, Thin Oven, Tesco*, 1 serving/125g				
210/168	3.4/2.7	30.8/24.6	8.1/6.5	2.6/2.1
Chips, Beefeater, Deep-Fried, McCain*, 1oz/28g				
71/253	0.9/3.3	10.6/37.7	2.8/9.9	0/0
Chips, Chippy, Deep-Fried, McCain*, 1oz/28g				
51/182	0.9/3	7.8/27.8	1.8/6.5	0/0
Chips, Chunky Oven, Harry Ramsden's*, 1 serving/150g				
185/123	4.2/2.8	29.9/19.9	5.4/3.6	2.4/1.6
Chips, Chunky, COU, Marks & Spencer*, 1 serving/150g				
135/90	2.4/1.6	26.4/17.6	2.6/1.7	2.3/1.5
Chips, Crinkle-Cut Oven, 5% Fat, McCain*, 1 serving/100g				
163/163	2.9/2.9	30.2/30.2	5.4/5.4	2.9/2.9
Chips, Crinkle-Cut Oven, Asda*, 1 serving/100g				
244/244	3.8/3.8	37/37	9/9	3/3
Chips, Fine-Cut, Frozen, Fried in Blended Oil, 1oz/28g				
102/364	1.3/4.5	11.5/41.2	6/21.3	0.7/2.4
Chips, Fine-Cut, Frozen, Fried in Corn Oil, 1oz/28g				
102/364	1.3/4.5	11.5/41.2	6/21.3	0.8/2.7
Chips, Homefries, Crinkle-Cut, Oven-Baked, McCain*, 1 serving/225g				
448/199	7.2/3.2	78.3/34.8	15.5/6.9	0/0
Chips, Homefries, Straight-Cut, Frozen, McCain*, 1 serving/200g				
282/141	4/2	52.2/26.1	8.8/4.4	0/0
Chips, Micro, McCain*, 1oz/28g				
54/194	0.9/3.3	7.6/27.3	2.2/7.9	0/0
Chips, Oven-Baked, McCain*, 1oz/28g				
48/173	0.8/2.8	8.2/29.3	1.4/4.9	0/0
Chips, Oven-Baked, Straight-Cut, New, McCain*, 1oz/28g				
51/182	1/3.6	8.8/31.4	1.3/4.7	0/0
Chips, Oven, BGTY, Sainsbury's*, 1oz/28g				
42/151	0.8/2.7	7.6/27.1	1/3.5	0.6/2.1
Chips, Oven, Cooked, Value, Tesco*, 1 serving/125g				
308/246	5.6/4.5	49.4/39.5	9.8/7.8	3.6/2.9

kcal serv/100g	prot serv/100g	carb serv/100g	fat serv/100g	fibre serv/100g
Chips, Oven, Crinkle-Cut, Sainsbury's*, 1 serving/165g				
297/180	5.4/3.3	48.7/29.5	9.1/5.5	4/2.4
Chips, Oven, Frozen, McCain*, 1oz/28g				
39/138	0.7/2.5	7.3/26.2	1.1/4	0.5/1.9
Chips, Oven, New, BGTY, Sainsbury's*, 1 serving/165g				
185/112	4/2.4	31.7/19.2	4.6/2.8	3.1/1.9
Chips, Oven, Steak-Cut, Asda*, 1 serving/100g				
153/153	2/2	27/27	4.1/4.1	2.5/2.5
Chips, Oven, Steak-Cut, Sainsbury's*, 1 serving/165g				
266/161	4.3/2.6	44.7/27.1	7.8/4.7	4.6/2.8
Chips, Oven, Steakhouse, Tesco*, 1 serving/125g				
165/132	3.4/2.7	28.4/22.7	4.3/3.4	2.1/1.7
Chips, Oven, Straight-Cut, 4% Fat, Healthy Eating, Tesco*, 1oz/28g				
35/124	0.6/2.3	6.1/21.8	0.9/3.1	0.5/1.9
Chips, Oven, Straight Cut, 5% Fat, Sainsbury's*, 1 serving/165g				
281/170	5.6/3.4	46.2/28	8.1/4.9	4.1/2.5
Chips, Oven, Straight-Cut, GFY, Asda*, 1oz/28g				
42/150	0.7/2.6	7.6/27	1/3.5	0.7/2.4
Chips, Oven, Straight-Cut, Reduced-Fat, Tesco*, 1 serving/100g				
127/127	2.3/2.3	22.7/22.7	3/3	2.1/2.1
Chips, Oven, Straight-Cut, Tesco*, 1oz/28g				
46/166	0.7/2.6	7.8/27.8	1.4/4.9	0.5/1.7
Chips, Steak-Cut Frying, Safeway*, 1 serving/125g				
289/231	4.1/3.3	33.9/27.1	15.1/12.1	2.8/2.2
Coleslaw, 50% Less Fat, Asda*, 1oz/28g				
17/61	0.6/2.1	1.9/6.8	0.8/2.8	0.3/0.9
Coleslaw, Aldi*, 1 serving/100g				
206/206	0.8/0.8	8.6/8.6	18.7/18.7	0/0
Coleslaw, BGTY, Sainsbury's*, 1oz/28g				
19/69	0.3/0.9	1.8/6.6	1.2/4.3	0.5/1.9
Coleslaw, Budgens*, 1 serving/50g				
103/206	0.6/1.2	4.8/9.5	9.1/18.1	1/2
Coleslaw, Classic, Marks & Spencer*, 1 pot/190g				
124/65	3.6/1.9	16.7/8.8	4.4/2.3	2.5/1.3
Coleslaw, Co-Op*, 1 serving/50g				
65/130	0.5/1	3.5/7	5.5/11	1/2
Coleslaw, Creamy, Asda*, 1oz/28g				
55/195	0.3/1	2.2/7.8	5/17.7	0.3/1

kcal serv/100g	prot serv/100g	carb serv/100g	fat serv/100g	fibre serv/100g
Coleslaw, Creamy, Healthy Eating, Tesco*, 1 serving/30g				
29/95	0.7/2.4	2/6.8	1.9/6.4	0.4/1.4
Coleslaw, Creamy, Sainsbury's*, 1oz/28g				
69/245	0.4/1.3	1.3/4.6	6.9/24.6	0.4/1.6
Coleslaw, Creamy, Tesco*, 1oz/28g				
52/186	0.3/1.1	2.1/7.6	4.7/16.8	0.4/1.5
Coleslaw, Finest, Tesco*, 1 serving/50g				
107/214	0.6/1.2	3.1/6.1	10.3/20.5	0.8/1.6
Coleslaw, GFY, Asda*, 1 serving/50g				
48/96	0.7/1.4	4.5/9	3/6	0.8/1.6
Coleslaw, Healthy Eating, Tesco*, 1 serving/100g				
85/85	1.3/1.3	7/7	5.8/5.8	1.6/1.6
Coleslaw, Healthy Living, Tesco*, 1 serving/60g				
51/85	0.8/1.3	4.2/7	3.5/5.8	1/1.6
Coleslaw, Reduced-Fat, Sainsbury's*, ⅓ pot/87g				
89/102	1/1.2	6.4/7.3	7/8	1.5/1.7
Coleslaw, Safeway*, 1 serving/75g				
128/170	0.5/0.7	5/6.7	11.7/15.6	0/0
Coleslaw, Sainsbury's*, ⅓ pot/75g				
108/144	1/1.3	5.1/6.8	9.4/12.5	1.3/1.7
Coleslaw, Tesco*, 1 serving/50g				
79/158	1.1/2.2	2.6/5.2	7.2/14.3	0.8/1.6
Croquette, Potato, Asda*, 1 pack/127g				
224/176	2.9/2.3	33/26	8.9/7	2.3/1.8
Croquette, Potato, Frozen, Tesco*, 1 croquette/30g				
58/193	1.1/3.7	6.9/23	2.9/9.7	0.3/1
Croquette, Potato, Sainsbury's*, 1 croquette/28g				
50/180	1.1/3.9	6.4/23	2.2/8	0.3/1
Croquette, Potato, Tesco*, 1 croquette/30g				
43/142	0.9/3	5.8/19.2	1.8/5.9	0.5/1.5
Dhal, Lentil, Patak's*, 1 can/283g				
156/55	7.9/2.8	26.3/9.3	2.8/1	2.8/1
Fries, Crispy Savoury Seasoning Southern, McCain*, 1 serving/100g				
179/179	2.8/2.8	26.4/26.4	6.9/6.9	0/0
Fries, Home Oven Chips, McCain*, 1oz/28g				
53/188	0.9/3.2	8.8/31.5	1.5/5.5	0/0
Gratin, Potato, Somerfield*, ½ pack/225g				
356/158	4.5/2	24.8/11	27/12	0/0

	kcal serv/100g	prot serv/100g	carb serv/100g	fat serv/100g	fibre serv/100g

Grills, Cauliflower Cheese, Dalepak*, 1 grill/94g

231/246	4.3/4.6	18.8/20	13.9/14.8	2.4/2.6

Grills, Vegetable, Dalepak*, 1 grill/85g

170/200	4.4/5.2	14.6/17.2	10.5/12.3	2.7/3.2

Mushrooms, Garlic, Breaded, Asda*, 1 serving/100g

173/173	5.7/5.7	17.9/17.9	8.8/8.8	0.9/0.9

Mushrooms, Garlic, Marks & Spencer*, 1 serving/100g

95/95	4/4	2/2	8.1/8.1	2.8/2.8

Onion Rings, Battered, Asda*, 1 serving/100g

343/343	3.8/3.8	31/31	22.7/22.7	1.7/1.7

Onion Rings, Battered, Sainsbury's*, 1 ring/12g

32/268	0.4/3.6	3.5/28.9	1.8/15.3	0.3/2.2

Onion Rings, Breaded, Iceland*, 4 rings/45g

132/293	2/4.4	15.4/34.2	6.9/15.4	1.2/2.7

Onion Rings, Oven-Crisp Batter, Tesco*, 1 onion ring/17g

40/236	0.7/4.2	4.2/24.8	2.3/13.3	0.4/2.5

Parsnip, Roast, Aunt Bessie's*, 1 serving/125g

206/165	2.8/2.2	18.6/14.9	13.4/10.7	6.4/5.1

Parsnip, Roasted, Marks & Spencer*, 1 serving/112g

134/120	2/1.8	16/14.3	7.2/6.4	0.9/0.8

Pie, Vegetable, Healthy Eating, Tesco*, 1 pack/450g

360/80	12.2/2.7	50/11.1	12.2/2.7	3.6/0.8

Potato, Farls, Marks & Spencer*, 1 farl/55g

79/144	2.3/4.2	18.6/33.8	0.2/0.4	2.6/4.7

Potato, Jacket, with Garlic, Mini, Asda*, 1 serving/65g

59/91	1.4/2.2	8.5/13	2.1/3.3	0/0

Potato, Mash, Cabbage & Spring Onion, COU, Marks & Spencer*, 1 serving/225g

180/80	3.8/1.7	26.6/11.8	5.6/2.5	4.3/1.9

Potato, Mash, Cabbage & Spring Onion, Sainsbury's*, ½ pack/225g

279/124	4.5/2	33.3/14.8	14.2/6.3	2.5/1.1

Potato, Mash, Creamy, Finest, Tesco*, ½ pack/250g

373/149	5/2	31/12.4	25.3/10.1	3/1.2

Potato, Mash, Fresh, Tesco*, 1 pack/400g

368/92	8.4/2.1	44.4/11.1	17.6/4.4	7.6/1.9

Potato, Mash, Fresh, with Butter, Sainsbury's*, ½ pack/225g

290/129	3.4/1.5	34.7/15.4	15.3/6.8	2.5/1.1

	kcal serv/100g	prot serv/100g	carb serv/100g	fat serv/100g	fibre serv/100g
Potato, Mash, with Carrot & Swede, COU, Marks & Spencer*, 1oz/28g					
	17/60	0.3/1	3.4/12.2	0.3/1.2	0.5/1.9
Potato, Mashed, Creamy, Fresh, Waitrose*, 1 serving/200g					
	164/82	3.8/1.9	28.4/14.2	3.8/1.9	2.2/1.1
Potato, Mashed, Fresh, Sainsbury's*, ½ pot/200g					
	192/96	4/2	29.2/14.6	5.6/2.8	2/1
Potato, Mashed, GFY, Asda*, ½ pack/200g					
	176/88	3.8/1.9	34/17	2.8/1.4	0/0
Potato, Roast, Baby, Finest, Tesco*, ½ pack/150g					
	149/99	5.4/3.6	22.7/15.1	4.1/2.7	2.1/1.4
Potato, Roast, BGTY, Sainsbury's*, 1 serving/100g					
	145/145	2.2/2.2	23.9/23.9	4.5/4.5	2/2
Potato, Roast, COU, Marks & Spencer*, ½ pack/150g					
	158/105	3.3/2.2	27.2/18.1	3.9/2.6	5/3.3
Potato, Roast, Crispy, Aunt Bessie's*, 1 serving/83g					
	154/185	1.9/2.3	19/22.9	7.7/9.3	1.5/1.8
Potato, Roast, Crispy, Cooked, Marks & Spencer*, 1 serving/85g					
	94/110	1.4/1.6	18/21.2	1.8/2.1	1/1.2
Potato, Roast, Frozen, Asda*, 1 serving/100g					
	188/188	2.6/2.6	22/22	10/10	0.8/0.8
Potato, Roast, Marks & Spencer*, ½ pack/150g					
	180/120	3.6/2.4	29.9/19.9	4.8/3.2	4.2/2.8
Potato, Roast, Safeway*, 1 serving/225g					
	407/181	7/3.1	63.7/28.3	13.7/6.1	5.2/2.3
Potato, Roast, Tesco*, 1 serving/100g					
	146/146	2.4/2.4	19.6/19.6	6.4/6.4	0.9/0.9
Potato, Skins, Loaded, Cheese & Bacon, Bird's Eye*, 2 skins baked/120g					
	236/197	7.9/6.6	25.9/21.6	11.2/9.3	2.5/2.1
Potato, Slices, Crispy, Marks & Spencer*, 1oz/28g					
	55/195	0.9/3.2	5.7/20.2	3.2/11.3	0.8/2.8
Potato, Waffles, Bird's Eye*, 1 waffle/56g					
	94/167	1.1/2	11.6/20.7	4.8/8.5	0.8/1.5
Potato, Wedges, Asda*, 1 wedge/40g					
	57/142	1.4/3.4	8.4/21	2/4.9	0.7/1.7
Potato, Wedges, Frozen, Tesco*, 1 serving/200g					
	262/131	4/2	44.8/22.4	7.4/3.7	3.6/1.8
Potato, Wedges, New York-Style, Healthy Eating, Tesco*, ½ pack/125g					
	124/99	2.9/2.3	20.5/16.4	3.4/2.7	1.6/1.3

kcal serv/100g	prot serv/100g	carb serv/100g	fat serv/100g	fibre serv/100g
Potato, Wedges, Savoury, McCain*, 1 serving/200g				
300/150	5.8/2.9	45.4/22.7	12.4/6.2	0/0
Potato, Wedges, Sour Cream & Chives, McCain*, 1 serving/100g				
132/132	2.4/2.4	24/24	4.1/4.1	0/0
Potato, Wedges, Spicy, Asda*, 1 serving/100g				
145/145	1.8/1.8	21.8/21.8	5.7/5.7	2.1/2.1
Potato, Wedges, Tesco*, 1 serving/110g				
135/123	3.3/3	20.2/18.4	4.6/4.2	1.7/1.5
Potato, Boulangere, Marks & Spencer*, ½ pack/225g				
180/80	6.3/2.8	35.8/15.9	2/0.9	2/0.9
Potatoes, Anya, Sainsbury's*, 1 serving/100g				
80/80	1.4/1.4	19.7/19.7	0.1/0.1	1/1
Potatoes, Dauphinois, Sainsbury's*, ½ can/200g				
176/88	3.6/1.8	21.8/10.9	8.2/4.1	1.2/0.6
Potatoes, Dauphinois, Finest, Tesco*, 1 serving/200g				
332/166	4.4/2.2	29.4/14.7	21.8/10.9	1.6/0.8
Ratatouille, Vegetable, Marks & Spencer*, 1 pack/300g				
135/45	6.9/2.3	7.5/2.5	9/3	6.3/2.1
Rosti, Potato & Root Vegetable, COU, Marks & Spencer*, 1 cake/100g				
85/85	1.6/1.6	13.3/13.3	2.7/2.7	1.5/1.5
Salad, Beetroot, Sainsbury's*, 1 tub/200g				
160/80	1.8/0.9	23.4/11.7	6.6/3.3	4.2/2.1
Salad, Bowl, French-Style, Way to Five, Sainsbury's*, 1 pack/264g				
103/39	1.8/0.7	11.1/4.2	5.8/2.2	5.8/2.2
Salad, Caesar, BGTY, Sainsbury's*, ½ bag/127g				
168/132	4.6/3.6	10.9/8.6	12.6/9.9	2.2/1.7
Salad, Caesar, Lower Fat, BGTY, Sainsbury's*, ½ pack/126.9g				
132/104	4.6/3.6	12.4/9.8	7.1/5.6	2.2/1.7
Salad, Green Side, Marks & Spencer*, 1 serving/200g				
30/15	1.8/0.9	5/2.5	0.4/0.2	0/0
Salad, Green Side, Sainsbury's*, 1 pack/200g				
28/14	1.6/0.8	4.2/2.1	0.6/0.3	1.6/0.8
Salad, Mediterranean-Style Side, Way to Five, Sainsbury's*, 1 serving/244g				
61/25	2.2/0.9	7.3/3	2.4/1	0/0
Salad, Mediterranean-Style, Asda*, ½ pack/135g				
22/16	1.4/1	4.1/3	0/0	0/0

kcal serv/100g	prot serv/100g	carb serv/100g	fat serv/100g	fibre serv/100g
Salad, Mixed Bean, Way To Five, Sainsbury's*, 1 can/270g				
227/84	14.6/5.4	36.5/13.5	2.4/0.9	10.3/3.8
Salad, Mixed Leaf with Olive Oil Dressing, Pizza Express*, 1 pack/240g				
326/136	2.2/0.9	5/2.1	33.8/14.1	1.7/0.7
Salad, Potato, Healthy Eating, Tesco*, 1 pot/250g				
218/87	5.5/2.2	30/12	8.5/3.4	2.3/0.9
Salad, Tuna Nicoise, No Mayonnaise, Shapers, Boots*, 1 pack/276.4g				
152/55	12.4/4.5	17.7/6.4	3.6/1.3	3.9/1.4
Samosas, Vegetable, Marks & Spencer*, 1 samosa/45g				
115/255	2.3/5.1	11.2/24.8	6.9/15.3	1.3/2.8
Samosas, Vegetable, Tesco*, 1 samosa/50g				
126/252	2.5/5	14.2/28.4	6.6/13.2	1.4/2.7
Seaweed, Crispy, Blue Dragon*, 1 packet/55g				
345/628	3.4/6.2	10.6/19.2	31.9/58	4.9/8.9
Stir-Fry, Chinese Chop Suey Veg, Sharwood's*, 1 pack/310g				
223/72	4.7/1.5	43.1/13.9	3.4/1.1	1.9/0.6
Stir-Fry, Chinese Mixed Vegetable, Sainsbury's*, 1 serving/150g				
75/50	2.6/1.7	7.1/4.7	4.1/2.7	0/0
Stir-Fry, Chinese Vegetable & Oyster Sauce, Asda*, 1 serving/150g				
93/62	2.9/1.9	12/8	3.8/2.5	0/0
Stir Fry, Chinese Vegetables, Tesco*, 1 serving/175g				
93/53	2.8/1.6	18.9/10.8	0.7/0.4	2.3/1.3
Stir Fry, Mushroom, 2 Step, Tesco*, ½ pack/180g				
34/19	4.1/2.3	3.8/2.1	0.4/0.2	1.3/0.7
Stir Fry, Noodles & Bean Sprouts, Tesco*, 1 serving/125g				
155/124	6.8/5.4	24.8/19.8	3.3/2.6	2.4/1.9
Stir Fry, Oriental Style Vegetables, Sainsbury's*, 1oz/28g				
17/62	0.4/1.5	1.5/5.2	1.1/3.9	0.4/1.5
Stir Fry, Thai Style, Tesco*, 1 pack/350g				
322/92	13.3/3.8	29.4/8.4	16.8/4.8	6.3/1.8
Vegetables, Mediterranean Style, Ready to Roast, Sainsbury's*, 1 serving/200g				
268/134	6.2/3.1	12.4/6.2	21.6/10.8	2/1
Vegetables, Roast, Marks & Spencer*, 1 pack/420g				
273/65	5.9/1.4	20.6/4.9	17.6/4.2	1.8/0.4
Vegetables, Roasted Winter, Tesco*, 1 serving/200g				
170/85	4.4/2.2	20/10	8/4	4/2

	kcal serv/100g	prot serv/100g	carb serv/100g	fat serv/100g	fibre serv/100g

Vegetables, Roasted, Italian, Marks & Spencer*, 1 serving/95g

219/230	1.7/1.8	6.7/7.1	20/21	1.6/1.7

Water Chestnuts, Amoy*, 1oz/28g

12/42	0.3/0.9	2.8/10.1	0/0	0/0

VEGETARIAN FOODS

Bacon, Quorn*, 1 rasher/30g

42/141	4.1/13.5	2.4/8.1	1.8/6.1	0.9/3

Bacon, Vegetarian, Rashers, Tesco*, 1 rasher/20g

47/237	4/19.9	2.9/14.5	2.2/11	1.2/6

Bacon, Vegetarian, Realeat*, 2 rashers/35.7g

99/275	10.1/28	9.6/26.6	2.2/6.2	0.6/1.7

Bolognese, Meat-Free, Asda*, 1 serving/229g

179/78	13.7/6	25.2/11	2.5/1.1	1.4/0.6

Bolognese, Meatless, Granose*, 1 pack/400g

400/100	32/8	32/8	16/4	0/0

Bolognese, Vegetarian, Marks & Spencer*, 1 pack/360g

360/100	16.2/4.5	45/12.5	12.6/3.5	7.6/2.1

Burgers, Chargrilled-Style, Vegetarian, Safeway*, 1 burger/57g

95/167	10.7/18.8	2.1/3.7	4.8/8.5	2.3/4

Burgers, Chilli Flavour Brown Rice & Tofu, Cauldron Foods*, 1 burger/75g

185/246	12.2/16.2	10.1/13.5	10.6/14.1	3.2/4.3

Burgers, Juicy Mushroom & Sweet Onion, Cauldron Foods*, 1 burger/87.5g

99/113	5.6/6.4	8.7/9.9	4.7/5.3	2.4/2.7

Burgers, Meat-Free, Asda*, 1 burger/60g

138/230	14.4/24	6.6/11	6/10	0.2/0.3

Burgers, Meat-Free, Sainsbury's*, 1 burger/57g

92/161	11.2/19.6	2.2/3.9	4.2/7.4	2.7/4.8

Burgers, Mushroom, Cauldron Foods*, 1 burger/87.5g

135/153	6.2/7.1	13.3/15.1	6.2/7.1	2.4/2.7

Burgers, Mushroom, Tesco*, 1 burger/87g

144/166	2.4/2.8	17.7/20.4	7/8.1	2.7/3.1

Burgers, Quorn*, 1 burger/50g

56/112	6.2/12.4	2.7/5.3	2.3/4.6	1.8/3.6

Burgers, Quorn*, New Improved, 2 burgers/100g

137/137	17.8/17.8	8.8/8.8	3.4/3.4	3.7/3.7

kcal serv/100g	prot serv/100g	carb serv/100g	fat serv/100g	fibre serv/100g
Burgers, Quorn*, Original, 1 burger/50g				
55/109	6/12	3.5/6.9	1.9/3.7	2.5/4.9
Burgers, Quorn*, Premium, 1 burger/81g				
96/118	9.2/11.4	5.8/7.1	4/4.9	2.8/3.5
Burgers, Quorn*, Southern Style, 1 burger/63g				
113/180	6.7/10.7	7.7/12.3	6.2/9.8	2/3.1
Burgers, Savoury Tofu, Cauldron Foods*, 1 burger/75g				
162/216	11.1/14.8	9.9/13.2	8.6/11.5	2.6/3.5
Burgers, Spicy Bean, Dalepak*, 1 burger/118g				
242/205	5.4/4.6	26.9/22.8	12.5/10.6	3.5/3
Burgers, Spicy Bean, Sainsbury's*, 1 burger/110g				
262/240	5.5/5	29.6/27.1	13.5/12.4	2.2/2
Burgers, Spicy Black Bean, Cauldron Foods*, 1 burger/88g				
158/180	9.5/10.8	11.8/13.4	8.1/9.2	4.5/5.1
Burgers, Spicy Vegetable, Asda*, 1 burger/56g				
108/193	1.9/3.4	11.2/20	6.2/11	0/0
Burgers, Vegeburger Mix, Realeat*, 1 serving/62.5g				
233/370	18.9/30	25.2/40	6.3/10	3.8/6
Burgers, Vegeburger, Herb & Vegetable, Realeat*, 1 burger/125g				
433/346	40/32	40/32	12.5/10	0/0
Burgers, Vegeburger, Linda McCartney*, 1 burger/59g				
79/134	13.3/22.6	1.7/2.9	2.1/3.6	0.9/1.6
Burgers, Vegetable, Captains, Bird's Eye*, 1 burger/48g				
96/200	2.3/4.7	12.2/25.5	4.2/8.8	1/2
Burgers, Vegetable, Organic, Tesco*, 1 burger/90g				
108/120	2.3/2.6	15.8/17.6	3.9/4.3	1.9/2.1
Burgers, Vegetable, Quarter Pounders, Dalepak*, 1 burger/114g				
251/220	5/4.4	23.7/20.8	15/13.2	3.1/2.7
Burgers, Vegetarian, Bean, Mexican-Style Quarter Pounders, Tesco*, 1 burger/101g				
215/213	4.3/4.3	25.3/25	10.7/10.6	2.8/2.8
Burgers, Vegetarian, Flame-Grilled, Linda McCartney*, 1 burger/60g				
80/134	13.6/22.6	1.7/2.9	2.2/3.6	1/1.6
Burgers, Vegetarian, Mushroom & Red Onion, Tesco*, 1 burger/78g				
105/135	3.7/4.7	14.5/18.6	3.6/4.6	1.1/1.4
Burgers, Vegetarian, Quarterpounders, Chargrilled, Tesco*, 1 burger/113.5g				
187/164	18.2/16	8/7	9.1/8	2.9/2.5

	kcal serv/100g	prot serv/100g	carb serv/100g	fat serv/100g	fibre serv/100g

Burgers, Vegetarian, Spicy Bean, Linda McCartney*, 1 burger/85g

190/223	3.7/4.3	22.3/26.2	9.5/11.2	2.5/2.9

Burgers, Vegetarian, Tesco*, 1 burger/56g

92/164	9/16	3.9/7	4.5/8	1.4/2.5

Cannelloni, Spinach & Wild Mushroom, Linda McCartney*, 1 pack/340g

381/112	16.7/4.9	47.9/14.1	13.6/4	5.8/1.7

Cannelloni, Vegetarian, Tesco*, 1 pack/400g

552/138	21.2/5.3	39.2/9.8	34.4/8.6	6/1.5

Casserole, Lentil & Vegetable, Granose*, 1 pack/400g

220/55	11.2/2.8	31.6/7.9	5.6/1.4	0/0

Cauliflower Cheese, Vegetarian, Safeway*, 1 serving/150g

138/92	7.1/4.7	7.8/5.2	8.7/5.8	2.1/1.4

Chilli, Meat-Free, Sainsbury's*, 1 pack/400g

308/77	16/4	16.4/4.1	20/5	20.8/5.2

Chilli, Vegetarian, Quorn, Tesco*, 1 pack/400g

340/85	17.6/4.4	60/15	3.2/0.8	8.4/2.1

Curry, Red Thai, Quorn*, 1 pack/400g

464/116	18.4/4.6	62/15.5	15.6/3.9	16/4

Curry, Vegetable with Pilau Rice, Linda McCartney*, 1 pack/339g

224/66	5.4/1.6	45.8/13.5	2/0.6	1.7/0.5

Cutlets, Nut, Goodlife*, 1 serving/88g

248/282	9/10.2	24.1/27.4	12.8/14.6	2.6/3

Cutlets, Nut, Grilled, Cauldron Foods*, 1 cutlet/87g

250/287	8.9/10.2	23.3/26.8	13.4/15.4	4/4.6

Enchiladas, Quorn*, 1 pack/400g

384/96	21.2/5.3	46.8/11.7	12.4/3.1	7.6/1.9

Falafel, Vegetarian, Organic, Waitrose*, 1 felafel/25g

55/220	2/8	5.8/23.3	2.6/10.5	1.9/7.6

Frankfurters, Vegetarian, Tivall*, 3 sausages/90g

220/244	16.2/18	6.3/7	14.4/16	2.7/3

Hot Dog, Meat-Free, Sainsbury's*, 1 sausage/30g

70/235	5.3/17.8	1.3/4.2	4.9/16.4	0.6/1.9

Hot Dog, Vegetarian, Tesco*, 1 sausage/30g

81/271	5.7/19	1.8/6	5.7/19	0.6/2

Hot Pot, Vegetable, Granovita*, ½ can/210g

202/96	6.3/3	25.2/12	8.4/4	0/0

Kiev, Vegetarian, Cheesy Garlic, Meat-Free, Sainsbury's*, 1 Kiev/123g

263/214	21.3/17.3	13/10.6	14/11.4	3.7/3

	kcal serv/100g	prot serv/100g	carb serv/100g	fat serv/100g	fibre serv/100g
Kiev, Vegetarian, Garlic Butter, Tesco*, 1 Kiev/142g					
	462/325	20.4/14.4	31.4/22.1	28.3/19.9	1.1/0.8
Kiev, Vegetarian, Garlic Butter, Tivall*, 1 Kiev/125g					
	366/293	18.9/15.1	13.5/10.8	26.3/21	3.3/2.6
Kiev, Vegetarian, Garlic, Safeway*, 1 Kiev/142g					
	423/298	18.7/13.2	28.8/20.3	25.8/18.2	1/0.7
Kiev, Vegetarian, Vegetable, Marks & Spencer*, 1 Kiev/155g					
	326/210	7.1/4.6	27.6/17.8	20.8/13.4	3.9/2.5
Lasagne, Quorn*, 1 pack/300g					
	249/83	12.3/4.1	29.7/9.9	9/3	3.9/1.3
Lasagne, Quorn, Safeway*, 1 pack/400g					
	360/90	19.6/4.9	41.6/10.4	12.8/3.2	6.8/1.7
Lasagne, Vegetable, Eat Smart, Safeway*, 1 pack/380g					
	266/70	13.3/3.5	41/10.8	4.9/1.3	5.3/1.4
Lasagne, Vegetable, Linda McCartney*, 1 pack/320g					
	374/117	22.4/7	45.4/14.2	11.2/3.5	6.1/1.9
Lasagne, Vegetable, Mediterranean, Linda McCartney*, 1 pack/320g					
	333/104	10.2/3.2	50.6/15.8	9.9/3.1	4.8/1.5
Lasagne, Vegetarian, Tesco*, 1 pack/430g					
	581/135	22.8/5.3	58.5/13.6	28.4/6.6	4.3/1
Margarine, Sunflower, Granose*, thin spread/7g					
	50/720	0/0	0/0	5.9/84	0/0
Mayonnaise, Vegetarian, Tesco*, 1 tsp/12g					
	89/738	0.2/1.5	0.1/0.8	9.7/81	0/0
Milk, Soya, Sweetened, Sainsbury's*, 1fl oz/30ml					
	14/45	1.1/3.6	0.9/2.9	0.6/2.1	0/0.1
Moussaka, Quorn*, 1 pack/400g					
	364/91	14.4/3.6	39.2/9.8	16.4/4.1	4.8/1.2
Mushroom, Escalope, Creamy, Vegetarian, Tesco*, 1 pack/300g					
	765/255	30/10	60/20	45/15	6/2
Nuggets, Meat-Free, Blue Parrot Cafe, Sainsbury's*, 1 nugget/18g					
	41/228	3.1/17.3	2.3/12.5	2.2/12.1	0.5/3
Nuggets, Vegetarian, Safeway*, 4 nuggets/80.1g					
	161/201	13/16.3	8.4/10.5	8.3/10.4	2.9/3.6
Nut Roast, Leek, Cheese & Mushroom, Organic, Cauldron Foods*, ½ pack/143g					
	343/240	18.9/13.2	18.9/13.2	21.3/14.9	5.9/4.1

kcal serv/100g	prot serv/100g	carb serv/100g	fat serv/100g	fibre serv/100g

Nut Roast, Tomato & Courgette, Organic, Waitrose*, ½ pack/142g

| 295/208 | 16.6/11.7 | 17.8/12.5 | 17.5/12.3 | 7/4.9 |

Nut Roast, Vegetarian, Tesco*, 1 serving/160g

| 218/136 | 8.6/5.4 | 18.2/11.4 | 12.2/7.6 | 3.2/2 |

Pasty, Vegetarian, Cornish, Linda McCartney*, 1 pasty/170g

| 420/247 | 8.8/5.2 | 43.4/25.5 | 23.5/13.8 | 2.6/1.5 |

Pâté, Brussels-Style, Quorn*, 1 pack/130g

| 150/115 | 14/10.8 | 7.4/5.7 | 7/5.4 | 4.4/3.4 |

Pâté, Deli, Quorn*, 1oz/28g

| 32/115 | 3/10.8 | 1.6/5.7 | 1.5/5.4 | 1/3.4 |

Pâté, Vegetarian, Spinach, Soft Cheese & Onion, Co-Op*, 1oz/28g

| 48/170 | 1.4/5 | 0.8/3 | 4.2/15 | 1.1/4 |

Pâté, Vegetarian, Yeast, Wild Mushroom, Granovita*, 1oz/28g

| 60/213 | 2.8/10 | 1.4/5 | 4.8/17 | 0/0 |

Pie, Cottage, Meat-Free, Sainsbury's*, 1 pack/400g

| 364/91 | 17.6/4.4 | 46.8/11.7 | 12/3 | 2.8/0.7 |

Pie, Cottage, Quorn*, 1 pie/300g

| 213/71 | 8.1/2.7 | 32.1/10.7 | 5.7/1.9 | 3.9/1.3 |

Pie, Cottage, Quorn, Sainsbury's*, 1 pack/450g

| 329/73 | 13.5/3 | 45.9/10.2 | 9.9/2.2 | 8.1/1.8 |

Pie, Creamy Garlic & White Wine Mushroom, Linda McCartney*, 1 serving/201g

| 412/205 | 7.4/3.7 | 43.2/21.5 | 23.3/11.6 | 10.7/5.3 |

Pie, Creamy Mushroom, Quorn, Sainsbury's*, 1 pie/134g

| 355/265 | 6.8/5.1 | 33.1/24.7 | 21.7/16.2 | 2.5/1.9 |

Pie, Quorn & Mushroom, Tesco*, 1 pie/141g

| 378/268 | 7.5/5.3 | 33.6/23.8 | 23.7/16.8 | 1.8/1.3 |

Pie, Quorn Cottage, Safeway*, 1 pack/400g

| 260/65 | 14/3.5 | 40/10 | 4.4/1.1 | 8/2 |

Pie, Vegetarian, Deep Country, Linda McCartney*, 1 pie/176g

| 444/252 | 12/6.8 | 48.6/27.6 | 23.4/13.3 | 2.5/1.4 |

Pie, Vegetarian, Shepherd's, Linda McCartney*, 1 pack/340g

| 317/93 | 15.6/4.6 | 47.3/13.9 | 7.1/2.1 | 5.4/1.6 |

Pie, Vegetarian, Vegetable Cumberland, Marks & Spencer*, ½ pack/211.1g

| 190/90 | 5.9/2.8 | 28.3/13.4 | 5.5/2.6 | 3.4/1.6 |

Pork, Ribsters, Quorn*, 2 ribsters/83.9g

| 99/118 | 13.4/15.9 | 4/4.8 | 3.3/3.9 | 2.4/2.8 |

kcal serv/100g	prot serv/100g	carb serv/100g	fat serv/100g	fibre serv/100g
Potato, Wedges, Spicy, & Garlic Dip, Linda McCartney*, 1 pack/300g				
366/122	7.8/2.6	45.9/15.3	16.8/5.6	9.3/3.1
Quorn, Goujons, with Chunky Salsa Dip, Quorn*, 1oz/28g				
57/204	2.9/10.4	4.8/17	2.9/10.5	0.8/3
Quorn Balls, Swedish-Style, in Chunky Tomato & Basil Sauce, Quorn*, 1 pack/400g				
296/74	32.8/8.2	20/5	9.2/2.3	8/2
Quorn Balls, Swedish-Style, Quorn*, 3 balls/50g				
72/144	11/22	2.7/5.4	1.9/3.8	1.6/3.2
Quorn Deli, Chicken-Style, Slices, Quorn*, 3 slices/33g				
36/108	5.6/16.9	1.3/4	0.9/2.7	1.1/3.2
Quorn Deli, Ham Flavour, Quorn*, 1 slice/20g				
26/130	3.9/19.3	1.2/6.1	0.6/3.1	0.6/3.1
Quorn Deli, Ham, Wafer Thin, Quorn*, 1 serving/18g				
23/130	3.5/19.3	1.1/6.1	0.6/3.1	0.6/3.1
Quorn Deli, Turkey Flavour with Stuffing, Quorn*, 1 slice/13g				
13/102	1.8/13.7	1.1/8.3	0.2/1.5	0.6/4.5
Quorn Escalopes, Garlic & Herb, Quorn*, 1 escalope/140g				
293/209	12.5/8.9	23.7/16.9	16.5/11.8	5.3/3.8
Quorn Fillets, Chargrilled Tikka Style, Mini, Quorn*, ½ pack/85g				
110/129	10.6/12.5	12.2/14.4	2/2.4	4.3/5
Quorn Fillets, Chinese-Style Chargrilled, Mini, Quorn*, 1 serving/85g				
115/135	10.3/12.1	13.3/15.6	2.3/2.7	4/4.7
Quorn Fillets, Garlic & Herb, Quorn*, 1 fillet/100g				
198/198	10.7/10.7	16.7/16.7	9.8/9.8	4.1/4.1
Quorn Fillets, Hot & Spicy, Quorn*, 1 fillet/100g				
176/176	10.9/10.9	14.7/14.7	8.2/8.2	6.4/6.4
Quorn Fillets, in a Mediterranean Marinade, Quorn*, 1 fillet/80g				
90/112	10/12.5	7/8.8	2.4/3	3.2/4
Quorn Fillets, in Breadcrumbs, Quorn, 1 fillet/94g				
184/196	10.3/11	13.3/14.2	10/10.6	3.6/3.8
Quorn Fillets, in White Wine & Mushroom Sauce, Quorn*, 1 pack/325g				
247/76	20.5/6.3	19.5/6	9.8/3	6.8/2.1
Quorn Fillets, Lemon & Black Pepper, Quorn*, 1 fillet/100g				
195/195	11.6/11.6	17.2/17.2	8.9/8.9	3.3/3.3
Quorn Fillets, Lemon & Pepper, Sainsbury's*, 1 fillet/100g				
198/198	11.6/11.6	16.9/16.9	9.3/9.3	3.8/3.8

	kcal serv/100g	prot serv/100g	carb serv/100g	fat serv/100g	fibre serv/100g
Quorn Fillets, Oriental, Sainsbury's*, 1 serving/294g					
	353/120	11.8/4	72.3/24.6	1.8/0.6	5.3/1.8
Quorn Fillets, Provencale, Morrisons*, 1 serving/165g					
	94/57	8.9/5.4	9.6/5.8	2.3/1.4	1.8/1.1
Quorn Fillets, Quorn*, 2 fillets/102g					
	88/86	13.4/13.1	5/4.9	1.5/1.5	5/4.9
Quorn Fillets, Thai, Quorn*, 1 serving/79.4g					
	85/107	11.8/14.9	4.8/6.1	2/2.5	2.8/3.6
Quorn Fillets, with a Crispy Seasonal Coating, Quorn*, 1 fillet/100g					
	197/197	8.8/8.8	18.4/18.4	9.8/9.8	3/3
Quorn Grills, Lamb Flavour, Quorn*, 1 frill/90g					
	104/116	10.3/11.4	9.4/10.4	2.9/3.2	3.8/4.2
Quorn Mince, Quorn*, 1 pack/300g					
	273/91	45/15	4.2/1.4	8.4/2.8	14.7/4.9
Quorn Nuggets, Quorn*, 1 nugget/20g					
	38/191	2.1/10.6	3.1/15.7	1.9/9.5	0.7/3.5
Quorn Nuggets, Southern-Style, Quorn*, 1 nugget/20g					
	39/197	2.4/12.1	3.1/15.7	1.9/9.5	0.7/3.5
Quorn Pieces, Quorn*, 1 pack/300g					
	276/92	42/14	5.4/1.8	9.6/3.2	14.4/4.8
Quorn Slices, Roast, with Sage & Onion Stuffing, Quorn*, ¼ pack/70g					
	47/67	5.3/7.5	3.4/4.9	1.3/1.9	2.1/3
Quorn Steaks, Peppered, Quorn*, 1 steak/98.2g					
	107/109	11.2/11.4	7.3/7.4	3.7/3.8	3.9/4
Quorn Steaks, Peppered, Sainsbury's*, 1 steak/95g					
	124/130	11.3/11.9	11.3/11.9	4/4.2	4.3/4.5
Quorn Chicken-Style Roast, Quorn*, 1oz/28g					
	30/108	4.7/16.9	1.1/4	0.8/2.7	0.9/3.2
Roast, Vegetarian, Chicken-Style, Tesco*, 1 serving/113g					
	214/189	25/22.1	5.4/4.8	10.2/9	1.9/1.7
Sausage & Mash, Quorn, Sainsbury's*, 1 pack/394g					
	339/86	15/3.8	43.3/11	11.8/3	2.8/0.7
Sausage & Mash, Quorn, Tesco*, 1 pack/400g					
	292/73	16.4/4.1	35.2/8.8	9.6/2.4	5.2/1.3
Sausage & Mash, Vegetarian, GFY, Asda*, 1 pack/400g					
	292/73	16.8/4.2	36/9	8.8/2.2	8.4/2.1
Sausage & Mash, Vegetarian, Safeway*, 1 pack/450g					
	450/100	24.6/5.5	40.2/8.9	21.2/4.7	8.2/1.8

kcal serv/100g	prot serv/100g	carb serv/100g	fat serv/100g	fibre serv/100g
Sausage & Mash, Vegetarian, Tesco*, 1 pack/410g				
435/106	18/4.4	41/10	22.1/5.4	8.2/2
Sausage Roll, Vegetarian, Linda McCartney*, 1 roll/51g				
133/260	5.6/10.9	11.8/23.1	7.4/14.5	0.8/1.6
Sausage, Cumberland, Grilled, Cauldron Foods*, 1 sausage/50g				
80/160	6.3/12.6	6.2/12.3	3.4/6.7	1.2/2.4
Sausage, Cumberland, Waitrose*, 1 sausage/50g				
80/160	6.3/12.6	6.2/12.3	3.4/6.7	1.2/2.4
Sausage, Honey Roasted Pepper & Dijon Mustard, Cauldron Foods*, 1 sausage/50g				
67/133	4.2/8.4	6/12	2.9/5.7	1.1/2.2
Sausage, Leek & Cheese, Organic, Cauldron Foods*, 1 sausage/41g				
80/194	5.9/14.5	4.6/11.2	2.1/5.2	0.7/1.7
Sausage, Leek & Pork, Style Flavour, Quorn*, 1 sausage/44g				
56/127	5.9/13.3	3.3/7.5	2.2/4.9	0.9/2.1
Sausage, Lincolnshire, Cauldron Foods*, 1 sausage/50g				
106/212	7.4/14.7	7.3/14.5	5.3/10.6	1.1/2.2
Sausage, Meat-Free, Asda*, 1 sausage/43g				
81/189	8.6/20	3/7	3.9/9	1.2/2.9
Sausage, Meat-Free, Premium, Realeat*, 1 sausage/50g				
71/142	7.4/14.8	1.9/3.7	3.8/7.5	1.5/3
Sausage, Mushroom & Herb, Waitrose*, 1 sausage/50g				
62/123	5.1/10.2	4.1/8.1	2.7/5.4	0.3/0.5
Sausage, Mushroom & Tarragon, Wicken Fenn*, 1 sausage/47g				
82/175	4.7/10.1	8/17	3.5/7.4	1.1/2.4
Sausage, Roasted Garlic & Oregano, Cauldron Foods*, 1 sausage/50g				
90/179	6.6/13.1	4.5/9	5.1/10.1	1.1/2.1
Sausage, Smoked Paprika & Chilli, Cauldron Foods*, 1 sausage/50g				
76/152	3.9/7.8	5.9/11.8	4.1/8.2	1.3/2.6
Sausage, Spinach, Leek & Cheese, Gourmet, Wicken Fen*, 1 sausage/46g				
92/201	4.7/10.3	7.8/17	4.7/10.2	0.9/1.9
Sausage, Sun-Dried Tomato & Herb, Linda McCartney*, 1 sausage/35g				
93/266	7.6/21.8	3.5/10.1	5.4/15.4	0.6/1.7
Sausage, Vegetarian, Hot Dog, Tesco*, 2 sausages/60g				
163/271	11.4/19	3.6/6	11.4/19	1.2/2
Sausage, Vegetarian, Linda McCartney*, 1 sausage/35g				
88/252	8.1/23.2	3/8.6	4.8/13.8	0.4/1.2

kcal serv/100g	prot serv/100g	carb serv/100g	fat serv/100g	fibre serv/100g
Sausage, Vegetarian, Quorn*, 1 sausage/42g				
47/111	5.6/13.4	2.5/5.9	1.6/3.8	1.1/2.6
Sausage, Vegetarian, Safeway*, 2 sausages/89.7g				
149/165	15.5/17.2	1.8/2	8.8/9.8	7.3/8.1
Soya, Mince, Dry Weight, Sainsbury's*, 1 serving/50g				
164/328	23.6/47.2	16.6/33.2	0.4/0.8	1.8/3.6
Soya, Mince, Organic*, 1oz/28g				
101/359	12.9/46	7.8/28	2/7	0/0
Soya, Mince, Unflavoured, Nature's Harvest*, 1 serving/100g				
345/345	50/50	35/35	1/1	4/4
Soya, Mince, with Onion, Sainsbury's*, ½ pack/180g				
122/68	9.7/5.4	14.4/8	2.9/1.6	3.2/1.8
Spaghetti Bolognese, Meat-Free, Heinz*, 1 serving/200g				
162/81	6.6/3.3	26.2/13.1	3.4/1.7	1.2/0.6
Spaghetti Bolognese, Meat-Free, Sainsbury's*, 1 can/400g				
280/70	13.6/3.4	48/12	3.6/0.9	4.8/1.2
Spaghetti Bolognese, Quorn*, 1 pack/400g				
292/73	22.8/5.7	37.6/9.4	5.6/1.4	9.6/2.4
Spaghetti Bolognese, Quorn, Sainsbury's*, 1 pack/450g				
347/77	22.1/4.9	53.6/11.9	5/1.1	8.1/1.8
Spaghetti Bolognese, Vegetarian, Tesco*, 1 pack/340g				
374/110	17.3/5.1	46.6/13.7	13.3/3.9	4.1/1.2
Spaghetti Carbonara, Quorn*, 1 pack/400g				
460/115	20/5	36.4/9.1	26/6.5	4.4/1.1
Stew, Vegetable & Dumplings, Linda McCartney*, 1 pack/340g				
384/113	8.5/2.5	46.6/13.7	6.1/1.8	1.7/0.5
Stir Fry, Quorn, Spicy Chilli With Vegetables & Rice, Quorn*, ½ pack/170g				
162/95	10/5.9	26.5/15.6	1.7/1	3.1/1.8
Streaky Strips, Meat-Free, Morningstar Farms*, 1 strip/8g				
28/348	0.9/11.5	1.1/13.4	2.2/27.6	0.3/3.9
Tikka Masala, Quorn, & Rice, Tesco*, 1 pack/400g				
364/91	13.6/3.4	55.6/13.9	9.6/2.4	6.8/1.7
Tikka Masala, with Rice, Quorn*, 1 pack/400g				
476/119	17.2/4.3	54/13.5	21.2/5.3	6.4/1.6
Toad In The Hole, Vegetarian, Aunt Bessie's*, 1 pack/190g				
481/253	24.9/13.1	37.8/19.9	25.8/13.6	2.3/1.2
Toad in the Hole, Vegetarian, Linda McCartney*, 1 pack/190g				
359/189	25.8/13.6	26.4/13.9	16.7/8.8	2.1/1.1

kcal serv/100g	prot serv/100g	carb serv/100g	fat serv/100g	fibre serv/100g
Toad in The Hole, Vegetarian, Meat-Free, Asda*, 1 toad/173g				
407/235	15.6/9	43.3/25	19/11	5.4/3.1
Toad In The Hole, Vegetarian, Tesco*, 1 pack/190g				
471/248	24.9/13.1	50.4/26.5	19/10	5.3/2.8
Toad In The Hole, Vegetarian, Tryton Foods*, 1oz/28g				
73/262	4.1/14.8	5.2/18.6	4/14.2	0.4/1.6
Tofu, Deep-Fried, Organic, Evernat*, 1oz/28g				
44/156	4.8/17.3	0.7/2.6	2.4/8.5	0/0
Tofu, Natural, Organic, Evernat*, 1oz/28g				
34/120	4/14.4	0.5/1.8	1.7/6.2	0/0
Tofu, Organic, Cauldron Foods*, 1oz/28g				
33/118	3.6/12.9	0.3/1.2	1.9/6.8	0.1/0.2
Tofu, Smoked, Organic, Evernat*, 1oz/28g				
36/127	4.6/16.3	0.2/0.8	1.8/6.6	0/0
Vege Roast, Chicken-Style, Realeat*, 1 pack/454g				
844/186	104.4/23	14.5/3.2	40.9/9	0/0
Vegetarian Mince, Safeway*, 1 pack/454g				
781/172	78.5/17.3	20.4/4.5	43.1/9.5	8.2/1.8
Vegetarian Mince, Vegemince, Realeat*, 1 serving/125g				
220/176	19.4/15.5	7.5/6	12.5/10	2.5/2

Make
www.thorsonselement.com
your online sanctuary

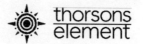